Informed
Decisions

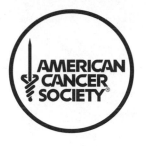

AMERICAN
CANCER
SOCIETY®

Informed
Decisions

THE COMPLETE BOOK OF
CANCER DIAGNOSIS, TREATMENT, AND RECOVERY

Gerald P. Murphy, M.D., Lois B. Morris,
and Dianne Lange

VIKING

VIKING
Published by the Penguin Group
Penguin Books USA Inc., 375 Hudson Street,
New York, New York 10014, U.S.A.
Penguin Books Ltd, 27 Wrights Lane,
London W8 5TZ, England
Penguin Books Australia Ltd, Ringwood,
Victoria, Australia
Penguin Books Canada Ltd, 10 Alcorn Avenue,
Toronto, Ontario, Canada M4V 3B2
Penguin Books (N.Z.) Ltd, 182–190 Wairau Road,
Auckland 10, New Zealand

Penguin Books Ltd, Registered Offices:
Harmondsworth, Middlesex, England

First published in 1997 by Viking Penguin,
a division of Penguin Books USA Inc.

10 9 8 7 6 5 4 3 2 1

Line drawings by David Rosenzweig

A NOTE TO THE READER
The ideas, procedures, and suggestions contained in this book are not intended as a substitute for consulting with your physician. All matters regarding your health require medical supervision.

Grateful acknowledgment is made for permission to reprint excerpts or adapt and use selections from the following works:
"How to Perform Skin Self-Examination," reprinted with permission of The Skin Cancer Foundation, New York, NY, Copyright 1992.
"Words for Describing Pain," from "The McGill Pain Questionnaire" by Ronald Melzack, Ph.D., 1970.
"My Life as a Runner with Cancer" from *The New York Road Runners Club Complete Book of Running* by Fred Lebow and Gloria Averbuch. Copyright © 1992 by Fred Lebow and Gloria Averbuch. Reprinted by permission of Random House, Inc.
"Exercises to Do in Bed" by Willibald Nagler, M.D.
"Metamorphosis" from "Beauty Tips for the Dead" by Judith Hooper. © 1992 Judith Hooper.
"Coping with Disappointment and Frustration" and "Don't Avoid It—Talk About It" from *Cancer and Hope: Charting a Survival Course* by Judith Garrett Garrison, MED, LSW, and Scott Sheperd, Ph.D. (CompCare Publishers, 1989).
"Single with Cancer" from *Cancervive: The Challenge of Life After Cancer* by Susan Nessim and Judith Ellis. Copyright © 1991 by Susan Nessim and Judith Ellis. Reprinted by permission of Houghton Mifflin Company. All rights reserved.
"Becky's Mom Has Cancer" from *An Almanac of Practical Resources for Cancer Survivors: Charting the Journey* by the National Coalition for Cancer Survivorship, Fitzhugh Mullan, M.D., and Barbara Hoffman, editors (Consumer Reports Books, 1990). Updated edition published October 1996 (Chronimed Publishing).
"To Die in Loving Arms" by Lois B. Morris, originally published in *Sunday Woman,* April 20, 1980.
"A Living Will," "Designation of Health Care Surrogate," and "Artificial Nutrition and Hydration" from "Artificial Nutrition and Hydration and End-of-Life Decision Making," 1994, reprinted by permission of Choice in Dying, 200 Varick Street, New York, NY 10014.

LIBRARY OF CONGRESS CATALOGING IN PUBLICATION DATA
Informed decisions : the complete book of cancer diagnosis, treatment, and recovery / Gerald P. Murphy, M.D.; Lois B. Morris; Dianne Lange.
    p.   cm.
  Includes index.
  ISBN 0-670-85370-4
  1. Cancer—Popular works.   I. Murphy, Gerald Patrick.   II. Morris, Lois B.   III. Lange, Dianne.
IV. American Cancer Society.
RC263.I624   1997
616.99′4—dc20   96-18319

This book is printed on acid-free paper.
∞

Printed in the United States of America
Set in Sabon
Designed by Cassell Design Group, Inc.

Consultants

Terry B. Ades, R.N., M.S., O.C.N., Director, Health Care Initiatives, American Cancer Society, Atlanta, GA.

Robert M. Beazley, M.D., Professor of Surgery, Boston University School of Medicine; Chief, Section of Surgical Oncology, University Hospital, Boston, MA.

Don Beerline, M.D., Chairman, Department of Pathology, Mount Diablo Medical Center, Concord, CA.

Foster Boyd, M.D., Retired General Surgeon and Past Chairman, National Service and Rehabilitation Committee, American Cancer Society, Atlanta, GA; Chairman, Cancer Committee, Clinton Memorial Hospital, Wilmington, OH.

Tony W. Cheung, M.D., Assistant Professor, Department of Medicine, Mount Sinai School of Medicine, New York, NY.

Grace H. Christ, D.S.W., Associate Professor, Columbia University School of Social Work, New York, NY.

Nessa Coyle, R.N., M.S., Director, Supportive Care Program, Department of Neurology Pain–Palliative Care Service, Memorial Sloan-Kettering Cancer Center, New York, NY.

Myles P. Cunningham, M.D., Clinical Associate Professor of Surgery, University of Illinois Medical College, Chicago, IL.

Jerome J. DeCosse, M.D., Ph.D., Professor of Surgery and Attending Surgeon, The New York Hospital–Cornell Medical Center, New York, NY.

Philip J. DiSaia, M.D., Dorothy Marsh Chairman in Reproductive Biology and Professor, Department of Obstetrics and Gynecology, University of California–Irvine, CA.

Robert C. Eyerly, M.D., Associate Surgeon, Geisinger Medical Center, Danville, PA; Clinical Associate Surgeon, Jefferson Medical College, Philadelphia, PA.

Harmon J. Eyre, M.D., Executive Vice President for Research and Cancer Control, American Cancer Society, Atlanta, GA.

Irving D. Fleming, M.D., F.A.C.S., Professor of Surgery, Department of Surgery, University of Tennessee Center for Health Sciences, Memphis, TN.

Lawrence Garfinkel, M.A., Special Consultant in Epidemiology and Statistics, American Cancer Society, New York, NY.

Gerald Haase, M.D., Clinical Professor of Surgery, University of Colorado School of Medicine, The Children's Hospital, Denver, CO.

George J. Hill, M.D., Professor of Surgery and Chief, Division of Surgical Oncology, University of Medicine and Dentistry of New Jersey–New Jersey Medical School, Newark, NJ.

Reginald Ho, M.D., Department Chief, Department of Oncology and Hematology, Straub Clinic and Hospital, Honolulu, HI.

Edward W. Humphrey, M.D., Emeritus Professor of Surgery, University of Minnesota, Minneapolis, MN.

George W. Jones, M.D., Professor of Urology and Surgery, Howard University Hospital and Medical School, Washington, D.C.

Rosaline R. Joseph, M.D., Professor of Medicine, Medical College of Pennsylvania, Philadelphia, PA.

Betsy Jubb, M.L.I.S., Librarian and Webmaster, American Cancer Society, Atlanta, GA.

Richard H. Lange, M.D., F.A.C.P., Chairman, Medical Affairs Subcommittee on Alternative and Complementary Methods of Cancer Management, American Cancer Society; Retired Chief, Nuclear Medicine, Ellis Hospital, Schenectady, NY.

John Laszlo, M.D., National Vice President, Research, American Cancer Society, Atlanta, GA.

Walter Lawrence, Jr., M.D., Professor, Surgical Oncology and Director Emeritus, Massey Cancer Center, Medical College of Virginia, Richmond, VA.

Edward R. Laws, Jr., M.D., F.A.C.S., Professor of Neurological Surgery and Medicine, University of Virginia, Charlottesville, VA.

Seymour H. Levitt, M.D., Professor and Chairman, Department of Therapeutic Radiology–Radiation Oncology, University of Minnesota Hospital and Clinic, Minneapolis, MN.

Virgil Loeb, Jr., M.D., Professor Emeritus of Clinical Medicine, Washington University School of Medicine, St. Louis, MO.

Matthew Loscalzo, A.C.S.W., Director, Oncology Social Work, The Johns Hopkins Oncology Center, Baltimore, MD.

LaMar S. McGinnis, M.D., Clinical Professor of Surgery, Emory University School of Medicine; Medical Director, Eberhart Cancer Center, Atlanta, GA.

Robert J. McKenna, Sr., M.D., Clinical Professor Emeritus of Surgery, University of Southern California, Los Angeles, CA.

Willibald Nagler, M.D., F.A.C.P., Physiatrist-in-Chief, The New York Hospital–Cornell Medical Center; Consultant, Rehabilitation Medicine, Memorial Sloan-Kettering Cancer Center, New York, NY.

Daniel W. Nixon, M.D., Professor of Experimental Oncology and Medicine, Medical University of South Carolina, Charleston, SC.

Darrell S. Rigel, M.D., Clinical Associate Professor, Department of Dermatology, New York University School of Medicine, New York, NY.

Eugene G. Roach, Ph.D., M.D., Clinical Associate Professor of Psychiatry and Medical Genetics, Indiana University School of Medicine, Indianapolis, IN.

Arlene E. Robinovitch, M.S.W., Oncology Social Work Consultant, Seattle, WA.; Retired Director, Patient Rehabilitation and Support Services, American Cancer Society, Atlanta, GA.

David S. Rosenthal, M.D., Professor of Medicine, Harvard Medical School; Henry K. Oliver Professor of Hygiene and Director of Harvard University Health Services, Cambridge, MA.

Richard W. Sayre, M.D., Chairman, Diagnostic Imaging, Mount Diablo Medical Center, Concord, CA.

Wendy S. Schain, Ed.D., Clinical Psychologist, Kensington, MD.

Leslie R. Schover, Ph.D., Staff Psychologist, Center for Sexual Function and the Cancer Center, The Cleveland Clinic Foundation, Cleveland, OH.

Robert J. Schweitzer, M.D., Clinical Professor of Surgery, University of California–Davis (East Bay); Associate Clinical Professor of Surgery, University of California–San Francisco; Surgical Oncologist, Summit Medical Center, Oakland, CA.

Naomi Stearns, M.S.W., Oncology Social Work Consultant, The Woodlands, TX.

Derrick Wheeler, National Vice President, Information Center, American Cancer Society, Atlanta, GA.

Writers

Betsy Anderson

Beryl Lieff Benderly

Diana Benzaia

Kathleen Doheny

Roberta Grant

Ann Greenberg

Maryann Hammers

Gretchen Henkel

Dianne Lange

Sarah Lansill

Jean McCann

Michael McCann

Lois B. Morris

Joan Duncan Oliver

Maura Rhodes

Mae Rudolph

Ron Schaumburg

Illustrations:

David Rosenzweig

PREFACE

To understand something is to take away some of the mystery and fear that surround it. Educating people about cancer, helping them understand what causes this disease and how it can be treated, has been part of the American Cancer Society's mission since the beginning. *Informed Decisions* marks another milestone in our effort, begun more than eighty years ago, to show people that they are not powerless against cancer.

As cancer emerges as the primary cause of death in this country—because cardiovascular illness is claiming fewer lives and men and women are living to an older, more vulnerable age—the delivery of health care is changing rapidly and sometimes alarmingly. Within a few years, 80 percent of Americans are expected to be receiving some kind of managed health care. Considering this trend, *Informed Decisions* can enhance the knowledge of today's consumers about the options for cancer care to which they are entitled.

Here are the facts—and the peace of mind that comes from having accurate, reliable information at a time when it is needed the most.

               — Harmon J. Eyre, M.D.
                  Executive Vice President for
                  Research and Cancer Control
                  American Cancer Society
                  January 1997

ACKNOWLEDGMENTS

We are immensely grateful to the 42 named consultants who have volunteered their time, knowledge, and expertise throughout all stages of this project. Their contributions and cooperation have made this book a remarkable collaboration. We take this opportunity, too, to credit Judith Unger, R.N., and Teresa Sims, R.N., O.C.N., B.S.N., for their efforts.

To the unsung heroes of the American Cancer Society National Home Office we extend our heartfelt appreciation. In particular, Rosemarie Perrin has been a constant conduit for information and a source of steady, practical, professional support. Special thanks, as well, to Harmon Eyre, M.D., and to all those who in their various roles have helped and smoothed our way: Harry Johns, Cynthia Currence, Carla Montgomery, Darlene Caron, Mary Joe Lang, and Mary Mize.

We sing the praises of our editor at Viking Penguin, Mindy Werner, who has provided expert guidance, sound judgment, and goodwill throughout. Hats off to Cynthia Achar, Roni Axelrod, Kate Griggs, Michael Hardart, Susan Hans O'Connor, and Jaye Zimet for the skills and talents they invested in this project. We wish to thank as well Ron Harris and Cassell Design Group.

Thanks are due to Barbara Lowenstein, our agent and champion, and to Genell Subak-Sharpe, who made the essential introductions.

Finally, we acknowledge the hard work of Raj Chowdhry, Sarah Lansil, and Daniel Horton. They kept the details checked, the faxes flowing, and the computers running.

Contents

INTRODUCTION

How to Use This Book

If you or someone close to you has cancer, you are a featured player in a drama of treatment and recovery over which you have much more control than you may realize. Indeed, at no other time in history have so many decisions concerning cancer care fallen so squarely on the shoulders of people with the disease and their families. And never has so much knowledge been available. The catch is that you need to know how to access it, weigh it, and arrive at a rapid determination of what is best for you.

The fact is, there is no "right way" that applies to everyone. Cancer is as many as 100 different diseases. And every person who has it, even two people with the same type of cancer at precisely the same stage, differs from every other.

It is the purpose of the American Cancer Society's *Informed Decisions: The Complete Book of Cancer Diagnosis, Treatment, and Recovery* to present all the information you need to make the critical choices that face you and to simplify the decision-making process. You will find that you have important opportunities to influence your care, recovery, and well-being.

Knowing about options in surgical techniques might help you spare a body part or essential function, for example. Learning of techniques to prevent or off-set side effects can help you enter treatment with much less fear. Understanding the precise stage of your cancer will enable you to choose among treatment recommendations with far more certainty. Knowing what questions to ask your doctors each step of the way will streamline the communication and decision-making processes. And learning what you can ask for, how to assert yourself, and whom to turn to will make it much more likely that you'll get what you need.

There are numerous ways to use the information in this book:

- to understand the options you have;

- to feel secure in your choice of health care professionals and treatment facilities;

- to comprehend the recommendations that your caregivers provide;

- to organize and evaluate the enormous amounts of data and details you will encounter at a time when you are least able to absorb them;

- to be specific in your questioning so you can get the information you need;

- to request additional therapies, services, or programs that may not have been offered to you;

- to collaborate with your health care team rather than to feel helpless and passive;

- to be sure you are receiving the best possible care;

- to be in control of what is happening to you;

- to alleviate fear and anxiety;

- to understand medical terms and concepts that health care professionals use to describe cancer and its treatment;

- to appreciate the current state of knowledge about cancer and grasp what is on the horizon;

- to be aware of the resources and services available to you and your family, even in this era of managed health care resources.

Decisions are hard to make, especially if they will influence the course and quality of your life, if they must be made quickly, and if you lack the expertise to choose wisely. This book will guide you, whether you are the person with cancer or a concerned family member or friend. Even if you choose to leave the decisions to others, you will have the information at hand to understand what is happening and why.

How the Book Is Organized

Some people will choose to read about the kind of cancer that is of concern to them and then to turn to the remaining chapters in consecutive order, or in whatever order interests them. Others may want to use the book as a reference, reading only those chapters that are relevant to them at the time.

Informed Decisions consists of seven parts and two appendices. You will find information about specific types or sites of cancer—breast, prostate, colon, pancreas, leukemia, lymphoma, and so on—in the last section, "An Encyclopedia of Common and Uncommon Cancers." As explained in the introduction to this section, Part VII provides details specific to each cancer, including diagnostic tests, typical treatments, investigational approaches, and special needs.

All the chapters in the preceding six parts pertain to everyone with any type of cancer. Consult these chapters for complete background information and advice about the details offered in the encyclopedia section. For example, specific chemotherapy regimens may be mentioned as standard treatments for a particular type of cancer. By referring to the chapter on chemotherapy (Chapter 17) you will learn everything you need to know about why and how that therapy is used and the effects it may have on you.

Almost every chapter provides tips on managing the emotions of, reactions to, and side effects of having cancer and being treated for it. Several chapters are devoted to coping issues as well. Being able to manage the experience in a positive way helps immeasurably to make people feel more empowered, comfortable, and in control of what is happening, and even to believe that they've come through the experience as better, stronger human beings.

Part I ("Is It Cancer?") consists of eight chapters that explain what cancer is and its terminology, signs and symptoms, screening tests and examinations, self-tests, and diagnostic procedures.

The five chapters in Part II ("Why Me? Why Now? What Now?") detail who is likely to get cancer and why. This section shows you where and how to get the help you need and how to evaluate recommendations. Here too is information on communicating with doctors and dealing with the health care system (including managed care), how many opinions to seek, and how to become involved with or develop a support network from the start.

All cancer treatment modalities, from the traditional to the experimental to the alternative, are the subject of the nine chapters in Part III ("Treatment Strategies"). You will learn how doctors decide on treatments, how each type works and how they work together, how to tolerate therapy most comfortably, and, of course, how to decide on what is the best course of action.

Obtaining the highest possible quality of life is the subject of Part IV ("Living the Best You Can with Cancer"). The 10 chapters cover everything from pain relief (so important we've devoted two chapters to it), to managing stress and depression, and living well with disabilities and limitations. Nutrition and exercise advice are offered. How cancer affects sexuality and body image, and how to restore intimacy and regain a good, strong sense of self are subjects of still other chapters. Finally, we detail the coping challenges and predictable psychological crises that individuals and families face and present strategies for dealing with them.

Part V ("Advancing Illness") explains metastasis and recurrence, offers approaches to diagnosis and treatment, and presents options for care, comfort, and well-being.

The two chapters in Part VI ("Special Needs") are devoted to children's cancers and to those that occur among people with AIDS.

Appendix I provides a large directory of resources, which lists organizations state by state and nationwide that can be of considerable help to people with specific types of cancer, to anyone who has cancer, and to families and friends. Among the many sources of help and information provided here are the chartered divisions of and the many programs sponsored by the American Cancer Society. Appendix II covers the world of cancer information and resources on line.

About the American Cancer Society

Represented in more than 3,400 communities throughout the country and Puerto Rico, the American Cancer Society (ACS) is a nonprofit health organization dedicated to eliminating cancer as a major health problem. This book is just one example of the many ways the American Cancer Society seeks to fulfill its mission: to save lives and diminish suffering from cancer through research, education, advocacy, and service. Funding is derived solely from the contributions of the public; the ACS accepts no funds from city, state, or federal governments. The American Cancer Society is the largest private source of cancer research dollars in the United States. Founded in 1913 by 10 physicians and five concerned members of the community, the organization is now represented by 2 million Americans. Most offer their time free of charge to the ACS to work to conquer cancer. Among these volunteers are the experts in the various areas of cancer research and treatment that we have brought together to bring you the state-of-the-art information in this book (see "Consultants," pages v–vi).

A Warning

There is one more important way that you can use the information provided in this book: to weigh the claims of new cures and breakthroughs reported in the media. Almost every day, newspaper and TV reporters proclaim an extraordinary discovery related to cancer: genes linked to various tumors, the possibility of a cancer vaccine, the dangers of an environmental pollutant, dietary preventatives, revolutionary new treatments, or new perils associated with existing treatments.

Very often the research that is reported is highly preliminary and requires further studies to verify or develop the new, headlined findings. Sometimes later studies that do not replicate the discoveries are not as "newsworthy" and fail to be widely reported, leaving the public with a false impression about the state of knowledge. Moreover, many of the truly revolutionary findings that make the news are breakthroughs in basic science that will take years, perhaps decades, to translate into treatments or cures. They do provide hope down the road, but they may not be as available as you might wish.

The need to create headlines and "sound bites" often leads to distortions of legitimate findings and confusion about what to do as a result. The day the National Cancer Institute released findings that showed that taking beta carotene supplements could increase the risk of cancer among smokers, media in many communities were blaring, "Beta carotene supplements may cause cancer!" This was an outright misrepresentation of the study's findings, which determined that the nutritional supplement neither helped nor harmed the nonsmokers in the lung cancer study who took it daily for 12 years. But it must have caused considerable alarm among people who had begun to take beta carotene after earlier studies suggested it might have some preventive benefit.

Chapter 1 in this book, and many other chapters, mentions areas of new research that are commonly reported in the news. Consulting these chapters will help you put what you read or hear into a realistic perspective.

...And an Invitation

This book reflects both the expertise of scientists and practitioners at the forefront of cancer research and treatment and the combined experiences of men, women, and children who have had the illness. We would like to invite readers— those with cancer, their families, health care providers—to contribute their thoughts, advice, suggestions, and decisions to readers of future editions of *Informed Decisions*. Write to Editors, *Informed Decisions*, P.O. Box 544, Shelter Island Heights, NY 11965. Share your experiences, to benefit all.

PART I

IS IT
CANCER?

WHAT IS CANCER?

This year about 1.4 million Americans will learn they have cancer. In an instant their lives will be turned upside down. Plans and concerns about almost every aspect of life—work, relationships, money, and pleasure—will be superseded by one question that often goes unspoken: "Am I going to die?" The answer, statistically speaking, is no. Of all those whose cancers are diagnosed today, more will survive than will die as a result of the disease. Of the estimated 10 million Americans living with cancer, about 7 million were treated five or more years ago and most are considered cured.

Considerable progress has been made in effectively treating some forms of cancer. For example, some types are usually curable. These include Hodgkin's disease, Ewing's sarcoma (a bone cancer), testicular cancer, Burkitt's lymphoma, rhabdomyosarcoma (muscle cancer), osteogenic (bone) sarcoma, Wilms' tumor (kidney cancer in children), and acute lymphocytic leukemia in children. Formerly, childhood cancers were almost always fatal; today about two of every three children with cancer appear to be cured. The death rate for people with cancer under 65 has also declined.

Regrettably, the mortality rate of older people is increasing, owing in large part to the numbers who are long-time smokers. Yet for cancers other than those related to tobacco, the outlook is also better for older Americans. It is important to understand, though, that the remarkable decline in heart disease means the elderly population is growing rapidly: Since people are living longer, they are more likely to develop cancer, and so the total number of new cases of cancer will increase unless there are dramatic breakthroughs in cancer prevention. Looking at the impact of cancer on the *total* population, we are experiencing the first sustained decline in the death rate from cancer since record-keeping began in the 1930s.

A New Attitude

Today many of those confronting cancer are learning that even when a *cure*—that is, ridding the body of all cancer cells permanently—is not possible, long-term survival is. In fact, cancer is increasingly being treated as a chronic condition like heart disease or diabetes. With prompt treatment, regular monitoring, and proper psychological and social support, there's a good chance that a person can live a productive life *with* the disease for many years.

The chapters of this book provide specific information to help you understand cancer and its treatment, get the best possible care, interpret what health care professionals tell you throughout the process, and make informed decisions about your own treatment and recovery. This chapter discusses the most basic question: What is cancer? As you'll see, the most fundamental notions about this disease have changed throughout history. With new knowledge has come much progress in treatment and recovery. We'll introduce some recent treatment advances, all of which are explored at greater length later in this book. Mostly, though, we address the basic science of this very common disease process.

If at this moment practical concerns are more pressing—such as where to find help or how to interpret diagnostic or treatment information or deal with side effects—you may want to turn first to the chapters that are immediately relevant to your needs.

The information in this chapter will provide some background for why cancer is treated the way it is now. As you read in the daily newspaper of new discoveries or see reports on television, this chapter will help you put them in context. Some of the basic science of cancer that seems esoteric today may be useful background for the headlines you will read tomorrow.

Changing Views

Medical historians say that the turning point in cancer treatment was the beginning of the twentieth century, when scientists began to look at life-threatening diseases as solvable problems. Several medical mysteries were unraveled at the time. Mosquitoes were identified as yellow fever carriers, lice were linked to typhus, a treatment for syphilis was found, and the first radical mastectomy was performed. Medical institutions became centers of research, and physicians started to organize and share their knowledge with each other.

The Long Search for a Cause

The common perception of cancer nearly a century ago was that it was a "wasting" disease like tuberculosis, the major killer of the day. That concept was so frightening that people hesitated even to say the word cancer aloud. But scientists were intrigued by this ancient scourge and were committed to finding its cause.

At that time, some researchers said that cancer was a natural result of aging. As cells degenerated, they thought, some became malignant. Others said cancer was hereditary, and investigations into genetics began. Some began to consider chemical links; and still others questioned whether viruses or bacteria were at fault. Finally, the "irritation" theory became popular, and researchers began trying to identify irritants—such as tobacco and coal tar—that would cause cancer in laboratory animals. Ultimately, though, these experts were forced to confront the fact that although all these factors might be involved, none of them invariably caused cancer. Not every animal or person exposed to an irritant or a particular chemical in the laboratory developed cancer, nor did all elderly people or everyone with a family history of cancer get it.

Scientists had to abandon the theory that cancer had a single cause. But there was enough truth in the beliefs and speculations of the time to support a range of misconceptions, some of which still persist. For example, despite the fact that scientists proved you couldn't "catch" cancer, many people continue to think of it as contagious. *It's not.* Irritation may play a role, but bruises or injuries *cannot* cause cancer. And although smoking doesn't always lead to lung cancer, this cancer used to be very rare before the widespread use of cigarettes. We now know for certain that smoking is linked to cancer.

Treatment Evolution

During these early years of cancer research, doctors were also investigating various therapies, ranging from electrical treatments to assorted "magic bullet" drugs. With the discovery of the x-ray, interest in radiation therapy peaked very early in this century. Unfortunately, the life-threatening dangers of the poorly controlled doses of radiation soon became obvious, and the therapy fell from favor. However, radium, which could deliver a consistent dose of radiation without many side effects, eventually came into more widespread use. But it was surgery—usually *radical* surgery, in which the tumor and a large area of tissue around it is removed—that became the primary treatment. Today surgery (though typically far less radical) remains the most effective curative therapy.

After World War II, research efforts to find a cure for cancer escalated dramatically. Radiation therapy and chemotherapy were refined (see Chapters 16, "Radiation," and 17, "Chemotherapy"), and surgery became safer (see Chapter 15, "Surgery"). Today each of these therapies continues to be fine-tuned, leading to more successful results and fewer complications.

Removing a Tumor. In recent years, surgery has taken a new course. Improved biopsy techniques and ways to see inside the body, such as computerized tomography (CT scan), magnetic resonance imaging (MRI), and ultrasound, have improved the accuracy and ease of diagnosis. Operating on someone just to look for a growth, called *exploratory surgery*, happens far less often than even a decade ago (see Chapter 8, "Diagnostic Tests"). The radical approach to removing cancer and preventing its recurrence is being replaced in many cases by operations that spare organs, limbs, and body functions. This type of surgery is often followed by other therapies (see Chapter 20, "Combination Treatments").

Chemotherapy Progress. Chemotherapy, treatment with anticancer drugs that are injected into the bloodstream or taken by mouth and circulated throughout the body, has been responsible for curing several types of child-hood cancer, Hodgkin's disease, and others. These drugs target critical meta-bolic processes within cancer cells and cause the cells to stop growing and eventually to die (see Chapter 17, "Chemotherapy").

Today there are new ways of countering some of the problems associated with chemotherapy. For example, sometimes chemotherapy initially causes the tumor to shrink but then the cells resist the drug(s) and cancer recurs. New drugs, specifically designed to prevent adaptive metabolic pathways from developing, have been partly successful. They prevent cancer cells from escaping the lethal effects of chemotherapy.

An exciting new approach to chemotherapy is the disruption of blood vessel formation in tumors so that they cannot grow. Another promising approach is selectively blocking a certain enzyme that makes cancer cells immortal (see "Planned Destruction" later in this chapter). Using chemother-apy in these innovative ways should have little or no deleterious effect on nor-mal cells, at least in adults. These are among the exciting experimental leads.

Looking into the Future

Today's new research frontier is *biological therapy*, the use of natural, bio-logical materials to stimulate the body's own cancer-fighting mechanisms. It is a promising way to destroy cancer cells (see Chapter 18, "Biological Therapies"). And looming on the horizon are some exciting possibilities of genetic engineering, such as developing a means to selectively destroy cancer cells regardless of where they are.

Research into the intricate link between mind and immunity, called *psy-choneuroimmunology*, is also under way. Some of these approaches are still in the early, basic science stage and are not likely to be practiced soon, but they are signs of progress and hope.

Cancer Is a Process

All the diseases we call cancer have one characteristic in common: the uncon-trollable growth and accumulation of abnormal cells. The development of these abnormal cells is actually a lengthy, progressive, multistep process called *car-cinogenesis* (see "A Step-by-Step Process," later). It starts with damage to one or more genes that eventually causes a cell to produce abnormal cells; it ends—sometimes years later—with the formation of a detectable tumor. Carcinogenesis may take 10 to 20 years from the time the first abnormal cells begin replicating to the point at which a person notices any sign or symptom of a tumor.

How Healthy Cells Behave

To understand an abnormal condition or process such as carcinogenesis, it's helpful to know how healthy cells behave. A normal cell divides, matures, dies, and is replaced by another in an orderly way according to a genetic pro-gram that is unique to that particular cell type (that is, skin, intestine, blood, etc.). As a cell grows, it takes its proper place among the other cells in its tissue of origin. And when the cell matures, it performs the task it is genetically programmed to do. Eventually it dies and is replaced by a new, younger cell. As the developing cells mature, one cell bumps up against a neighboring one, molecular messages are relayed and received, telling the young cell that it's time to stop growing.

Cellular Disorder

When a cell has been transformed into a cancer cell, however, its offspring—the *daughter cells*—no longer follow biological rules. They often divide more rapidly than they should. Their growth is disorderly, and they never mature properly. Their offspring, in turn, are similarly abnormal and have a tendency to become even more disorderly. These wayward cells tumble over each other, piling on top of neighboring cells and eventually form a mass or tumor. (Some types of cancer cells don't divide so much more rapidly than normal, but they do fail to die on schedule.)

Cancer cells that don't know when to stop dividing and/or when to die are described as *immortal*. They can also destroy normal surrounding tissues and often spread throughout the body, which is a hallmark of *malignancy*.* The tumor and the cells that extend from it are called *malignant*. The person in whom these events are happening is said to have *cancer* (see Chapter 2, "The Language of Cancer").

Eventually, if the disruptive growth of the cancer cells is not controlled *and* the abnormal cells extend to adjacent areas or spread (*metastasize*) to form tumors elsewhere in the body, the affected organs and systems cannot continue their vital functions (see Chapter 33, "Metastasis and Recurrence"). Unless the proliferation of cancer cells is arrested, the body cannot survive.

The Body Fights Back

Since genetic alterations or mutations occur throughout life, everyone is at some risk of getting cancer. Whether a malignancy eventually occurs, however, will depend on your body's own defenses. Some of these anticancer mechanisms are genetically programmed in specific white blood cells, some rely on other body systems, and some have yet to be discovered.

Immunity

The immune system, for example, is a kind of built-in search-and-destroy system. Cancer cells have molecules on their surfaces called *antigens*. Scientists believe that when immune cells circulating in the bloodstream detect these "foreign" antigens, they destroy the cancer cell. Occasionally, though, cancer cells escape detection. Some researchers think cancer cells do this by reducing the number of exposed antigens that can signal the immune system or by camouflaging them.

---

* Some of the terms that appear in italics throughout this chapter will be used repeatedly throughout this book. Others may appear in other literature you may encounter as you read about cancer elsewhere. Often, too, you will hear or read these terms in news reports of cancer research breakthroughs.

To illustrate just how important healthy immunity is, consider the high cancer risk among people who lack normal immunity because of certain drugs or such diseases as AIDS. These *immunocompromised* people have almost 200 times more malignancies than the general population (see Chapter 36, "AIDS-Related Cancers"). Learning how the immune system responds and what might stimulate it into action sooner or more forcefully is also an area of intense investigation (see Chapter 18, "Biological Therapies").

Planned Destruction

All cells are equipped with controls designed to prevent them from making too many copies of themselves or flawed ones. For example, cells are programmed to die after a certain number of replications. This is an important part of the normal aging process. Recently, it was discovered that every time a cell divides, some *DNA*, or deoxyribonucleic acid (the body's basic genetic material), is lost from the tips of its chromosomes. Eventually, when the cell starts to make abnormal copies, these tips—and their extra DNA—are nearly depleted, and the chromosomes become unstable. Consequently, the cell cannot duplicate itself; it ages and dies. (Cancer cells, in contrast, produce an enzyme—*telomerase*—that replaces the lost portion of the chromosome tips, which makes the cells immortal.) It is now also known that specific genes may produce chemicals that cause abnormal cells to die as they should.

Of course, it is also possible for anticancer mechanisms to fail and actually cause cancer. For instance, in a healthy cell, *tumor suppressor genes* play a role in maintaining normal cell growth. In recent years, researchers have learned that cancer may occur when these protective genes are inactivated and the process that leads to tumor growth is not suppressed.

It's been estimated that about 50 percent of all cancers—including breast, colon, and lung cancer—may be linked to mutations in a tumor suppressor gene known as p53. Since its discovery, ten other tumor suppressor genes have been identified. Researchers are trying to replace the defective gene and thereby stop the growth of cancer cells.

Prevention

One active area of research is the prevention of cancer once the carcinogenic process has started. For example, some cancers are preceded by an accumulation of abnormal (though not malignant) cells in what is called a *precursor lesion*. If a precursor lesion can be detected and removed, cancer will probably be prevented.

Clinical trials are under way to determine the effectiveness of *chemoprevention*—that is, using certain agents to prevent the evolution of a precancerous cell into a malignant one. For instance, researchers are trying to determine whether certain antioxidants, such as retinoids, vitamin E, and beta carotene, may prevent some cancers. Aspirin and nonsteroidal anti-inflammatory agents, such as ibuprofen, are being evaluated to learn if they can suppress cancer by inhibiting the proliferation of abnormal cells.

Today some of the genetic mutations that set the stage for cancer are rapidly being identified, such as for the hereditary forms of breast and colon cancer. Scientists expect to build on that knowledge and to devise treatments for reversing the mutation and/or halting carcinogenesis well before cancer cells proliferate and invade healthy tissue.

The Cancer Puzzle: What Makes a Cell Go Wrong?

The question that has intrigued physicians since Hippocrates, who named the disease *karkinos* (the Greek word for crab), is, "How does it happen?" The ancient Greeks believed an excess of one of the four bodily humors, black bile, was to blame. This idea persisted for 1,500 years. When the black-bile theory was finally put to rest, seventeenth-century doctors pinpointed abnormalities in the network of lymph nodes and vessels. With advances in the microscope, researchers could examine cells very closely for the first time.

By the 1950s, when the specialty of molecular biology began, scientists first began scrutinizing cells' DNA and the *genes* it contains.

Genetic Traces

The period from the late 1970s through the early 1980s was a time of major breakthroughs in understanding what cancer is and how it happens. For example, researchers discovered that as DNA molecules from a cancer cell were replicated and their information passed along to subsequent generations of cells, genes that actually induce cancer—called *oncogenes*—went along with them. It's now known that genetic flaws or mutations in critical portions of DNA activate oncogenes and may start the cancer process. Over time, as cells divide, more and more mutations occur. The discovery of oncogenes was a very important advance in understanding the origin of cancer.

Growth Factors

There are also mechanisms on the cell's surface that convey signals to the biological machinery within it and regulate the cell's activities. When erroneous messages are sent or a cell fails to receive and transmit a signal correctly, its growth and development are affected. Called *growth factors*, the various chemical messengers responsible for such communication constitute an intriguing subject for study.

Unlike healthy cells, tumor cells do not appear to respond properly to growth factors, and scientists are attempting to learn why this normally carefully regulated system fails.

There have also been some important advances based on using specific growth factors to enhance cancer therapies. For example, some growth factors stimulate the bone marrow to produce normal blood cells, and these growth factors have been used to replenish blood cells when they have been depleted by the toxic effects of chemotherapy. As a result a person can tolerate larger doses of anticancer drugs.

The concept of blocking other growth factors that stimulate the growth of cancer cells is also being studied as a way of enhancing the effects of some

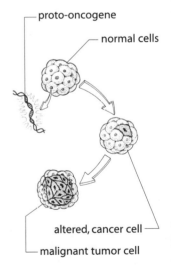

proto-oncogene

normal cells

altered, cancer cell

malignant tumor cell

How Cancer Begins
For unexplained reasons, a proto-oncogene in the cell's DNA becomes a cancer gene and causes the cell to behave abnormally and reproduce uncontrollably. The multiplying cancer cells form a tumor.

anti-cancer drugs (see Chapter 18, "Biological Therapies"). Besides this, new drugs to block blood vessel formation in tumors, gene therapy, and other innovations are being developed in an effort to prevent and cure cancers.

A Step-by-Step Process

Carcinogenesis is believed to take place in three stages: initiation, promotion, and tumor formation.

Initiation

During the *initiation* phase, some critical mutating event, usually involving an oncogene, alters a single cell's genetic programming, transforming it into a cell that will reproduce abnormal versions of itself.

The initial damage done or the cause of the mutation may be inherited or it can be acquired over time by exposure to cancer-causing chemicals, viruses, or radiation. Such change is irreversible. Some of these initiators have been identified; others remain a mystery. Certain viruses can be involved—such as hepatitis B, Epstein-Barr, and some papilloma (wart) viruses. Some chemicals have been implicated, such as hydrocarbons in tobacco, asbestos, and benzene. Moreover, large doses of radiation from repeated x-rays, excessive radon exposure, or proximity to nuclear accidents can be a cause (see Chapter 10, "Cancer Causes and Risks").

In many forms of cancer, more than one altered gene is required to transform a healthy cell into a malignant one. Depending on whether the initiating event is a single mutation caused by radiation or multiple events, this transformation process may take many generations of cells before cancer is set in motion. Thus, depending on where the cell comes from and the initiation event, it may take as few as three years or as many as 20 before the next phase begins—if it ever does. During this quiet time, the cell is *latent*.

Promotion

The second step, which increases the likelihood of carcinogenesis, is called *promotion*. Some carcinogens (such as the many found in tobacco) are both initiators and promoters, and some, particularly dietary factors like fat, act only as promoters. In either case, promoters do not damage the gene, as initiators do, but they are believed to affect how the genes' messages are expressed, or how they direct cells' behavior. And their effects are potentially reversible. If scientists are able to learn how to use this information, it may be possible to delay or prevent cancer by interfering with tumor promotion. In other words, although it may be impossible to prevent the initial mutation, it may be possible to interfere with the tumor promotion phase of carcinogenesis.

Different carcinogens, or cancer-initiating and/or promoting factors, regardless of when they exert their effects, vary in power. Some are very weak, perhaps too weak even to set the stage for cancer. Others, such as aflatoxin (a toxin that comes from a mold found in certain foods, such as contaminated peanuts) are exceptionally potent. Finally, a substance that is a pure promoter may have no effect on cells that have not already undergone initial genetic mutation.

We are all exposed to potential carcinogens every day, from the air we breathe, the food we eat, the sunlight we enjoy, and sometimes the work we do or the hobbies we pursue. Yet most of us do not get cancer (see Chapter 10, "Cancer Causes and Risks"). A great deal of research is under way to understand this natural resistance. It may be possible, for example, to use what is learned to interfere with carcinogenesis early enough to prevent cancer. Natural antioxidants in foods—such as vitamins C and E and beta carotene (which becomes vitamin A in the body)—may destroy a certain kind of oxygen molecule called a "toxic singlet" that is known to cause genetic damage.

Tumor Formation

Unlike healthy cells, cancer cells don't know their limits. Their feedback mechanisms have gone awry, and they pile up on top of each other haphazardly, forming masses, and develop blood vessels of their own. Other natural biological substances such as growth factors and hormones (like the sex hormones estrogen and testosterone) may also stimulate their development, as in the case of breast and prostate cancer, respectively. At some point, a tumor becomes large enough to be detected by examination or with tests. Or it may create problems or symptoms that prompt a person to seek medical attention.

Early, tiny, localized tumors (meaning those that have not yet extended into nearby regions or metastasized to other parts of the body) are called *in situ* cancers. A surgeon may detect them and remove them before they evolve further, or they remain small and insignificant even without treatment.

Cancer Differences

Cancer seems to find some organs more hospitable than others (see the box entitled "Leading Sites of New Cancer Cases and Deaths—1996"). Sex and age differences also seem to influence who gets what type (see Chapter 9, "Who Gets Cancer?"). In any event, once carcinogenesis begins, the tumor will develop, grow, and possibly metastasize at a pace that varies, depending on the type of cancer cell and who has it. The American Joint Commission on Cancer has established a system, called the TNM classification system, for classifying all types of cancer (see Chapter 2, "The Language of Cancer"). Just as there are risk factors that increase a person's chances of developing cancer in the first place, there are also factors—many of which remain undiscovered—that influence a person's hopes for recovery.

Today's Advances

It has taken almost 2,000 years for scientists to go from thinking black bile was the cause of cancer to unraveling the mysteries of DNA. Clearly the work is still incomplete. Yet there is excitement in almost every field of biological research because we are on the brink of learning what the many pieces of the puzzle are *and* how they fit together. Fortunately, each basic discovery also

Leading Sites of New Cancer Cases and Deaths—1996

Age-Adjusted Cancer Death Rates, Females by Site, US 1930-92

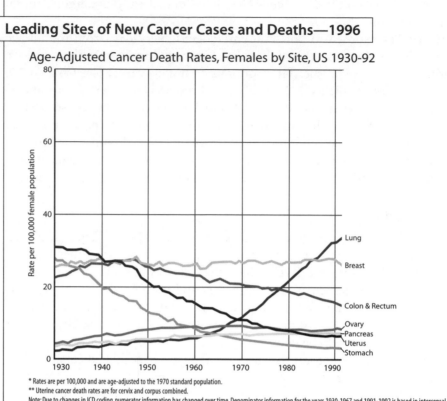

* Rates are per 100,000 and are age-adjusted to the 1970 standard population.
** Uterine cancer death rates are for cervix and corpus combined.
Note: Due to changes in ICD coding, numerator information has changed over time. Denominator information for the years 1930-1967 and 1991-1992 is based in intercensal population estimates, while denominator information for the years 1968-1990 is based on postcensal recalculation of estimates.

Age-Adjusted Cancer Death Rates, Males by Site, US 1930-92

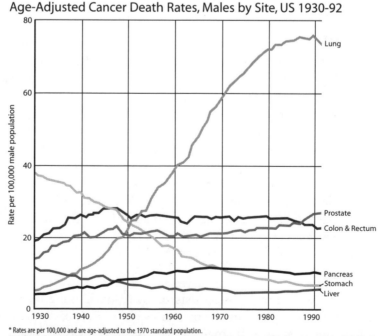

* Rates are per 100,000 and are age-adjusted to the 1970 standard population.
Note: Due to changes in ICD coding, numerator information has changed over time. Rates for cancer of the liver are particularly affected by these coding changes. Denominator information for the years 1930-1967 and 1991-1992 is based in intercensal population estimates, while denominator information for the years 1968-1990 is based on postcensal recalculation of estimates.
Source: Vital Statistics of the United States, 1995

Source: American Cancer Society, *Cancer Facts & Figures—1996*

aids scientists who are developing new treatments. So although a cure for all cancers is probably in the distant future, cures for certain types, ways to slow cancer's progress, and treatments to extend a person's lifespan *with* cancer and improve the quality of his or her life are continually emerging.

Disease-fighting *monoclonal antibodies*—antibodies that seek out cancer cells—are being studied as both diagnostic tools and delivery systems that can carry anticancer drugs directly to the target. Other biological therapies—such as interferon, vaccines, and biological response modifiers—are also being fine-tuned and tested. New classes of drugs and treatment combinations are being studied in medical centers and universities throughout the world (see Chapter 21, "Investigational Treatments").

Techniques that allow more aggressive chemotherapy than ever before, such as bone marrow transplant, are well on their way to becoming more available. Genetic therapy and drugs that selectively destroy the blood supply of malignant tumors are among the novel approaches to attack cancer. Drugs that inhibit cells that have become resistant to standard chemotherapy are also in the experimental stage and are likely to become very important for treating cancers that are now incurable.

Living Well with Cancer

Simultaneous to these efforts, the importance of not only living longer but living well has become a top priority among both caregivers and scientists, as it always has been for people with cancer. Drugs and psychological techniques that make the side effects of chemotherapy more tolerable are now available (see Chapter 17, "Chemotherapy"). For instance, it is now commonplace to use medications and relaxation techniques to prevent severe nausea and vomiting after high-dose chemotherapy. Not long ago, patients often had to suffer through the treatment and dreaded it as much as they did the cancer.

There has been a change in managing pain, making this greatly feared aspect of cancer tolerable for most people with medication and mind/body therapies (see Chapters 24, "Pain Relief," and 25, "Coping with Stress, Fear, Anxiety, and Depression"). The importance of support groups and better coping strategies is being recognized, and ways to measure their impact scientifically are being evaluated (see Chapters 13, "Your Support Network," and 31, "Coping Strategies"). Both physical symptoms due to the cancer and stress, anxiety, and depression can be managed. When they are, life improves immeasurably.

Information about new treatments and how to participate in research studies accessible to everyone is widely available (see Chapter 21, "Investigational Treatments"). Regardless of how aggressive you choose to be in seeking treatment, today you have more options than ever before. Now you can make choices suited to your individual physical condition, your emotional needs and comfort level, and the feelings and concerns of those close to you. Living with cancer is a serious, demanding challenge, but the resources for coping well and maintaining an acceptable quality of life are here. This book will help you make the decisions that suit you best, every step of the way.

The Language of Cancer

Each of the different cancers is as unique as a fingerprint in its growth and development, likelihood of spreading, the way it affects the body, and the symptoms it produces. Most of the language that describes cancer relates to these distinctions.

Although medical terminology is used primarily among professionals to communicate many specific details concisely, it is helpful for the layperson to understand the terms in a general way. This helps to comprehend a diagnosis and is invaluable when seeking information about a particular cancer. Although the language medical professionals use is often unwieldy, there is an order and precision to the jargon.

CANCER ✔ BASICS

Cancer Vocabulary

A *tumor* is any abnormal growth. A new growth is also called a *neoplasm*.

A benign neoplasm is slow growing, doesn't spread or invade surrounding tissue, and doesn't usually recur when removed. It may become malignant.

A *malignant* neoplasm invades surrounding tissue and spreads to other parts of the body. When it is removed it may recur if cancer cells have spread to surrounding tissues.

The suffix "-oma" refers to a tumor or neoplasm that may be benign, as an "adenoma," or malignant, as an adenocarcinoma.

Adjectives are sometimes used to describe a cancer more specifically (for example, "small-cell neuroendocrine carcinoma").

Some cancers are named for the person who discovered them or first described them, such as Ewing's sarcoma or Warthin's tumor.

Cancer Classification

Because cancer growth and development have so many phases, physicians use terms that specify where the cancer is and the type of tissue involved. Other terms and categories describe the extent of disease.

Tissue Types

The simplest system categorizes cancer according to the type of tissue it affects.

- The most common cancers, accounting for 80 to 90 percent of cases, are carcinomas, which originate in *epithelial* tissue. Epithelial tissue is found throughout the body; it includes the skin and the covering and lining of organs and internal passageways, such as the gastrointestinal tract. Most carcinomas affect organs that secrete something, such as the breasts, which are capable of producing milk, or the lungs, which secrete mucus.

- Carcinomas are divided into two subtypes: *adenocarcinoma*, which indicates a cancer that develops in an organ or gland, and *squamous cell carcinoma*, which refers to a cancer that originates in the skin. (However, *melanoma* also affects skin.)

- *Sarcoma* refers to cancer that begins in connective tissue such as bones, tendons and cartilage, muscle, and fat.

- *Leukemias* are cancers of the bone marrow and lymph system, which make blood.

- *Myeloma* is cancer that originates in the plasma cells of bone marrow.

- *Lymphomas* develop in the glands or nodes of the *lymphatic system*, a network of vessels, nodes, and organs (specifically the spleen, tonsils, and thymus) that purify body fluids and produce infection-fighting white blood cells, or *lymphocytes*. One class of lymphoma is known as *Hodgkin's disease*; all others are called *non-Hodgkin's lymphomas*.

- Tumors of nerve tissue are named after the specific type of cell they affect. For instance, cancer of a nerve cell known as the *glial cell* is called *glioma*. A tumor on the covering of the brain, the *meninges*, is labeled a *meningioma*.

Cancer Site

The body part in which cancer first develops is known as the *primary site*. A cancer's primary site may determine how the tumor will behave; whether and where it may spread, or metastasize; and what symptoms it is most likely to cause. The most common primary sites of cancer are the skin, lungs, colon, rectum, breast, uterus, mouth, and bone marrow.

A cancer is always described in terms of the primary site, even if it has spread to another part of the body. For instance, advanced breast cancer that has spread to the lymph nodes under the arm and to the bone and lungs is always considered breast cancer. To convey the extent of the cancer, a doctor might say this is "a primary tumor of the breast with regional metastases to the axillary lymph nodes and systemic spread to the bones and lungs."

Tumor Grade

Once a tumor has been detected, some or all of it can be removed for microscopic examination. One thing the pathologist tries to determine is how closely the cells resemble healthy, mature cells. Such cells are said to be *differentiated*. Cancer cells that do not look like their healthy counterparts are called *undifferentiated*, *anaplastic*, or, because they often look like very immature cells, *primitive*. *Carcinoma in situ* describes cells that are beginning to become abnormal but are not a definite invasive cancer. It is the earliest stage of cancer. Actual growths or tumors made up of undifferentiated cells are probably somewhat advanced, because they grow more rapidly than the differentiated, healthy, mature cells.

Information on the cells' characteristics is used to label, or *grade*, tumors and is important in determining how the cancer should be treated and how successful treatment may be. High-grade tumors are usually fast growing, aggressive, and undifferentiated. There are some variations on how tumors are graded, but in general there are four classifications, based on how closely they resemble the tissue from which they developed:

- Grade I tumors are 75 to 100 percent differentiated.

- Grade II tumors are 50 to 75 percent differentiated.

- Grade III tumors are 25 to 50 percent differentiated.

- Grade IV tumors are under 25 percent differentiated.

Staging

Cancers are further classified according to *stage*. *Staging* is useful to describe how far a cancer has progressed based on the size of the primary tumor and on whether and where it has spread. There are five cancer stages, labeled 0 to IV. Depending on the type of cancer, stages are sometimes further subdivided, such as IIA and IIB. Simply put, a cancer in its early stage will probably be small and confined to its primary site. In advanced stages it will be large and will have spread to lymph nodes or other structures.

There are different ways to determine the stage of a cancer, depending on its type. Some cancers may be easily staged with physical examination and laboratory tests; others require surgery.

The TNM System

Cancers are often classified and staged according to the *TNM system* of the American Joint Commission on Cancer, which looks at three aspects of a cancer.

- *T* indicates the size of a primary tumor and whether it has begun to invade nearby tissues and structures, such as blood vessels, bones, nerves, and organs.

- *N* refers to whether lymph nodes have been affected by the primary tumor and, if so, how large the metastases are.

- *M* signifies whether a cancer has spread to other organs and the extent to which metastasis has occurred.

Each of these letters is assigned a subscript, a number that defines the extent to which a primary tumor has grown, invaded lymph nodes, and metastasized.

The TNM system defines stages of cancer in terms of specific combinations of the three groupings just described. The details at each stage vary according to the type of cancer. In other words, there is a definitive TNM classification for lung cancer that may differ from the specifics of the TNM classification for prostate cancer. (See TNM staging for specific cancers in the Encyclopedia section.) For example, a primary Stage I tumor of the breast is a T1 N0 M0 growth. This means that the tumor is less than 2 centimeters in diameter (T1), has not metastasized to the lymph nodes under the arm on the same side as the primary site (N0), and has not spread elsewhere in the body (M0).

From Cell to Tumor

The stages of the TNM system represent a natural progression of cancer. All cancers are thought to develop from a single abnormal cell, which divides into two abnormal cells, which divide into four abnormal cells, then eight, then 16, then 32, and so on. Some cells divide fairly slowly; others divide rapidly. The rate at which cancer cells grow is called *doubling time*. It is thought that the doubling process must occur 30 times—which can take months, even years—before a tumor can be detected. At this point it will contain about 1 billion cells and will be large enough to be felt or seen on an x-ray or with an imaging procedure.

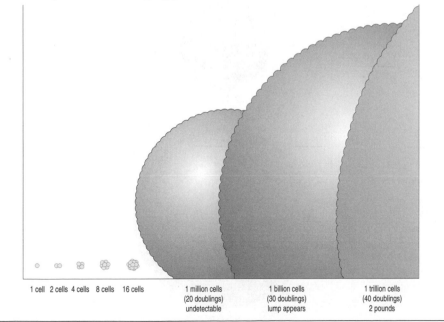

1 cell 2 cells 4 cells 8 cells 16 cells

1 million cells
(20 doublings)
undetectable

1 billion cells
(30 doublings)
lump appears

1 trillion cells
(40 doublings)
2 pounds

Tumor Sizes

Centimeters may be hard to visualize. The size of a quarter is a helpful comparison. Tumors are typically measured in centimeters, sizes that are sometimes hard to visualize. These circles will give you a rough idea of how large some tumors are relative to a quarter.

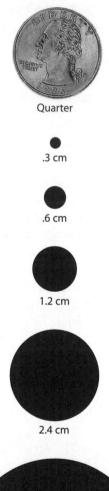

Quarter

.3 cm

.6 cm

1.2 cm

2.4 cm

4.8 cm

SIGNS AND SYMPTOMS

Cancer is a progressive disease. It goes through many stages, producing an array of symptoms along the way. Some symptoms occur early and are caused by a tumor growing within an organ or structure. If a cancer spreads, it may produce entirely new symptoms as other organs, structures, and systems become involved. As the immune system fights to rid the body of malignant cells, still other symptoms arise.

How a Tumor Grows

Tumor cells need a blood supply to bring them fresh nutrients and carry away wastes. The process by which a tumor links up with the bloodstream is called *vascularization* or *angiogenesis*. It is believed that the tumor secretes a substance known as *tumor angiogenesis factor (TAF)*, which induces nearby blood vessels to produce new capillaries that grow toward the tumor and finally connect with it.

Side Effects of Tumor Growth

As the tumor becomes vascularized, it begins to grow rapidly and puts pressure on nearby organs, nerves, and blood vessels. This pressure creates some of the earliest warning signs of cancer, especially when a tumor is in an area of the body with little room for expansion. For instance, even a small tumor in the brain can cause headaches by pressing on blood vessels and nerves.

Growing tumors can also erode blood vessels. This usually results in bleeding from an orifice near the tumor. A common example is blood in the stool caused by a tumor rupturing blood vessels in the colon.

A developing tumor also can affect how the body functions by obstructing an organ. For example, a growth in the esophagus, the passageway between the throat and stomach, may cause *dysphagia*, or difficulty swallowing.

Whether a tumor prompts the warning signs that bring a person to seek early medical attention often depends on its location. For instance, one of the early signs of pancreatic cancer is a yellowing of the skin, or *jaundice*. This occurs when the growth, even while very small, blocks the nearby bile duct. However, if there is no blockage, jaundice is unlikely. In this case, the tumor may grow quite large before causing another symptom, such as pain, which occurs when the tumor presses on the back. Breast cancer is an example of a malignancy that rarely causes early symptoms. That's why screening tests such as breast self-exams and mammography are so important (see Chapter 5, "Screening for Cancer").

Cancer Spread

As the tumor grows, it pushes on the cells of healthy structures so aggressively that it squeezes through tiny spaces between cells and, like a plant in fertile soil, takes root. Tumors may release enzymes that weaken and destroy tissue, making invasion easier. Whenever a new growth springs up, it may produce new symptoms that can draw attention to the cancer.

The Body Goes to War

The immune system has been likened to an elaborate military force. It is made up of several components, each with a different and highly specialized function. These include cells known as *monocytes* and *macrophages*, which circulate throughout the body. These cells identify cancer cells and process that information in a way that will activate other defensive components of the immune system, such as the *T-* and *B-lymphocytes*. These lymphocytes, which are found in the lymph nodes, spleen, and bloodstream, actually destroy foreign cells. A subgroup of these cells—the *T4*, or *T helper*, cells— does not destroy enemy cells directly but helps the T- and B-lymphocytes and the macrophages to carry out their functions.

Another major component of the immune system consists of the *natural killer*, or *NK*, cells. The role of these cells in the immune response to cancer is being clarified, but it appears that they help kill tumor cells.

As the immune system battles cancer cells, the consequences of this internal war may become obvious. For instance, the person may suffer from weight loss and body wasting, or *cachexia*. These hallmarks of cancer result because the immune response uses so much energy. People with cancer also may find they are more susceptible to infectious diseases as the immune system directs much of its energy to killing the cancer.

Cancer Symptoms

Silent cancers usually aren't so silent. Often early symptoms are ignored because the person either is frightened by their implications and refuses to seek medical advice or does not recognize them as warning signs of cancer. That's why it's important to know what some of the symptoms of cancer are. They include unexpected weight loss, fever, fatigue, pain, changes in the skin and hair, and a special group of symptoms called *paraneoplastic symptoms*, which are caused by the abnormal production of hormones.

Weight Loss

Ultimately, most people who develop cancer experience weight loss and a related condition, cachexia, which refers not only to the loss of fat and muscle, but also to the wasting away of organs. The heart, liver, and brain are usually spared the effects of cachexia.

Sometimes weight loss is an early sign. The scale may register 5 pounds less within two weeks, or 10 pounds less in a month or so, without dieting or increased exercise. Such loss of weight is most likely when a cancer affects a part of the digestive system, such as the pancreas, stomach, or esophagus. Early weight loss has also been associated with Hodgkin's disease and cancer of the kidney and lung.

A number of aspects of cancer are believed to contribute to weight loss and cachexia. Some tumors directly affect the function and efficiency of the digestive system, often by preventing the body from absorbing all the nutrients it needs from food. In addition, most tumors, particularly those that have vascularized and are expanding rapidly, appear to grow independently of the host, drawing fat, protein, and carbohydrates from healthy tissue.

A growing tumor also turns up the calorie-burning thermostat: Not only do the cancer cells use large amounts of energy as they divide and the tumor vascularizes, but the immune system also requires energy, which further accelerates the metabolism. This increase in energy expenditure is compounded by the fact that people with cancer often don't feel like eating and so don't increase their calorie intake to meet the increasing metabolic demands of their body. This loss of appetite may be caused by nausea induced by certain toxohormones released by the tumor; it may also be a side effect of cancer treatments, such as chemotherapy (see Chapter 26, "Food and Nutrition").

Fever

About 70 percent of people with cancer experience fever, particularly if the disease directly affects a component of the immune system, such as the lymph nodes. People with Hodgkin's disease, for instance, have an elevated temperature about a quarter of the time. Their fever fluctuates, going up to 100 or 101 degrees and then returning to normal. Fever commonly occurs with liver cancer and in the presence of secondary tumors, such as metastatic carcinomas of the lung, kidney, pancreas, and gastrointestinal tract.

Activation of the immune system almost always triggers fever: It's just one sign that the body is fighting off sickness. In addition, tumors may give off *pyrogenic*, or fever-inducing, substances. Fever is also a symptom of a secondary infection and if it is very high may cause sweating, malaise, and even confusion.

Fatigue

Weight loss and cachexia can cause weakness and fatigue. Usually fatigue is not a significant symptom until a cancer is fairly advanced, unless the person is experiencing chronic blood loss. (Often stomach or colon cancer causes blood loss.)

Pain

Pain is a symptomatic wild card. It may result from many aspects of the disease. Most often, discomfort suggests advanced disease. Usually it's the result of the destruction of healthy tissue by a tumor, infection, pressure on or stretching of internal organs and other structures, or the obstruction of an organ.

Yet pain can be among the first signs of certain cancers. For instance, sarcomas are often painful early on; testicular cancer can cause pain in the scrotum; bladder cancer can make urination painful; certain lung tumors can cause pain in the arm, shoulder, and upper back and chest on the side where the growth is located. Growths that are confined to small spaces, such as the brain, the eye, or the sinuses, may cause pain by pressing on nearby blood vessels or nerves.

The location of cancer pain does not always reveal the location of the tumor. Because the body is linked by a network of nerves that feed into the same system for interpretation by the brain, pain in one part of the body may be perceived as originating in another. This phenomenon is known as *referred pain*. For example, pain produced by a tumor of the esophagus is often felt in or near the shoulder, and stomach cancers often cause pain in the chest.

Although the pain of advanced cancer can be intense and persistent, progress in pain management now means that unremitting suffering is not inevitable (see Chapter 24, "Pain Relief").

Skin Clues

Cancer can cause dozens of visible signs. Some of the most obvious are cancers of the skin. A skin tumor often starts as a small growth that eventually ulcerates, bleeds, and doesn't scab over and heal. A mole that is malignant, such as melanoma, usually exhibits subtle but significant changes. It may go from having a definite border to looking as if it is spreading in all directions. It may change color, grow larger, or both.

Although rare, a metastatic growth on the skin can result from a primary tumor of the lung, breast, colon, ovary, stomach, or kidney. Such a growth on the skin is usually a firm, flesh-colored, reddish or bluish nodule, and is located near the site of the primary tumor. Sometimes these tumors arise on the scalp and cause patchy hair loss.

Among the other signs of cancer that appear on the skin are

- darkening of the skin, or *hyperpigmentation*. This usually occurs under the arm or on the lower back, neck, or groin and has been linked to cancer of the gastrointestinal tract, uterus, prostate, ovary, and kidney.

- reddening of skin, or *erythema*. This can be a manifestation of lymphoma or leukemia or gastrointestinal, breast, lung, or cervical cancer.

- itching, or *pruritus*. This is common in Hodgkin's disease and other lymphomas, as well as in carcinomas of the pancreas, stomach, and brain. Itching may occur with cancer of the ovary or adrenal gland.

- excessive hair growth, or *hirsutism*.

Other Symptoms

Some cancer symptoms are direct results of neither the primary tumor nor a metastatic growth. Rather, they occur because cancer causes the overproduction of hormones, or the tumor itself produces and secretes substances called *toxohormones* that may have far-reaching effects on other organs, such as the liver, thymus, and spleen. The problems that result are called *paraneoplastic symptoms*. Hyperpigmentation, for example, is thought to be due to the excess production of melanocyte-stimulating hormone (MSH). Fever may result from the release of a pyrogenic substance from a tumor. Toxohormones most likely have a role in cachexia.

It is also suspected that cancer tumors release toxic substances that affect the neurologic and muscular systems, a phenomenon called *carcinomatous neuromyopathy*. This condition affects about 7 percent of those with cancer and usually occurs with cancers of the lung, ovary, stomach, prostate, breast, colon, and cervix.

The most common manifestation of carcinomatous neuromyopathy is muscle weakness and wasting. Nerves may be stripped of their protective covering, the *myelin sheath*, and be seriously damaged. Some people develop a condition that resembles a muscle-weakening disease called myasthenia gravis.

The Emotional Response

Cancer is a serious, frightening, and life-threatening disease. Most people realize that once it is diagnosed, the road to recovery may be long and painful. The word cancer elicits images of nauseating chemotherapy, surgery, disfigurement, hair loss, weakness, and pain. People respond psychologically and emotionally to the threat of this disease much as they have to other crises in their lives (see Chapter 31, "Coping Strategies").

Can Your Mood Be a Cancer Symptom?

By influencing hormones and brain chemicals, numerous physical illnesses can produce anxiety and depression. Of the cancers that can produce such symptoms, pancreatic cancer seems to be the most common. In many cases, symptoms of depression, anxiety, insomnia, and feelings of impending doom appear before any physical symptoms. Since cancer of the pancreas often produces no bodily symptoms until the illness is quite advanced, mood changes could be an important early warning sign.

Pay attention to depression, anxiety, or other emotional symptoms that seem to appear from nowhere. Like most of the other early-warning signs of cancer, the mood symptoms could also indicate a number of other problems, or nothing at all. If your unusual depression or anxiety doesn't go away within a few weeks, see your doctor.

SPECIAL

CONCERNS

INFORM

YOURSELF

When to See a Doctor

A good rule of thumb when trying to decide whether to make an appointment with your doctor is to ask yourself if the symptom has been bothering you for a while. Symptoms that linger—even those that are only a mild annoyance—are especially important cancer warnings. Although they may turn out to be false alarms, it is best to have these symptoms checked.

Since it is impossible to remember all the possible symptoms of the 200 different cancers, the American Cancer Society has established the following seven symptoms that are common cancer clues.

1. **A change in bowel habits or bladder function**. Chances are you are at least vaguely aware of when and how often you move your bowels and how often during a normal day you need to urinate. A change in either routine might be a sign of cancer: Chronic constipation or, conversely, long-lasting diarrhea may indicate cancer of the colon or rectum. See a doctor about these symptoms immediately, because waiting until the constipation becomes so severe that even laxatives don't help or stools become pencil thin often means allowing the cancer to become dangerously advanced.

   You should also see a doctor immediately if you notice blood in your stool.

   See your physician if passing urine is painful or difficult or if blood appears in your urine. These are potential signs of prostate or bladder cancer.

2. **Sores that do not heal**. Cancers of the skin may bleed and resemble sores that never heal. They can crop up anywhere on the body, including the genitals. Such sores may also form in the mouth and should be evaluated as soon as they are noticed; this is particularly true of people who smoke, chew tobacco, or frequently drink alcohol, because their use of these cancer-causing substances boosts the chance that the lesions in their mouths may be malignant.

3. **Unusual bleeding or discharge**. Unusual bleeding can occur in early or advanced cancer. Coughing up blood is a sign of lung cancer. A woman who has vaginal bleeding between periods or anytime after menopause should see a physician immediately. Cancer of the lining of the uterus (the *endometrium*) or of the cervix can cause vaginal bleeding. Blood in the stool may indicate cancer of the colon or rectum or both. Blood in the urine can mean cancer of either the bladder or the kidneys. A bloody discharge from the nipple may be a sign of breast cancer.

4. **Thickening or lump in the breast or elsewhere**. Many tumors can be felt through the skin, particularly in the breast, testicles, or soft tissues of the body. You can also sometimes feel lumps in certain lymph glands, such as the axillary nodes under the arm. The best way to catch these palpable cancers is by performing regular self-exams (see Chapter 7, "Examining Yourself"). In general, any thickening or

lump should be reported to your physician promptly: You may detect a primary tumor in an early, operable stage, before it has vascularized or metastasized.

5. **Indigestion or difficulty in swallowing.** These two symptoms are also known as *dyspepsia* and *dysphagia*, and they may indicate cancer of the esophagus, stomach, or *pharynx* (the tube connecting the mouth with the esophagus). Usually by the time these symptoms occur, the cancer is fairly advanced, so you should seek medical attention immediately.

6. **Recent change in a wart or mole.** Warts or moles that change color, lose their definite borders, or grow should be seen by a physician immediately. The skin lesion may be melanoma, a malignancy that is often curable if attended to early.

7. **A nagging cough or hoarseness.** If you develop a cough that lingers for two weeks or more, see a physician. Along with persistent hoarseness, this may be an indication of a malignancy of the lung, *larynx* (voice box), or thyroid. It often suggests an advanced stage of cancer.

The Power of Denial

Denial is the most common response to the suggestion of cancer. Many who notice something amiss in their bodies often attempt to make sense of the symptoms or find some less serious cause. "That nagging cough is just part of a bad cold," they might say. Or, "I'm constipated because I haven't had time to eat right lately." Or, "That headache won't go away because my workload is so intense right now."

They deny that something serious might be wrong, and because many of the warning signs of cancer mimic symptoms of less serious illnesses, or even of stress, it is easy to postpone a checkup.

Other Common Reactions

Some people are as frightened of the loss of independence that goes with serious illness as they are of sickness itself. They hate the thought of being weak or helpless and dependent on family, friends, and doctors. They may also be afraid of what their disease will mean to others: A woman may fear that losing a breast to cancer will affect her husband's feelings for her. A young parent may worry about how his or her children will deal with the realities of the disease. Rather than denial, some people respond with guilt, anger, or depression. And some panic.

Timing Is Critical

Most of the time these reactions serve as delay tactics. It isn't until a symptom arises that seriously interferes with day-to-day life that some are spurred into action. Pain is a major motivator for seeking medical help, for instance.

The problem with putting off medical care, of course, is that time is of the essence when it comes to fighting cancer. As this chapter explains, cancer waits for no one. With the passage of time it grows, vascularizes, and metastasizes. On the other hand, it is quite possible to stop many tumors before they have time to do lasting damage. That's why it is important to understand how cancer grows, the stages it goes through, and the way it causes symptoms. That knowledge can help even the most fearful person act and get help.

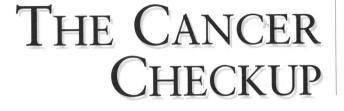

THE CANCER CHECKUP

For most of human history people have gone to healers and doctors when they felt sick. But as the practice of medicine has become more
sophisticated, we have learned how to detect serious illness even before symptoms occur. Early detection and intervention is one of our most effective tools
to contain health care costs and save lives.

Avoiding possible causes of illness, such as smoking, which increases the
risk of lung cancer and heart disease, is known as *primary prevention*.

Too Scared to Get Tested?

Many people do not go for routine screening tests because they are afraid
to find out that they have cancer. Although screening tests are obviously
performed to detect disease, the vast majority of people screened are free
of illness. Normal test results are an enormous relief from the nagging anxiety that comes from avoiding the screening. Indeed, for those at normal or
high risk of various cancers, the best way to escape worry and concern is to
have the tests regularly.

Detecting life-threatening illness as early as possible offers the greatest
opportunity for survival with the best quality of life. Cancer doesn't stop
developing just because you aren't ready to deal with it. What you don't
know *can* hurt you.

If you think that psychological barriers such as fear of cancer or fear of
its recurrence are preventing you from having a recommended test, talk to
your friends, family, and certainly your physician. The support and encouragement of others you care for and respect can be a great facilitator in helping you take loving care of yourself.

SPECIAL

CONCERNS

Equally important is *secondary prevention*, that is, detection of disease when it probably can be cured. The first and oldest early-detection method consists of a health history and physical examination in a medical setting: the *cancer-related checkup*.

Supplementing the checkup are numerous *screening tests* used to detect abnormalities in people who have no symptoms or who don't recognize a symptom as being associated with cancer. Chapter 5 lists specific tests and their recommended intervals.

Guidelines for Everyone

To help healthy people and their doctors decide which early detection methods best suit their individual needs and how often they should be examined, the American Cancer Society, after much research, has established cancer-related checkup guidelines. These guidelines are useful for people at average and high risk (see Chapter 10, "Cancer Causes and Risks"); they are not intended for those who already have signs or symptoms of cancer.

One reason the ACS established guidelines for early detection was to ensure that everyone—those cared for by private physicians as well as those

INFORM
YOURSELF

If Your Doctor Doesn't Follow the American Cancer Society Guidelines

Guidelines are recommendations, not rules. Some physicians believe that some tests should be done more or less often than the ACS suggests, and the interval with which they are done may vary, depending on your health and family history. Although most physicians reported in a 1989 study that they emphasized early cancer detection more than they had five years earlier, they varied considerably in how often they performed tests recommended by the ACS in people who have no symptoms.

If you've never had a "cancer-related checkup," it may be because your doctor calls it something else. Or, rather than schedule a visit specifically to conduct all the tests and examinations, your physician may give you different parts of the checkup when you come in at other times for other health problems.

But doctors can overlook some tests or wrongly assume that another physician is doing them. For instance, your general practitioner may assume that your dentist examines your mouth, tongue, and throat as part of your annual dental checkup. If you are a woman, your doctor may assume that you see a gynecologist regularly for a Pap smear and pelvic examination.

To take responsibility for your own health (and be a health-conscious consumer), ask your doctor about all aspects of the cancer-related checkup and whether you should have the different tests and examinations at the intervals suggested by the ACS. If your physician believes that other intervals are appropriate, find out what he or she suggests. If your doctor tells you the test is unimportant in your case, ask why. If you are unsatisfied with the explanation, get a second opinion.

who rely on government-funded facilities and programs—receives the same standard of care. Many other professional medical organizations make their own recommendations, and not all groups agree, particularly with regard to tests for detection. This book presents primarily the ACS guidelines.

Since epidemiological information is continually being updated and new tests are being developed and evaluated, the ACS periodically reviews and, if necessary, revises its guidelines. To check if there have been any recent changes in the guidelines that appear in this book, call the ACS at 800-ACS-2345.

The Cancer-Related Checkup

The ACS recommends a cancer-related checkup every three years for asymptomatic men and women 20 to 39 years of age and an annual exam for those age 40 and older. (Since the risk of cancer increases with age, the frequency of checkups also increases. If you are at high risk for certain cancers, you may receive a more frequent checkup at the discretion of your physician.)

The cancer-related checkup consists of a discussion of your health history and personal risk factors, a physical examination, and screening tests. It also offers the health care provider an opportunity to teach self-examinations of the breasts, testes, and skin (see Chapter 7, "Examining Yourself").

The checkup may be performed by your primary health provider—usually a general practitioner, a family practitioner, an internist, or a gynecologist. Some women may visit their family doctor for all aspects of the checkup except the breast and pelvic exams, and have those two exams done by their gynecologist. Sometimes a nurse practitioner may perform some aspects of the checkup. *Screening tests* are an essential part of the cancer-related checkup.

Health History and Counseling

The checkup begins with a review of family and personal health histories. The doctor asks about your prior illnesses and those of close family members—siblings, parents, aunts and uncles, and grandparents. A history of cancer in any first-degree relative (parent, sibling, or children) is especially important.

Next comes a review of your lifestyle, focusing on any factors that may increase the risk of cancer (see Chapter 9, "Who Gets Cancer?"). The higher the risk, the more frequent certain screening tests should be.

This review of hereditary and lifestyle factors that may influence the development of cancer should serve as the basis for health counseling during the examination about personal-risk factors—such as tobacco use, sun exposure, sexual practices, other environmental or occupational exposures, and role of diet and nutrition in developing cancer. For example, if you eat few fruits and vegetables, the physician or nurse might explain that a diet low in fiber increases the risk for colorectal cancer.

The Physical Examination

The physical examination relies on the doctor's ability to observe and feel, or *palpate*, different body parts and organs and thereby identify variations from normal size, surface texture, and sensitivity. A particular benefit of this examination is that it involves no risks because only inspection and touch are involved.

The Oral Cavity. Focusing a light into your mouth, the doctor inspects and feels the lips, gums, tissues lining the mouth, the hard palate on the roof of the mouth, the tongue, and the throat. (Dentures are removed before the examination.) The physician looks for abnormalities in color, moisture, surface texture, and symmetry and for areas of thickening, sores, or discharge. After observing tongue movement, the doctor depresses the tongue with a flat instrument to see the back of the mouth and throat.

The Thyroid Gland. The thyroid is a butterfly-shaped gland located at the base of the neck, in front of the larynx or voice box. It secretes a hormone that controls many aspects of metabolism.

The doctor observes the front of the neck for any swelling. Asking you to take a sip of water, the physician watches for any abnormal movement in the neck. Then, usually standing behind you, he or she gently manipulates the structures in your neck and palpates the front and side surfaces of the thyroid gland, noting any tenderness, discomfort, or nodules.

The Lymph Nodes. The *lymphatic system* is a network of vessels throughout the body that carry fluid called *lymph* away from muscles, joints, deep layers of the skin, and organs. Round or bean-shaped nodules called *lymph nodes* or *glands* are located at certain junctures. Waste products, bacteria and other microorganisms, and cancer cells that have spread into the tissue surrounding a tumor are filtered at these nodes. Many illnesses, particularly infections, can lead to temporarily swollen lymph glands. Cancer spread may be suspected when nodes remain enlarged with no sign of an infection.

Lymph nodes are located throughout the body, including behind the knees, around the elbows, on the spine, around the lungs and aorta, and in the gastrointestinal system. However, the nodes can be effectively palpated only in three areas where sufficiently large masses of them occur: in the neck, under the arms (*axilla*), and in the groin. The neck nodes are palpated as part of the thyroid examination, and the axilla nodes are checked as part of the breast examination in women. The doctor feels the nodes with the fingertips, using a circular motion. Normal nodes are movable, soft, and not tender.

The Skin. A thorough skin examination requires the removal of clothing so that every inch of the body can be examined. Some doctors have you stand and turn slowly for the examination; others perform it while you recline and have you turn as needed. In people at high risk for skin cancer, particularly those with many moles, photographs may be taken for comparison in following years. In addition to simple observation, the physician usually spreads the buttocks to view inner skin, and raises a man's testicles or spreads a woman's legs to examine the genital area.

Many doctors use an ABCD mnemonic (memory aid) as a guide for spotting malignant melanoma, the most severe type of skin cancer. These lesions tend to

- (A) be **A**symmetrical.

- (B) have irregular **B**orders.

- (C) vary in **C**olor from one area to another.

- (D) have a **D**iameter greater than 6 millimeters (that is, larger than about one-quarter of an inch).

The physician also looks for any sore that has been present for more than three weeks that bleeds, oozes, or crusts; any irritated red patches that may or may not itch or hurt; any change in long-standing "beauty marks" or moles, such as elevation, darkening of color, swelling, tenderness, or pain. Any new pigmented lesions will be evaluated carefully, and other types of skin cancer will be looked for, too.

The Female Pelvis. The pelvic examination is used to detect cancers of the female reproductive system, specifically the ovaries, endometrial lining of the uterus, cervix, vagina, and vulva. Unfortunately, a pelvic examination is not highly effective in detecting these cancers in their early stages. (The exception is cancer of the cervix, which can be detected by a Pap smear.) Despite the limitations of this examination, it is recommended because it poses no risks and is one of the few methods available for cancer detection of a woman's reproductive organs.

A woman should avoid sexual intercourse for 24 hours before a pelvic examination, and douching and any medication, including vaginal contraceptives, should be avoided for three days before the test. Immediately before the procedure she should urinate and, if necessary, move her bowels. After removing her clothing from the waist down, the woman reclines on a special examining table that has stirrup supports to keep her legs raised and spread.

First, the doctor visually inspects the external genitalia: the vulva, labia majora and minora, clitoris, and anal region, looking for any sores, swellings, or other abnormalities. Then he or she palpates the lymph nodes in the groin (*inguinal* lymph nodes).

Next the vagina and cervix are inspected using a speculum, a metal or plastic instrument with two paddlelike extensions. The speculum is lubricated and inserted into the vagina, and the paddles are opened to expose the inside walls of the vagina and the cervix. After a visual inspection in which the physician looks for abnormal discharge, sores, erosion, or growths, a Pap smear (see Chapter 6, "Routine Tests") may be performed.

The third part of the pelvic is the *bimanual examination*. The doctor uses gloved hands to palpate the internal pelvic organs in the following manner: The lubricated index and middle finger of one hand are inserted into the vagina while the other hand is placed on the abdomen. By pressing the fingers and hand together, the doctor can palpate the size, shape, and position of the uterus and ovaries and may be able to detect abnormal masses.

The final segment of the pelvic is the *recto-vaginal exam*. One gloved finger is inserted in the vagina and another is inserted into the rectum. Again, as the fingers press together over the back wall of the vagina and the front wall of the rectum, the doctor can feel local structures and abnormalities.

The Rectum and Prostate. The rectum is the last 5 or 6 inches of the colon or large intestine and the anus. The *prostate* is a walnut-sized gland that surrounds the urethra in men. It secretes a fluid that contributes to the seminal fluid expelled during ejaculation. These structures can be evaluated by a digital rectal examination.

Men are usually examined either while standing and leaning over the exam table or while reclining on their left side with their knees drawn up. Women are examined in the same position used for a pelvic or, as with men, while reclining on their left side.

The doctor inserts a single gloved, lubricated finger into the rectum and rotates it slowly to feel for any growths, tumors, or other abnormalities. In men, the finger is also moved to palpate the prostate gland, located in front of the rectum, checking for asymmetry, hardness, or protrusions from the gland's normally smooth and rubbery surface.

The Breasts. In women, breasts contain 15 to 20 glandular lobes surrounded by fatty tissue. Each lobe has a duct that opens on the surface of the nipple. Male breasts lack lobes. When breast cancer does occur in men, which is rare, it is usually in the tissue covering the chest muscle.

Examination of a woman's breasts begins with the woman sitting or standing with her hands on her hips. The doctor visually observes the breasts, looking for any marked unevenness, imbalance, or abnormal breast contour and for unusual nipple position, discharge, retraction (or pulling inward), and skin changes, such as puckering, dimpling, discoloration, or scaling. Movement and change in the breasts are further observed as the woman slowly raises her arms over her head and then lowers them and presses her palms together at waist level. Women with large breasts also may be asked to lean forward.

SPECIAL CONCERNS

Physical Examination: Does It Hurt?

None of the physical examinations recommended in the cancer-related checkup should cause pain or serious discomfort. Although the doctor often applies a very firm hand when palpating an organ or area, this pressure should not make you wince. If you feel pain or tenderness, speak up—it could be an important warning sign.

Mild discomfort during a pelvic examination may derive from your own level of tension, as well as from the physician's lack of dexterity. If you can relax your vaginal and rectal muscles, and the doctor works quickly but gently, the only sensation should be moderate pressure. Try to relax by breathing slowly and deeply during the examination.

Many people feel squeamish about the digital rectal examination. The examination should not be painful, because the doctor's entering finger is far smaller than the size of typical exiting bowel movements. Entry may be easier if you bear down, as if moving your bowels, but then try to relax for the few seconds it takes for the examination.

Then the doctor palpates both breasts, usually with the middle three fingers of both hands, first with the woman sitting up and then again in a reclining position with her arms over her head. The doctor will gently squeeze each areola, the pigmented area around the nipple, to check for nipple discharge and will raise the woman's arms to feel the lymph nodes in the armpits.

The Testicles. The egg-shaped *testicles* are the male reproductive glands that produce sperm and male sex hormones, such as testosterone. The two testicles hang outside the body in a small pouch called the *scrotum*, located below and behind the penis.

The testicular exam is relatively brief. With the man standing, the doctor observes the genital area, looking for any signs of swelling or other abnormalities. Then the doctor raises the scrotum, observes the underlying skin, and palpates lymph nodes in the groin and along the upper inner thigh. Using both hands, all surfaces of each testicle are palpated for any lump, thickening, or other abnormality. The doctor also notes any significant differences in the size, weight, and firmness of the testicles.

5

SCREENING FOR CANCER

Screening usually means testing everyone in a segment of the population to detect a disease. For example, a screening test may be recommended for everyone in a certain age group, or it may be done on an individual basis regardless of age. For example, if your family members have had a particular cancer, you may be tested more frequently for abnormalities associated with the disease than someone without such a history.

The cancer-related checkup is considered a general screening examination, but tests are also available that can detect specific cancers, often before symptoms develop. When cancer is detected at such an early stage, it is much more likely to respond to treatment and not spread.

Many screening tests are performed in conjunction with the cancer-related checkup, but they may be done at any time—in a doctor's office, at health fairs, at work, or in special clinics. Physicians may perform some tests, but most can be done by nurses or technicians with special training. Few health insurance plans or government-funded programs cover all screening tests. Health maintenance organizations, which often focus on preventive health care, may be more likely to provide low-cost screening tests. Some tests are offered periodically at little or no cost by employers or community centers, sometimes subsidized by health organizations and foundations.

Who Should Be Screened?

The basic principle of secondary prevention is that *all* adults, regardless of whether they are at risk, should be screened periodically for early cancer detection. However, screening tests also have special value for people at high risk for certain cancers. These include those who

- have a family history of cancer, such as women whose mothers, grand-mothers, aunts, or sisters have had breast cancer, or those whose first-degree relatives have had colorectal cancer.

- have had disorders that predispose them to certain cancers, such as a *dysplastic nevus*, a skin growth that increases the risk of malignant melanoma.

- have been exposed to carcinogens, such as those whose occupations put them in contact with known cancer-causing or cancer-promoting chemicals or other substances.

- have already had one cancer, in which case screening tests can help detect a recurrence of the same cancer and check for other cancers for which they may be at higher risk. For example, women who have had breast cancer are at increased risk of cancer in the other breast as well as cancer of the endometrium and colon.

Thus, although most members of the general public are advised to follow the American Cancer Society guidelines, those at higher risk for any reason should discuss with their doctor whether more frequent physical examinations and/or screening tests are needed and what other tests not routinely recommended might be added to their cancer checkup.

Accuracy of Tests

No screening test is 100 percent accurate. Some may not detect a cancer and thereby produce a *false-negative* result. Others may wrongly signal an abnormality, giving a *false-positive* result. Either inaccuracy, of course, can cause significant problems.

A person with a false-negative result may be falsely reassured that he or she is healthy. (This is why it's so important to pay attention to symptoms when they do occur, regardless of recent screening test results.) Conversely, a person with a false-positive test may be unnecessarily alarmed and subjected to costly and uncomfortable diagnostic tests.

Since the most important criterion for a screening test is its accuracy, scientists, public health officials, and health care organizations must carefully evaluate a test's sensitivity and specificity when deciding on a recommendation. These terms describe the ability of a screening or diagnostic test to detect an abnormality.

Sensitivity means the test's ability to identify a disease when one is present. A highly sensitive test yields few false-negative results, whereas a relatively insensitive one will often fail to diagnose disease. Sensitivity is expressed as a percentage of people with the disease who have accurate positive results or a percentage of true positives. For example, sensitivity of Pap smears varies enormously, from 60 to 99 percent, depending on how carefully the woman follows pretest instructions (see page 44), how well the test is done, and the expertise of the cytotechnologist analyzing the smear. That means for every 100 women who are told there is no indication of cancer on

Can a Screening Test Tell If You Have Cancer?

Most screening tests cannot tell whether you have cancer. Rather, they indicate an abnormal condition that may be caused by cancer—among other things—or that may be a precursor to cancer.

A positive result on a screening test indicates a variation from the expected result, suggesting a higher probability of cancer. This is different from *detection*, which is the actual discovery of an abnormality in a person who may or may not have symptoms.

A positive screening test requires a more complete diagnostic evaluation. Further tests are performed to find the cause of the positive result and determine whether cancer is present. A *diagnosis* confirms the presence and location of a specific type of cancer.

their Pap smears, anywhere from one to 40 will have a false-negative result—that is, from one to 40 will be falsely reassured that they are free from the abnormalities that may signal cancer.

Specificity is a measure of a test's ability to exclude a disease when it is not present. In other words, specificity measures a test's ability to identify people who are free of the disease. A highly specific test should yield few false-positive results; a nonspecific test will mistakenly diagnose disease where none exists. Specificity is expressed as a percentage of people without the disease who have negative results or a percentage of true negatives.

The specificity of Pap tests has been estimated at 99 percent. Thus, out of every 100 women who were told the smear indicated cancer, only one will not have the disease.

Is the Test Worth the Cost?

One of the most difficult criteria to analyze is cost–benefit. The principle of cost–benefit ratios demands that the cost for screening large numbers of people and the cost of follow-up tests and subsequent early intervention yield an economic benefit—that is, the costs to society of screening and follow-up must be lower than those incurred by not screening and simply treating the disease after it causes symptoms and is diagnosed by traditional methods.

Cost to Society

When the ACS conducted extensive epidemiological studies in 1980 to weigh the costs and benefits of screening for various cancers, it concluded that the benefits outweigh the overall costs for screening for cancers of the breast, cervix, and, to a lesser extent, colon.

Since benefit includes an analysis of long-term survival, cancers whose course appears unaffected by early detection are not subject to routine screening. For example, currently the only way to detect lung cancer is by chest x-ray, an expensive test that also involves exposure to radiation. Studies suggest that by the time lung cancer is detectable on x-ray, it is usually too late to extend or save the person's life. So chest x-ray was excluded from the recommended procedures when the screening guidelines were first established in 1982.

ACS Recommendations

Summary of American Cancer Society Recommendations for the Early Detection of Cancer in Asymptomatic People

Test or Procedure	Population		
	Sex	Age	Frequency
Sigmoidoscopy, preferably flexible	M & F	50 and over	Every 3-5 years
Fecal occult blood test	M & F	50 and over	Every year
Digital rectal examination	M & F	40 and over	Every year
Prostate exam*	M	50 and over	Every year
Pap test	F	All women who are, or have been, sexually active, or who have reached age 18 should have an annual Pap test and pelvic examination. After a woman has had three or more consecutive satisfactory normal annual examinations, the Pap test may be performed less frequently at the discretion of her physician.	
Pelvic examination	F	18-40 Over 40	Every 1-3 years with Pap test Every year
Endometrial tissue sample	F	At menopause if at high risk†	At menopause and thereafter at the discretion of the physician
Breast self-examination	F	20 and over	Every month
Breast clinical examination	F	20-40 Over 40	Every 3 years Every year
Mammography†	F	40-49 50 and over	Every 1-2 years Every year
Health Counseling and Cancer Checkup§	M & F M & F	Over 20 Over 40	Every 3 years Every year

* Annual digital rectal examination and prostate-specific antigen should be performed on men 50 years and older. If either is abnormal, further evaluation should be considered.

† History of infertility, obesity, failure to ovulate, abnormal uterine bleeding, or unopposed estrogen or tamoxifen therapy.

‡ Screening mammography should begin by age 40.

§ To include examination for cancers of the thyroid, testicles, prostate, ovaries, lymph nodes, oral region, and skin.

INFORM YOURSELF

Personal Costs

Although a test may not be considered cost effective for society as a whole—either by the government, insurance companies, health care plans, or national professional organizations—your own analysis of what is beneficial personally may lead to a different conclusion. Recommendations for society in general need not prevent you from choosing to have a particular test. However, in most cases, unless you have symptoms, it is unlikely that the test will be covered by health insurance or a health care plan. Few policies cover checkups or ACS recommended screening tests, and insurers are even less likely to reimburse for tests that are not recommended.

INFORM

YOURSELF

Where to Have Your Screening Test

Among the many variables that can influence the accuracy of a screening test are who performs the test; who interprets it; the training, experience, and skill of the tester and the interpreter; and the effectiveness of the technology used. For example, a gynecologist who does clinical breast exams every day is likely to be better able to find and interpret any abnormalities than an internist who deals with a wider range of illnesses.

Before undergoing any screening test, ask about the training and experience of those who will perform the test and interpret its results.

ROUTINE TESTS

The following tests form the battery of routine screening tests currently recommended by the American Cancer Society.

Fecal Occult Blood Tests

The fact that colorectal cancers and polyps (small growths), which may lead to cancer, often bleed intermittently provides the basis for tests that detect blood or the breakdown products of blood in the feces.

Several types of tests are available for detecting fecal occult blood. All involve techniques that identify *hemoglobin*, a component of blood.

Guaiac-impregnated cards, or cards containing other chemicals, are based on a simple biochemical reaction. When fecal material is smeared on the card and a special chemical is added, the material foams and changes color. The color depends on whether hemoglobin is present, which would indicate that there is blood in the stool. This is the most widely used test and is available for home use.

Quantitative tests are also widely used. These are based on the breakdown of hemoglobin into components called *porphyrins*, which can be mixed with a substance that makes them glow. This type of test requires laboratory interpretation.

Immunoassay tests are complex and involve mixing fecal material with a hemoglobin antibody that has been tagged with a marker. If hemoglobin is present, a reaction occurs in which antigens in the feces become attached to the antibodies, which allows them to be measured. This test's complexity, cost, and need for laboratory interpretation have prevented its routine use.

Factors That Affect Results

Although the least expensive, quickest, and most commonly used tests for blood are guaiac based, they frequently yield false results because of diet and other factors that affect the intestinal tract. Therefore, the following foods, drugs, and vitamins should be avoided for three days before testing: all beef and lamb; raw fruits and vegetables; excess amounts of vitamin C–containing foods, such as citrus fruits and juices, or vitamin C tablets in excess of 250 milligrams per day; and aspirin and other drugs that irritate the gastrointestinal tract.

The guaiac-based tests have a high incidence of false-positive results: Many people may show a positive result but be cancer-free. Therefore, when a person has a positive result, physicians first suspect a dietary factor and repeat the test. If the second test is negative, it too is repeated, to confirm that it is a true negative. When either the second or the third test is positive, a sigmoidoscopy (see later) is recommended.

The quantitative porphyrin tests are unaffected by diet and may be more sensitive. However, they are not as specific for lower gastrointestinal bleeding as the guaiac-based tests.

Shortcomings

Unfortunately, because most malignancies bleed only intermittently, a fecal occult blood test can be positive one day and negative the next, which means that cancer can be easily missed. Therefore, whether fecal occult blood testing saves lives in the general population is controversial. Nonetheless, for the individual who has a true positive that detects colorectal cancer in its earliest stages, prompt treatment can be lifesaving.

Recommendations

The ACS recommends a fecal occult blood test for men and women age 50 and over every year. People with a family history of colorectal cancer; chronic inflammatory bowel disease; familial polyposis syndromes; a history of prior colorectal, breast, endometrial, or ovarian cancers; or a history of adenomas of the large bowel may require testing at an earlier age.

Sigmoidoscopy

Sigmoidoscopy is the most specific and sensitive test for colorectal cancer. A *sigmoidoscope* is a cylinder-shaped instrument (*endoscope*) that is inserted into the rectum and gently passed upward into the lower part of the bowel for direct observation of that lower portion of the colon. The extent of the examination depends on the type of endoscope used, either rigid or flexible and varying in length from about 10 to 24 inches. (Since 1992 the ACS has recommended that a flexible scope be used.) If any polyps or other suspicious areas are observed during the examination, a small instrument can be inserted through the scope to retrieve a sample of tissue from the suspected abnormality for microscopic examination (see Chapter 8, "Diagnostic Tests").

Accuracy

Because tissue samples can be removed and analyzed, sigmoidoscopy is quite accurate. Its sensitivity is largely determined by the reach of the instrument.

About 30 percent of colorectal cancers are within reach of the short, rigid sigmoidoscope. The slightly longer, flexible sigmoidoscope can reach nearly 50 percent of such cancers, and the longest flexible scope can reach another 10 percent. (In contrast, the much longer colonoscope, typically used as a diagnostic rather than as a screening tool, can reach 95 percent or more of colorectal cancers.)

Recommendations

The ACS recommends sigmoidoscopy, preferably using a flexible scope, for men and women age 50 and over every three to five years. The exact interval should be based on the advice of the family doctor.

Those with a family history of adenomatous polyposis or inflammatory bowel disease should receive earlier screening with a flexible sigmoidoscope. In fact, the ACS considers people with long-standing inflammatory bowel disease syndromes to be at high risk for colorectal cancer.

Colonoscopy, examination of the colon with an endoscope, is not recommended for screening purposes, but it may be advised at 5- to 10-year intervals beginning at ages 35 to 40 in people at high risk of colon cancer. This includes those with first-degree relatives who have a history of a hereditary type of colorectal cancer or who developed colorectal cancer when they were 55 or younger.

Mammography

Mammography is a type of breast x-ray that has proved to be the most effective means of detecting breast cancer early. It is especially helpful in identify-

---

Sigmoidoscopy: Does It Hurt?

A flexible sigmoidoscope not only makes the procedure more comfortable than when a rigid sigmoidoscope is used but enables visualization of more of the lower bowel, making the examination more effective. If you are scheduled for sigmoidoscopy, ask in advance if a flexible scope will be used. If the answer is no, you may want to have another physician do this examination. The ACS now includes the term *preferably flexible* in its recommendation.

During the procedure you will feel pressure and the urge to defecate. However, if you have followed instructions properly for preparation (such as repeated enemas to empty the bowel), there will be no feces to pass. When air is pumped into the bowel to enlarge it for viewing, you will feel some discomfort or cramps similar to gas pains.

As usual in any situation that causes anxiety, attempts to relax—using visualization techniques or listening to music with a headset—will make the test easier to bear (see Chapter 25, "Coping with Stress, Fear, Anxiety, and Depression"). It lasts 10 to 15 minutes at most. If you think you will be particularly anxious, ask your physician about giving you a tranquilizer or mild sedative ahead of time.

If you experience any residual soreness, a warm bath can be very soothing.

SPECIAL
!
CONCERNS

ing small and/or deep tumors that cannot be felt by a clinical exam or self-examination. It is also useful for evaluating lumps or suspicious areas discovered during self-examination or a clinical breast exam.

Preparation

There is no special preparation for the x-ray, except to shower or bathe the night before or on the morning of the test and not to use any deodorant, powder, cream, or other substance on your breasts or underarm area that day. These products can appear on the film and obscure the image.

Clothing is removed from the waist up. One breast is placed on a flat plastic plate while another plate presses against it, flattening the tissue so it is of uniform thickness. Squeezing to the point of pain is unnecessary.

One to three x-rays of two different views of the breast are taken, which requires a few minutes. The procedure is repeated on the opposite breast.

Radiation Risks

Modern, *dedicated* mammography equipment (meaning it is used only for breast x-rays) that is well maintained is safe and uses very low levels of radiation (usually about 0.1 to 0.2 rad). Theoretically, if 100,000 45-year-old women received a 0.2-rad dose to their breasts, there would be one life lost as a result of the exposure. The benefits are much greater. In that same group, 150 breast cancers would be detected.

In 1992 Congress passed the Mammography Quality Standards Act, which made mammography the only medical test to be regulated by the government to ensure its quality. Only accredited facilities are allowed to perform the test. To be accredited, a breast center, radiologist's office, or clinic must have dedicated mammography equipment, the personnel performing the x-ray must be licensed or certified, the doctors interpreting the mammograms must be certified, and the x-ray and film-processing equipment must be inspected annually.

SPECIAL

CONCERNS

Mammography: Does It Hurt?

Some women avoid mammography because friends have told them it hurts when the breast is squeezed during the x-ray procedure. If mammography is done properly—and at the appropriate time in your menstrual cycle—discomfort when the breast is pressed onto the x-ray plate should be minimal for most women. Of course, individuals may vary in their perception of the procedure. And, in a small percentage of women with especially dense breasts, mammography can be painful.

Because your breasts are likely to be most tender just before or during your menstrual flow, try to schedule your appointment for the week after menstruation. If your cycle suddenly changes, don't hesitate to reschedule the appointment.

Accuracy

Mammography is not infallible, which is why self-examination and clinical breast examinations must also be done regularly. It's been estimated that 10 to 15 percent of cancers can be palpated but not seen on mammograms.

Accuracy depends on reliable equipment, careful positioning during the x-ray, and interpretation by a radiologist experienced in reading mammograms. But in the best of circumstances, visualization of suspicious areas can be problematic. Dense breasts, for example, which are common in younger women, may be difficult to visualize. Since breast implants may obscure a suspicious lesion, women with silicone or saline implants should seek radiologists who are experienced in performing mammography on augmented breasts.

Recommendations

The ACS recommends that cancer screening with mammography begin at age 40. From 40 to 49, a mammogram is recommended every one to two years. After the age of 50, annual mammograms are advised.

Current subjects of debate include whether women under 50 should have mammograms and whether a baseline mammogram is useful. Critics point out that mammograms in younger women are more likely to be inaccurate.

Another argument is that screening women in their 40s has not produced a significant decrease in mortality, so that the widespread use of mammography in women without symptoms and not at high risk is unwarranted. The ACS disagrees. We say that the studies suggesting mammograms are ineffective are flawed. In addition, the period during which the women were followed was too short for cancer to develop to detectable size. The ACS data from the Breast Cancer Detection Demonstration Project confirm that the reductions in the mortality rate in women 40 to 49 years old receiving clinical examination and mammography and in women 50 years old and older are the same.

Women at high risk for breast cancer should discuss screening intervals with their physicians.

Pap Test (Papanicolaou Smear)

A *Pap test* or *Pap smear* involves removing cells from a woman's cervix and examining them under the microscope to determine the presence and extent of abnormal cells. It is named after Dr. George N. Papanicolaou, the researcher who developed the technique more than 60 years ago. The test is usually performed during a complete pelvic examination (see Chapter 4, "The Cancer Checkup").

The vagina is held open by the paddles of a speculum and a cotton swab or tiny spatula or brush is swept across the cervix to remove some cells. The specimen is then smeared on a glass slide, which is sprayed with or dipped in a preservative and sent to a laboratory. A cytotechnologist usually examines the cells for abnormalities, but recently this procedure has been automated and computerized screening is becoming more widely available. The chief value of these automated screening devices is a reduction in the false-negative rate.

Preparation

To help ensure the test's accuracy, intercourse should be avoided for 24 hours before the exam and douching and any medications, including vaginal contraceptives, should be avoided for three days before the test. Since the test cannot be done during menstruation, it's best to have it between the twelfth and sixteenth days of the menstrual cycle.

Accuracy

False-negative Pap test results are not unusual (see Chapter 5, "Screening for Cancer"). A woman can improve her chances of obtaining an accurate result by following the preceding directions, but most false-negative results are due to factors beyond her control: poor technique in obtaining the smear and laboratory errors. It is helpful to inquire about the laboratory to which specimens are sent. It should be certified by the American Society of Cytologists, the College of American Pathologists, or both.

SPECIAL

CONCERNS

If You've Been Affected by DES

DES, or diethylstilbestrol, is a synthetic form of estrogen that was prescribed between 1941 and 1971 to many pregnant women to help prevent miscarriage, a use for which it has since been shown to be ineffective.

Tragically, some babies exposed to DES in the womb, as well as their mothers, developed serious problems in later life. Among these problems is a higher risk of vaginal and cervical cancer in DES daughters, of testicular cancer in DES sons who have undescended testicles, and of breast cancer in DES mothers.

If you know or suspect that you have been exposed to DES, discuss more frequent screening with your physician. Some experts recommend that DES daughters have a complete annual gynecological evaluation from a physician experienced in DES screening; follow-up visits may be needed more often, depending on findings at the first checkup. The examination should include Pap smears of the vagina and cervix, and use of an iodine-staining technique of the vagina and cervix to detect cell abnormalities.

Depending on the results of this examination, a *colposcopy*, a closer examination of the cervix through a magnifying instrument, may be needed as well as a biopsy to provide a sample of cervical tissue for laboratory examination.

DES sons should get a baseline examination of the testes from a urologist, practice regular testicular self-examination (see Chapter 7, "Examining Yourself"), and return to the physician if any lumps or other abnormalities are encountered.

DES mothers should do a breast self-examination every month and have mammograms as recommended by their gynecologist.

Because of the estimated eight- to nine-year *lead time* before precancerous changes evolve into invasive carcinoma, almost all false-negative results can be caught at an early stage by repeat testing within one to three years.

Recommendations

The ACS recommends that all women begin having annual Pap tests at the onset of sexual activity or at age 18, whichever occurs first. After a woman has had three or more consecutive satisfactory normal annual examinations, the Pap test may be performed less frequently at the discretion of the physician. Testing should continue throughout life, even though the test is less reliable in older women. The absence of estrogen stimulation, which occurs after menopause, can cause atrophy and inflammation that may be confused with cell abnormalities. Consequently, there is a higher incidence of false-positive and false-negative results in older women. When a woman who no longer menstruates has a positive result, some physicians advise a short course of estrogen therapy followed by a repeat Pap test. In this way unnecessary diagnostic tests may be avoided if the original test was false positive.

Endometrial Tissue Sample

Experts believe that endometrial cancer, which has become much more common than it once was, is now the most common female genital cancer.

An *endometrial tissue sample* (or biopsy) involves the removal of a small piece of *endometrium*, the lining of the uterus, through a suction tube or with a spoonlike cutting instrument called a *curette*.

The older curette technique is like a mini-D&C, which refers to *dilation* (opening of the cervix) and *curettage* (scraping of the endometrium with a curette). Just one quick swipe retrieves enough tissue for laboratory analysis. However, the curettage method is likely to cause more bleeding than the suction approach and carries a greater risk of uterine perforation.

With the newer suction technique, a tube so thin that dilation of the cervix usually is not required is inserted through the cervix and threaded up into the uterus. The tube is attached to a suction device that removes a small tissue sample.

Preparation

There is no special preparation for an endometrial tissue sample. Although a painkiller may be prescribed, no anesthesia is given for either technique.

Accuracy

The suction endometrial biopsy is estimated to provide 95 percent accuracy in ruling out cancer of the endometrium. The accuracy of the curette method is comparable.

Recommendations

The ACS recommends that endometrial tissue sampling be done at menopause in women at high risk—that is, in women with a history of infertility, obesity,

Does Endometrial Biopsy Hurt?

Endometrial tissue sampling can be uncomfortable. However, the degree and duration of pain vary markedly, depending on the technique used.

The older curette technique is more painful. The swipe of the curette knife can cause a searing pain, and cramping may last for a half-hour or so afterward.

With the suction method women report that they feel a momentary heavy pressure—like a punch from the inside—and mild to moderate cramps briefly.

Discomfort can be alleviated considerably by taking a nonsteroidal anti-inflammatory drug, such as ibuprofen, a half-hour before the procedure. Not only is the drug an effective painkiller, but it reduces cramping. Listening to music also helps provide distraction and relieve anxiety (thus relaxing your muscles), so bring along a headset (see Chapter 25, "Coping with Stress, Fear, Anxiety, and Depression").

To protect yourself further, ask your doctor which technique will be used beforehand. If it's the curette approach, ask why. Most gynecologists believe that the suction method can give information of equal value with less discomfort and less risk of bleeding and uterine perforation.

failure to ovulate, abnormal uterine bleeding, estrogen therapy (when not given with progesterone), and tamoxifen therapy. After that the physician and woman should discuss how often it should be done in her particular case.

In asymptomatic women, endometrial biopsy should not be done until menopause and then only in women at high risk for this type of cancer. Subsequent endometrial tissue sampling depends on the woman's risk.

PSA (Prostate-Specific Antigen) Test

Some prostate cancers grow rapidly, metastasize, and lead quickly to advanced illness, but many never cause symptoms and are only discovered incidentally at autopsy. Although prostate cancer is curable when treated early, a survey by the American College of Surgeons shows that about 25 percent of all diagnoses are late.

Until the 1980s, the digital rectal examination was the only technique available to screen men for prostate cancer. Now, the *prostate-specific antigen (PSA) test* has proved effective. It has been in widespread use since 1985.

The PSA involves drawing a blood sample from a vein in the arm. The blood is analyzed in a laboratory to determine the level of PSA, a substance that is produced by certain cells in the prostate. No special preparation is needed. However, since ejaculation can temporarily raise PSA levels by as much as 40 percent, men should avoid sexual activity for two days prior to the test.

Accuracy

PSA may increase in the presence of *benign enlargement of the prostate (BPA)* or inflammation of the prostate (*prostatitis*), and it may be elevated when cancer is present. However, 40 percent of men with prostate cancer do not have an elevated PSA.

Recommendation

The ACS recommends an annual PSA, along with digital rectal examination (DRE), beginning at age 50.

Men in high-risk groups, such as African-Americans or those with a family history of the disease, may start at a younger age. Generally, men with a life expectancy of at least 10 years after detection may benefit from the test.

There is some controversy about the recommendation because studies have not yet shown that PSA screening decreases prostate cancer mortality rates. Long-term research studies are under way to resolve this. However, most prostate cancers should be treated when detected; and with early treatment prostate cancer can be cured.

Other Screening Tests

In addition to the routine and recommended screening tests previously discussed, other tests are available to screen for different types of cancer. Some are controversial, and some are appropriate only for those at high risk for certain cancers.

Lung Cancer

Considerable debate centers around screening for lung cancer. It is one of the most devastating of all malignancies, because by the time lung cancer is

---

If Your Doctor Does the Exam Differently

The methods of performing the screening examinations in this chapter are recommendations by the ACS and/or experts in medical specialties. The instructions your doctor gives you on how to prepare for a test and the way he or she performs a particular examination may differ slightly from what you read here and elsewhere.

To reassure yourself, discuss the screening examination with your doctor. You might bring a copy of the information you have read when you have your checkup and share it with him or her. Don't be hesitant to ask questions about how to prepare for a test, particularly if you receive no instructions when you make your appointment. The office or clinic nurse will be able to tell you what you need to do or avoid. If you are not satisfied with the instructions you get or have questions that the nurse cannot answer, ask to speak to the doctor.

If you think that an aspect of the examination has not been done or has been performed differently from what you expected, ask why. Usually there is a logical explanation that will set your mind at ease. If you are still not satisfied, consider having the test or examination repeated elsewhere.

SPECIAL

CONCERNS

detectable on x-ray, it is often too late to prevent mortality. The two tests that have been put forward as potential screening procedures are the chest x-ray and sputum analysis. When the ACS conducted extensive evaluations and cost-benefit analyses to develop its screening guidelines, the results for these tests were disappointing. X-ray diagnosis in people without symptoms only seemed to generate a *lead-time bias*—that is, although the time from detection to death was lengthened, the outcome remained the same.

The use of *sputum cytology*, in which sputum is analyzed for abnormal cells in a manner similar to that done for Pap smears of the cervix, presents different problems. A coughed-up sputum sample provides a collection of cells that can come from anywhere in the lung. Although *dysplasia* (abnormal cells) and lung cancer can be detected much earlier than with x-ray, subsequent attempts to find exactly where the cells came from and to detect the cancer can be very tedious and costly. Sputum testing of large numbers of asymptomatic people was not found to reduce mortality from lung cancer either. No organization recommends screening for this disease.

Nonetheless, if the site of abnormal cells detected by sputum analysis can be found and treatment instituted, the results for an individual can be lifesaving. So although these tests are not cost-effective for mass screening, they may be beneficial for individuals who know they are at high risk for lung cancer because of family history, occupational exposure to carcinogens, or a history of smoking.

Bladder Cancer

The traditional examinations of cells in urine are not reliable for detecting bladder cancer. However, those who have had *transitional cell carcinoma* (a type of cancer that is easy to treat but that often recurs) should discuss the potential of *flow cytometry* with a *urologist* (a physician who specializes in disorders of the urinary tract). In this procedure, which is far more sensitive than normal urine tests, a urine sample is examined to evaluate the DNA of bladder cells shed into the urine. Those with a strong family history of bladder cancer also might wish to consider such testing. A test for bladder tumor antigen has recently become available and it appears to be effective for detecting recurrent, low-grade bladder cancer.

Ovarian Cancer

CA 125 (*carbohydrate antigen*) is a substance found in blood that was initially thought to be a tumor marker specific to ovarian cancer. There was great hope that a way had been found to detect this cancer early and save lives. Unfortunately, this has not proved to be the case. Scientists have determined that CA 125 may be elevated with benign as well as malignant ovarian lesions and that numerous other conditions—pregnancy, endometriosis, fibroid tumors, and pelvic inflammation—may also raise CA 125 levels. Thus, the test is not recommended for screening for ovarian cancer. Rather, the blood test seems to be more useful to follow patients known to have the disease: If the CA 125 level returns to a normal or undetectable level after treatment, it's a good indication that the treatment has been effective. If the level does not drop or lowers and then rises again, residual or recurrent disease is probable.

Women with a family history of ovarian cancer or who are at high risk for other reasons, such as they have breast, endometrial, or colon cancers or know they carry the breast cancer susceptibility gene (BRCA1), might want to discuss periodic CA 125 screening with their doctors. Such women might also ask about periodic ultrasound evaluations. (This procedure uses sound waves to provide images of internal soft tissue.) (For information on other blood tests for cancer, see Chapter 8, "Diagnostic Tests.")

Looking at Genes

Genetic analysis is an area of intense research interest. For example, researchers have isolated genes associated with a familial form of colorectal cancer. They believe that up to 95 percent of those with the gene will eventually develop cancer of the colon. In those found to have the gene, screening for colorectal cancer could be more frequent and more scrupulous, markedly raising the odds that their malignancies could be detected and treated at a curable stage.

Similarly, another gene indicates that a woman has an 85 percent chance of developing early-onset breast cancer. Yet another gene is believed to be involved in the development of carcinoma of the lung.

Despite the seemingly beneficial potential of genetic markers for cancer risk, their use is ultimately likely to be mired in controversy. Although many might consider it a boon to know in advance of their higher risk so that they could ensure scrupulous monitoring and early treatment, others might not want to know.

Furthermore, the question of who beyond the individual is entitled to that information is debatable. Many fear that health and life insurers might use such data to deny coverage to those at higher risk or that potential employers would avoid hiring anyone who might face a devastating illness. Indeed, the National Institutes of Health has established a working group to explore the ethical, legal, and social implications of genetic testing.

Do You Need Extra Tests?

If you have a family history of a particular cancer or if your lifestyle, environment, or occupation has exposed you significantly to a carcinogen, you may be at high risk for a type of cancer for which routine screening is not recommended.

If you want a test that is not routinely recommended, your physician should explain the costs, risks, and benefits of the procedure under the principle of informed consent.

If you want such a test but your physician disagrees with your choice, you have two options: The doctor may proceed with the test after explaining his or her misgivings, or the doctor may refuse to perform the test and you can seek a second opinion.

SPECIAL

CONCERNS

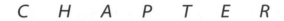

EXAMINING YOURSELF

In addition to the examinations and screening tests provided by health care professionals, you can easily do a self-examination for various types of cancer. The following can be done at home.

Breast Self-Examination

Breast self-examination (BSE) is the only self-examination formally recommended by the American Cancer Society as part of its guidelines for detecting cancer early in people with no symptoms. Although no studies demonstrate conclusively that BSE saves lives, breast growths are often first detected by hand. Thus, all women 20 and older should examine their breasts monthly as a routine health habit.

The major risk of BSE is that a woman may believe that self-examination can replace a clinical breast examination or mammogram. A woman may miss a tumor that a physician or nurse can feel or that will appear on an x-ray. Frequent examination also increases the likelihood that small lesions, which might have come and gone between professional examinations, will be reported to the physician and prompt unnecessary medical testing.

Some women experience considerable anxiety when they examine their breasts for cancer. If this anxiety results in a woman being unable to do monthly self-examinations or not doing it thoroughly, more frequent clinical breast examinations may be necessary.

Testicular Self-Examination (TSE)

Young men at high risk for testicular cancer are sometimes encouraged to practice testicular self-examination (TSE) regularly. However, the usefulness of this screening test by all men is controversial, because the cancer is rare. Those at high risk include men whose testes did not descend into

How to Perform Breast Self-Examination

You should perform a BSE every month, a few days after menstruation ends, when the breasts are at minimum fullness, so that you become familiar with the usual appearance and feel of your breasts and are better able to detect any changes from your normal state. Postmenopausal women should examine their breasts at the same time each month.

Stand in front of a mirror and look at your breasts while your hands are at your sides; then examine them with your hands raised above your head, then with your hands on your hips. Do you notice anything unusual? In most women one breast is slightly larger than the other, but you should look for differences in shape, for a flattening or bulging in one but not the other, or for skin puckering.

Watch for any reddening or other abnormality of the nipples, any hardness or changes in shape or size. Unless you are pregnant or nursing, there should be no nipple discharge even upon light squeezing. Any soreness of the nipple should be investigated by your physician.

Raise your hands above your head; then lower them and place your hands on your hips. Do you notice any irregular changes in the movement and shape of your breasts during and after such movement?

Next, lie down. Raise your right arm above your head and rest it on a pillow behind you. Use your left hand to gently explore your right breast, using the pads of the three middle fingers. Move your hand in small circles around the breast, applying gentle pressure, until the entire breast is covered. After you check the right breast, repeat the procedure on the left side. Any thickening, lump, or other abnormality should be reported to your physician.

Breast Self-Examination
By making small circular motions along a particular grid, you can examine the entire area from collarbone to below the breast and from the breastbone to the armpit. It's best to use the same method each time. Some women prefer to do a breast self-exam in the shower; soapy hands glide easily over wet skin.

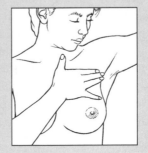

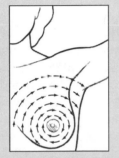

The exam can be done in a circular pattern,

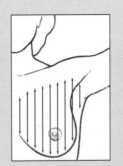

up and down in vertical strips,

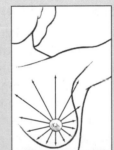

or in wedges, radiating from the nipple outward.

How to Perform TSE

Testicular self-examination should be performed monthly to enable you to become familiar with the usual appearance and feel of your testes so that you can detect any changes from your normal state.

The best time to perform a self-exam is during or after a warm bath or shower, when the scrotal skin is most relaxed. Although the two testicles are encased in a single scrotal sac, each should be examined separately. Hold the testicle between your thumbs and fingers with both hands and roll it gently between your fingers. Then stand in front of a mirror, holding your penis out of the way, and observe the testicles.

You are looking for any hard lumps or nodules or any change in the size, shape, or consistency of your testes. If you notice any abnormalities, see your doctor promptly. Also call your doctor if you experience any other signs of testicular cancer, such as a dull ache or a sensation of dragging and heaviness in the lower abdomen, groin, or both.

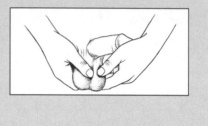

the scrotum until after the age of 6 or who continue to have one or both testes undescended.

Unlike most women, who are knowledgeable about BSE, many men are not aware of TSE. Although this may reflect a generally lower level of health awareness among men than among women, it also may be because young men deny that they are at risk for any health problem, particularly one that might affect their concept of manhood.

Since early testicular cancer usually does not produce pain or other markedly noticeable symptoms that a man might attribute to malignancy, careful self-examination could be expected to increase the odds of early detection. However, little research is available to document the potential benefits or risks of the procedure. For this reason the ACS has made no formal recommendations on TSE.

Skin Self-Examination

Although the ACS has made no formal recommendations on skin self-examination (SSE), the Skin Cancer Foundation suggests that such examinations begin in childhood so that individuals learn to perform SSE by their teens. The Foundation currently advises self-examination every three months, which should supplement an annual skin examination by a physician, though the frequency of this recommendation may change in the near future.

Oral Self-Examination

Some doctors and dentists recommend oral self-examination (OSE) to people at high risk of oral cancers because of a history of smoking or tobacco

How to Perform Skin Self-Examination

Skin self-examination should take place with all clothes removed, in a well-lighted room, and in front of a full-length mirror. You should have a hand mirror so that you can see the back of your body.

You will slowly examine every visible area of your skin, including body crevices, between your legs, under your arms, and under the hair on the back of your neck.

The first time you do SSE it may be useful to draw a rough sketch of your body, front and back, and to note the locations of any moles or skin lesions you have, as well as their size and color. Then refer to your sketches to check for changes.

You can use the ABCD method described in Chapter 4, "The Cancer Checkup," though this technique applies mainly to screening for malignant melanoma. The following guidelines recommended by the Skin Cancer Foundation will help you scrutinize your body for all types of skin malignancies. Look for

- any skin growth that increases in size or becomes pearly, translucent, tan, brown, black, or multicolored

- any mole, birth mark, beauty mark, or brown spot that changes color, increases in size or thickness, changes texture, has irregular borders, or is bigger than the size of a pencil eraser and appears after age 21

- any spot or sore that continues to hurt, itch, crust, scab, erode, or bleed, or any open sore that does not heal within three weeks.

- If you observe any of these changes, call your doctor for a prompt appointment.

The illustrations below will help you notice a suspicious lesion that may be skin cancer.

Examine your face, especially the nose, lips, and mouth, and the front and back of the ears. Use a hand mirror or floor-length mirror or both to get a clear view.

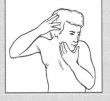

Thoroughly inspect your scalp, using a blow dryer and mirror to expose each section to view. Get a friend or family member to help, if you can.

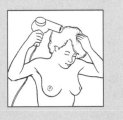

Check your hands carefully: palms and backs, between the fingers, and under the fingernails. Continue up the wrists to examine both the front and back of your forearms.

Standing in front of the full-length mirror, begin at the elbows and scan all sides of your upper arms. Don't forget the underarms.

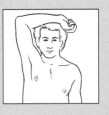

Next focus on the neck, chest, and torso. Women should lift breasts to view the under-side.

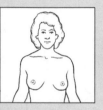

With your back to the full-length mir-ror, use the hand mirror to inspect the back of your neck, shoulders, upper back, and any part of the back of your upper arms you could not view earlier.

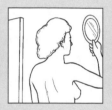

Still using both a hand mirror and a full-length mirror, scan your lower back, buttocks, and backs of both legs.

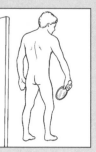

Sit down; prop each leg in turn on a stool or chair. Use a hand mirror to examine the genitals. Check the front and sides of both legs, thigh to shin; ankles, tops of feet, between toes, and under toenails. Examine soles of feet and heels.

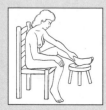

chewing or certain prior tissue abnormalities in the mouth.

Knowledge about OSE is extremely limited and difficult to do. No research is available to document the potential benefits or risks of the procedure.

Home Fecal Occult Blood Tests

Some doctors recommend that people at high risk for colorectal cancer do a home test for fecal occult blood occasionally. Nonetheless, research has shown that most fail to follow this advice.

Two of the same tests available in doctors' offices—the guaiac-impregnated cards and the quantitative tests based on the breakdown of hemoglobin into porphyrins (see Chapter 6, "Routine Tests")—also are available for home use. The former are widely available in pharmacies and their results are immediately evident to users who follow directions on the packages. The lat-ter are less widely available and are more apt to be given to patients by their physicians for home use. The quantitative tests require that the fecal sample, once it is obtained and stored as directed, be mailed to a commercial labora-tory for analysis. The report is usually then sent to the person's physician.

Whether these tests help reduce deaths is unclear. In the absence of research documenting the accuracy of the tests, the ACS can make no recommendations.

DIAGNOSTIC TESTS

Many signs and symptoms of cancer resemble those of other conditions. Weight loss and abdominal pain can be caused by stomach cancer or an ulcer. Pink or reddish urine can be caused by kidney cancer or a kidney infection. A positive fecal occult blood test can indicate a variety of intestinal problems. The only way to confirm—or rule out—cancer as the cause of a suspicious symptom is to undergo diagnostic testing.

The specific tests that are ordered depend on a number of factors, including symptoms, location, type of the suspected tumor, and preferences of the physician and person being tested.

Approaches to Testing

The term *work-up* is often used to describe the evaluation and testing process. It begins with a complete medical history, during which the physician asks about current symptoms or illnesses, past illnesses, medical background of relatives, medications, home and work environment, and lifestyle choices that may affect health, such as smoking.

A physical exam follows the medical history. If possible, the physician will palpate the affected area.

Why Do Doctors Order So Many Tests?

In many cases the doctor will order more than one test because no single exam supplies all the information required both to confirm a cancer diagnosis and to determine the best treatment options.

The most definitive diagnostic test is a *biopsy*, the removal of a piece of tissue for microscopic evaluation. A tissue sample can be easily retrieved from a tumor near the body's surface, but if the mass is inaccessible, an imaging exam that enables a tumor to be located precisely and visualized may be ordered before the biopsy can be done.

Besides confirming cancer, a biopsy (explained in detail later in this chapter) provides information about the tumor, including its type, classification, *grade* (the degree of abnormality of the tumor cells; see page 16), potential *aggressiveness* (how quickly it may spread) and other information that may help determine the best treatment. Imaging tests help determine the tumor's size and whether it has spread. This information allows physicians to *stage* the tumor, and/or the extent of its growth, an important step in planning treatment and determining probable outcome; see page 16.

After treatment has begun, further tests are usually ordered to see how the disease is responding to therapy.

An Elimination Process

The least costly and/or invasive tests are done first. For example, to detect a mass that cannot be felt, the physician can order an ultrasound exam. This test is relatively inexpensive, safe, painless, and noninvasive. Then, if the situation warrants it, the doctor may order more costly imaging procedures, such as computerized tomography or magnetic resonance imaging exams. (These tests are described later in this chapter.) Finally, if a mass is found, the most definitive test, a biopsy of the mass, is done.

QUESTIONS TO ASK

Is This Test Necessary?

When diagnostic tests are ordered, ask your doctor these questions:

- Why are you recommending this test? What will you learn from it?
- What are the alternatives to the test? Do any less invasive or less costly procedures provide the same information?
- What are the possible side effects, complications, or risks of the test?
- What are the risks of not having the test?
- Will I be hospitalized? For how long? Can the test be done on an outpatient basis?
- How much will the test cost? Is it covered by my health insurance or health care plan?
- Does a certified technician or a board-certified physician perform the test? Does a board-certified physician interpret and evaluate the test results?
- Where will the test be performed? Will it be done at a hospital with a certified laboratory, accredited by the College of American Pathologists?
- When will I get the results? How accurate will they be? Who will explain the results to me?
- What further tests will be necessary if the results are positive? What if they are negative?

Combined Tests

The following hypothetical situation shows how diagnostic tests work together to provide a complete picture.

If you show signs of jaundice and complain of weight loss, abdominal pain, and nausea, a physician will take your medical history and perform a physical exam. If pancreatic cancer is suspected, several tests may be ordered.

First, *ultrasonography* may be recommended to visualize the pancreas. This procedure uses sound waves to create a computerized image of the interior of the body. However, in some cases ultrasonography doesn't provide sufficient information. If any suspicious areas are visible on ultrasound, a *computed tomography (CT) scan* may be ordered. A CT image is clear and provides more information than ultrasonography, but it is expensive and may not be done initially.

If a mass in the pancreas is detected on the ultrasound or CT scan, it must be checked for malignancy. A *fine-needle aspiration biopsy (FNAB)*, in which a needle is inserted into the suspicious mass and a minute amount of tissue or individual cells are removed, is the simplest, least invasive, and least expensive type of biopsy.

Needle biopsies are usually performed on easily accessible tumors, but sometimes they are also used on tumors of deep organs such as the pancreas. They may be combined with ultrasound and CT scans.

An *endoscopic biopsy*, removal of a sample of tissue through an *endoscope*, a flexible, cylinder-shaped instrument, may also be recommended. An *incisional biopsy* is the surgical removal of a portion of the mass. An *excisional biopsy* is removal of the entire mass.

Imaging Examinations

Conventional x-rays have been available for almost a century. They are the most familiar, inexpensive, and accessible imaging exams. For some forms of

What Is This Test Like?

QUESTIONS TO ASK

Studies show that diagnostic tests may be less stressful if you know exactly what to expect. Here are some questions to ask so that you'll be prepared.

- What happens during the test? What will I feel, see, smell, and hear during the procedure?
- Is the test invasive? That is, will anything be inserted or injected into my body?
- Is any part of the test painful or uncomfortable?
- Can anything be done to prevent or lessen the discomfort? Will I be given a sedative or local or general anesthesia?
- How long does the test take?
- Does this test have any side effects or complications?

cancer, such as breast cancer, an x-ray (mammogram) is the preferred diagnostic method.

Newer imaging exams, such as CT scan, magnetic resonance imaging (MRI), and ultrasound are based on computers. In most body regions they provide more information than standard x-rays and can detect tumors not seen on an x-ray.

Using imaging techniques, a physician can sometimes pinpoint the location of a suspicious mass, even if it is deep within the body. Often a biopsy needle can be directed precisely to the mass or suspicious lesion, thus avoiding exploratory surgery. However, even the most sophisticated imaging exams cannot distinguish between benign and malignant tumors with certainty, so further diagnostic tests may be required.

After a diagnosis is made, imaging exams may be used to stage the disease. Following treatment, they may help determine whether therapy has been successful.

A certified technician, physician, or radiologist performs imaging exams in a physician's office, outpatient facility, or hospital. A *radiologist* (a physician who specializes in imaging techniques) usually interprets the exams.

Conventional Radiography

Because x-rays are painless, quick, easily accessible, and relatively inexpensive, and require little, if any, preparation, they are often used for the initial evaluation.

X-rays are high-energy beams of radiation that, when passed through the body, create shadows on a sheet of film, called a *radiograph*. A radiograph is commonly referred to as an *x-ray* or *film*. The x-rays pass through soft tissue more readily than through dense tissue, such as bone. Since the soft tissue absorbs fewer x-rays than dense tissue, it is darker on the film, whereas bones are white.

Tumors are usually denser than the tissue that surrounds them, which can make them noticeable on the radiograph or x-ray.

Contrast Studies. To improve and increase the information obtained from conventional x-ray techniques, air or a dye such as iodine or barium may be used as a *contrast medium* to outline, highlight, or fill in parts of the body.

X-rays with a contrast medium can be used to detect large tumors deep within the body, such as in the kidneys, liver, pancreas, and brain.

Depending on the dye and the part of the body examined, the contrast medium may be introduced in the following ways:

- by enema, as in a *barium enema*, which is used to study the large intestine and rectum.

- swallowed, as in an *upper G.I. (gastrointestinal) series,* used to study the upper digestive tract.

- injected into an artery or vein, as in an *intravenous pyelogram (IVP),* which is used to study the kidneys and urinary tract.

Getting a Safe, Accurate Test

Ask your doctor the following questions to prepare for a diagnostic test.

- Should I curtail my activity, restrict my diet, or refrain from smoking, alcohol, or caffeine before the test or immediately afterward?
- Should I decrease the dose or stop taking over-the-counter or prescribed medications, such as aspirin, vitamins, painkillers, or oral contraceptives?
- Will I be able to drive myself home after the test?
- When will I be able to resume my usual activities?

Tell your doctor if you

- are pregnant or think you may be.
- currently have any illness.
- have had a serious illness in the past.
- have taken any prescription or over-the-counter medications, including contraceptives, hormones, vitamins, aspirin, laxatives, or cough medicine within the past few days, weeks, or months.
- have any allergies.
- have a pacemaker.
- had surgery to repair an aneurysm.
- have any metal clips, pins, or implants in your body from surgery or any metal fragments in your eyes from accidents.
- smoke.
- have not had adequate rest lately.
- feel nervous, anxious, or upset.
- are claustrophobic.

- inserted through a catheter into a natural opening or a small incision, as in a *hysterosalpingogram*, in which dye is injected into the uterus through a slender tube that has been passed through the vagina and cervix into the uterus to study that organ and fallopian tubes.

A special diet, enema, or other preparation measures may be required when a contrast medium is used. Eventually, the material will be eliminated by the body.

These tests may be uncomfortable. Dye may cause a burning sensation and nausea. However, the discomfort is usually brief and sedatives may be administered before certain tests. Barium enemas may cause cramping and a strong desire to expel the fluid.

Most contrast studies involve little risk, including risk of allergic reaction, but complications can occur when a dye is used.

If you have a history of allergies or sensitivity to iodine or seafood (which is high in iodine) or any medication, tell the radiologist. The test may still be done with a different dye and medication that reduces the chance of an allergic reaction.

A few contrast studies are considered high-risk procedures because the dye can induce a stroke or cause nerve damage. For most people the risk of a serious complication is less than two in 100 procedures. High-risk contrast media studies include

- *cerebral angiogram* (also called *arteriogram*), an x-ray of the blood vessels in the neck and brain, which requires injecting dye into neck arteries.

- *coronary angiogram*, an x-ray of the heart and surrounding arteries in which dye is injected into the heart chambers.

- *pulmonary angiogram*, an x-ray of the blood vessels of the lungs in which dye is injected into pulmonary arteries.

It is important that these procedures be performed by skilled and experienced technicians and physicians.

Safer, less invasive tests—such as CT scan, ultrasound, or nuclear scan—may substitute for some contrast studies.

Digital Radiography

Instead of using film, *digital radiography* converts x-ray images to electronic data that can be viewed on a monitor and stored on computer disks. The technique allows specific areas of the image to be enlarged, and the contrast of the image can be adjusted to allow greater visibility, thus reducing the need

SPECIAL

CONCERNS

Is Radiation Risky?

Radiation can damage cells, causing them to reproduce abnormally. Usually the damaged cells simply die or the body's immune system destroys them with no ill effects. The risk of diagnostic x-rays causing enough damage to induce cancer is far outweighed by the diagnostic benefits, especially when using modern equipment that emits low doses of radiation.

But since the effects of even low-level radiation are cumulative and the the risk of cancer grows with the amount of radiation a person is exposed to over a lifetime, x-rays should not be done indiscriminately.

If your physician recommends that you have an x-ray, you can minimize the amount of radiation exposure by taking the following steps:

- Have your x-rays done in a medical school, hospital, or office of a board-certified radiologist, where x-ray machines are more likely to be regularly calibrated and inspected and skilled, accredited personnel perform the exams.

- Ask for your x-ray report and keep track of x-rays you have had to avoid repeating the same exam. Many doctors accept x-rays taken by others.

- Stay still when the x-ray is being taken to avoid a blurred image, which will require a repeat exam.

- Before having an x-ray, be sure to tell the physician if you are pregnant or think you may be.

for contrast media and the amount of radiation required for a clear image. Most large hospitals have digital radiography equipment.

Computed Tomography (CT) Scan

The CT scan is a sophisticated x-ray procedure that creates clear cross-sectional (front-to-back) images of internal structures and offers much more information than conventional x-rays. Also, unlike a conventional x-ray exam, which directs one broad x-ray beam over an area, a CT scan is produced by numerous pencil-thin rays passing through the body from various angles and levels.

While you lie on a table, a scanner rotates around you and directs thousands of x-ray beams at a particular region of your body. A computer generates a two-dimensional picture from these images (also called *sections* or *slices*). Individual slices are displayed on a computer screen.

A technician usually performs a CT scan, and a radiologist evaluates the results. No hospitalization is required. The image may clearly show a tumor's size, shape, volume, and location.

The test does take some time, usually about 30 minutes to one hour, but it is painless, although there may be some discomfort when holding still in certain positions for a long time. An intravenous dye may be used to provide contrast. Fasting or an enema may be necessary before the test.

A disadvantage of the test is its cost, which may run six to 10 times that of a conventional chest x-ray. The radiation exposure is similar to that of a conventional x-ray.

The technique has some limitations. Very small tumors may not be visible, and the scan may not show how far the cancer has spread, particularly if no mass has developed.

Magnetic Resonance Imaging

One of the newest imaging techniques, *magnetic resonance imaging (MRI)* uses radio waves and a strong magnetic field to penetrate the body and generate high-quality, two-dimensional images of almost every organ in the body. MRI can provide views from all directions. The procedure is especially useful for areas that are difficult to visualize with standard x-rays, such as the brain, spinal cord, pelvis, and musculoskeletal system. Indeed, almost all body parts can be visualized, and new applications are being developed every day.

An MRI image has better contrast than a CT scan, and even very small tumors can be detected early. The MRI also distinguishes between tumors and cysts.

Despite its advantages, MRI does have limitations. It doesn't detect *calcifications* (tiny calcium deposits that can signal cancer in the breast tissue) as clearly as a CT scan or conventional x-ray. Even more important, MRI is more expensive than CT and not as widely available.

An MRI takes about an hour. It is painless, but because the test requires complete enclosure in a narrow, tubular machine, it can be uncomfortable, even frightening for some people. Children and those who are very large or claustrophobic may have difficulty lying still for the time required. Some people complain of the continual loud thumping and pounding of the machinery.

Some facilities offer "open-air" MRI, which alleviates the feeling of claustrophobia. This newer design has open sides, no pounding noise, and can accommodate very large people. However, open MRIs are not widely available, and because they are less powerful they do not produce the clearest image.

MRI is usually not recommended for pregnant women. Anyone wearing a pacemaker or who has internal clips, metal implants, joint replacements, and other medical devices or who has metal fragments in the eye may be unable to have an MRI because the strong magnetic field can disrupt or dislodge the devices or fragments.

MRIs are very costly and may not be covered by your insurance or health plan.

Nuclear Medicine

Nuclear medicine involves the use of radioactive substances, called *radionuclides* or *tracers*, to create images of organs and detect masses in areas that are not visualized by standard x-ray.

The radionuclides are administered orally or intravenously. A machine (called a *rectilinear scanner*, *gamma ray camera*, or *scintiscope*) produces a two-dimensional image, or scan, showing how and where the radioactive compound travels in the body and where it accumulates. Radionuclides appear on the scan as spots of light.

Depending on the organ being scanned and type of radionuclide used, a

TIPS & ADVICE

Having an MRI?

Before having an MRI tell your doctor

- if you cannot comfortably lie flat.
- if you are severely claustrophobic.
- if you are pregnant or think you may be.
- if you have any medical devices, such as a cardiac pacemaker, aneurysm clip, implants, or hearing aid.
- if any metal shrapnel is in your body from an old war wound or an auto accident or any metal fragments in the eye.
- if you have any tattoos (some tattoos contain metallic particles).

To prepare for an MRI exam do the following:

- Do not wear any makeup because some products contain metallic particles.
- Do not wear a watch or belt. (It's best to remove street clothes and ask for a surgical gown.)
- Remove all personal possessions, such as car keys, wallet, and credit cards.
- Practice relaxation techniques to quiet claustrophobia or other feelings of anxiety (see Chapter 25, "Coping with Stress, Fear, Anxiety, and Depression").

tumor may be detected as an area of either increased radioactivity (a "hot spot") or decreased radioactivity.

A very small tumor cannot be detected through a nuclear scan, nor can the scan distinguish between tumors and cysts.

Although nuclear medicine procedures do not provide as much detail as CT or MRI scans, they can provide information unavailable from other scans and are easily accessible and less costly.

The procedure, which causes little discomfort, involves about as much radiation exposure as conventional x-rays. The scanning machine emits no radiation, and most of the radioactive substance introduced into the body is eliminated within a day or so.

Ultrasonography

Ultrasonography, or diagnostic ultrasound, is effective, painless, noninvasive, readily available, and relatively inexpensive. The procedure involves no radiation and is considered safe enough to examine fetuses during pregnancy. Consequently, it is sometimes recommended as the initial diagnostic method, particularly when a positive screening test raises a suspicion of cancer.

Ultrasound uses sound waves and their echoes to create a picture of the interior of the body. A microphone-like instrument, called a *transducer*, that emits and receives sound waves is passed over the part of the body being examined. The echo patterns are converted to a detailed computer image that is viewed on a monitor.

In most cases, little preparation is required for an ultrasound. Depending on the organ being examined, it may be necessary to fast overnight, take a laxative, have an enema, or consume large quantities of water before the test. It is usually performed on an outpatient basis in a hospital because only certain specialists have ultrasound equipment in their offices.

Ultrasonography, which can differentiate cysts from solid masses, can visualize soft tissues that don't show up well on x-rays, so it is often used to detect tumors in the liver, pelvis, and abdominal area. The procedure has also been used to detect prostate cancer and, along with mammography, to determine if a breast lump is a cyst or a solid mass. It may also be helpful in guiding needle aspirations or needle biopsies.

Ultrasound cannot penetrate bone or gas-filled spaces, so it is ineffective for detecting tumors in the brain, lungs, or intestines. It is also inaccurate when used in obese people, because fat can interfere with the sound waves.

The long-term effects of ultrasound are unknown, but no harmful effects have been detected.

Blood Tests

Blood tests are easy to perform, usually inexpensive, and virtually risk-free. The blood sample is obtained by a lab technician, nurse, or doctor inserting a needle into a vein and is relatively painless. The only preparation may be the need to fast for several hours.

Blood tests fall into one of two categories: *nonspecific* and *specific*.

INFORM

YOURSELF

Blood Tests for Cancer

Everyone hopes that someday a simple, inexpensive blood test will reveal whether a person has cancer. Since cancer is actually a hundred different diseases, it's unlikely that one test will screen all types of malignancies. However, tests can now detect certain molecules, often a type of protein, produced by specific types of cancer. These molecules are called *tumor markers*.

Tumor markers are most useful to monitor the effectiveness of treatment, to follow the course of a disease, or to detect recurrent disease. They can also help predict the stage of the disease, since the higher the tumor marker level, the greater the likelihood that the disease has metastasized. With a few exceptions tumor markers are not widely used to screen or diagnose disease because noncancerous conditions can sometimes produce a positive result.

Some of the most common tumor markers are the following:

- *Carcinoembryonic Antigen (CEA)*. This substance is elevated in the blood of people with colorectal, gastrointestinal, kidney, stomach, breast, pancreatic, liver, and lung cancers. Cigarette smoking and several benign disorders also cause elevated CEA levels. The test is not specific enough for diagnosis, but it is used to detect tumor recurrence or to monitor treatment of colorectal cancer.

- *Carbohydrate Antigen 125* (CA 125). About 80 percent of women with ovarian cancer have elevated levels of this antigen in their blood. CA 125 is also often elevated in endometrial, pancreatic, stomach, and colorectal cancers, especially with invasive, widespread malignancies.

  But a high level is not proof of cancer, because CA 125 is elevated in women with endometriosis, pelvic inflammatory disease, ovarian cysts, and other benign gynecologic disorders. Even menstruation and early pregnancy can elevate CA 125.

  A low CA 125 level does not exclude malignancy. Only about half the women with stage I ovarian tumors have elevated CA 125 levels. Therefore, the test is not reliable for detecting early-stage ovarian cancer. It is most valuable when combined with a careful pelvic exam and ultrasonography or when used to detect recurrent disease.

- *Carbohydrate Antigen 19-9* (CA 19-9). This antigen is elevated in cancers of the gastrointestinal tract, including the colon, pancreas, or stomach. The test is usually conducted in conjunction with the CEA test.

- *Carbohydrate Antigen 15-3* (CA 15-3). This antigen is elevated in women with breast cancer, especially when the cancer has spread. The test is most often used to stage the tumor, monitor treatment, and detect recurrence.

- *Prostate-Specific Antigen (PSA)*. This antigen, produced by the prostate gland, is elevated in men with prostate cancer. However, benign disorders such as *prostatitis* (an inflamed prostate) or an enlarged prostate and recent ejaculation also cause elevated PSA levels. In addition, the PSA test is not sensitive enough to detect all prostate cancers and may miss about a third of them.

The PSA test is most valuable when combined with a digital rectal exam. Together, the two tests find about a third more cases of prostate cancer than either test alone. If the PSA test results are abnormal, ultrasonography is recommended to determine if a tumor is present. The PSA test is also used to follow and monitor men who are being treated for prostate cancer.

- *Human Chorionic Gonadotropin (HCG).* Pregnant women normally have high levels of this hormone, but when it remains high in the months after delivery, it is a strong indication of a rare condition called *trophoblastic malignancy.* Cancers of the testicles and ovaries and some lung tumors can also cause elevated HCG levels.

- *Alpha-Fetoprotein (AFP).* Elevated levels of this substance can indicate chronic hepatitis B or cirrhosis as well as pancreatic, stomach, or liver cancer. The higher the AFP level, the greater the likelihood of cancer, so an abnormal AFP level should be followed with an ultrasonography exam. When used along with HCG, AFP can also be used to detect testicular cancer or monitor its treatment.

- *Adrenocorticotropic hormone (ACTH).* This hormone, produced by the pituitary gland, may be elevated in lung or pituitary tumors.

- *Alkaline phosphatase.* This enzyme is elevated in liver cancer and in bone and gallbladder diseases, cirrhosis, and hepatitis. Birth control pills and some hormones, tranquilizers, and antibiotics can also raise this enzyme level. The test for this enzyme is not specific.

- *Plasma proteins.* Elevated levels and abnormal kinds of plasma proteins are found in multiple myelomas, hepatomas, and brain tumors in children.

Nonspecific blood tests, such as a blood count or liver function tests, reflect overall health and general organ functions. They may reveal an abnormality that could be the result of a number of conditions.

Specific blood tests, on the other hand, can point to abnormalities that are primarily associated with cancer. These tests measure substances, called tumor markers, that may be a product either of a tumor or of the body in response to a tumor.

Cytology

To obtain a *cytologic smear*, cells are scraped or brushed from an area by a physician or nurse and then examined under a microscope by a pathologist (a physician who specializes in the changes in tissues and organs of the body associated with disease) or a cytology technician to determine if the cells are malignant. Any body fluid may also be examined cytologically.

A *Papanicolaou test* (more commonly called *Pap smear*), in which cells are swabbed from the cervix and examined for cancer, is the most familiar cytological test. (See Chapter 6, "Routine Tests.") Sputum, scrapings from the mouth and tongue, and breast fluid extracted through the nipple can also be studied cytologically.

Smears are painless and relatively inexpensive. However, analysis results are not always accurate. Pap smears, for example, have a false-negative rate of up to 40 percent. The false-positive rate is much lower. The accuracy of a cytologic smear depends on the sample preparation and skill and experience of both the person obtaining the sample cells and the technologist or pathologist examining them.

Therefore, although cytologic smears are valuable screening devices, a final diagnosis cannot be made on the basis of these tests. A biopsy is necessary to confirm a diagnosis.

Biopsy

A *biopsy* is the removal of tissue from a suspicious mass or lesion for microscopic examination. Since it provides the most accurate analysis of cells, it is considered the gold standard of diagnostic tests. When cancer is confirmed, the tissue sample may also provide information that will affect the treatment plan.

The tissue may be obtained through needle aspiration, through an endoscope, or by surgical removal. Depending on how the tissue is removed, the location and size of the tumor, and the amount of tissue taken, the biopsy may be done in a physician's office, an outpatient surgical facility with local anesthesia, or a hospital under general anesthesia.

A pathologist examines the removed cells and/or tissue. The accuracy of the interpretation depends on the skill and experience of both the surgeon obtaining the tissue sample and the pathologist. Both should be board-certified to ensure they are specialists.

Complications may include discomfort and pain, excessive bleeding, infection, or scarring.

Needle Biopsies

The simplest, least invasive, and least expensive way to obtain a tissue sample or a small amount of fluid from a suspicious mass is through a fine needle (called a *fine needle aspiration*).

Needle biopsies are usually performed on easily accessible tumors, but they can also be used on tumors of deep organs such as the pancreas or liver, thus dramatically reducing the need for exploratory surgery. A simultaneous imaging test may help visualize the needle placement, ensuring that it reaches the precise location of the tumor. There is always a risk, however, that the needle will miss a very small tumor, causing a false-negative diagnosis. Placing the needle in a large and/or indistinct lesion is also difficult. If not enough tissue is withdrawn for an accurate diagnosis, a second procedure may be necessary.

A *core needle biopsy* uses a wider needle to retrieve a larger tissue sample.

There may be some discomfort when the needle is inserted into the skin and again when it enters the tumor. Local anesthesia or sedation is often used.

On a superficial, easily felt tumor, such as one in the thyroid, it may take

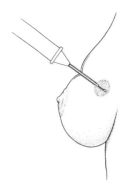

A bit of tissue from a breast lump can be obtained by using a special needle. This *needle biopsy* can be done in a doctor's office under local anesthesia.

only 15 minutes to obtain a tissue sample. On the other hand, if the tumor is located deep within the body, it may be more difficult to place the needle precisely, and the procedure may take an hour or more. Ultrasound or CT imaging is usually needed to guide the needle placement.

Surgical Biopsy

Removing tissue from a suspicious mass during surgery is the most invasive and expensive method of obtaining tissue. Surgery involves some risk of complications, such as excessive bleeding and infection, and general anesthesia involves risk as well. Postoperative pain and discomfort can occur, and hospitalization is costly.

Despite these disadvantages, a surgical biopsy allows more tissue to be removed more precisely than is possible during a needle or endoscopic biopsy. And with more tissue to analyze, the pathologist can make the most definitive diagnosis possible.

Surgical biopsies fall into two broad categories: incisional and excisional. *Incisional biopsy* is the removal of a piece of the suspicious mass. If malignancy is confirmed, the entire tumor is removed later in another operation. Incisional biopsies involve the remote risk that cancer cells, if present, may scatter into normal tissue and cause cancer spread. This is called *cancer seeding*. It is rare but it can happen in both incisional and needle biopsies.

Excisional biopsy is removal of the entire tumor, preferably along with a margin of surrounding normal tissue. The goal is to establish a diagnosis and cure the disease simultaneously. Excisional biopsies are usually performed on small, easily accessible tumors that have not begun to spread and do not include vital tissue. For example, an entire suspicious skin lesion or lump in the breast may be removed at once.

Tissue may be prepared for examination by *frozen sections* or permanent specimens. A frozen section is obtained during surgery and prepared within minutes while the person is on the operating table. The surgeon removes tissue from the tumor and immediately sends the sample to a pathologist. The pathologist quickly freezes the tissue in a special machine, slices it into ultra-thin sections, places it on slides, stains it, and examines it under a microscope. The pathologist then makes a diagnosis and reports it to the surgical team.

If cancer is confirmed and the tumor can be removed, it is excised immediately. Because the biopsy, diagnosis, and surgery all take place at one time (*one-step procedure*), frozen sections most often eliminate the need for a second operation (*two-step procedure*). A disadvantage of the one-step procedure is that freezing distorts the cells, making analysis difficult. Therefore, a diagnosis based on a frozen section involves a small risk of error. A skilled and experienced pathologist can diagnose a frozen section with more than 98 percent accuracy. (To verify the accuracy of the frozen-section diagnosis, tissue is also examined as a fixed-tissue specimen the following day.)

A two-step procedure means that the biopsy and tumor removal take place at different times. A permanent, *fixed tissue* specimen is prepared for the biopsy. Tissue processed this way is placed in a special preserving solution, embedded in paraffin, sliced, placed on a slide, stained, and sectioned during a time-consuming procedure that yields a high-quality slide and a diagnosis with 99 percent accuracy. However, the process takes one or more days. This means if cancer is confirmed and is operable, a second operation is necessary.

A two-step procedure allows time for further testing and second opinions, though. Moreover, you can participate in decisions about immediate treatment. However, if the tumor is deep inside the body, a second major operation may be too risky, and a one-step procedure may be preferable.

If a one-step procedure is preferred or is only a possibility, the surgeon should explain all the options in advance and obtain appropriate patient consent (see Chapter 15, "Surgery").

Bone Marrow Analysis

Bone marrow aspiration is removal of contents of the bone marrow for laboratory analysis. It is done to diagnose leukemia and other cancers as well as such blood disorders as anemia. The test can also determine if cancer has spread to the bone marrow from elsewhere.

After the skin and tissue surrounding the area to be penetrated by the needle are anesthetized, a long needle is inserted into the bone. Typically, the hip bone, pelvis, or breastbone is used. Fluid from the bone marrow (a soft substance at the center of the bone that produces blood cells) is withdrawn and examined microscopically.

A bone marrow biopsy is usually performed in conjunction with a bone marrow aspiration. With the needle still in place, the physician removes tiny fragments of bone along with the fluid.

Bone marrow aspiration and biopsy are virtually risk-free and take less

QUESTIONS
TO ASK

Before Having a Biopsy

Always clarify the reasons for a biopsy. Ask any questions about the technique and how the sample will be handled well before the actual procedure begins. You might ask your doctor:

- Are you going to biopsy a portion of the tumor or remove it completely? Why?
- If you biopsy just a portion of the mass, will I need another operation to remove the entire tumor?
- Will the biopsy be examined as a frozen section or permanent specimen? Why?
- Can the mass be needle-aspirated? If not, why not?
- Will the biopsy be examined by a board-certified pathologist?
- Will the report be confirmed by a second pathologist? (This is a common but not universal practice.)
- Will you consult personally with the pathologist(s)?
- Will the biopsy leave a scar? Where will it be?

than an hour to perform in a doctor's office or hospital. However, even though sedatives and local anesthetics are given, the procedure can be painful. A sharp jolt and a sensation of intense pressure can be felt when marrow is withdrawn. The puncture site may be bruised and tender for a few days.

The tests are performed by a physician and the tissue is examined microscopically by a pathologist or *hematologist* (a physician who specializes in blood disorders).

Endoscopy

If the tumor is in an inaccessible internal organ, an *endoscopy* may be recommended. This allows the outside or inside surfaces of the organs to be viewed directly. Tissue from organs can also be removed through the endoscope for biopsy.

An *endoscope* is a lighted, cylinder-shaped magnifying instrument narrow enough to pass through one of the body's natural openings, such as the nose, mouth, anus, urethra, or vagina or through a small incision that can be made almost anywhere (sometimes called "Band-Aid" surgery because the incision is small enough to be covered by a small bandage).

A surgeon can see deep inside the body and, with the aid of an attached brush or cutting instrument, remove tissue samples for biopsy. Some endoscopes have a tiny camera built onto the tip that transmits sharp images to a television monitor.

Endoscopy is often recommended to evaluate an abnormality detected on an x-ray or other exam. It may also be used before surgery to pinpoint the exact site of a tumor.

There are many different types of endoscopes, all of which can be identified by how they are used. For example, a *cystoscope* is used to inspect the urinary tract; a *colonoscope* is used to examine the colon; and a *bronchoscope* is used to look inside the lungs.

Depending on the type of endoscope and the part of the body being examined, a special diet or enema may be required. The procedure may be performed on an outpatient basis in a physician's office, or it may require an overnight stay in the hospital. Recuperating time varies according to the procedure.

Some endoscopies are uncomfortable, but they are usually not painful, especially with anesthesia or a sedative. Many people are exhausted after an

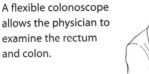

A flexible colonoscope allows the physician to examine the rectum and colon.

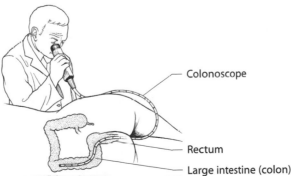

Colonoscope

Rectum

Large intestine (colon)

endoscopic procedure and might want to curtail some activities for a while.

Complications of endoscopy include the rare risk of perforation of the area being examined, infection, and excessive bleeding.

Exploratory Surgery

Exploratory surgery allows a physician to inspect internal organs directly to evaluate a mass and, if necessary, obtain tissue for further study. Depending on what is found, the surgeon may estimate how far the disease has spread, remove lymph nodes that may be affected, and obtain fluid and tissue samples.

The operation, which usually follows imaging exams and other diagnostic tests, is performed in a hospital by a surgeon.

Surgery always involves some risk and chance of complications, such as excessive bleeding and infection. General anesthesia, which is usually required, also involves risks.

Hospitalization for several days may be necessary, and recovery may require weeks. Postoperative pain and discomfort are common.

QUESTIONS

TO ASK

Diagnosis by Surgery

Before undergoing surgery, ask your doctor these questions:

- Describe the procedure you are recommending. What will be done and why?

- Why is this surgery necessary?

- What are the risks of this procedure, and how likely are they?

- What are the possible side effects and complications?

- Can I arrange to have my own blood drawn and stored in advance in case I need it?

- Is the procedure covered by my insurance or health care plan? How will I be billed? Will I receive separate bills from the hospital, surgeon, anesthesiologist, pathologist, and radiologist?

- Are there any other diagnostic tests that can be performed instead of surgery?

- Will a board-certified surgeon who specializes in oncology perform the procedure?

- How experienced is the physician in performing this type of operation?

- How long will I be hospitalized? How long will the recovery period be? When can I return to my daily routine?

Why Me?
Why Now?
What Now?

WHO GETS CANCER?

At least since the ancient Greeks, physicians, patients, and family members have pondered the question of why some people get cancer and others don't. Nearly 300 years ago an Italian physician, Bernardino Ramazzini, attempted the first scientific answer. The disease didn't strike entirely randomly, he observed; rather, personal characteristics and lifestyle choices seemed to increase a person's chances of getting it. He noticed, for example, that breast tumors occurred more commonly in nuns than among other women. He wrote in 1700 that the nuns' special susceptibility arose from "disturbances of the uterus" brought on by "their celibate life." Today *epidemiologists* (scientists who study the frequency and distribution of diseases within populations and the factors that influence those patterns) know that childless women, not only those who remain celibate, are more likely to get breast cancer than are women with children.

Sixty years later, John Hill of London reported a cluster of cancers among users of snuff, a form of tobacco. Fifteen years after that, another London practitioner, Percival Pott, noted the high rate of scrotal cancer among chimney sweeps, whose own slang recognized that the distinctive genital "soot-wart" was widespread in the trade. And in 1795 Samuel Thomas von Soemmering, an anatomist at the University of Mainz in Germany, observed that "carcinoma of the lip occurs most frequently where men indulge in pipe smoking."

In the two centuries since, many observers have noticed relationships between occupations, behaviors (such as smoking or eating particular foods), and individual characteristics (such as a person's age or gender) and the increased likelihood of getting cancer. These accumulated, systematic observations have contributed to the now quite sophisticated science of epidemiology.

Epidemiologists do not seek out the organic causes of disease. Rather, they search for the factors that appear statistically linked to a person's risk of becoming ill and provide important clues for other scientists investigating the causes of the illness. Discovering that lung cancer occurs more frequently among smokers, for example, led to research that eventually identified the chemicals in cigarette smoke that damage lung cells.

Cancer Links

This chapter discusses the factors that epidemiologists have identified as strongly influencing whether a person gets cancer. These include age, gender, geography, environmental conditions (e.g., diet, exercise, smoking, and exposure to pollutants and radiation), racial membership, economic standing, and family history. By examining the associations between all these factors and cancer, clues to how and why the illness develops continue to surface. None of these, however, or even any combination of them, accurately predicts an individual's fate. Statistics deal in large numbers, not in life histories. Still, some associations are strong enough to convince scientists that each of these basic factors taps into something fundamental about the nature of cancer. (See Chapter 10, "Cancer Causes and Risks.")

Age

With a handful of exceptions, cancer is a disease of aging and is vastly more likely to strike in the middle or later years than in childhood, youth, or young adulthood. Indeed, experts unanimously cite age as the single most important risk factor.

The median age of diagnosis is 67; two-thirds of cancer deaths occur after age 65. So as our population ages, and deaths from other causes diminish— as have stroke and heart attacks over the past several decades, for example— more and more Americans will live long enough to develop cancer.

Several factors seem to make older people more susceptible. Immune function declines with age, one theory suggests, so people may lose some of their earlier ability to fight off malignancies. Or, another theory proposes, *free radicals,* highly reactive molecules formed as a byproduct of normal cell functioning, damage the body's cells a million or more times a day. Though natural bodily defenses repair much of this harm, that ability declines with time. The damage may therefore accumulate to the point where it leads to cancer. Or there may be some other significant difference between young and older tissue, argues a third theory. According to a fourth theory, the high cancer rate of the later years is due to the simple fact that older people have lived longer. This allows more time to be exposed to carcinogens and enough time—often several decades—for many cancers to develop.

Whatever the reason, malignancies that originate in the *epithelial cells* (the layer of cells that line vital organs) rarely strike before the age of 30. In general, the rates of lung, colorectal, and prostate cancer rise steadily through a person's 30s, 40s, 50s, and beyond, leveling off or even dropping a bit at extremely advanced ages. Female reproductive cancers that originate in the epithelium of the breast, ovary, and uterus increase sharply at menopause. Among nonepithelial cancers, such as multiple myeloma and chronic lymphocytic leukemia, rates increase with age.

Another, smaller peak in cancer incidence occurs among children under 5. However, whether this symmetry at each end of life represents the lingering influence of factors present before birth or a less than maximally efficient immune system at the beginning and end of life remains unclear. Nonetheless, Wilms' tumor, a kidney malignancy; retinoblastoma, an eye cancer; neuroblastoma, a nerve cancer; and some types of leukemia generally attack children under the age of 5. Cancer accounts for 10 percent of childhood deaths.

Fewer than 10,000 of the nation's annual half million cancer deaths occur in those under age 35, and only about 55,000 people between 35 and 54 die of cancer in any year. But at age 55 the threat begins to rise sharply. More than a quarter of a million people between the ages of 55 and 74 die of cancer each year. The remaining 180,000 cancer deaths occur in those over 75.

Gender

At every age, males run a greater cancer risk than females; in 1996, an estimated 764,300 new cancers were diagnosed in men, as compared to 594,850 in women. The genders also diverge in the cancers that strike them. Reproductive cancers have been rising in both sexes in recent years. With the exception of skin cancer, prostate and breast cancers are the most common malignancies in men and women. Recently breast cancer incidence rates have leveled off and breast cancer death rates have decreased 5 percent. Breast and prostate cancers now rank as the second largest cancer killers of their respective sexes.

Lung Cancer. The genders' incidence patterns differ sharply for lung cancer, which peaked and began to fall among men in the mid-1980s but which continues to rise sharply among women. A rare disease until the early years of this century, lung cancer began its steep climb among men in the 1930s and 1940s, reaching an age-adjusted mortality rate of more than 80 per 100,000 before it began to slow. Women's lung cancer rate only began to accelerate in the mid-1960s, overtaking the then largest killer, breast cancer, in 1987. It now kills 41 women per 100,000 each year, and among women over 54 the climb shows no signs of abating in the next few years. Among women between the ages of 35 and 54, however, mortality rates are level or declining slowly.

This divergence mirrors the genders' differing experiences with smoking as well as the several decades the disease takes to develop. Smoking became popular among men in the early decades of this century, but women adopted the habit in large numbers only during and after World War II, producing a several-decade lag for the disease to develop in women. The drop in the male death rate began two decades after the epoch-making surgeon general's report of 1964, which for the first time officially linked smoking to lung cancer.

The higher rate of cancer deaths in men from other cancers may also represent differences in lifestyle, including greater exposure to cancer-causing chemicals on the job.

Reproductive Cancers. New breast cancer diagnoses surged in the 1970s, when then First Lady Betty Ford broke a long-standing taboo by speaking publicly of her mastectomy, soon to be followed by a similar surgery acknowledged by Happy Rockefeller, wife of then Vice President Nelson Rockefeller.

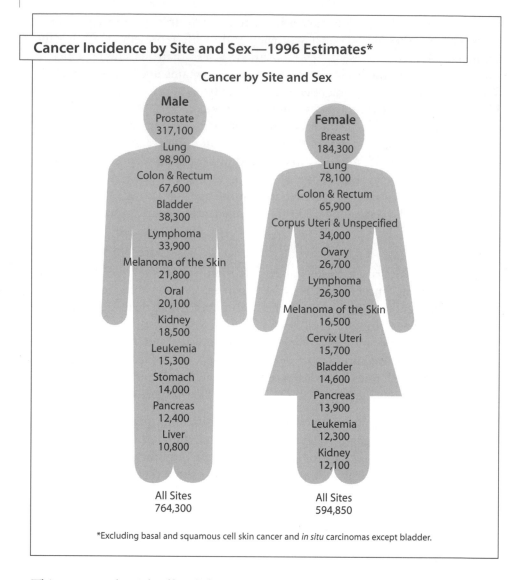

Cancer Incidence by Site and Sex—1996 Estimates*

Cancer by Site and Sex

Male

Prostate
317,100

Lung
98,900

Colon & Rectum
67,600

Bladder
38,300

Lymphoma
33,900

Melanoma of the Skin
21,800

Oral
20,100

Kidney
18,500

Leukemia
15,300

Stomach
14,000

Pancreas
12,400

Liver
10,800

All Sites
764,300

Female

Breast
184,300

Lung
78,100

Colon & Rectum
65,900

Corpus Uteri & Unspecified
34,000

Ovary
26,700

Lymphoma
26,300

Melanoma of the Skin
16,500

Cervix Uteri
15,700

Bladder
14,600

Pancreas
13,900

Leukemia
12,300

Kidney
12,100

All Sites
594,850

*Excluding basal and squamous cell skin cancer and *in situ* carcinomas except bladder.

This unprecedented official frankness and the attendant immense publicity made the topic of breast cancer acceptable in polite conversation and prompted millions of women to have mammograms—many for the first time.

The jump in tumors discovered mirrored the jump in women screened. As mammography technology improved during the early 1980s, public consciousness of the technique also climbed, as did the number of newly discovered breast cancers. Meanwhile, the baby boom generation began to enter midlife, inflating both the number of women of prime breast cancer age and the number of new cases. Despite the 4 percent increase a year in breast cancer between 1980 and 1987, its annual incidence has leveled off at about 110 new cases per 100,000 women. This is possibly due to the surge in mammography and increase in detection of very-early-stage tumors in the preceding few years.

The incidence of prostate cancer, the major male reproductive malignancy, has also been rising dramatically in recent years. Most experts believe this can be attributed to the test for prostate cancer, prostate-specific antigen (PSA), which now permits earlier diagnosis (see Chapter 6, "Routine Tests").

Economics and Race

Low socioeconomic standing and membership in a racial minority, factors often closely related in the United States, strikingly increase the risk of developing and especially of dying from cancer. African-American men, for example, have the highest cancer rates of any population group in this country, and their rate of prostate cancer is among the highest in the world. In addition, African-Americans experience lower five-year survival than whites for most major cancers. In 1991 the mortality rates were 228 for blacks and 170 for whites per 100,000; the incidence rates were 439 for blacks and 406 for whites. Native Hawaiians come next among racial groups, followed distantly by Japanese, Chinese, Hispanics, Filipinos, and Native Americans, whose rate is the lowest of any group.

Differences in genetic susceptibility may account for some of these divergences, but differences in lifestyle are clearly important. When African-Americans are matched with whites by income and educational level, cancer rates among whites are consistently higher, except for cervical, prostate, and stomach cancers. Whites in the lowest socioeconomic group, furthermore, have 20 percent more cancer than whites in the highest group, with cervical cancer four times as common among poor women and larynx and esophageal cancers—both related to high tobacco and alcohol use—twice as common among poor men.

As routine Pap smears and the increasing frequency of hysterectomies have drastically decreased cervical cancer among women receiving adequate medical care, the influence of education and financial resources becomes more obvious. People without adequate medical care do not have access to and therefore cannot benefit from early detection. Many believe a cancer diagnosis is fatal and may not know that many cancers are curable if caught early. Thus, they often fail to recognize the potentially life-saving importance of early detection, believing instead that finding a cancer sooner merely prolongs the time of suffering with the knowledge of impending death.

Upper-income individuals, though their overall cancer rate is lower, still suffer disproportionately from malignancies of the breast and uterus. This may reflect in part a cultural pattern of delayed childbearing, which increases the risks of these cancers.

Environment

In epidemiology, environment refers not only to the natural world but to every outside influence on the body. Thus, to say that environmental factors account for cancers doesn't mean that epidemiologists exclusively blame industrial chemicals seeping into drinking water or wastes contaminating the air. Rather, it means that cancers may arise from countless outside forces, including diet, viruses and other microorganisms, x-rays and other sources of radiation, tobacco, alcohol, and substances encountered in the home or workplace. Currently, the evidence for the role of these factors is very limit-ed. Many of these influences are considered aspects of a person's lifestyle. A single environmental factor, for example, accounts for 30 percent of all can-cer deaths. This major killer is tobacco, which affects both smokers and non-smokers who breathe the second-hand cigarette smoke. Diet, especially when it is high in animal fat and low in green and yellow vegetables, may account for another 35 percent of cancers. Reproductive and sexual behavior—includ-ing the number of sexual partners, exposure to viral infections, and age at which a woman first gives birth—may account for another 7 percent. Occupational exposures to chemical carcinogens contribute to about 4 per-cent of cancers. Factors that meet the popular definition of "environmental," such as air and water pollution, radiation from radon gas and other natural-ly occurring radioactivity, and exposure to sunlight, also have an effect.

Geography

Incidence rates vary drastically among countries. Melanoma, for example, is 155 times as likely to strike a resident of the Australian province of Queensland as a citizen of Osaka, Japan. Cancer of the nose or pharynx is 100 times more frequent in Hong Kong than it is in southwestern England. Prostate cancer is 70 times as likely to afflict an African-American living in Atlanta as any man living in Tianjin in China.

Although genetic influences may play a role in these differences, studies of international migration strongly suggest the importance of lifestyle (includ-ing diet), environmental quality, and even whether people die of other dis-eases before they reach the relatively advanced age when cancer becomes common. When Japanese immigrate to Hawaii and California, for example, their incidence rates of bowel and breast cancers come to resemble the American rate rather than the Japanese pattern.

Geography also affects cancer rates within the United States, although its role is less pronounced than it is among countries. For example, the District of Columbia has a cancer death rate almost twice that of Utah. Delaware, the state with the highest cancer death rate, exceeds Utah's rate by 61 percent. Indeed, the strikingly high death rates from lung cancer among East Coast men in the 1960s highlighted the danger from the asbestos used in shipyards in the area during World War II. An elevated oral cancer death rate among southern women drew attention to the danger of cancer caused by using snuff.

Family History

Group characteristics and environment do not explain all cancers, however. Genetic propensities also contribute. In a few striking cases, particular can-cers are clearly hereditary. These include the eye cancer retinoblastoma, the colon cancer associated with familial adenomatous polyposis, the thyroid cancer of Siple's syndrome, and the various malignancies of the Li-Fraumeni syndrome. In other cases families show a strong tendency to develop certain cancers. A history of several cancers, including breast and colon cancers, among close relatives is a strong risk factor.

Patterns and Trends

Tracking trends in incidence and mortality yields important information about cancer. The stunning rise of lung cancer in this century, for example, mirrored both the growing popularity of smoking and the habit's deadly effect. The current drop in lung cancer among men but not among women reflects the success of past antismoking campaigns, aimed mainly at men, and the importance of stepping up campaigns aimed at women. The precipitous fall of cervical cancer, once as common a killer as breast cancer, testifies to the importance of widespread access to the Pap smear. The corresponding drop in stomach cancer, though harder to explain, indicates an important change in the food supply. Some experts suggest that more refrigeration of foods or less consumption of smoked or salted foods is responsible.

Discouraging though the incidence rates of cancer appear, epidemiology has tracked some areas of progress. For example, between 1960 and 1963, only 39 percent of Caucasian cancer patients and 27 percent of African-Americans lived

Are You at Risk?

Many people believe that cancer is becoming more common in the United States than it used to be. This perception is not accurate. Except for lung cancer, which has risen steeply for 60 years and continues to rise among women, age-adjusted incidence rates have not risen significantly. In other words, the *proportion* of the people of a given age who get a particular cancer remains stable. As the population ages, however, more people move into the older, more cancer-prone age groups. As the immense baby boom generation advances into middle age, for example, the number of women in age groups more susceptible to breast cancer has risen, along with the number of breast cancer cases.

Also creating the impression of rising rates are improvements in detection, which reveal cancers that would formerly have remained undetected. The number of diagnosed breast cancers rose dramatically between 1982 and 1986, for example, as more women underwent mammography and more early-stage cancers were discovered that once would have gone undetected for several more years. Since 1987 incidence rates have dropped, possibly because many of the cancers that would have been detected after 1987 had already been discovered. Although firm conclusions must await further research, some experts believe that the rate of breast cancer has not decreased but that only the time at which the cancers are discovered has changed.

Although cancer rates may not be on the rise, there is much you can do to reduce your own personal risks and those of your family, such as breaking bad habits (for example, smoking) that are known to be linked to cancer and incorporating healthy behavior, such as exercise, into your lifestyle. The specific risk factors are the subject of Chapter 10, "Cancer Causes and Risks."

INFORM

YOURSELF.

five years after diagnosis. But 23 years later, between 1986 and 1991, those numbers increased to 58 percent and 42 percent, respectively.

In some cases, particularly the childhood cancers, progress has been spectacular. In 1960–1963, the percentage of children surviving five years after acute lymphocytic leukemia stood at a dismal 4 percent; by 1986–1991, it had reached 77 percent. Today 90 percent of children with Hodgkin's disease survive five years, as opposed to half 50 years ago.

Despite this progress, much remains to be done. The nation's largest cancer killer, lung and bronchial cancer, claims the lives of 87 percent of its white victims and 89 percent of its black ones within five years of diagnosis, the overwhelming majority in the first year. And the discrepancy between the races in both incidence and survival rates for many cancers remains altogether too large.

CANCER CAUSES AND RISKS

Cancer is a complicated disease that science does not yet fully understand. Nonetheless, researchers have identified enough factors that appear to be involved to suggest some strategies that may help prevent cancer or reduce the risk. This chapter outlines these known risk factors and clarifies the often confusing notion of risk.

Some experts believe that as many as 80 percent or more of cancers in the United States can be prevented. But preventable in theory does not necessarily mean avoidable in real life. For example, millions of smokers have kicked the habit in order to reduce their chances of developing lung cancer. But who would recommend that all women have their first child before age 18 or that no one spend time outdoors in the daytime, steps that would cut the incidence of breast and skin cancers, respectively? Nor are most Americans likely to become vegetarians, although a meatless diet might also reduce certain types of cancers. To say that cancers are theoretically preventable, therefore, means only that they arise from *risk factors,* many of which come from outside the body and are to some extent within individual control.

What Risk Means

In everyday parlance, *risk* implies an inherent danger, like that of skydiving or driving while drunk, but scientists mean something different when they use the word. Indeed, they often use the word *risk* to refer to things that appear safe, such as working outdoors, delaying childbearing, or even belonging to a particular family.

Statistical Risk

With regard to cancer, risk is a statistical association between a particular factor and the chance of contracting the disease. Thus, people who are exposed to a lot of sun run a higher than average risk of developing skin cancer. Women who have their first child after age 30 or who have no children at all are at a higher risk for breast cancer. Those who eat lots of fat may have a higher risk of colon cancer. And a woman related to someone who has had a breast malignancy has a higher chance of developing one as well. Statistical risks can be *voluntary*, like lighting up a cigarette, or *involuntary*, like breathing the air in a room full of smokers.

By identifying associations of this kind, epidemiologists discover clues to the causes of cancer and help individuals and society at large decide what measures might offer protection. Knowing that a family history of colon cancer increases risk, for example, has encouraged researchers to seek (and ultimately to find) a gene related to certain types of the disease. This awareness has also served as a warning to individual family members that they may need closer medical surveillance to spot tumors early.

Risk Doesn't Predict

Even though people may use their awareness of specific risk factors to guide their behavior, it's important to remember that statistical odds say nothing about particular people or their fates. Risk statistics do not predict which individuals will fall ill. Many cancers, furthermore, occur in people with no known risk factors, whereas many people at high statistical risk escape the disease altogether. That is, risk indicates an increased probability, not a prediction.

Fear of Cancer

People's perceptions of danger do not always match the true level of the hazard. Even though one in 10 smokers develops lung cancer, millions of people continue to puff away, either undeterred by the fact that stopping would lower their risk or not caring. On the other hand, a great deal of media attention has been paid to the potential cancer risk of living near high-tension electrical power lines or utility substations. Yet, after years of deliberation, the American Physical Society, representing the world's largest group of physicists, said it could find no scientific evidence that the electromagnetic fields radiating from the power lines cause cancer.

Fearful Behavior

Although many Americans fear cancer more than any other disease, some studies suggest that people more readily accept risks that they choose voluntarily, like smoking, than they do risks imposed on them without their consent, like air pollution. This may explain why people greatly overestimate the proportion of the nation's cancers that arise from involuntary exposure to industrial chemicals and pollution. Although some environmental factors do pose serious hazards to people working in particular industries or living in certain areas, these represent only a small portion of Americans' total cancer risk. Rather, those elements of lifestyle like smoking, diet, and reproductive practices that are theoretically changeable but deeply embedded in people's habits account for the great majority of cancers.

A rational view of risk must be at the heart of any sensible prevention program. Indeed, research shows that the less people know about cancer, the more they fear it. And fearful people are less likely to take effective action to protect their health, especially to follow guidelines for early detection of cancers that are most easily treated before they produce noticeable symptoms (see Chapter 5, "Screening for Cancer"). A practical approach to cancer prevention thus demands an understanding of what does and does not cause the disease and an awareness that there remain many unknown factors.

Searching for Causes

Cancer occurs when a group of cells escape from the normal controls that ordinarily regulate their growth and begin to multiply in an aggressive, unruly fashion (see Chapter 1, "What Is Cancer?"). A full-fledged malignancy represents not one but a series of events in which something went seriously wrong with the body's control mechanisms.

This interaction of factors explains why scientists can rarely pinpoint a single cause for any cancer, just as it is impossible to say, for example, which of many factors "caused" a riot. There must be a precipitating incident; an atmosphere that encourages, or at least does not discourage, the spreading violence; the failure of the police to contain the disturbance; and even weather favorable to large numbers of people rampaging through the streets. Each of these "causes" may be necessary, but none is sufficient by itself.

In the same way, the very fact that only some of the people exposed to most cancer-causing agents develop the disease proves its multistep nature. If there were a single, or simple, cause, then everyone, or nearly everyone, would fall ill. But more than nine smokers in 10 do not die of lung cancer, and many of the people who survived the atomic attacks on Hiroshima and Nagasaki, perhaps the heaviest such dose of cancer-causing radiation known to history, remain cancer-free.

Further complicating the search for causes is the fact that a condition associated with a particular cancer may not cause it but merely indicate another, underlying cause. For example, the incidence of breast cancer is higher in women who bear children later in life. Late childbearing and the increased risk of breast cancer may therefore be due to an underlying factor, possibly an estrogen imbalance in the body that facilitates the growth of malignancies.

Even if researchers could clarify all the relationships in a cancer process, additional obstacles would remain. Because cancers generally take years, even decades, to develop, the task of tracking down what specific exposure disrupted the cells' replicating machinery is made even more difficult. Some factors, furthermore, act synergistically; that is, one condition amplifies another's power. Thus, smokers who also are exposed to asbestos develop cancer more readily than do smokers who are exposed only to tobacco.

Carcinogens, Promoters, and Enhancers

Despite all these provisos, science has clearly and strongly implicated exposure to certain factors in the development of tumors. First are a number of agents that cause a cell to alter its growth in a cancerous direction: chemicals like benzene; viruses like the human papilloma virus; and radiation from nuclear reactions, x-ray machines, or ultraviolet rays from the sun. These are called *carcinogens,* and they may act either by directly affecting the cell's growth-regulating genetic material (DNA), in which case they are called *genotoxic,* or by damaging other parts of the cell.

Cancer *promoters* cannot by themselves cause a change in the cell's DNA, but they can aid and abet an alteration or injury when it does take place. Both synthetic chemicals, such as fluorocarbons and PCBs, and natural chemicals, such as the body's own bile acids or sex hormones, can be cancer promoters.

Cancer *enhancers* are passive conditions that favor the development of cancer. For example, compounds called nitrites, sometimes used as food preservatives, are not in themselves carcinogens but can turn into the carcinogen nitrosamine in the stomach. Of course, whether or not that carcinogen is capable of affecting normal cell growth depends on the presence of many other factors and conditions. Some are known, some are unknown; some are controllable and some are not. Again, it is important to remember that many people who are exposed to genotoxic carcinogens or cancer promoters or both never develop cancer.

SPECIAL

CONCERNS

Can Emotions Make You Sick?

For some years now, the suspicion has been growing that the mind may play a role in influencing who gets cancer. One popular theory suggests that emotional states like depression can encourage the growth of a malignancy. Another holds that stress and negative feelings suppress the immune function, which is believed to be crucial to preventing the disease.

A veritable industry now churns out books, articles, tapes, lectures, and workshops dedicated to the proposition that positive emotions, thoughts, and attitudes can keep cancer at bay and even defeat it should it strike.

Some psychological researchers seek the traits that add up to a "cancer-prone" personality. Others map mental strategies to defeat malignancies. In fact, some of the more extreme mind-body approaches come perilously close to "blaming the victim" for either becoming sick or failing to conquer an aggressive, potentially fatal disease. Others more circumspectly observe that social support seems to help many people cope with the severe stress of having cancer and undergoing its treatment.

The scientific verdict on this work is mixed. Although some studies support a relationship between mental factors and either the onset or course of cancer, others do not. Critics, furthermore, discount as poorly designed some of those studies claiming a connection. Recent large, well-designed studies have found no relationship between emotions and cancer onset. Some doctors see a person's emotional state playing a possible role in influencing the disease's progression. But there's one way that emotions can affect cancer risk more directly: Smoking, drinking, and other behaviors known to be linked to cancer often represent an attempt to cope with stress or depression.

Major Risk Factors

According to informed estimates, three-quarters of all cancers in the United States arise from tobacco and alcohol use, diet, and reproductive and sexual behavior. Contrary to most people's perceptions, exposure to occupational and industrial hazards and pollution probably accounts for fewer than 10 percent of cancer cases. Although no direct link has been established between a sedentary lifestyle and cancer, researchers are evaluating whether exercise might reduce cancer risk by enhancing immunity, shortening the time food passes through the intestine, and altering hormone levels.

Tobacco

Lung cancer, which strikes smokers nearly 20 times as often as nonsmokers, overwhelmingly results from cigarette smoking. Cancers of the mouth, pharynx, larynx, esophagus, bladder, kidney, and pancreas also are related to smoking. In the case of organs along the airway—including the mouth, esophagus, pharynx, larynx, and lungs—direct exposure to smoke is to blame. The many chemicals contained in cigarette smoke also enter the bloodstream, circulating to distant organs and thus affecting the kidney and bladder and other organs.

Pipes and cigars, though less likely to cause lung cancer, are implicated in tumors of the mouth, throat, and lip. More than 200 years ago, smokeless tobacco (snuff and chewing tobacco) was tied to mouth cancer. More recently, scientists have established that *passive smoking*—inhaling cigarette smoke of others without smoking oneself (*environmental tobacco smoke*)—also increases the risk of developing lung cancer.

Alcohol

Alcohol works in partnership with tobacco, increasing the chances that smokers who also drink will develop mouth, pharynx, larynx, and esophageal cancer. Although there is some evidence that alcohol is a carcinogen, it actually is a co-carcinogen because it seems to make tobacco carcinogens more harmful. In addition, drinking heavily enough to bring on liver cirrhosis causes changes in the tissues that can increase the risk of liver cancer.

Studies have revealed an association between alcohol consumption and breast cancer, but the mechanism for this link cannot be explained.

Diet

The lifestyle factor that has received the most attention in recent years is diet. In fact, evidence suggests that about one-third of the 500,000 cancer deaths each year that occur in the United States is due to dietary factors. These include types of food, food preparation methods, portion sizes, food variety, and overall caloric balance.

Fat, Fiber, and Cancer. A high-fat diet has been associated with an increased risk for cancer of the colon and rectum, prostate, and endometrium. The relationship between dietary fat and breast cancer is much weaker. It is believed that a high-fat diet is a cancer promoter, with numerous theories to explain the effects of fat. For instance, fat seems to be involved in the production of free radicals (see Chapter 9, "Who Gets Cancer?"), which play a role in many types of cancer. A high-fat diet also increases the flow of bile acids in the intestine, and bile acids are cancer promoters in the colon.

By looking at the percentage of dietary fat comprising the total number of calories typically consumed in various parts of the world and the incidence of cancer in those countries, some parallels have become clear. For instance, there is a high incidence of cancers of the breast, prostate, colon, pancreas, ovary, and endometrium in Western countries but a low incidence in Japan and other places where much less fat is consumed. The Eskimo people in the Arctic eat a lot of fat, but it is primarily from fish, which produce mostly omega-3 fatty acids. This type of fat actually protects against cancer and heart disease. But when the diets of people in these countries become more Westernized, their cancer rate increases. In addition, animal studies have shown that reducing the percentage of fat calories also diminishes the incidence of cancer.

Fiber plays a preventive role in some of these fat-associated cancers, though the exact mechanism is unknown. For example, people in the Finnish countryside eat a lot of fat, mainly in dairy foods, yet the rate of colon cancer in Finland is low. Researchers think that because Finns consume so much bran fiber—which, among other things, decreases the concentration of bile and fatty acids in the colon—their cancer risk is low. Insoluble fiber (such as oat bran) is thought to reduce the risk of colon cancer.

Obesity, which typically is a consequence of eating too much fat, also increases the risk of cancer at several sites: colon and rectum, prostate, breast (among postmenopausal women), endometrium, and kidney.

CANCER

BASICS

Foods That Prevent Cancer

The American Cancer Society recommends eating a variety of fruits and vegetables, for several reasons. One is that they are rich sources of fiber, which appears to lower the risk of some cancers. Fruits and vegetables also contain specific nutrients that seem to prevent the changes that lead to cancer. For example, they contain vitamins C and E, which eliminate carcinogens such as nitrosamines, and vitamins A and carotenoids, the so-called *blocking agents* that reduce the action of carcinogens. Beta carotene, vitamin E, and selenium are antioxidants; that is, they counteract free radicals, which appear to cause changes in cells that lead to cancer. In addition, some studies show that other specific substances in fruits and vegetables, such as the sulfur compounds in garlic, have an anticancer effect. Antioxidant supplements have not demonstrated a reduction in cancer risk.

Although minerals don't receive as much attention as vitamins do, several studies have found that potassium, calcium, and magnesium help reduce the risk of cancer of the stomach and bladder.

Additives and Preparation Methods. Certain substances added to foods or methods of preparing foods can either cause or promote cancer. There are an estimated 2,300 "flavoring agents" in foods, about half of which are synthetic. The U.S. Food and Drug Administration systematically evaluates these additives, and although several of them, including flavoring and coloring agents, have been banned, some experts believe that a more comprehensive survey is needed.

But so-called natural methods of preserving foods are not necessarily safer. For example, pickled, cured, and smoked products appear to promote stomach cancer, possibly because of the nitrates and nitrites used in curing as well as other compounds produced during smoking and pickling. It has been suggested that the sharp decrease in stomach cancer during this century may be largely the result of refrigeration; that is, Americans no longer eat so many preserved foods.

Polycyclic aromatic hydrocarbons (PAHs), which are established carcinogens, are formed when meats are charcoal-broiled, and some research has shown that PAHs are formed when foods are smoked or fried. However, it is not known whether they can cause cancer in humans.

Pesticides and Herbicides. Scientific evidence supports the health benefits and cancer-protective effects of eating fruits and vegetables. Although pesticides and herbicides can be toxic in high doses, current evidence is insufficient to link pesticides in foods with an increased risk of any cancer.

Natural Carcinogens. Although naturally occurring carcinogens do not present much of a problem in the United States, they do exist. One of the most notable is *aflatoxin,* which is produced by a mold that grows on grains and nuts stored in hot, humid conditions. It is one of the most potent liver carcinogens known and contributes to the high rates of that cancer in Africa.

Although much attention has been paid to single food additives and preservatives, many epidemiologists now believe that perhaps more attention should be focused on dietary habits than on particular chemical carcinogens.

New Recommendations. In 1996 the ACS revised its nutritional guidelines to lower cancer risk suggesting a diet that includes a high proportion of plant foods (fruits, vegetables, grains, and beans), limited amounts of meat, dairy, and other high-fat foods, a balance of caloric intake and physical activity, and limited alcohol consumption. Women at an unusually high risk of breast cancer might consider not drinking any alcohol.

Sexual and Reproductive Behavior

People's choices regarding sexuality and reproduction affect their own and their children's cancer risk in a variety of ways.

Circumcision. At the beginning of life, for example, the decision to circumcise a boy may reduce both his and his future partner's cancer risk. Cancer of the penis is 100 times more common in Jamaica than in Israel, where both Jews and Muslims are universally circumcised. The female sexual partners of circumcised men also face a lower risk of cervical cancer than do those whose partners are uncircumcised. Whether this is due to the practice of circumcision or to poor hygiene has not been established. Some authorities believe that human papilloma virus, which is sexually transmitted and associated with cervical cancer in women, is responsible.

Promiscuity. Because exposure to the sexually transmitted human papilloma virus has been implicated in cervical cancer, having many sex partners and becoming sexually active early also raises women's risk of contracting the disease.

Delaying or Avoiding Childbearing. Women who don't have children or who have them later in life are at increased risk for both breast and ovarian cancer.

Infectious Agents

Viruses. Because viruses can invade and alter cells' genetic material, viral infections are implicated in some cancers. The Epstein-Barr virus, for example, is associated with Burkitt's lymphoma, a tumor found mainly among children in Africa. The hepatitis B virus is responsible for much of the liver cancer that causes death around the world. The human papilloma virus that causes genital warts may play an important causative role in cervical cancer. The human T-cell leukemia virus, a close relative of the virus that causes AIDS, is associated with a type of leukemia found most often in the Caribbean and Japan. And the AIDS virus is associated with a cancer known as Kaposi's sarcoma and some types of lymphoma.

Medical Treatments

Ironically, some of the treatments that doctors use to restore health can increase the risk of cancer. For example, some of the drugs used in chemotherapy to fight cancer are themselves carcinogenic. Immunosuppressive drugs used in conjunction with organ transplants reduce the body's ability to fight off malignancies. The accumulated radiation from diagnostic x-rays and radiation therapy can damage cells, and when that damage is extensive, it may cause cancer.

The estrogen replacement therapy used by many postmenopausal women may promote endometrial cancer. The artificial estrogen diethylstilbestrol, or DES, was widely prescribed to pregnant women in the 1950s and 1960s to prevent miscarriage. But this treatment also unwittingly exposed these women's daughters to cancer of the vagina. There has been speculation that DES use by a mother increases her son's risk of testicular cancer.

Family Characteristics

A number of the most common cancers, including breast, colon, ovarian, and uterine cancer, recur generation after generation in some families. In addition, certain other conditions that tend to occur in families may predispose those affected to specific cancers. Finally, a few rare cancers, such as the eye cancer retinoblastoma and a type of colon cancer, have been linked to specific genes that can be tracked within a family. In some cases, such as the very rare Li-Fraumeni syndrome, particular genes make family members susceptible to a wider variety of malignancies.

Although it is extremely helpful to know your genetic heritage, it's also important to keep in mind that environmental influences may outweigh the risks inherent in your family tree.

Occupation

Scientists have identified a number of occupations that expose workers to carcinogens. Though they are not responsible for a large percentage of malignancies, occupational exposures can pose very great dangers to people in particular lines of work.

Industries whose workers may face increased cancer risks include transportation, chemicals, rubber, shipbuilding, hairdressing and cosmetology, agriculture, electric equipment manufacture, and health care. Such industrial materials as asbestos, petroleum, benzene, styrene, solvents, dyes, cadmium, lead, cotton and wool dust, the disinfectant ethylene oxide, radioisotopes, flame retardants, and organic pesticides may all contribute to cancers. In addition, exposure to radon, x-rays, and other types of ionizing radiation may increase the risks.

Environment

Carcinogenic contaminants are widespread in the environment.

Radiation. An unknown but substantial number of homes and office buildings contain invisible, radioactive radon gas, which is implicated in lung cancer. Some experts say as many as 10,000 cases of lung cancer per year are associated with radon exposure.

Sunlight. Ultraviolet light poses a decided danger, especially to light-skinned people. This hazard increases as one approaches the equator. At the latitude of

---

Shaking the Family Tree

To create a resource that will be useful to you and your relatives, assemble the following facts about your parents, siblings, grandparents, aunts, and uncles. Keep in mind, though, that many factors—environmental as well as inherited—are involved. Being aware of your genetic heritage can help your physician tailor a preventive health care plan for you. Make a chart that indicates the following information about your relatives:

- cause of death—that is, the cause given on the death certificate;
- serious illnesses, including age of onset;
- health habits, such as smoking and drinking.

If elderly relatives are reticent about discussing cancer, a taboo subject a generation or two ago, explain how the information will help you. Next, make sure to let your doctor know your findings and share them with those relatives who may also be affected.

INFORM

YOURSELF

Common Cancer-Causing Chemicals

In 1989 the National Toxicology Program identified 20 substances that are carcinogenic when they are eaten or inhaled or come in contact with the skin. Many of them have been banned from manufacture in the United States. Those remaining are the following:

- *Arsenic and certain arsenic compounds.* Although arsenic is no longer made in the United States, arsenic compounds are used in a variety of products imported into this country and pose a risk to workers in those industries outside the United States. Arsenic is present in some pesticides and herbicides and is used in glass and ceramic manufacture and metal smelting. People who eat meat from livestock fed arsenic drugs or arsenic-containing additives may consume trace amounts. Drinking water may be contaminated in areas where pesticides are used. Arsenic may also be inhaled in areas near pesticide and glass factories or in cigarette smoke. Arsenic is linked to several malignancies, including cancers of the liver, lung, and skin.

- *Asbestos.* Even though the use of asbestos is being phased out, the mineral fiber is so widespread that workers in several industries—particularly construction and demolition—are exposed to it. The general public may be exposed if they live or work in buildings where asbestos has been used. In 1989 the Environmental Protection Agency announced a six-year plan to eliminate 84 percent of the asbestos products made in the United States. Asbestos is associated with lung cancer and mesothelioma, a type of cancer that affects organ linings.

- *Azathioprine.* Azathioprine is a drug used to treat autoimmune diseases and is prescribed to people receiving organ transplants. Workers in the pharmaceutical industry and in hospitals also may be exposed. Azathioprine is linked to non-Hodgkin's lymphomas and skin cancer.

- *Benzene.* Benzene is a chemical widely used in the manufacture of other chemicals, plastics, paints and paint thinners, and adhesives and as a gasoline additive. It also is present in car exhaust and cigarette smoke. Benzene increases the risk of leukemia.

- *Bis (chloromethyl) ether* and *technical-grade chloromethyl methyl ether.* These ethers are used in plastic manufacturing and have been linked to lung cancer, particularly oat-cell carcinomas.

- *Butanediol dimethylsulfonate (Myleran).* A drug used for leukemia and a blood condition called polycythemia, Myleran may actually lead to other blood disorders, including leukemia.

- *Chlorambucil (Leukeran).* A drug used to treat leukemia, lymphomas, and other cancers, Leukeran may in turn increase the risk of leukemia (see Chapter 17, "Chemotherapy").

- *Chromium* and *chromium compounds*. Chromium is a metal used in the protective coating on cars and in the tanning and manufacture of textiles, paint, and food, as well as in water treatment. (Not all forms of chromium are carcinogenic.) Exposure to chromium is mainly an occupational hazard for workers, who are at increased risk of several cancers, including lung cancer.

- *Conjugated estrogen*. This may be prescribed following removal of the ovaries, to treat breast and prostate cancer, and to replace the estrogen no longer produced by a woman's body after menopause. It may increase a woman's risk of endometrial cancer.

- *Cyclophosphamide (Cytoxan, CTX, Endoxan, Neosar)*. Cyclophosphamide is a widely used anticancer drug (see Chapter 17, "Chemotherapy"). Workers in the pharmaceutical industry and health care professionals as well as patients receiving one of these drugs are at a greater risk for leukemia and other cancers such as bladder cancer.

- *Diethylstilbestrol (DES)*. DES is an estrogen-like hormone used to treat advanced breast and prostate cancer, menopause symptoms, and various reproductive problems. In the past, DES was also used to prevent miscarriage and in animal feed as a growth promoter. When taken during pregnancy, it may increase the risk of a particular type of cancer of the vagina or cervix in daughters exposed in utero and possibly testicular cancer in sons.

- *Methoxsalen with ultraviolet A therapy* (PUVA). PUVA is a combination treatment used for skin conditions like vitiligo, psoriasis, and mycosis fungoides. It increases the risk of squamous cell carcinoma of the skin.

- *Mustard gas*. A gas used in chemical warfare, mustard gas may lead to cancer of the respiratory tract.

- *2-Naphthylamine*. A chemical used in research laboratories, 2-naphthylamine is associated with bladder cancer.

- *Thorium dioxide*. Thorium dioxide is used in the manufacture of ceramics and incandescent lamps, in magnesium alloys, and as a source of nuclear energy. Before 1945 it was used in x-ray imaging. This radioactive substance is associated with several cancers, including cancer of the liver and kidney.

- *Vinyl chloride*. A flame-retardant widely used in industry, vinyl chloride is also the parent compound of *polyvinyl chloride* (PVC), a plastic resin used in many products, such as containers, electrical insulation, water and drain pipes and hoses, flooring, windows, credit cards, and video disks. Workers in any of these industries are at the greatest risk, as they handle the products. However, vinyl chloride is also released into the air near the manufacturing plants and may affect others in the community. New car owners also are exposed to high levels from products used in car interiors. No level of vinyl chloride is considered safe, and exposure is linked to several cancers, including lung, liver, and brain cancers and lymphomas.

Philadelphia, sunlight accounts for an estimated 40 percent of the melanomas and 80 percent of the squamous and basal cell carcinomas in Caucasians.

Pollution. Although the major air pollutants, as defined by the U.S. government, do not show strong links to cancer, asbestos (which was widely used as insulation from the 1950s to the 1970s) is a well-established carcinogen. Some studies suggest that the chlorination of water may account for a small rise in cancer risk. But probably the main danger from pollution arises when dangerous chemicals used in industry escape into the surrounding environment. It's been estimated that 1 percent of cancer deaths are linked to air, land, and water pollution.

SPECIAL

CONCERNS

Relative Risk: Living with a Familial History of Breast Cancer

Research on women at genetic risk for breast cancer—those with a mother or sister who have had the disease—shows that this family legacy can significantly affect their emotional well-being and health behavior.

Anxiety about her increased risk may interfere with a woman's willingness to carry out the early detection procedures—monthly breast self-exams and regular mammograms and clinical breast exams—that offer the best chance of finding a cancer in its early, most treatable stages.

The emotional impact of a relative's cancer can be great, depending on a woman's experience with the disease. It can range from the severe, continuing, and debilitating distress that often afflicts daughters who as children or early adolescents watched their mother die from breast cancer to the occasional anxiety generally experienced by those who as adults had a mother or sister survive the disease.

Both the stage and the outcome of the mother's or sister's illness seem to influence the high-risk woman strongly. In general, the younger the high-risk woman is and the more serious the disease's consequences are for her relatives, the greater and longer lasting the emotional impact will be. Thus, the very women who need the most vigilant surveillance—those at the highest risk for the most aggressive premenopausal tumors—often suffer the most paralyzing fear.

GETTING HELP FOR CANCER: WHO, WHAT, WHERE, AND HOW

From diagnosis to treatment to recovery, cancer care can involve a legion of health care professionals who provide a range of specific skills. The places where care is offered can also vary widely, from the physician's office to a hospital, from a specialized cancer care center to your own home.

Among all these people and places is an extraordinary breadth of expertise and technology to meet your medical, emotional, and practical needs and those of your family. Finding out what options are available and orchestrating these many resources into a functioning system can be a challenge. As more care providers become involved, the need to communicate effectively with them grows even more important.

Knowing the who, what, where, and how of cancer care places you in the best position to make effective decisions about treatment and rehabilitation. To this end, this chapter addresses the following questions:

- Who provides treatment? How do you evaluate their expertise? How are these caregivers organized? What constitutes a treatment team, and who coordinates the team's efforts? What is your role as the person with cancer?

- Where is cancer care provided? How do you assess hospitals to ensure that you will receive complete, high-quality care?

- How can care providers, patients, and family members achieve real teamwork?

- What techniques ensure good two-way communication between professionals and the people in their care?

The Team Concept

Until the last few decades, cancer care was a relatively straightforward process. Perhaps during a routine visit to the family doctor, someone might report a disturbing symptom or the physician might detect a troubling sign of disease. The

INFORM

YOURSELF

Getting the Best Cancer Care from Managed Care

Increasing numbers of people receive medical care through health maintenance organizations (HMOs) and similar managed care plans designed to control health care costs. Typically these plans require that each person be cared for by a primary physician, the "gatekeeper," through whom all referrals to specialists must be made. The specialists usually must also be members of the plan.

The push to control costs has also led to guidelines for the treatment of illnesses and referral to specialist care that in some cases severely restrict the consumer's choices. The doctors in the managed care plan may be limited in what they can do or recommend on their patient's behalf, and a case manager's approval of any recommendations is often required. Some plans offer financial incentives to their doctors to keep costs down, a controversial policy that may be at odds with the best quality of care.

Although not-for-profit HMOs have existed for years, no system is yet in place to assure that this rapid shift to for-profit managed care delivers the diagnostic, treatment, and long-term recovery opportunities to everyone with cancer. Many state governments are beginning to regulate some HMO practices.

The American Cancer Society feels an obligation to assist the managed care industry in understanding the requirements for appropriate care. The ACS is collaborating with numerous medical specialty organizations related to cancer care, patient advocacy groups, and insurance organizations, among others, to develop care and treatment guidelines and accountability practices.

Here's what you can do now to get the most out of your managed care plan:

- Insist on knowing how cancer is managed in your plan. What are the plan's restrictions on your choices of doctors, including specialists? Will you have prompt access to an oncologist?

- Ask about limitations to screening, diagnostic tests, and treatments.

- Does the plan offer access to investigational treatments?

- Are your doctor or others in the plan experienced in detecting and treating cancer generally or your type of cancer particularly? Ask whether the primary care doctors have specific training in cancer diagnosis and are required by the plan to stay abreast of new developments.

- Does the plan allow its primary care physicians to refer you to doctors outside the network or to specialized facilities if necessary? For example, if your child has cancer, does the health plan permit referral to a specialized pediatric cancer center?

- Will all decisions be yours? Will all options be presented to you?

- During the course of your illness, does your primary doctor have to approve treatments, procedures, or tests, or can a specialist assume the role of principal caregiver?

- Will you have access to a team of care providers in many disciplines— for example, medical, surgical, and radiation oncologists—to help plan your treatment and facilitate recovery?

- Can you get rehabilitation, counseling, supportive services, and adequate pain relief as needed?

The more you know about the current standard of care for your particular cancer, the better you will be able to assert your needs and insist on state-of-the-art treatment. Although not all the answers to all your questions may be to your liking—for example, the HMO may delay referrals to necessary specialists—you will have information you need in order, perhaps, to change plans. Certainly you will have grounds for informed complaint, to the primary care doctor, to the managers through the plan's grievance procedures, to the benefits manager at work, or to your state insurance regulatory board, if need be. And by all means, seek the help of your local American Cancer Society unit (see Appendix I, "Resources"). Patient advocacy is one of our most important missions.

person was then referred to a specialist. If cancer was detected, the only treatment available was surgery (and, later, radiation or chemotherapy). After the procedure, the person usually would be sent home—with fingers crossed.

That scenario has changed with advances in treatment, with the development of the medical specialty of oncology (cancer care), and a vastly greater appreciation of the many needs of the person with cancer and his or her family. Health concerns are only part of the picture, however: People with cancer need help for psychological, social, financial, and occupational concerns as well. From diagnosis through recovery, the best cancer care today requires far more expertise than any single caregiver can provide. Thus, many professionals, paraprofessionals, and even cancer survivors who serve as volunteers are involved, often as soon as treatment begins, each contributing expertise as particular needs arise.

Increasingly, experts in cancer care recognize that the person with cancer is best served when all these many helpers function as a unified team, managed by one professional team leader. The reasoning is that by working together, people with the illness, their loved ones, and their caregivers can pool all their strengths and resources to achieve a common goal: survival that offers the highest quality of life for the longest amount of time.

This unity of care and caregivers—in which someone is always available to assess everyone's individual needs and see that they are met—is the ideal scenario. Some hospitals and cancer centers do have formal teams to coordinate and provide care, and many oncologists have at least some of the necessary caregivers on their staffs. Most common, however, is the informal network of care providers and resources to whom your doctor refers you or that you discover through other sources, such as cancer survivors, the American Cancer Society, other organizations, and books such as this one.

You should be aware, however, that some insurance companies and prepaid or managed health plans discourage the input of more professionals than *they* deem essential to cancer care.

Selecting a Care Coordinator

Most people are best served by a doctor whom they trust who coordinates their care or at least advises on the process and helps evaluate the results. Otherwise, patient and family will likely be overwhelmed by the numbers of professionals with whom they become involved over the course of the illness.

Identifying who will serve this role of care coordinator may be the most important early decision in managing your illness.

Some people prefer to work with their primary physician: the general practitioner, family practitioner, internist, gynecologist, pediatrician, geriatrician, or primary care provider in a health maintenance organization whom you consult when earliest symptoms arise or who discovered signs of cancer in a checkup. The primary physician can help choose an oncologist to manage the cancer treatment, who will keep him or her informed throughout the treatment. This physician is often in the best position to provide continuing care, as he or she is likely to have known you before the symptoms emerged and will be involved in your health care after the active cancer treatment ends. This long-term perspective can be extremely valuable in making the most appropriate choices during treatment and recovery.

Your primary physician may offer to assume this adviser role or agree to provide such a service when asked. But not everyone has a regular doctor, and indeed, that doctor may not be comfortable serving in that capacity.

For many people, oncologists assume the physician-coordinator role, and their practices are set up to provide many types of services. Of course, they won't necessarily have the detachment from their role of providing your cancer care directly. Still, oncologists are informed about the latest treatments, are aware of the multifaceted needs of people who have cancer, and are familiar with the resources available for follow-up care.

Regardless of who assumes the role of professional adviser or coordinator, it is essential that you, the patient, feel comfortable with the choice. If your team leader seems cold and uninvolved or if you are made to feel less like a human being and more like a collection of symptoms, you may need to find someone else to take charge.

When making a decision, it is important to consider your coordinator's qualifications, indeed those of all your caregivers. Suggestions for evaluating physicians' qualifications and behavior, and other factors to consider before committing your care to a person or facility, are provided later in this chapter.

Who's on the Team: An Overview

If you have a physician adviser or team leader, that person will remain constant throughout your illness and recovery. Other cancer care professionals and support personnel come and go as your needs change throughout your illness and recovery. Often most of the team is replaced as the process moves from diagnosis to different treatments or to different care settings.

What's *Your* Role on the Cancer Team?

For the team to provide the best care for you throughout your illness and recovery, you should view yourself as the team's star player—but not necessarily its coordinator or manager. That role you should consider delegating to your chosen physician adviser.

As the key team member, you will decide which procedures or treatments offer you the best chance for recovery and the highest quality of life, after others provide information, describe alternatives, and make recommendations. Your authority is to say yes or no or to grant another member of the team (possibly a family member or close friend) the authority to make such decisions for you.

Do not think that to be a "good" team player you must either be exceedingly active in your care, participating in even the most minor decisions, or remain passive and let those in authority have their way. Everyone has his or her own way of coping with the crisis of illness (see Chapter 31, "Coping Strategies"). As long as your style does not prevent you from proceeding— by denying that you are really sick, for example, or by insisting on collecting opinions long after all options have been determined, or by accepting only those caregivers who tell you what you want to hear—you should function in the way that works best for you.

Some people cope by taking control of all their care and learning about every detail. As soon as they hear the diagnosis, they do as much research as time allows into the types of care and physicians and facilities available to provide it. They seek multiple opinions from different specialists until they find one whose philosophy fits their own. Other people, however, feel better relying on the advice of the expert or experts to whom they have entrusted their care. They may feel ill equipped to absorb all the details needed to make major decisions and are satisfied to let others evaluate the technicalities and present them with recommendations from which to choose.

No matter what role feels right for you, you *always* have the right to state your needs, express your preferences, and obtain the information you require for making informed decisions—indeed, that is your responsibility. A diagnosis of cancer often makes people feel that their bodies—even their entire worlds—are out of control. Recognizing that it is appropriate for you to take an active part in medical decisions may help restore a sense of power over the situation, which can be therapeutic in its own right.

Diagnosis

Cancer may be suspected first by a primary care physician, by a specialist to whom you go for care of distressing symptoms in a particular part of your body or for treatment of a separate condition, or perhaps by a doctor in a hospital in which you are being treated for a medical emergency. This "first-line" doctor will either order diagnostic tests or make a referral to one or more specialists who can provide these tests. When the test results are available, the physicians involved will confer and, if necessary, consult with other experts.

Unless a care coordinator is already in place, the primary care physician—the person you tend to think of as "my doctor"—is generally the appropriate person to discuss the diagnosis with you. For example, a man suspected of having prostate cancer may be referred to a urologist, who specializes in the genitourinary system, for diagnostic tests. If the diagnosis is indeed cancer, the urologist may accept responsibility from then on, may collaborate with the primary physician, or may refer the man to yet another specialist, such as an oncologist.

In any event, no matter who is "in charge" of the case, it is reasonable to expect all physicians who have participated to be available to answer questions.

Treatment

Once the diagnosis is confirmed, the focus will shift to designing the treatment plan. If you are going to work with a physician team leader, now is the time to select him or her.

Most commonly, some combination of surgery, radiation, and chemotherapy is recommended, and the choices you make will determine which physicians will become involved next. In many cases, the treatment begins in a hospital. Depending on how the hospital is organized, inpatient care will be coordinated by an attending physician, resident physicians (doctors who are completing advanced training), and other members of the medical staff.

Depending on your needs during treatment, other professionals may be brought in at the request of the attending physician. For example, a nutritionist may be consulted about your diet while undergoing chemotherapy, or a psychiatrist may be called in to help evaluate and treat depression.

Many hospitals also offer the services of a social worker or a nurse to respond to personal problems, help address complaints, and, if necessary, direct cancer patients and their families to appropriate sources of help in dealing with insurance companies and other practical tasks. Nurses or social workers also may serve as leaders of discussion or support groups and provide education. Another important person is the discharge planner, again a nurse or a social worker, who coordinates plans for your return home to make sure needed services or equipment will be available.

Depending on the type of cancer involved, the treatment may continue for an extended time following your discharge from the hospital. Cancer survivors usually make follow-up visits to one or more of their physicians. Nurses working in clinics or physicians' offices frequently administer chemotherapy. Home care nurses, respiratory or other therapists, social workers, or other providers may provide help in the home or in a private or clinic office.

Rehabilitation and Recovery

Recovery from the illness and from any side effects of the treatment requires a new or expanded team of cancer care professionals. These may include specialists in regaining the use of muscles that have been weakened, adjusting to the loss of body parts, and coping with the tasks of life and the practical and emotional consequences of illness. Care is often given in the home or coordinated through available resources in the community.

For those who wish it, social workers, psychologists, psychiatrists, and psychosocial or psychiatric nurses provide supportive care for individuals or groups. Organizations of cancer survivors provide useful information and support and sometimes political activism. Social workers affiliated with hospitals or voluntary organizations offer needed assistance in locating community health and social service organizations and in gaining placement in a rehabilitation center, among many other services. Alternative medical practitioners may be an important resource for those who wish to supplement their ongoing, standard care.

Advanced Illness

Recurrent or advancing illness calls forth many of the professionals who took part in the earlier diagnosis and treatment. Treatment may now be provided in specialized research centers where experimental treatments are available. Experts in pain management (including psychiatrists, psychologists, behavioral medicine specialists, social workers, anesthesiologists, and nurses) may be called in for consultation. Hospice care professionals offer practical help, comfort, and care for those who are approaching death and for their families.

Types of Medical Doctors

People being treated for cancer encounter numerous types of physicians throughout all phases of their cancer care. The following is a guide to medical doctors and their specialties:

- To earn a medical degree and a license to practice, physicians complete four years of college plus four years of medical school and, in most states, an additional year of internship. Physicians with this basic level of training are often referred to as *generalists* or *general practitioners* (GPs).

- Many physicians undergo one to five years of additional training to become *specialists*. About two dozen specialties are recognized by the American Board of Medical Specialties.

- In recent years family medicine has developed into a specialty of its own; those who complete the additional training are usually called *family practitioners.*

- Collectively, GPs, family practitioners, and doctors who specialize in pediatrics, obstetrics/gynecology, geriatrics, and internal medicine (known as internists) are considered to be *primary care physicians.* The term *primary care* reflects the fact that these doctors are usually consulted first when a medical need arises. For instance, an obstetrician/gynecologist is often the physician a woman sees for her primary care. Subscribers to health maintenance organizations (HMOs) and other prepaid health plans are usually required to visit a primary physician before receiving a referral to a specialist.

- Doctors who pass qualifying tests administered by a panel of fellow physicians are known as *board-certified specialists*. Some qualified and experienced specialists, however, do not elect to apply for board certification (see page 104 for more on this).

- An oncologist specializes in cancer care. A *medical oncologist* provides chemotherapy, hormone therapy, and other nonsurgical, nonradiation treatments. Medical oncologists often serve as the primary or coordinating physician for people with cancer. A *radiation oncologist* specializes in using radiation to treat cancer, and a *surgical oncologist* performs operations to diagnose and remove cancer. As their titles indicate, *gynecologic oncologists* and *pediatric oncologists* subspecialize in treating women's and children's cancers, respectively. Many of an oncologist's functions are also provided by specialists in other areas.

Other Physician Specialists

Virtually any type of medical or surgical specialist may be involved directly with cancer care or indirectly if you have additional health problems. Some of these specialists include the following:

- *Radiologists* specialize in the use of x-rays, ultrasound, computed tomography (CT scans), magnetic resonance imaging (MRI), and other medical imaging techniques.

- *Hematologists* specialize in blood disorders and are consulted in cases of cancer of the blood, bone marrow, and lymph system.

- *Neurologists* specialize in disorders of the brain and central nervous system.

- *Pathologists* study tissue samples to determine the type and extent of disease.

- *Gastroenterologists* specialize in disorders of the digestive system.

- *Endocrinologists* specialize in disorders of the glands (thyroid, adrenal, and so on) of the endocrine system.

- *Dermatologists* specialize in diseases of the skin.

- *Nephrologists* specialize in kidney disorders.

- *Anesthesiologists* specialize in administering anesthesia during surgical procedures; they may also be consulted for pain relief.

- *Physiatrists* specialize in physical medicine or rehabilitation medicine, which in cancer care generally means the diagnosis and treatment of a physical disability.

- *Psychiatrists* specialize in mental health and mental disorders; in cancer care, psychiatrists are consulted in regard to symptoms—including depression, anxiety, confusion, and dementia—that frequently occur in people with cancer, sometimes as a direct physical result of the disease.

- *Urologists* specialize in disorders of the urinary system and the male genitourinary system.

- *Obstetricians/gynecologists* specialize in diseases of the female reproductive system. Obstetricians deliver babies.

About Surgeons and Their Specialties

Surgeons are doctors who receive additional training in operating on the body for diagnostic and treatment purposes.

- *General surgeons* or *surgical oncologists* perform surgical diagnostic procedures to determine the location and extent of disease. They also remove tumors and, if necessary, the surrounding tissue. Some of the specialists listed earlier, such as obstetricians/gynecologists, also are trained in surgical techniques.

- Some other surgical specialties encountered in cancer care are *thoracic surgery* (chest); *reconstructive/plastic surgery* (reconstruction of removed or injured body parts and correction of appearance); *neurosurgery* (brain and nervous system); *orthopedic surgery* (bone and connective tissue).

About Nurses

Nurses are vital members of the cancer team and are crucial to the planning and delivery of daily care. They educate patients about their illness, administer medications, monitor responses, manage side effects, sometimes run support groups, and generally administer the treatment plan. Often the most accessible caregivers on the team, nurses are the people to whom the patient frequently turns first to identify problems and find solutions to a range of medical, emotional, and social problems.

Nurses are found in all cancer care settings. Ambulatory care nurses, who work in outpatient clinics or offices, often prepare and administer chemotherapy. In the hospital, nurses tend to your immediate needs in addition to administering many treatments. Nurses also care for patients in their homes or in hospices.

Nurses have different degrees of training and experience:

- *Registered nurses* (*RNs*) have earned an associate degree (two years) or a bachelor's degree (four years) in nursing from a school accredited by the National League for Nursing and have passed a state licensing exam. They monitor patients' conditions, provide treatment, and help those with cancer and families adjust physically and emotionally to illness.

- *Nurse practitioners* have additional training in primary care and share many tasks with physicians, such as taking patients' histories, conducting physical exams, and administering (and, in some states, prescribing) medications.

- *Clinical nurse specialists* have a master's or other advanced degree and specialize in the direct care of patients in specific areas, such as cancer care, heart surgery, or problems associated with aging. They usually work in institutions such as hospitals or long-term care facilities.

- *Oncology-certified nurses* are clinical specialists in cancer care. They have passed certification and licensing exams qualifying them to administer chemotherapy, manage side effects, administer pain-control medications, handle emergencies, and provide long-term care and support. In large facilities, some oncology-certified nurses, like some physicians, subspecialize in such areas as breast cancer or radiation oncology.

- *Nurse anesthetists* pass a national certification test and a state licensing test and are qualified to administer anesthesia to patients undergoing surgery and to monitor vital signs during and after the operation.

Assisting nurses in their duties are *licensed practical nurses (LPNs)*, who have had one year of nursing education and who provide limited routine care under the supervision of physicians or registered nurses; and *nurses' aides,* who train for a few months to meet patients' needs such as changing linen and giving baths.

Other Members of the Cancer Care Team

In addition to doctors and nurses, numerous other health care professionals provide help during illness and recovery.

The Medical Support Team

All the following people must be specially trained and often licensed, depending on the state's requirements. Anyone with doubts about a provider's qualifications should ask for proof.

- *Radiation technologists* assist radiologists in diagnostic and therapeutic services.

- *Dietitians/nutritionists* design optimal meal plans to improve recovery. Because cancer can affect appetite and treatment can trigger nausea and vomiting, nutritional counseling is often essential.

- *Physical therapists* (sometimes called *physiotherapists*) work with the body to restore strength, function, flexibility, and muscle tone.

- *Speech therapists* work with people who have lost the ability to speak or to speak clearly.

- *Occupational therapists* work with people who have become disabled, to help them relearn how to perform daily activities.

- *Respiratory therapists* provide inhalation treatments, deep suctioning, oxygen, and other techniques to aid or strengthen breathing.

- *Enterostomal therapists* teach people how to care for ostomies.

The Psychosocial Support Team

Although they are not licensed to prescribe medication, the following professionals may offer counseling services:

- *Psychologists,* who hold a Ph.D. or Ed.D. degree (those with a master's degree also may provide some services), address personality issues, relationship problems, emotional issues, and other psychological concerns. They often suggest behavioral or cognitive approaches to dealing with pain and the side effects of cancer treatment.

- *Social workers* have a degree in social work (B.S.W., M.S.W, or D.S.W.) and in most cases must be licensed or certified by the state in which they work. They are trained to help people with cancer and their families deal with a range of emotional and practical problems related to the illness and its treatment, such as child care, finances, emotional issues, family concerns and relationships, transportation, and problems with the health care system.

  Some social workers (*oncology social workers*) specialize in cancer-related problems. They counsel people concerning fears, answer questions about diagnosis and treatment, locate care facilities and community service programs, lead support groups, and help people and families overcome communication problems and other relationship issues. Social workers may be involved in care during the hospital stay, but they also may seek clients on an outpatient basis in hospitals and clinics, through social service agencies, and in private practice settings.

Choosing and Evaluating Care Providers

Informed consent is critical to today's health care system. The term usually refers to the permission you give to a doctor or hospital to administer medications or to carry out procedures after you receive information about their risks and benefits. Informed consent also relates to your selection of the caregivers themselves. You and your family have the right to know about the training, expertise, and philosophy of treatment of those responsible for delivering care. If you do not feel comfortable with the answers, you have the right to look elsewhere.

Often, however, people are intimidated by the health care system, regarding doctors as all-knowing, all-powerful beings whose word is law. You may hesitate to ask "dumb" questions for fear of taking up the doctor's valuable time. Furthermore, if the physician has an unpleasant manner or prescribes a course of treatment you find objectionable, you may feel you have no right to protest or to request another approach.

To get the best out of the health care system, you often need to act like a consumer, asking questions, exploring alternatives, and demanding quality.

Finding a Doctor

Many people already have a relationship with at least one primary care physician, often the doctor who first discovers evidence of cancer. To find a specialist in cancer diagnosis and treatment, that doctor will supply the names of colleagues in the area. Members of HMOs or similar health plans may be assigned to a primary care physician or may be asked to select one from a list.

Usually, the members of these plans need written referrals from their primary caregiver before they can see a specialist.

To conduct your own search, two important resources are the toll-free telephone information number of the American Cancer Society (800-ACS-2345) and the National Cancer Institute (NCI) Cancer Information Service (800-4-CANCER). The NCI is the federal government's principal agency for research on cancer prevention, diagnosis, treatment, and rehabilitation and for dissemination of cancer information. A call to your local American Cancer Society chapter will yield helpful information as well (see Appendix I, "Resources"). Some hospitals advertise numbers to call for referrals, although such services include only those physicians who have admitting privileges at that facility.

Many libraries carry the *Directory of Medical Specialists,* which lists those physicians who have had additional training and who have passed special qualifying tests. Anyone who has the time or expertise to research specialized on-line consumer databases such as Medline (available through some computer networks and at larger libraries) might look for those doctors who have published journal articles on specific types of cancer or whose work is most often cited. To simplify this process, a trip to a medical library can be helpful. The NCI also maintains an on-line computer database called PDQ, or Physician Data Query, and can provide information from it for callers to the Cancer Information Service toll-free line (see Appendix II, "Cancer Information On Line" for more specific information). Among other things, the database contains a directory of 10,000 physicians whose practices center on cancer treatment.

State, county, and local health departments or medical societies maintain lists of doctors. A call to the department of oncology or internal medicine at a major medical school or teaching hospital in your area is another option.

Asking friends or family members who have had experience with cancer for names of doctors who have been helpful to them is yet another approach.

Assessing Your Doctor's Qualifications

You should never commit yourself to a doctor's care before determining that he or she is qualified and able to deliver the type of care you require. A simple but effective strategy is just to ask your doctors about their qualifications; for a list of questions, see page 105.

- Board certification indicates that a doctor has been trained in a certain specialty and has chosen to take certification exams given by peers. To maintain their certification, physicians must undergo continuing education after passing the exam. Specialists who have reached a higher plateau of achievement are rewarded with the title of Fellow.

  Doctors need not be board certified to become specialists and to achieve a high level of accomplishment in their careers. Increasingly, however, they do seek these additional qualifications. To find out whether a physician is board certified, call the American Board of Medical Specialties, at 800-776-CERT.

Qualifying Questions

- Are you board certified?
- What is your specialty? Do you have a subspecialty?
- What training have you had in treating my type of cancer?
- How long have you been in practice?
- How many patients with my illness have you treated in the past year?
- Are you or others in your practice involved in clinical trials of new treatments?
- What are your office hours?
- How can you be contacted outside those hours?
- Who supervises your patients when you are on vacation?
- What hospitals are you affiliated with?
- Which hospital do you prefer to admit your cancer patients to? Why?
- May I tape-record our conversations so that I can review the details later? May I bring someone with me to appointments?
- Who besides you will be on my care team?

- Experience is an essential clue. Years in practice are one measure, but the number of procedures performed or people treated for cancer also is significant. You should ask about the doctor's patient load, percentage of cancer patients, and the types of cancer he or she is experienced in treating. Because physicians doing research usually have published their findings in medical journals, you might ask for copies of articles in order to learn about their philosophy and approach.

- Consider the nature of the doctor's practice. A solo practice means that patients see the same physician on each visit, which provides continuity. A group practice, on the other hand, may offer more resources, expertise, and availability of care. A multispecialty group includes doctors with different areas of knowledge, whereas a single-specialty group may have more experience in a particular field.

- Hospital affiliations are important. Because doctors can send patients only to those facilities where they have admitting privileges, people seeking treatment should know where they will go for surgery or other care.

- A teaching affiliation, especially with a prestigious medical school, may indicate that the physician is a respected leader in the field. Academic physicians who maintain practices often are in close touch with experts around the country and may be well versed in the latest therapies.

- A physician's reputation is less easily evaluated. Sometimes asking others in the community can reveal a doctor's standing.

Evaluating Practice Style

- Are appointments easy to make? Is your physician readily available if he or she is needed before the next appointment?

- Is the office environment clean and comfortable, conveying a sense of both efficiency and concern?

- Does the doctor's staff treat you courteously and respectfully?

- Is the doctor reasonably punctual? Does he or she apologize for any long waits?

- Do examinations and conversations take place in private? Do they seem rushed?

- Does your doctor appear open to the contributions of other health professionals, such as social workers, nurses, home care providers, or physical therapists? Will he or she make referrals?

- Do nurses and other assistants seem well trained? Are they willing to take time to answer your questions and to provide instruction and education as needed?

- Does the office staff help with insurance documents? Are they willing to negotiate terms of payment?

- Are phone calls returned quickly?

- Are the results of lab tests reported promptly?

Other Factors Related to Choosing a Physician

Assuming that your physician's qualifications are adequate, you now will want to consider other factors in your choice of caregiver.

- Location is important, especially when dealing with a long-term illness like cancer. Doctors whose offices are hard to get to, or hospitals that are inconvenient, may add an unnecessary complication.

- Length of time in practice can be relevant. Newly trained physicians may have little hands-on experience treating a particular type of cancer, although they may be more aware of modern techniques of cancer diagnosis and treatment than are some doctors who trained years ago. On the other hand, since medical oncology has been a recognized specialty only since 1973, many doctors who do not identify themselves as oncologists per se have nevertheless had decades of experience treating people with the disease.

- Style of practice can be difficult to assess unless you already have been under that doctor's care. Nonetheless, certain elements quickly convey a sense of the physician's style, as noted in the box at the top of this page.

- A doctor's personal manner is perhaps harder to quantify than his or her practice style, although it may be even more relevant—especially if the doctor is serving as your care coordinator. A good communication style is critical. Empathy may not always be obvious, but concern, understanding, and support should be readily evident. For the doctor-patient relationship to succeed, most people need a doctor who will take time to answer questions and to recognize that for anyone with cancer, learning about the disease is an essential part of making informed treatment decisions.

How you weigh each of these various factors is an individual matter, but remember that doctors are human and that few can live up to the ideal image some people have of them.

Do You Have to Like Your Doctor?

TIPS & ADVICE

It helps, but it's *trust* that is essential. A lovable person can be a poor caregiver, and a seemingly uninterested doctor can be quite able. Your focus needs to be on getting well, and so if you believe that your physician's skills will serve that purpose, that's good. If you also like the doctor, that's a bonus.

An exception, perhaps, is the physician who serves as your care coordinator. A strong bond between you and the person guiding your recovery can be potent medicine. Empathy can also be transformed into advocacy. The physician who cares about you as a person will make sure that everything possible is being done on your behalf.

Because several doctors may be involved at various stages of your illness, the odds are slim that all of them will meet all of your needs. When dealing with physicians on the team other than the physician adviser, confidence in their ability is probably more important than rapport. Evaluating physicians ahead of time to the extent possible should help weed out those you simply cannot work with.

If you find that an uncomfortable relationship with a certain provider is interfering with your care, speak up. Talk to the physician, head nurse, social worker, or other team member you trust and express your concern. Sometimes the problem is merely one of communication.

Sometimes the difficulty results from expecting too much from one person. It is not uncommon to pin all hopes for cure, information, professional support, and 24-hour-a-day concern on the doctor and then to feel disappointed when he or she does not come through in some way. When evaluating a problem with any doctor, always consider whether there is someone else on your care team, or in your doctor's office, who can come through for you in ways that your doctor necessarily cannot.

If the issues between you and your doctor run deeper, however, switching caregivers, though sometimes difficult, is always an option.

In sum, you don't have to like all your doctors, but you do have to trust their strategy for your recovery.

Care Settings

Depending on the specifics of the case, cancer diagnosis and treatment take place in a variety of settings and facilities. Threading your way through this maze can sometimes be bewildering and discouraging. Knowing what to expect—and where to expect it—can help reduce your anxiety and enable you to take full advantage of the services offered.

During the diagnostic phase, the process usually begins in a primary care physician's office. Pap smears, biopsies, and certain other procedures and lab tests may be done here. If other or more tests are needed, you may be referred to a specialist's office, a diagnostic facility (such as a radiology office), or, in some cases, a hospital.

Once the diagnosis is confirmed, the care team or the physician in charge develops the treatment plan, which may begin with a stay in the hospital. Fortunately today, many people with cancer spend comparatively little time there. Advances in medicine and technology mean that more types of surgery and other procedures can be delivered on an outpatient basis. For example, many chemotherapy regimens are now administered and monitored in doctors' offices or clinics. Also, the advent of managed care has meant tighter controls on hospital admissions and lengths of stay.

Which facility is used depends on a number of factors. As mentioned, the physician must have admitting privileges at a hospital before he or she can send patients there. Also, people who subscribe to certain HMO plans may use only those hospitals authorized by the insurer.

Types of Hospitals

A National Cancer Institute (NCI)–designated *comprehensive cancer center* is a hospital (or a unit within a community or teaching hospital) dedicated to research on and treatment of this disease only. These centers offer high-quality, up-to-date care, provide a range of support services, and are involved in basic and clinical research and training. They also participate in the NCI's high-priority clinical trials. The NCI has granted comprehensive status to 27 facilities around the country (see Appendix I, "Resources"). Generally, these comprehensive cancer centers are especially appropriate for second opinions, consultations in complicated cases, or for new, often experimental treatments not available elsewhere. Most people with cancer, however, begin their diagnostic and treatment journey elsewhere, especially if they live far from any of the comprehensive cancer centers.

Some hospitals call themselves comprehensive but are not in fact NCI-designated facilities. All hospitals that have been named by the NCI are nonprofit institutions.

The National Cancer Institute–designated *clinical cancer centers* are similar to comprehensive centers but offer somewhat fewer services. Instead, they mainly investigate new forms of treatment and engage in clinical trials. Currently, 17 institutions have achieved this designation (listed in Appendix I, "Resources"). Like the comprehensive cancer centers, clinical cancer centers are nonprofit.

Again, note that not all facilities that call themselves cancer centers or clinical cancer centers have necessarily been approved by the NCI. Lacking this designation does not mean that they provide inadequate care; it does mean that such a hospital or cancer center (which may advertise itself in the popular media) should be evaluated on its own merits.

Community hospitals with a clinical oncology program or cancer unit often provide highly competent care, although they may not offer treatment involving high-tech devices or high-risk procedures. But in recent years, community hospitals have become increasingly important care sites, owing to the rising numbers of cancer specialists, easier access to up-to-the-minute cancer research databases, and other developments.

Teaching hospitals have residency and fellowship programs for training new physicians. The best are teaching hospitals directly attached to medical schools. Others may be affiliated with (but not controlled by) medical schools and may have less extensive facilities. Still others have residency programs but no connection with a medical school.

As a rule, teaching hospitals provide a wide range of quality care, in part owing to the leading clinicians, researchers, and educators on their staffs. Because of the hospitals' teaching role, patients are seen by many physicians; they get a lot of attention but also must endure a good deal of extra poking, prodding, and interviewing.

Government-supported (public) hospitals, such as Veterans' Administration (VA), city, county, or state hospitals, chronically suffer from low funding. Some may not offer state-of-the-art cancer treatment, whereas others may have excellent cancer programs. These hospitals and programs must be evaluated individually.

Proprietary (for-profit) hospitals, sometimes owned by the physicians who work there, vary widely in their services. Some prefer to treat patients with less serious, shorter-term, more profitable conditions. Others have excellent cancer programs. Each hospital and program must be evaluated individually.

Nonhospital Treatment Settings

In many areas, diagnostic and treatment services are offered in so-called free-standing outpatient centers, meaning that they are not housed in hospitals. These may be privately run, for-profit centers or affiliated with nonprofit institutions. The facilities and care vary, so each must be evaluated on its own merits.

Home Care. Following discharge from a hospital or conclusion of treatment in a freestanding center, some types of care, such as intravenous infusions or feeding via a tube, may be administered by nurses or therapists who come to your home. Home care is becoming a more popular alternative, since it allows people with cancer to be treated in comfortable, convenient, and familiar surroundings. Furthermore, in many cases, home care costs far less than treatment delivered elsewhere. (See also Chapter 34, "Supportive Care.")

Hospice Care. Sometimes the disease has advanced to such an extent that treatment is concentrated primarily on maintaining comfort. In such cases, the hospice may become the care setting, or more likely, hospice care may be

How Can You Determine the Quality of Cancer Care at a Treatment Setting?

QUESTIONS

TO ASK

Ask whether the cancer diagnosis and treatment program offered there has been approved by the *Commission on Cancer* of the *American College of Surgeons.* If it is, you'll know that it meets stringent standards and offers total cancer care, including lifetime follow-up. You also will know that no matter whether you receive your treatment in a large internationally known or a small local setting, its ability to deliver quality cancer care is constantly under scrutiny.

Not limited to surgeons, the commission includes members from about 30 professional organizations who set guidelines for cancer diagnosis and care. At this writing, more than 1,300 large and small hospitals and treatment facilities nationwide, from NCI-designated facilities to community hospitals to freestanding diagnostic and treatment centers, have applied for and received the commission's stamp of approval. Although they represent only about 20 percent of the general hospitals in the United States, they in fact currently are treating about 70 percent of those newly diagnosed with cancer. A similar number of hospitals also are attempting to meet the approval standards for their cancer programs.

An approved cancer program must provide specific state-of-the-art diagnostic and treatment services in all medical disciplines that a person with cancer may require. Each facility must also try to follow up every patient treated there, to ensure that each receives continuing care and, of course, to detect recurrences or new cancers as early as possible. In addition, rehabilitation services and patient and family education are available through all these cancer programs.

The program's leadership consists of representatives from all health care disciplines involved directly or indirectly with cancer patients at that location. Among their responsibilities are monitoring and evaluating patient care, which includes maintaining a database on care and outcomes. Many of the programs share these data with the National Cancer Data Base, which monitors treatment and outcome patterns regionally and nationally for some 40 types of cancer. (The American Cancer Society can give you a copy of the *National Cancer Data Base Annual Review of Patient Care,* which reports on varying types of cancer each year: telephone 800-ACS-2345.)

In each facility, a tumor board, also consisting of representatives from a range of cancer care disciplines, meets weekly to confer on individual cases and, if possible, improve care. There is never a charge to patients for this multidisciplinary consultation process (see Chapter 12—"How Many Opinions Do You Need?"—for more on tumor boards).

These are only the minimum requirements. The commission also encourages approved programs—which it regularly reviews and recertifies—to offer prevention, screening, nutritional counseling, community outreach, and support services.

For a list of all Commission on Cancer–approved programs, write the American College of Surgeons at 55 East Erie Street, Chicago, IL 60611-2797.

provided at home. This type of care is designed to help people with cancer, as well as their families, during the final stages of the illness (see Chapter 34, "Supportive Care"). The few freestanding hospice facilities are usually connected to a hospital.

Evaluating Hospitals

The easiest way to assess a quality hospital informally is by determining which well-respected doctors work there. Good physicians are seldom affiliated with substandard hospitals. After you have selected skilled doctors whom you trust and respect, the choice of a hospital usually follows automatically. Probably the simplest way to evaluate a hospital is to ask physicians in the community what they think of it.

At the very least, a quality hospital is accredited by the Joint Commission on Accreditation of Healthcare Organizations (JCAHO; 708-691-5632). Accredited hospitals are listed in the *American Hospital Association Guide to the Health Care Field,* found in many public libraries. Surprisingly, about one hospital in four fails to earn accreditation. Although accreditation does not necessarily indicate expertise in cancer care, approval by the American College of Surgeons Commission on Cancer does (see box page 110).

Services and Facilities. The extent and variety of services available in a facility is a key criterion. The best hospitals offer

- A postoperative recovery room;
- An intensive care unit;
- Anesthesiologists;
- A pathology lab, diagnostic lab, and blood bank;
- Round-the-clock physician staffing;
- A tumor board;
- Social work services;
- Respiratory therapists, physical therapists, and the like;
- Advanced diagnostic and therapeutic equipment (CT scans, radiation therapy, etc.).

Other Factors. As mentioned, the choice of a hospital depends in large part on the physician you select and where he or she has admitting privileges. When you are offered a choice of hospitals at which your doctor treats patients or when you are deciding among physicians, you should consider other factors. For example, hospitals with more than 500 beds tend to be somewhat bureaucratic, but they often provide more services and have more experience dealing with cancer of various types. As a rule, hospitals with fewer than 100 beds lack the facilities for complete and adequate cancer care.

Assuming they offer equivalent levels of care, a hospital close to home is usually preferable to one far away. Sometimes the best treatment strategy is to arrange a consultation at a distant comprehensive cancer center, followed by the delivery of care in a local facility.

You might want to choose a hospital because of a certain policy, such as whether or not children are allowed to visit. Such seemingly minor details can take on enormous importance to the person with the disease and the family.

TIPS & ADVICE

Overcoming Obstacles to Communication

There are many techniques for overcoming—or, better yet, preventing—barriers to communication. Rather than waiting for providers to sharpen their skills in this area, if you want the best care, consider how you can improve the lines of communication.

- Decide how much information you want to be told directly and at what level of detail. Let members of your care team know. If you don't tell them, they are apt to take their cue from how you seem to be communicating with them. For example, if you ask, "I don't have cancer, do I?" your doctor may conclude that you are not ready to hear the truth.

- Establish who else should be told what information about your illness and treatment and at what level of detail: a family member, friend, or whomever.

- Take notes, record conversations, bring another person along with you. Record conversations over the phone as well. Researchers have found that tape-recording medical conversations can improve a person's ability to understand treatment, especially concerning tests and their results. Inform all parties that you will be recording the conversation.

- Don't withhold information from your caregivers.

- If you don't understand something, ask that it be repeated, rephrased, or explained. You might say, "I'm having trouble grasping what you said—would you mind telling me again, and could you put it another way?" Another tactic is to repeat what was said and ask for confirmation: "Let me see if I have it right. You're saying that…"

- Ask questions—lots of them.

- Prepare questions ahead of time, asking the most important ones first.

- Arrange for office visits or phone calls that allow adequate time for discussions. Tell your doctor at the beginning of the visit that you have questions. If you still have questions at the end of the visit, say so and schedule another appointment or phone call to address them.

- Assess your attitudes to see whether they are interfering with your treatment: Are you angry, hostile, afraid? If so, express your emotions directly: "I'm afraid of what might happen." "I'm angry at being kept waiting so long." Doing so will help clear the air and keep your treatment from getting sidetracked.

- Be aware that your doctor isn't the only source of information. Ask questions of office staff, nurses, or other specialists caring for you. Emotional and practical issues may be best addressed by social workers or psychologists. Identifying which members of the team can answer which questions, and how they can be reached, is a vital part of the treatment plan.

Communicating with Caregivers

Good communication is crucial to good care. People with cancer need to feel they can speak openly and honestly with their doctors and other providers. Caregivers too must be able to talk to patients clearly and directly.

Talking, though, is only one part of effective communication. The other part is listening. The best doctors are those who give their full attention to what's being said: They ask questions to fill in blanks; they don't interrupt; and they resist making judgments before the whole story has been told. By the same token, people undergoing care need to listen carefully so they can understand the nature of their disease and treatment and make informed decisions each step of the way.

Obstacles to Communication

Even in ideal circumstances, good communication can be hard to achieve, and in a medical crisis, the obstacles to communication multiply:

- Fear—of disease, of treatment, of outcome—can interfere with your ability to think clearly or hear what is being said. Fear of what the answer might be can also prevent you from asking or even remembering important questions.

- The amount of detailed medical information can be too much to absorb and remember.

- Many people stand in awe of their doctors, resisting the urge to question what they're told.

- Some people remain silent because they lack self-confidence, believing that their questions are stupid or that they will be unable to understand the answers.

- Many doctors contribute to the problem by using technical terms.

- The need for many players on the health care team, located at different sites and possessing varying levels of expertise, increases the risk of miscommunication.

How Many Opinions Do You Need?

It is far simpler to take the advice of your primary care physician and get going with the recommended treatment than to seek a second opinion. You'll have to find a consulting physician—maybe more than one—and get an appointment. You'll need to obtain copies of laboratory tests and pathology and radiology reports and sometimes actual slides and x-rays. You may have to travel long distances, and then, of course, there's the matter of cost. But second opinions are common, for many reasons.

It is a good idea to get more opinions whenever you feel uncertain of the advice you have been given or you do not yet feel equipped to make a decision. But there are other medical and psychological reasons for seeking consultations before, during, or even after treatment. Here we review these reasons and discuss the issues involved in the process.

When and Why to Get a Second Opinion

For some cancers, doctors agree on well-established and proven treatments, but for others, expert opinions about the treatment of choice differ. And even when everyone acknowledges that a particular approach is likely to arrest the cancer, questions may arise about your ability to tolerate the treatment's immediate and long-term side effects or how it will affect your quality of life in the long run. For these reasons cancer specialists suggest second opinions, and reassurance that the treatment option selected is the right one may mean three or four consultations.

Is the Diagnosis Correct?

Confirmation of a diagnosis itself occasionally requires a second opinion. This may mean having a second pathologist review slides or another radiologist look at x-rays or other images to be certain the diagnosis is accurate.

Risks Versus Benefits

Many people seek another opinion to help them choose among their physician's suggested options or to learn about other possibilities. Because therapies that are successful in eradicating cancer can have long-lasting consequences such as infertility, changes in appearance, or the need to wear an ostomy bag, the benefits of a particular treatment always must be balanced against its drawbacks. Different therapies present various advantages and disadvantages, which you must weigh against your life stage, career needs, family demands, hopes, and dreams. Therefore, even though two therapies may present equal opportunities for eradicating the cancer, they may have far different effects on your life. Consequently, you need to gather as much information as possible before you make any decisions.

Second Opinions During Treatment

Seeking additional opinions is not always a decision to be made before treatment. You may wish another opinion in the midst of treatment if the tumor is not responding as expected. Or you may want a consultation at the end of a particular course of treatment to assess the need for further therapy.

Taking a Riskier Route

Diagnosed with rectal cancer in 1979, Irene, then 55, was adamant that she did not want a colostomy (removal of a portion of her colon; waste leaves the body through an opening in the abdomen and is collected in an attached bag), even though this surgery presented the least risk. After two physicians in her rural Kentucky town recommended colon resection and colostomy, she widened her search to metropolitan areas. She called major cancer centers to find out about alternative recommendations and finally found a surgeon in Minneapolis who would do conservative laser surgery, leaving her bowel functions intact. The doctor, however, made Irene accept one condition before he would treat her: She had to promise to return for yearly follow-up visits to ensure that the cancer had not spread. She agreed and in subsequent years underwent two additional laser surgeries, which would not have been necessary had her colon been removed. "Even though I didn't enjoy going back for surgery," Irene recalls, "I got what I wanted: freedom from a colostomy bag, and, lucky for me, disease-free survival for nearly two decades now!"

Lucky for her is right. This choice may not have been appropriate for a person who wanted the greatest chance for complete recovery. Although Irene's original surgeons tried hard to convince her that people can and do lead good lives with a colostomy bag, Irene was determined.

CASE HISTORIES

TRUE STORIES

Second Opinion Checklist

A second opinion is a good idea if

- you want to confirm your primary cancer physician's recommendation;
- your physician is not an oncologist;
- your physician is not experienced in treating your type of cancer;
- you want reassurance that you are getting the most current treatment;
- you are concerned about the side effects and/or long-term effects of the recommended treatment;
- you are interested in experimental therapies;
- you have trouble communicating with your physician;
- you have read about treatments with which your physician is not familiar;
- your physician has not asked about your lifestyle, family demands, and/or professional commitments and desires;
- the recommended treatment interferes with the way you lead your life and you want to know if there are other options;
- you are not confident of your physician's knowledge, experience, or judgment;
- you feel uncomfortable with your physician's recommendation.

Is There Time?

Arranging appointments, consulting with other physicians, and perhaps having additional tests takes time. Yet some people fear that if they delay, their condition may get worse. In the past, many physicians and patients believed that time was of the essence, but as more has been learned about how cancer develops, most experts agree that in most cases, getting more opinions does not create dangerous delays.

As one oncology nurse puts it, "The first thing I tell a patient is to do nothing." What she means is that people need time to adjust to the shock of being told that they have cancer. Then, as soon as they can think clearly, they can take the necessary action. With an illness as serious as cancer, you and your family need to feel confident that you have made the right decision.

...Or Are You Wasting Time?

Seeking endless consultations, postponing treatment indefinitely, or refusing to make any decisions at all does waste time, however. Indeed, seeking more and more opinions may mask an underlying fear of making the wrong choice and avoids getting down to the business of being treated. Continuing to seek opinions can also be a way of "wishing" that you will find a doctor who will say only what you want to hear.

Setting a date to talk over your options with your primary care physician or a coordinating physician is one way to make sure that the opinion- and information-gathering process will be efficient and productive.

Cost

At one time, health insurance companies required second opinions in an attempt to curtail costs, and they paid for the consultation. Unnecessary tests and surgery, the companies reasoned, would be avoided by having physicians serve as a check on one another. But second opinions did not lower costs, so many insurers stopped requiring them. Consequently, most consultations today are at the request of patients and/or on the advice of physicians and often must be paid for by the individual. Even for members of health maintenance organizations, seeking second opinions can be expensive, as members who consult physicians that do not belong to the HMO must pay for these visits themselves.

Some physicians, however, do not charge as much for a consultation as for a first visit, since much of the initial work-up, including laboratory and imaging tests, has been done. In any case, the fee for the consultation should be discussed when the appointment is made so that there will be no surprises.

Finding the Right Consultant

Your primary physician or oncologist is the best place to begin a list of other specialists in your community. Most doctors are accustomed to furnishing names of potential consultants and are not defensive or insulted when asked for recommendations. An independent search is another option. For information on how to do this, see Chapter 11, "Getting Help for Cancer: Who, What, Where, and How."

Although some physicians will provide a second opinion only if you have been referred by another doctor, most will.

How Far to Go?

Conflicting and highly technical data about cancer and your particular diagnosis can be overwhelming. In the first few weeks after his diagnosis, Isaac, then 38, who had a rare form of leukemia, was eager to learn everything he could about his illness. On the recommendation of his primary care physician, he consulted two major research centers about bone marrow transplantation. After he had found a marrow donor and chosen a center for the transplant, however, he found that all the statistics relating to his prognosis and chances for long-term survival only made him more anxious. Since transplant was his best chance for cure, once the treatment began, Isaac chose not to investigate every conceivable side effect or long-term consequence. He had learned enough to give his informed consent for the procedure; he felt confident that he had made the right decision and asked that his family not continue to explore every possible scenario or complication.

CASE HISTORIES

TRUE STORIES

In the Hospital

Getting other opinions while in the hospital is a bit more difficult, because you are physically confined and may be limited to consulting with a physician associated with that hospital. Also, the admitting physician usually must order a consultation if it is to be done in the hospital.

However, most hospitals—even smaller community hospitals with an organized cancer program—have a *tumor board,* a team of experts representing several medical disciplines. The primary physician presents the patient's case to this group of specialists and uses their collective expertise in designing a treatment plan.

For example, a radiologist on the tumor board may review a patient's x-rays and scans. A pathologist may review the pathology slides and use a projection microscope to discuss his or her findings with the other physicians. A surgeon, an oncologist, and other specialists also participate in the discussion. And, depending on the hospital, a psychologist or social worker may be part of the group. In large teaching hospitals, medical students and junior staff members attend as well, since the tumor board meetings serve an educational purpose.

In nonacademic settings, such as a small community hospital, the physician presenting a case—particularly if he or she is a general practitioner or family practitioner—usually delegates the management of the cancer patient's care to the appropriate specialist. Occasionally, the primary care physician oversees the treatment prescribed by an oncologist.

According to the American College of Surgeons, tumor board conferences "should focus on problem cases as well as on pretreatment evaluation, staging, treatment strategy, and rehabilitation." Although the conference is usually confidential, the physician presenting a case may be willing to share with you the salient points of the discussion and the rationale for the treatment recommendations.

The Logistics of Consultations

The more you know about your cancer and the issues that are important to you and your family, the more you will learn from the consultation. Being prepared also enables you to use efficiently the limited amount of time you have with the consulting doctor and ensures that you ask the necessary questions. Therefore,

QUESTIONS TO ASK

Who Knows Best?

The most important question to ask when making an appointment with a consulting physician is, "Do you have experience treating my type of cancer?"

Keep in mind that oncologists can have *subspecialties*—that is, they may also be, for example, surgeons, gynecologists, urologists, or radiologists. Even if you don't choose to be treated by a subspecialist, it's wise to consult one for a second opinion. This subspecialist may work with the primary cancer physician to design a treatment plan.

When Opinions Conflict

One physician may advocate treating your cancer with a combination of radical surgery or radiation and/or aggressive chemotherapy. Another may prefer a more conservative approach, such as limited surgery with or without radiation afterward. Based on current studies and their own experience, both specialists' opinions may be equally valid, but their disagreement puts you in a quandary. How can you decide which is best?

At this point, an oncologist should be able to explain to you the pros and cons of each approach. Your primary care physician can help you weigh the advantages and disadvantages of the conflicting recommendations. But you should not feel forced to make a decision until you have adequate information.

TIPS & ADVICE

when seeking a second opinion, prepare for the visit by completing and reviewing your research. You could ask a friend or family member to do the background research if you are unable to do it.

Along with gathering brochures, books, and other printed material, talking with other health care professionals—nurses and social workers, for instance—is helpful. Some people also seek out others with cancer to talk about their experience with a specific treatment.

If all the pertinent records are in your primary care physician's office, copies can be sent to the consulting physician. It may also be helpful, as some cancer advocacy groups recommend, to obtain your own copies of all medical records. Copies of x-rays and laboratory results may be expensive, but complete, up-to-date reports facilitate the consultation process.

During the visit, the consulting physician reviews your history, laboratory tests, and imaging examinations. Additional tests may be ordered if needed. Finally, the physician will offer his or her recommendations. The same advice given when discussing the diagnosis with the original doctor applies here: Take notes or use a tape recorder and bring a friend or family member (see Chapter 11, "Getting Help for Cancer: Who, What, Where, and How").

The consulting physician sends a written report to the referring physician and/or directly to you.

Comfort and Confidence

Trust is an intangible component of the relationship between you and your physician, and it must be factored into the final decision-making process. You must feel confident that your physician's advice is truly the best option.

People with cancer can expect to have a range of emotional responses to treatment recommendations, but whatever the end result, feeling reasonably comfortable with the treatment decision is essential. As Irene's story on page 115 indicates, some people feel more at ease with a treatment that has somewhat high risks but offers an opportunity to pursue life goals, such as having a family. Others prefer the choice that offers the best chance of survival, even though

Going with the First Opinion

Mike, 50, was diagnosed with Hodgkin's disease in the early 1990s. He did not seek a second opinion regarding treatment for his cancer because he said he felt "fairly comfortable" with the treatment recommended by his primary physician. "The cancer specialist came highly recommended," Mike recalls, "and I liked his whole demeanor and the way he explained things clearly to me. I more or less just put myself in his hands. He had given me the prognosis, which I was really pleased with, and I was ready to get involved in the treatment and get on with getting well."

Now, healthy and almost five years in remission, Mike is satisfied with the choice he made. "The doctor told me he had never given anyone such a large dose of chemotherapy, but I tolerated it well. My constitution was pretty strong. That and the fact that I got so much chemo make me pretty relaxed in terms of making it to the 60-month mark. I was lucky to have found the right professional, and I just went with that gut feeling."

the side effects could affect the quality of life more severely. Rarely are there "perfect" solutions, and the ultimate decision must always be a personal one.

By seeking second opinions, you and your family can ensure you've done all you could to participate in the information-gathering and decision-making process. On the other hand, if comfort means trusting the first opinion, even without consulting anyone else, then that is an option as well.

YOUR SUPPORT NETWORK

No one is born knowing how to deal with serious illness or how to solve the emotional and practical problems it creates. Nor are most people equipped to cope with these matters on their own. For these challenges, beginning at the time of diagnosis, the support of other people—family, friends, colleagues, religious groups, those who have or have had cancer, and/or helping professionals, and advocacy organizations—is paramount. Together, medical and social support systems address not just the disease but also the needs of the whole person.

Studies have long shown that men and women who have strong bonds with others endure crisis best. Because many people do not have family or community ties, fortunately a support network can be assembled to address the complex issues that arise. Such resources benefit everyone with cancer, regardless of the number of people in their lives.

Support takes many forms, depending on the people or group providing it. It can be as basic as someone offering a ride to the physician's office or help with the shopping. Or it may mean having someone with the same illness share information about treatment and recovery. Often support means participating in a group of people in similar circumstances among whom it's safe to vent your deepest feelings. It can mean a place to turn for advice and information. Whatever the purpose for which you seek support, it will fulfill the basic urge to remain connected to human society—a connection that, in itself, may actually promote healing (see "Does Social Support Affect the Course of Cancer?," page 124).

Those who benefit from others' assistance discover ways in which they can help others in turn; such reaching out restores a sense of self-worth and self-esteem. Cancer is a life crisis and one that nobody would willingly seek out; still, many people discover that the experience presents an opportunity to rediscover the importance of life and connections to other people and even to society as a whole.

This chapter describes the support network and ways of using it to achieve the highest quality of life during treatment and recovery. It also offers advice to those who want to help people with cancer. The "Resources" appendix at the end of this book provides more information about particular organizations and services and how to get in touch with them.

Why Is Social Support Important?

Dealing with cancer can produce enormous stress not only for those with the disease but for everyone who cares about them. Roles and relationships—indeed, your whole outlook on life—change suddenly and dramatically. You and your family must wrestle with social, physical, and financial upheaval and may experience fear, anger, guilt, and hopelessness, among other powerful feelings (see Chapters 31, "Coping Strategies," and 32, "Issues for Families and Friends").

When the diagnosis is first made, you and your loved ones may feel as if your lives are collapsing and you have lost all control over your future. During your treatment, you may continue to feel frightened and exhausted as you struggle to cope with the changes in your body, the side effects of the treatment, the complexities of the health care system, the financial impact of the disease, and the challenge of maintaining healthy relationships with your family and friends. After the treatment ends, even though you may still be grappling with the long-term consequences of a devastating disease, you will no longer have the daily hands-on care of physicians and nurses, and so you may feel as if you have been set adrift, even abandoned.

Taking an active step such as creating or tapping into a support network can provide a sense of empowerment that results when you recognize and resolve to conquer these and other challenges.

Making use of the people in your own life as well as the support and self-help groups, advocacy organizations, and helping professionals described in this chapter can lead to additional positive results:

- *Counteracting fear.* Being diagnosed with cancer and treated for it can be extremely frightening, and it may be difficult for you to share your feelings with family, friends, and even caregivers. Participating in a support group of people in similar circumstances, for example, can help you realize that your emotions are natural and that it's safe to express them. In turn, feeling normal reduces fear, which helps you cope more effectively with pain and other symptoms.

- *Reducing isolation.* Having a serious illness can be very lonely, even for those with many people in their lives. You may find that some people, out of fear or ignorance, may not know how to be helpful or may even withdraw from you. Or despite being surrounded by healthy family, friends, and colleagues, you may feel profoundly alone in your experience and reluctant to share what you're really going through. Helping professionals and/or a group of others who understand the experience can alleviate this sense of ostracism and isolation. Group experiences can also lead to new friendships built on mutual concern and caring.

- Outside support can also *counteract the isolation* that occurs even in well-meaning families, who may attempt to "protect" you by not talking about your illness. As Chapter 32 ("Issues for Families and Friends") explains, underlying such conspiracies of silence may be the desire of family members to insulate themselves from their own overwhelming feelings and reactions to having to deal with a crisis. Over time, family members may cease to communicate and may become cut off, just when they need one another most. A group support or counseling program may offer problem-solving strategies for such situations.

- *Helping keep your spirits up.* People in your extended support network can help you recognize the signs of declining mood and encourage you to stay connected to others and to get appropriate help. (For information on depression and cancer, see Chapter 25, "Coping with Stress, Fear, Anxiety, and Depression.")

- *Encouraging you to take good care of yourself.* Someone who feels that people understand and care is more likely to try to stay healthy by eating well, getting enough sleep, exercising, and so on. The influence of others also helps discourage destructive habits, such as smoking or drinking alcohol, that can damage the body and slow the recovery process.

- *Helping the whole family.* So much attention may be focused on the person with cancer that the well members of the family, especially children, may feel neglected. Recruiting extended family members or close friends to take over some responsibilities can provide great relief. In addition, support groups and counseling for families address their own special concerns, fears, worries, and practical problems.

- *Providing practical information.* Support and self-help groups are forums in which to share knowledge and strategies that can promote effective coping. This information can include advice on dealing with health care professionals and questions to ask; managing pain and side effects; even where to go to get hats, hairpieces, and prostheses at the best price.

- *Finding out about treatment sources and services and protecting your rights.* Helping organizations often can connect people to relevant clinical trials, sources of funding, and information about how to preserve insurance coverage, deal with managed care, and prevent illegal discrimination at work.

Making the Most of Your Own Informal Support Network

Informal support comes from family, friends, neighbors, social acquaintances, colleagues, and coworkers—the people you probably turn to first in times of trouble or in whose presence you ordinarily feel comfortable or safe. Given the immense disruptions that cancer can cause in your life, tapping into this network can help you maintain some normalcy in your life. For example, a

CANCER

BASICS

Does Social Support Affect the Course of Cancer?

In the mid-1970s a group of researchers at Stanford University, led by psychiatrist David Spiegel, organized support groups for women with metastatic breast cancer. After a year, they found that those who had participated in the group experienced less anxiety, depression, and pain compared with women who received the same medical care but who did not take part in a group.

More surprising results came a decade later, when the researchers followed up on these same women. They found that those in the support group lived an average of 18 months longer than the women who had not been in a group. Although this was a small study, the results suggest that although social support is by no means a cure for cancer, it may in fact affect the body's ability to fight the disease.

Scientists are a long way from proving conclusively that social support can change the course of illness and enhance longevity. Since Spiegel's work, several studies exploring this question have reported conflicting results. Nonetheless, some evidence suggests that participating in a support group, combined with good medical treatment, may contribute to recovery.

For example, a serious illness such as cancer causes the body to experience high levels of chronic stress. To mitigate the effects of stress, the body secretes certain hormones, but over time the constant production of stress hormones can lead to physical and mental complications, such as elevated heart rate, reduced immune function, and mood changes. Studies suggest that contact with other people reduces stress, thereby lowering the levels of stress hormones and reducing the risk of damage (see Chapter 25, "Coping with Stress, Fear, Anxiety, and Depression").

Psychiatrist Fawzy Fawzy and colleagues at the University of California at Los Angeles studied people with melanoma who underwent a six-week program of intensive education and emotional support. They found that the immune systems of these people—specifically the natural killer cells, thought to be involved in conferring resistance to cancer—functioned better compared with the immune systems of those who did not take part in a support group.

Much more research is needed to determine which forms of social support offer which benefits, to which people, and with which form of the disease. Even so, as David Spiegel notes in *Mind/Body Medicine*: "Evidence is mounting that social support in general and self-help groups in particular enhance our ability to cope better with physical illness" (see also Chapter 31, "Coping Strategies").

cancer survivor who belongs to a square dance club might get tremendous support simply from attending the club's weekly gatherings even if he or she can't participate fully in the activity.

Family and friends can help in any number of ways, depending on their abilities and interests. In practical terms, they can provide child care, act as a "call broker" to handle phone calls from concerned people, arrange transportation, or assist with the cooking, housecleaning, shopping, or other errands (see "Some Support Dos and Don'ts for Those Who Want to Help," page 131). You could ask them to look up books or articles in the library or to walk your dog. Ask for what you need. Many people are happy to find out there's something that you want that they can do for you.

Informal support has some limitations. Loved ones may become overwhelmed by the changes in family life and by their concerns about you. Also, if you typically conceal your needs because you don't want to be a "burden" to others, you may push away the support you really want.

Spouses or partners are usually the most important part of the informal support network, but research shows that one out of four people with cancer has serious communication problems with these significant others. The majority of those reporting such problems are women, who often state that they want to talk openly about their fears and anxieties but that their husbands tend to discount such feelings (see Chapter 32, "Issues for Families and Friends").

Another reason not to seek all your support from an informal network is that during a crisis not everyone can come through in ways that you would like. Although you might appreciate their efforts, members of the square dance club, for example, may not feel comfortable visiting a casual acquaintance in the hospital. Similarly, squeamish people may not be the ones to ask to do library research about your disease.

Getting the Formal Support You Need

Formal support, which is provided or overseen by people trained in the task, is not a replacement for informal support. Instead, it complements the informal network in a number of ways. Types of formal support include support and self-help groups, psychotherapy and counseling and other professional help, religious institutions, political and advocacy organizations, and coordinated volunteer efforts.

Formal support is often given in a group setting. Even the most thoughtful and loving friends or relatives cannot offer the same type of empathy and help as can people who, like you, are also walking the path of survivorship. For this reason, since the mid-1970s, participation in groups consisting of people with the same illness has been an increasingly recognized element of the recovery process.

Support and self-help groups enable the exchange of information, which increases the participants' knowledge, dispels myths, and helps people cope with the intricacies of the health care system. Some also serve as advocacy organizations for people with cancer: raising public awareness of the disease and the rights and needs of people who have it; campaigning for funding in support of research; and lobbying for changes in the health care system.

Perhaps most important on a personal level, groups offer an opportunity for their members to voice their concerns openly and honestly and, in doing so, to come to terms with their illness. People with cancer often dread a recurrence of the disease and must come to grips with their mortality. They fear the changes their bodies are undergoing, including disfiguring surgery or unseen internal damage. They worry that they will be abandoned by their caregivers, by society, and even by their loved ones. The stories of struggle and survival exchanged in a group help the participants recognize the reality—and the validity—of their own deepest feelings.

It must be stressed, however, that groups are not a substitute for medical treatment. Any group that contradicts or otherwise interferes in any way with ongoing treatment should be avoided.

Educational/Informational Workshops or Groups

Often sponsored by hospitals, educational groups inform their participants about various aspects of cancer. Typically they are led by a professional or a layperson or both and offer lectures or other types of presentations followed by a question-and-answer session. Their goal is to discuss the facts of the disease; they usually are not a forum for emotional sharing. As a rule, people with cancer are encouraged to attend along with concerned family members. Compared with the face-to-face encounters of support groups, educational workshops offer relative anonymity. Family members and others close to you can usually attend as well.

Research published in a cancer journal in the early 1990s underscores the importance of such mutual participation. People with cancer and their significant others were invited to watch an educational program together. The program conveyed the message that coping with chemotherapy can be difficult and emphasized that everyone with cancer needs support in finding ways to manage any side effects. The researchers found that watching the program together enhanced the ability of couples who participated in the study to talk about the disease and its treatment and that effective communication in turn raised the self-esteem of the person with cancer.

Support Groups

Support groups fall into two categories: those that are organized and run by one or more professional facilitators and those that are organized and run by the members themselves, usually referred to as self-help groups. In both cases, the focus is on the day-by-day adjustment to living with a serious illness.

Professionally Led Support Groups. Professionally led support groups serve people with certain types of cancer or with other specific needs. For example, there are groups for parents of children with cancer, for women with breast cancer, for people in advanced stages of the disease, or for bereaved family members. Other groups might be tailored to adolescent survivors, outpatient chemotherapy recipients, people undergoing long-term hospitalization, or at-risk populations (such as daughters of women with breast cancer).

Some groups are open only to people with the disease; others welcome family members and significant others. So much variety means that at least in large metropolitan areas, you can usually find a group whose participants' situation closely resembles your own. The leaders of such groups might be social workers, nurses, psychologists, physicians, or other health professionals.

Some groups charge fees to cover costs of the meeting room and to reimburse professional leaders, but many groups are subsidized by health care facilities or national organizations and so do not charge.

Self-Help Groups. Also referred to as peer-support networks, self-help groups differ from support groups principally in that they do not involve professional leaders and may concentrate more on practical, how-to issues. They also are operated (indeed are often founded) by the members themselves. Sometimes advisers such as oncology social workers are consulted on strategies for group leadership and development, but for the most part the agenda is set and carried out by the members.

Self-help groups may welcome people with any kind of cancer, with specific cancers, or with particular rehabilitative needs. For example, ostomy groups include people with intestinal disease, such as colon cancer, who have had surgery that requires them to wear special bags to collect body wastes. Laryngectomy groups are available for those whose voice boxes have been surgically removed. Depending on their constituency, groups might address practical problems (managing the ostomy bag, for example, or relearning ways of speaking), or they might deal with the emotional aspects of recovery.

Some self-help groups are local units of national organizations and are affiliated with medical institutions, and others are grassroots groups meeting in homes, churches, or community centers. Self-help groups are usually free, although they may collect voluntary contributions to defray costs.

Group Factors to Consider

The group you'll end up choosing depends on your own needs and interests, as well as on what is available in your community. As a rule, however, the more alike the people in the group are, the more quickly its members will find cohesion and the better able they will be to supply mutual aid.

Many people feel more comfortable addressing private issues if their groups are limited to their own sex and to similar diagnoses. For example, women recovering from breast surgery commonly have concerns about the changes to their bodies, their feelings of femininity, and the impact of the disease on their sexuality. Similarly, men recovering from prostate cancer may feel more comfortable in groups limited to men, where they can discuss more freely their concerns about impotence or incontinence.

In sum, some groups are formed on the basis of the type of cancer, the stage of the disease (new diagnosis, treatment, recovery, advanced), or the treatment modality (surgery, transplant, chemotherapy, etc.), whereas other groups include only those people sharing certain traits such as age (children, young adults, elderly, for example), culture (Hispanic, African-American, Native American, and so on), or relationship status (married, single, parents of children with cancer, children of parents with cancer).

Groups offer a variety of structures. Some meet weekly, twice a month, or monthly for sessions lasting one to two hours. Some, particularly those that are education oriented, run for a specified length of time (such as six weeks). Others are open-ended and operate as long as people are interested in attending. A group might be open (new members are welcome to join any time) or closed (membership is restricted to those who attend the first session). Many groups work best with perhaps six to eight members, although group sizes range from a handful of people to nearly 40; the larger groups tend to be more structured.

Groups for Family Members

Although many groups are open only to people with the illness, others invite family members to take part either with the person who is ill or on their own. In support or self-help groups organized around the issues and challenges facing the loved ones of people with cancer, they have an opportunity to share

INFORM

YOURSELF

Is Group Support Right for You?

Whether you are alone and need a sense of community or are surrounded by others, as long as you are curious about your illness and are eager to learn ways of managing it, group support may be ideal for you.

Although some people may be reticent to share their intimate thoughts and feelings with people whom they do not know well, participation does not mean you *must* talk. Indeed, a well-facilitated group puts no pressure on its members to open up. Even if you are shy in groups, you can gain much from just listening.

When deciding whether to take part in a group, consider the following:

- Attend one or two group meetings on a trial basis. If you don't find it useful, you don't have to go back.

- You may prefer the focus and direction offered in support groups led by professionals. Or you may enjoy the camaraderie and peer support available in a self-help group. If you find both approaches valuable, consider joining one of each. Tell the facilitator of the professionally led group if you also are participating in a self-help group.

- Groups that have an open structure generally allow participants to choose whether or not to attend a particular session.

- Groups don't always focus on feelings. Often a lot of solid information, including survival strategies, is exchanged.

- You have the "right to remain silent." Remember, though, that others may benefit from what you have to say.

- If you have specific needs you want addressed, you should bring them up. You might want to share your concerns with the group's leaders or organizers and tell them what you hope to get from the group.

- Consider taking part in educational workshops, where you can listen but won't be called on to speak or discuss your emotions. Keep in mind that such workshops are primarily for learning, not sharing.

- If you decide not to join a group just now, you can always change your mind. Keep any information you have gathered about group support. At a later stage of recovery, you may decide to give groups another look.

their concerns about diagnosis and treatment, vent their own feelings, share their experiences caring for and communicating with someone with cancer, and discover strategies for meeting needs of the entire family. Groups for young children of people with cancer can teach them about cancer and allow them to ask questions and express their feelings in a safe place.

Psychotherapy and Counseling

People with cancer and their families who are severely upset by their struggle with the disease may benefit from sessions with a mental health professional. The type of care provided in such cases is generally called *supportive psychotherapy,* in which the therapist or counselor helps facilitate coping rather than personality change. Psychotherapy can be delivered in a group or individually, or with one or more family members taking part. Therapists are skilled in recognizing the fundamental issues in a problem and exploring approaches to resolving them. The cost of psychotherapy may not be covered by insurance or other health plans.

Private sessions offer the chance to express feelings and thoughts that may not emerge in other formal or informal settings. Those in individual therapy also have the full attention of the professional for the length of the session. The confidentiality and objectivity available in therapy can be valuable, and a skilled therapist can offer feedback and suggest coping strategies.

Joint therapy sessions, in which couples or other family members participate, provide an opportunity for airing concerns in a focused way. For example, marital conflicts often are put on hold while the couple deals with the needs of treatment and recovery. In time, however, those conflicts may reemerge and require the attention of a therapist. Similarly, families organized to "protect" themselves against the reality of cancer (through silence, avoidance, or denial) may need guidance in ending the secrecy and reopening the lines of communication. Children may benefit from therapy to help them deal with the changes in the family structure caused by a serious illness. In joint sessions, the therapist serves as a moderator who can keep the discussion on track and help resolve emotions that get in the way of effective dialogue.

Mental health professionals also evaluate and treat severe distress (such as anxiety and depression) and help teach specific techniques that will help you better tolerate the symptoms, side effects, and long-term consequences of treatment (see Chapter 25, "Coping with Stress, Fear, Anxiety, and Depression").

The social work department at the hospital at which you are being treated can provide counseling, therapy, and/or referrals to trained, licensed psychotherapists who are skilled at treating people with cancer.

Organized Volunteer Visitation

One kind of formal support is volunteer visitation, such as the American Cancer Society's Reach to Recovery and CanSurmount programs (see Appendix I, "Resources"). In such programs, people who are recovering or who have recovered from cancer—sometimes referred to as "veteran patients"—are trained to interact on a one-to-one basis with other people who have the disease. Volunteers may visit people in their homes or in hospitals to provide understanding, encouragement, educational materials, and rehabilitation counseling. Such direct contact with caring, sympathetic people who know what you are going through and who have been trained to address your needs can make a world of difference in the quality and course of your recovery.

Religious/Spiritual Support

Seeking the support, either formally or informally, of your faith or religious community can provide solace and strength and help you adjust to your illness and changed circumstances.

Most religious institutions provide pastoral counselors for people in need. Besides offering spiritual guidance, such counselors are often in close touch with community and volunteer organizations offering services such as transportation or Meals on Wheels. Some religious communities may even help raise funds on your behalf.

Finding Sources of Support

The "Resources" appendix at the end of this book lists numerous organizations to consult. In addition, the following people and organizations should be able to tell you what is available in your area:

- Local chapter of the American Cancer Society.

- Oncologists or other physicians on your team.

- Social workers in the hospital's social work or social service department.

- Clinic or hospital nurses.

- Hospital chaplain.

- Local YMCA, YWCA, or YMHA.

- Local United Way information and referral services.

- Church or synagogue.

- Community centers and senior centers.

- State, county, or United Way family agencies and community mental health centers.

- National Self-Help Clearinghouse. This organization provides a listing of peer-support services available in your area. If you write for this list, state the type of self-help group you are looking for and enclose a self-addressed, stamped envelope. The address is 25 West 43rd Street, New York, NY 10036.

- American Self-Help Clearing House. Offering information similar to that of the National Self-Help Clearinghouse, this organization also publishes and distributes *The Self-Help SourceBook: Finding and Forming Mutual Aid Self-Help Groups.* See Appendix I, "Resources," page 660.

- The Internet. Modern computer technology has provided a new source of support for people with cancer. Not only can you get information via the

Some Support Dos and Don'ts for People Who Want to Help

TIPS & ADVICE

- Suggest specific ways of helping. Instead of saying, "Is there anything I can do?" say, for example, "I'm going to the supermarket this morning. If you'd like to give me your list, I can pick up some things for you." Or even, "I'm roasting a chicken and I'll bring it over." You might say, "I have to drop some things off at the library. Would you like me to see if they have any new mysteries?"

- One of the best things you can do is simply to be there. This may mean visiting someone in the hospital or at home, but even more important, it means being there emotionally: listening, avoiding judgments, responding to the person's needs at that moment. Even if you are a casual acquaintance, knowing that you care is extremely important. Sometimes a quick call or note will do. If you are unsure whether a hospital visit would be welcome, call first.

- The support you offer should be based on your relationship. For example, if you have never spent time with the person's children, your offer to "keep the kids for a few hours" may not be appropriate. If you hate driving, offering transportation may make both of you uncomfortable. If you haven't seen the person for a long time, don't expect deep emotions to be revealed in your conversation.

- Remember the others in the family. Sometimes the best thing you can do is to help the spouse or the children.

- Be sensitive to the person's situation. Don't bring a huge houseplant to someone living in a tiny apartment; don't bring food without first knowing tastes or dietary preferences.

- Give the person an out by suggesting alternatives: "I'd like to drop by for a few minutes. Is this afternoon okay, or would tomorrow be better?"

- Don't be offended if your offer of help is rejected. The person may have someone else to handle that need or may get genuine benefit out of doing a certain task himself or herself.

- Resist the temptation to tell the person you are trying to help about other people you know who have had serious illnesses or to question his or her medical treatment.

- Don't be afraid to discuss cancer directly, but follow the person's lead. If he or she changes the subject, respect that.

- Be aware of your own needs. Are you offering to visit because you want to make the person with cancer feel better, or because you want to make yourself feel better?

- Don't overdo it. Calling every day may be a burden to the person in recovery.

- Read Chapter 32, "Issues for Families and Friends."

Internet—the "superhighway" that spans the globe via computers with telephone connections—but you also can tap into a community of others who are ready and willing to talk with you about the disease. If you belong to an on-line service such as CompuServe, America Online, or Prodigy, search its contents for information and services dealing with cancer. CompuServe, for example, offers special medical databases that you can search electronically. It also provides the Cancer Forum, in which people with cancer answer one another's questions and share concerns. If you have direct access to the Internet, search the World Wide Web for cancer-related sites around the world. *The Self-Help SourceBook: Finding and Forming Mutual Aid Self-Help Groups* includes information on finding self-help on line. You should be aware, of course, that anyone can put any information on the Internet, so you must consider the source when evaluating the content. See Appendix II, "Cancer Information On Line."

TREATMENT STRATEGIES

PRINCIPLES OF TREATMENT

Decisions concerning how best to treat a cancer are based on many aspects of a person's life, but the main concern and primary goal is choosing what will work. What will obliterate the tumor? What will rid the body of any wandering cancer cells? And what will prevent the cancer from returning?

In some cases, such as a small, localized skin cancer, the treatment choice is clear, for surgical removal is effective. The treatment of other cancers, however, is still being evaluated. For example, some physicians may recommend that a small malignancy in the prostate of an elderly man be treated by radiation alone. Other physicians might argue that removing the prostate is the best approach. And still others might suggest more radical surgery, regardless of the man's age.

How far you want to go in understanding your treatment options and how involved you want to be in treatment decisions you alone must decide. This chapter provides a general overview of the conventional and experimental approaches to cancer therapy. The following chapters give more detailed information about specific treatments. If you choose to rely on your doctor to make all the decisions, this overview may be sufficient (although the individual chapters contain information that will help you prepare for and tolerate each type of treatment). But if you decide to take a more active part in the decision-making process, this chapter is the foundation for understanding the other chapters in this section.

The Aims of Treatment

Cancer treatments are based on the following principles:

- to remove all known tumor;

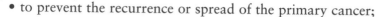
- to prevent the recurrence or spread of the primary cancer;
- to balance the likelihood of a cure of the cancer against the side effects of the treatment.

If the cancer has recurred or is growing rapidly, the principles for treatment shift slightly to include

- a direct, antitumor approach to controlling the cancer as long as possible;
- the treatment and relief of symptoms if all reasonable curative approaches have been exhausted.

Assessment of the Cancer

Although you will have already undergone many tests for purposes of diagnosis, new or repeated tests may now be needed to determine the tumor's characteristics and the extent of disease (see Chapter 8, "Diagnostic Tests"). This additional testing phase may take one or two weeks and can include blood tests, x-rays, a CT scan, and even surgery to obtain additional tissue samples.

Critical questions your doctor is attempting to answer in order to plan treatment are: How aggressive is the cancer? (That is, how likely is it to grow and spread rapidly?) What is the extent of the cancer at the present time?

CANCER

BASICS

Cancer Cell Tests

Cancer cells may be subjected to several tests at the time of diagnosis that reveal how similar they are to normal cells and whether they are fast-growing or slowly developing tumors.

A new laboratory technique for analyzing cells, called *flow cytometry*, is used to measure how many pairs of chromosomes the cells' DNA contains. If a cell has a normal number of chromosomes, it is said to be *diploid*, which means that it is not especially aggressive. Cells that have an abnormal number of chromosome pairs are called *aneuploid*. This is an indication of extremely disrupted DNA and is a sign that the tumor is aggressive.

Another test of a tumor's aggressiveness is a measurement of the cancer cells' *S-phase fraction* (SPF). This number indicates the percentage of diseased cells in the "synthesis" phase of their division cycle. If the number is high, a great percentage of the cells are in the S-phase and are dividing rapidly, indicating that the tumor is growing quickly. A low SPF is characteristic of a slow-growing tumor.

There is some debate among cancer specialists about the value of these tests, and studies are under way to evaluate their prognostic value. Meanwhile, other tests are being developed. Some measure the quantity of particular growth factors, and some search for the expression of certain genes or particular mutations. The tests may be done on tissue obtained by biopsy or samples from a removed tumor.

Cancer specialists evaluate aggressiveness using the following indicators:

- the seriousness of the signs and symptoms;
- how long the cancer has been present;
- how much time has elapsed between the initial diagnosis/treatment and any subsequent recurrence or relapse.

How Treatment Is Planned

When weighing the options, the physician considers such factors as the following:

- The type and stage of the cancer;
- Your general health;
- Quality of life for you and your family;
- Your financial status, insurance coverage, and managed care options;
- Logistics of travel for treatment;
- Effectiveness of the therapy;
- Side effects of the therapy.

Cancer Stages

The method of treatment your doctor recommends depends on where the cancer is, its size, whether or not it has spread, and how aggressive it is known to be. Oncologists consider these characteristics—known as the type and stage of cancer (see Chapter 2, "The Language of Cancer")—in selecting treatment options.

Overall Health

Your health status can be the determining factor in how aggressively the cancer will be treated. Among the many factors that the physician evaluates are:

- *Age.* The general rule has been that children and young adults tend to handle the stress of aggressive treatments better than older people do, but recent studies suggest that many elderly people can tolerate such treatments.
- *General activity level.* Active people may be better able to cope with various therapies than can those whose activity is limited. One system for assessing activity is called *performance status* (PS), which rates activity on a scale from 0 (normal) to 4 (bedridden).
- *Condition of specific organs and systems.* Kidney, heart, and lung function must be assessed before the treatment begins. Certain chemotherapeutic agents can damage these organs, and radiation therapy to the chest can affect lung function. Also, older people may have other serious illnesses.

Personal and Quality-of-Life Issues

To tailor the treatment to your individual needs, and to help you make the right choice considering all the circumstances of your life, doctors must ask many personal questions, and both you and your family need to air your hopes and concerns. Don't be surprised if your doctor wants to know: What are your hopes and dreams at the time the illness is diagnosed? How will the various treatments affect, for example, plans for marriage or hopes for bearing children? How will you take care of young children or other family members? Is extending life worth a great risk to you? Are you frightened of cancer treatments and apt to reject the suggestions most likely to help? Do you have a strong support system?

Financial Status

In a perfect world the issue of finances would not be such a crucial part of health care. However, in these times of shrinking insurance coverage, larger copayments for third-party reimbursements, restrictive health plans, and life circumstances that sometimes catch people without adequate health insurance, expense is a factor. For most people, though, whether they have cover-

T I P S   &
A D V I C E

Talk About It!

The period between diagnosis and the beginning of the treatment is one of uncertainty and ambiguity. Feelings of isolation, vulnerability, helplessness, and fear are common. The most valuable coping skill at this time is communication: Talk to your family, your doctor, your close friends. No concern is too insignificant for discussion.

The reason for airing your feelings is not just to "get them off your chest." Rather, many important decisions must be made right now, and emotions can distort your ability to determine what is best for you. For example, like many people, you may fear that the treatment of cancer is worse than the disease. Indeed, you may become so frightened that you decide you would rather let the cancer take its course than try to combat it. Sharing these terrors can clear the air: Your doctors will be able to give you up-to-date information and help you separate the actual from the imagined risks and benefits; your family members too will feel better prepared. Most important, you will be able to choose a course of action that you will not regret later.

You are less likely to have second thoughts about such important decisions if you make clear all your priorities—to yourself, your family, and your doctors—before embarking on a particular course of treatment. Likewise, informing your doctors and significant others about what you want from life now and in the future will let everyone know exactly where you stand. Your physician will be able to determine a treatment plan that you will find acceptable, and the other people in your life will be in a better position to support you (see Chapter 31, "Coping Strategies").

age for a given treatment will be a deciding factor. Cancer treatment can be financially devastating to a family, so information about treatment costs, insurance coverage, and health plan particulars must be obtained, and how the family plans to meet the uncovered costs needs to be discussed.

Logistics of Treatment

Sometimes the type of therapy recommended is appropriate for all reasons except one: You cannot get to the hospital or clinic. This is a common problem for elderly people who live alone or for people who must travel long distances to treatment centers where more advanced options are available or to research institutions for experimental therapies. For instance, the distant travel and long-term hospitalization often required for a bone marrow transplant can put enormous strains on a family's resources.

Will the Treatment Work?

Your doctor may offer you one or more treatment options based on the therapies' track record in large clinical trials, current reports in the scientific literature, the most up-to-date standard of care, and his or her own training and experience. In some cases, the likelihood of a treatment curing your particular kind of cancer is well established. In others, the odds of cure are still under study. Along with knowledge of the healing potential of the various options, your physician also weighs specific information about your particular type and stage of cancer and your physical condition. For example, you may not be able to tolerate the most effective therapy for your condition because you are in a poor physical state.

Because every person's cancer is unique, exactly how your tumor will respond to any therapy is not entirely predictable. Doctors balance the pros and cons of many treatment possibilities, narrowing the possibilities down to those they believe have the best chances of extending your life.

Treatment Away from Home

If you are considering a treatment that requires traveling a significant distance, you may want to discuss the following questions with your physician or the hospital or clinic social worker:

- How frequent are the treatments, and how much time does each one take?
- Will I be able to return home immediately after receiving treatment?
- Is any transportation, such as a shuttle bus, provided by the clinic or hospital?
- Is any financial aid available for me or my family when long-term hospitalization is necessary? (For instance, some treatment centers offer to spouses and relatives low-cost housing adjacent to the hospital so that they can be nearby.)

QUESTIONS

TO ASK

Side Effects

Some cancer treatments have uncomfortable, sometimes toxic, side effects. The more common ones, such as hair loss and nausea following chemotherapy, are temporary, and new antinausea drugs have made chemotherapy treatment much more comfortable. However, some side effects last longer and may be permanent. The possible loss of 30 percent of lung function after massive radiation doses for a person preparing for a bone marrow transplant, for instance, must be weighed against the consequences of less intensive therapy.

Conventional Approaches to Treatment

When considering different treatment approaches, it is helpful to keep in mind the general principles discussed at the beginning of this chapter: to remove all the primary tumor, if possible; to prevent its recurrence; and to preserve the integrity of your organs, physical functions, and immune system as much as possible.

Most cancer treatments include surgery to remove a tumor and often radiation or chemotherapy as well. Seventy to 85 percent of all people with cancer receive some combination of treatments, as either the primary therapy or the therapy for a recurrent tumor.

It is believed that a combined approach best prevents the recurrence of cancer. Cancer specialists believe that reducing, by radiation or chemotherapy, the number of cancer cells in certain tumors before surgery may reduce the possibility of its spread or recurrence (see Chapter 20, "Combination Treatments").

Surgery

Most people with cancer have surgery, whether it is to obtain a biopsy, to determine the stage of a particular cancer, or to remove a growth and perhaps some of the surrounding tissue. Many surgeries for early tumors are curative, determining both the stage and removing the tumor in one procedure.

The recovery and adjustment period after surgery depend on how large the tumor is, where it is located, and how much normal tissue must be removed along with the malignancy. Sometimes the surgery is so extensive that it affects the function of certain organs and interferes with normal life. In this case, you will need rehabilitation and some adjustments in your daily life. Occasionally, the surgery is disfiguring, and you will benefit from psychological help to adjust to the change.

Most serious and/or long-term or permanent effects can be predicted, so considering them is part of the decision to have surgery or not. In the event that the extent of the surgery is unknown beforehand, talking about all possible outcomes is part of the informed-consent process.

Chemotherapy

Chemotherapy is a *systemic* treatment, since it attacks cancer cells wherever they are in the body. Malignant cells divide more rapidly than do most normal cells, and chemotherapy works by destroying cancer cells during their

Informed Consent

Discussing the risks and benefits with the surgeon is part of a process called informed consent, which is a legal standard that means a person has been told enough about the risks and benefits of a treatment or procedure to decide whether he or she wants to proceed. If the person cannot sign a written consent form, permission can be granted by the court. (Informed consent is required before you undergo any cancer treatment, as discussed in each of the following chapters in this section.)

INFORM

YOURSELF

dividing phase when they are more vulnerable. Unfortunately, however, the cells of some organs (such as hair follicles and the lining of the stomach and intestines) also divide rapidly, so these organs are susceptible to the side effects of the anticancer drugs.

More than 50 anticancer drugs are now in use. They are given by mouth or injected into muscle or directly into the bloodstream. Chemotherapy is used alone as a definitive treatment for cancers such as Hodgkin's disease, in combination with another approach such as surgery, or as an *adjuvant* therapy (meaning that it is "added" before or after surgery or radiation therapy) to deal with any known or suspected spread of the primary tumor.

People receiving chemotherapy often receive a combination of drugs, with some designed to target the malignant cells at specific points in their division cycles. Using drugs in combination in this way helps minimize the toxic side effects.

The maximum chemotherapy dosage is based on the amount needed to destroy cancer cells versus the amount of damage that the rapidly dividing healthy tissues in the body can sustain.

Radiation Therapy

About 60 percent of people with cancer receive some sort of radiation therapy during their treatment. Like surgery, radiation therapy is considered a local treatment. A precise dose of radiation is targeted to a specific tumor to eradicate the cancer cells while sparing the surrounding healthy tissue. Radiation damages the diseased cells' DNA, making them less able to reproduce. Because cancer cells divide more quickly than do those of healthy tissue, they are more vulnerable to radiation, just as they are to anticancer drugs.

Radiation may be used alone, as the primary therapy, or following surgery, as a way of eliminating any stray cancer cells in the area and preventing the local recurrence of a tumor.

The equipment used to deliver radiation therapy has become quite sophisticated in the last 20 years, allowing tumors deep within the body to be targeted without damaging the surrounding tissues. Dosages are calculated according to the tumor's sensitivity to radiation and the normal, adjacent tissue's ability to tolerate exposure to radiation.

Experimental Therapies and New Approaches

Some people initially choose to try an experimental treatment, especially when they have a type of cancer that has not responded well to conventional therapies. Other physicians recommend this option only for treating recurrent cancer or advanced disease.

Experimental therapies are studied in *clinical trials*—studies that are usually carried out in connection with a medical school or in one of the NCI's comprehensive cancer centers. Clinical trials are designed to incorporate the best available care with new approaches in cancer treatement.

Some of the following therapies are better established than others; that is, the results of some studies are promising enough that they may already be considered "conventional" treatment for certain cancers although still under study for others.

Immunotherapy

The objective of immunotherapy is to "turn on" the body's own defense against cancer cells. Among the many agents currently being tested are *biologic response modifiers (BRMs)*, which include monoclonal antibodies, interferons, interleukin-2, and colony-stimulating factors (CSFs) (see Chapter 18, "Biological Therapies"). These agents are not without temporary side effects. CSFs, for example, cause fatigue, fever, rashes, and diarrhea. (See Chapter 18, "Biological Therapies.")

Bone Marrow Transplant

At first, bone marrow transplant (BMT) was used primarily for leukemia and lymphoma, but now it is being studied as a supportive therapy for people undergoing high-dose chemotherapy for solid-tumor cancers, such as breast cancer (see Chapter 19, "Bone Marrow Transplant").

The idea is to replace the bone marrow that has been damaged by chemotherapy or radiation with whole bone marrow or, in some cases, immature blood cells from bone marrow taken from a healthy person. This ability to transplant bone marrow makes it possible for you to receive high doses of anticancer agents that otherwise would be fatal.

The process, however, is difficult, and some of the side effects may be life-threatening and can create long-term, even lifelong, problems. Also, like their policies for other experimental treatments, many insurance companies' and managed care plans will not pay for bone marrow transplants for certain types of cancer.

Gene Therapy

If the cancer is triggered by a genetic defect, and scientists believe that some cancers are, then finding and correcting the defective gene is less damaging and more cost effective than chemotherapy. Gene therapy consists of delivering genes via viruses to human cells, where they can redirect the genetic messages, thereby replacing the malignancy message with a normal one.

Chemoprevention

Scientists are eager to develop ways to prevent cancer. Most studies of chemoprevention involve *prophylactic*, or preventive, drug therapies given to people at risk for a specific cancer. For example, a study is evaluating the use of Retin-A (tretinoin), which is related to vitamin A, to prevent skin cancers in people who have already had a number of them removed.

The Right to Choose

Physicians are trained to heal. But most cancer specialists would agree that the wishes of the person they are treating also must be honored. For example, Sarah, 83, was told she had advanced pancreatic cancer. When she learned that her cancer was fast moving and aggressive, she requested that her doctor not treat the cancer itself but rather help her to remain as comfortable as possible. She discussed her decision with her family, who initially wanted her to put up more of a "fight." They all spoke with hospital social workers and a psychiatrist, and all ultimately agreed her decision was well thought out. Sarah made final legal arrangements for her property, spent time with her children and grandchildren, and stayed at home for the duration of her illness.

Sometimes it is appropriate not to undergo treatment or to direct the treatment toward relief of the symptoms only, such as when a person has already been treated unsuccessfully or when disease has advanced so far that it cannot be cured.

In cases like these, there are legal issues that must be addressed by everyone involved. When the disease is advanced or the cancer has progressed and all treatment possibilities have been exhausted, it is important to establish the wishes of the person with cancer. For instance, a "Do Not Resuscitate" order must be in the medical chart if life-saving or life-support steps are not to be taken. Although the legal requirements vary from state to state, the law generally requires a signed document (a so-called living will and/or power of attorney for a family member) specifying the patient's wish to stop attempts at curative treatment (see Chapter 34, "Supportive Care").

CASE HISTORIES

TRUE STORIES

15

C H A P T E R

SURGERY

Surgery is the surest way of removing a visible tumor or cancer cells that have invaded a discrete area. Surgery also is the oldest form of cancer treatment and, for many types of malignancies, the most successful way to achieve a cure.

About 60 percent of people with cancer have some type of operation. For many, it offers a way to investigate the problem, because despite all the diagnostic tests available to visualize body organs, a direct view sometimes is the only means of confirming that a tumor is present. Also, surgery allows a doctor to retrieve a tissue sample to examine under the microscope when it is not possible to obtain a sample by other methods. At the same time, the surgeon can evaluate the extent of cancer in a process called staging (see Chapter 2, "The Language of Cancer").

Surgery can also be restorative, meaning that an operation can restore the person's appearance or the function of an organ or body part damaged by disease or its treatment.

Finally, surgery may be necessary to relieve pain and treat complications that are causing uncomfortable symptoms.

This chapter explains when surgery is necessary, what it can accomplish, and what someone with cancer can do to optimize his or her recovery.

The Evolution of Cancer Surgery

Documents from ancient Egypt indicate that tumors were being removed as long ago as 1600 B.C. However, it wasn't until the early nineteenth century that modern cancer surgery first was practiced, when a Kentucky surgeon, Ephraim McDowell, successfully excised a 22.5-pound ovarian tumor from a woman who went on to live for 30 more years. Removal of the cancer became a more practical option later in the decade with the introduction of general anesthesia, which was used for the first time in 1846 during an operation to treat a cancerous gland in the mouth. Not long after, in 1867, the principles of *antisepsis* (providing a germ-free environment) were established, significantly lowering the risk of infection from surgery.

Of course, there has been considerable progress in all aspects of surgery since then. Today, surgeons sometimes use lasers instead of scalpels to gain access to a tumor, they can see inside the body with tiny cameras, and may rely on automatic stapling devices rather than on hand-sewn stitches to close a wound. There have also been significant improvements in postoperative care, including pain management, infection prevention, and the replacement of lost fluids and nutrients.

Surgery to remove cancer has evolved into a specialty, surgical oncology. Surgical oncologists are skilled in removing tumors and restoring function to organs and systems that may be compromised by cancer surgery. They also are familiar with other therapies such as radiation therapy and chemotherapy and often work with medical and radiation oncologists as a team.

Informed Consent

Even though surgery can accomplish so much, opening the body to the outside environment and inserting instruments into it is a serious invasion. Therefore, surgery is not a step to be undertaken without careful deliberation and discussion of its advantages and disadvantages. Anesthesia also entails some risks, and postoperative discomfort is inevitable. Death is always a potential, though often small, risk.

The physical inactivity that follows surgery can create problems as well. Thus, anyone deciding to have an operation should be fully aware of *all* the risks of the procedure and why, despite those hazards, surgery is recommended.

Informed Consent for Surgery

A written consent form must be signed before surgery is performed. It contains a statement about the operation and its risks and benefits, such as

- the reason you are having the surgery (is it to cure you, to relieve symptoms, and/or as part of another type of treatment?);
- the chances that the operation will achieve this goal;
- the risk of disfigurement, disability, or death;
- the benefits and risks of not having the surgery;
- any available alternative treatments.

It is important that you read and understand each of these issues, that you not just sign on the dotted line. If you are feeling too nervous before the surgery to concentrate fully on the form, have a family member or close friend go over it carefully with you.

INFORM

YOURSELF

In some states, physicians of breast-cancer patients are required by law to inform women of all their treatment options in addition to surgery and provide them with a written summary on medically acceptable treatment alternatives. State legislatures are considering similar disclosure laws with regard to prostate cancer.

Why Surgery?

Usually surgery is recommended to achieve one or more goals.

Preventive Surgery

One of the most common examples of preventive or *prophylactic* surgery is removal of a *precancerous* lesion, an abnormal area that is likely to become malignant over time. For example, certain abnormalities in the cells of the cervix are detectable on a Pap smear (see Chapter 6, "Routine Tests") and can be removed under local anesthesia with a cutting instrument called a curette, removed with a scalpel (*conization*), vaporized with a laser, or frozen with liquid nitrogen (*cryosurgery*).

In addition, certain benign diseases are considered risk factors for cancer, such as ulcerative colitis, an inflammatory condition of the large intestine. Forty percent of people with diffuse colon involvement due to ulcerative colitis ultimately die of colon cancer. Since removing the colon significantly lowers this risk, a few people choose to live with a colostomy, a surgically created opening through which their intestinal waste exits their body, rather than live with the fear of developing cancer. Likewise, some women with several risk factors for breast cancer, including a mother or sister with breast cancer, may benefit from a prophylactic mastectomy, removal of the breast. This is a very controversial procedure, however, and it does not guarantee that the woman will not develop cancer in the small amount of tissue remaining in her chest or underarm when the mastectomy is subtotal (see "Breast Cancer" in the Encyclopedia).

Diagnosis and Staging

The most definitive way to diagnose cancer is to remove a sample of tissue and examine it. This procedure is called a biopsy (see Chapter 8, "Diagnostic Tests"). Sometimes this can be done by inserting a needle into the suspicious area, but at other times, the only way to gain access to it is through an operation that allows the surgeon to inspect the internal organs directly and to obtain a tissue sample for biopsy at the same time.

Surgery also is often the only way to determine how advanced a cancer is and whether it has spread from the primary site to other parts of the body. *Surgical evaluation staging* entails examining the internal organs. An example is the *laparotomy*, which involves opening the abdomen and looking at the liver, spleen, and other organs. Some diagnostic tests, such as ultrasound, may be done with the organs thus exposed.

A less invasive procedure is a *laparoscopy*. A laparoscope, fitted with a tiny camera, is inserted through a small incision in the abdomen, and images of the organs are projected onto a video screen. In both cases, tissue may be removed for *postsurgical staging* by a pathologist in the laboratory.

After a cancer has been treated, *retreatment staging*, also known as *second-look surgery*, allows doctors to determine how successful the therapy has been. In this operation, surgeons reexamine the affected organs to make sure there are no more cancer cells in the primary site, and they also look for metastatic cells in nearby areas.

Treatment

The surgical treatment of cancer involves removing, or *resecting*, the tumor to cure the disease. Typically, an area of normal-looking tissue surrounding the tumor, a *margin*, also is removed to ensure that no cancer cells remain in the immediate vicinity. Because tumor cells commonly spread via the lymphatic system, nearby lymph nodes may be examined and/or excised as well.

The trend in recent years has been to remove as little tissue as possible in order to spare body parts. For instance, a surgeon treating breast cancer may excise only the tumor and a margin of tissue around it rather than perform a complete mastectomy. Radiation therapy often follows to destroy any undetected cells in the breast. After that, chemotherapy is an option (see Chapter 20, "Combination Treatments").

Surgery alone is curative in about 30 percent of patients with all types of cancer.

Cytoreductive Surgery

Sometimes a tumor is so advanced that it cannot be removed entirely. For example, malignant cells can invade the area around the primary tumor so extensively that too much tissue would have to be removed for the organ to function properly. In this case, a doctor may consider *cytoreductive surgery*, removing as much of the cancer as possible and then treating the remaining cells with radiation therapy, chemotherapy, or both.

Cytoreductive surgery is highly controversial because it rarely cures the disease. Indeed, many experts feel it should be undertaken only if there is a good chance that some other form of treatment will be able to destroy the residual cancer cells.

Removing Metastases

Removing cancer cells that have migrated from the primary tumor can be a step toward cure, especially for those cancers that do not respond well to chemotherapy. This is particularly true if the primary tumor has been completely removed and the metastatic cells have settled in only one spot. For instance, colon cancer often spreads to the liver, and removing a solitary metastasis from this organ can lead to a cure in about 25 percent of cases.

Metastatic cells in the bone, liver, lungs, and brain from various primary sites may occasionally be removed successfully, increasing the odds of a cure.

Emergencies

Cancer can lead to life-threatening conditions, such as infection, hemorrhage (internal bleeding), and obstruction of the breathing passages or urinary or intestinal tract. Surgery can correct these situations and may also restore function to an injured organ or body part and relieve discomfort.

Palliation

Palliative surgery attempts to correct a problem that is causing discomfort. It is not intended to cure the cancer. For instance, a tumor in the abdominal area may grow so large that it presses on and blocks a portion of the intestine, interfering with digestion and causing pain and/or vomiting. *Debulking surgery*, which removes a large portion of the tumor, may relieve the blockage. Or an operation that allows an obstruction to be bypassed may relieve symptoms and allow vital life processes to continue. All or a portion of a tumor that presses painfully on a nerve may be removed.

Surgery to implant devices that aid other therapies is considered palliative. For instance, the vomiting and poor appetite that sometimes accompany chemotherapy deplete the body of nutrients. Therefore, it is sometimes beneficial to insert feeding tubes directly into the stomach.

Surgery also is used to implant catheters into veins for chemotherapy injections to avoid multiple needle sticks (see Chapter 17, "Chemotherapy").

Another facet of palliative surgery is removing organs that secrete certain tumor-stimulating hormones. This *ablation surgery* is done most often on women with a type of aggressive, incurable breast cancer, which is stimulated by the female hormones produced by the ovaries. An *oophorectomy* (removal of a woman's ovaries) is an attempt to slow the progress of the disease. Similarly, a man with prostate cancer may undergo an *orchiectomy* (removal of the testicles).

Controlling Complications and Diabilities

Sometimes a treatment that cures the cancer causes other problems that make surgery necessary. For example, radiation to the colon or small intestines may cause a narrowing of a portion of the intestines as many as 10 years later. The strictures interfere with digestion and require surgical correction.

Merely removing a tumor is not enough. To many experts, a treatment is truly successful only if it restores bodily function and/or appearance. Many reconstructive operations involve relatively new techniques. For instance, arms and legs left stiff or lifeless after surgery may be partially remobilized by loosening scar tissue or transferring muscle to these limbs. Breast reconstruction has become increasingly sophisticated as well. Breasts can be rebuilt with implants or with tissue taken from the woman's abdomen or back. New types of continent ostomies allow people greater control and freedom (see Chapter 28, "Managing Disabilities and Limitations").

The Operation: Before, During, and After

Most operations include preoperative testing and preparation; the actual surgery, which requires some type of anesthesia; and a recovery period. In

QUESTIONS

TO ASK

Questions to Ask Your Doctor

Before undergoing surgery, you will want to find out all you can about the benefits, risks, and side effects of the operation. Answers to the following questions will help you feel comfortable about your decision:

- Why am I having this operation? What are the chances of its success?
- Is there any other way to treat this cancer?
- Are you certified by the American Board of Surgery?
- Is the hospital where the operation will be performed accredited by the Joint Commission on Accreditation of Healthcare Organizations or by the Commission on Cancer of the American College of Surgeons?
- How many operations like the one you are suggesting have you done? Are you experienced in operating on my kind of cancer?
- Exactly what will you be doing—and removing—in this operation? Why?
- How long will the surgery take?
- What can I expect after the operation? Will I be in a great deal of pain? Will I have drains or catheters?
- How will my body be affected by the surgery?
- How long will it take for me to recover? Will any of the effects be permanent?
- Other than my cancer, am I healthy enough to tolerate the stress of the surgery and the anesthesia?
- How long will I be in the hospital after the surgery?
- What are the potential risks and side effects of this operation? What is the risk of death or disability as a result of this surgery?
- What will happen if I choose not to have the operation?
- What are the chances that the surgery will cure my cancer?

addition to these physical phases, there also are emotional issues to consider, such as anxiety about the surgery and its aftermath. Knowing what to expect can help alleviate some of your fear and nervousness.

Planning the Surgery

The surgical team must make many decisions before operating, such as what type of anesthesia to use; the size, location, and extent of the incision; whether it will be possible to remove all of the tumor or only a part of it; whether to use stitches or staples to close the incision; and whether or not to perform an ostomy, breast reconstruction, or other restorative procedures. Each consideration is a potential topic for discussion, depending on how involved in the planning you want to be.

Several tests are necessary to determine your general health and ability to withstand the rigors of surgery and recovery, and some tests are needed to assess the cancer.

In preparation for a major operation, the surgeon must determine whether you have any medical conditions such as diabetes, hypertension (high blood pressure), heart or lung disease, or an infection. Urine analyses, blood tests, chest x-rays, and electrocardiograms to evaluate heart function usually reveal any serious ailments.

The older a person is, the more comprehensive the preoperative testing will be, since the conditions that can interfere with recovery are more common later in life. If possible, certain medical problems are treated before surgery. For example, antibiotics can combat an active infection; hypertension may respond to medication. Chronic illness such as heart disease or diabetes can affect the anesthesia used. Often a specialist in that particular condition consults with the treatment team and is available during the surgery and immediately afterward in case of an emergency.

There are some things you should do before surgery to help it go smoothly. If you smoke, stop—at least for the time being. By clearing your lungs of smoke before your surgery, you diminish the chances of developing lung and breathing problems afterward. Likewise, avoid junk food and eat a well-balanced diet, because good nutritional status helps recovery.

Preparing for Surgery

Depending on the type of operation you are going to have, your body will be prepared (or *prepped*) inside and out to ensure that the surgery and recovery from anesthesia go smoothly.

Cleaning the Skin. To cut down on the risk of infection, the hair must be removed from the area surrounding the incision site. In the case of abdominal surgery, the entire abdomen, genital area, and upper legs may be shaved; for a brain operation, the head is shaved. You will shower or bathe the night before surgery. A technician or nurse will clean your skin with antiseptics the day before surgery, and the surgeon will repeat the procedure in the operating room.

Emptying the Digestive Tract. Because surgery interferes with digestion, your digestive tract must be emptied before the operation; therefore, you cannot eat or drink anything for about 12 hours beforehand. You may be advised to have a light dinner the night before your operation and then to eat nothing else. An empty stomach also prevents your vomiting food particles that could be inhaled into your lungs during the immediate recovery period. When surgery involves the colon, the bowels cannot handle the movement of waste material for several days after surgery. Therefore, you will be given a laxative, and your colon will be cleaned out with enemas the day or night before surgery.

Rest. It helps to have a good night's sleep before an operation. But since you may well be nervous, your doctor may prescribe a sleeping pill.

Special Preparations. For surgery on the digestive tract, a tube may be inserted through your nose into your stomach to keep it and your bowels empty and free of gas. Although stomach tubes do not hurt when inserted, this is usually done after you have been anesthetized.

A *catheter* (a thin, flexible tube) is often placed into the bladder to keep it empty during surgery. A doctor or nurse may insert the catheter before or during surgery.

Blood Transfusions and Fluid Balance. You may receive a blood or plasma transfusion before, during, and/or after surgery, depending on the type of operation and your condition. The blood you receive may come from a donor, in which case it is thoroughly tested for viruses and bacteria, such as those that cause AIDS, hepatitis, and syphilis. You may also store your own blood before surgery. This is called *predeposit autologous donation* and may be permitted as long as you do not have a serious heart condition or are *anemic* (have an insufficient number of red blood cells). Up to four units of blood may be collected five or six weeks before surgery. In a procedure called *hemodilution*, blood is taken to the operating room just before surgery and transfused during or after the operation.

The body can recover from the trauma of surgery when the blood contains healthy amounts of its various components, such as water, salt, sugar, protein, potassium, calcium, and vitamins. To keep these substances in balance, you may receive some or all of them intravenously before and/or after surgery.

Anesthesia

Anesthesia temporarily makes the body unable to feel pain. Typically, an *anesthesiologist* (a doctor who specializes in anesthesia) administers the drugs and monitors your vital signs—pulse, heart rhythm, and breathing rate—during the surgery and observes you after the operation while you regain consciousness. Anesthesia may also be administered by a *nurse anesthetist*, who has received special training and works under the direction of a doctor.

Local Anesthesia. Minor surgery, such as the retrieval of cells near the skin's surface for biopsy, requires numbing only the area involved, or *local anesthesia*. A drug to temporarily deaden the nerves supplying the area is injected near the site. You remain awake and usually feel little more than some minor pressure.

Another type of local anesthesia is called *topical*, in which a numbing agent is sprayed or painted onto the skin's surface or a mucous membrane such as the throat.

Regional Anesthesia. When it is necessary to interfere with sensation in a larger part of the body without affecting consciousness, a *regional anesthetic* or *nerve block* is used. For example, an anesthetic agent injected into the fluid surrounding the spinal cord can numb the pelvic region and legs for surgery on the lower body. The drug may be given in a single injection or continuously through a small catheter placed under local anesthesia directly into or near the spinal canal. Although you remain awake, usually you will receive medication to help you relax.

There are several types of regional anesthesia. *High spinal* anesthesia is used when organs in the middle or upper stomach are being treated. A *low spinal*, or a *saddle block*, is used when the surgical site is the rectum or genitals. An epidural, or *caudal* anesthesia, is injected into the area outside the spinal cord.

General Anesthesia. The purpose of general anesthesia is to put you to sleep so that surgery can be performed. It may be administered via a face mask through which an anesthetic gas flows. As you inhale the gas, it gradually enters the bloodstream, where it is carried to the brain. Or the anesthetic is injected directly into the bloodstream, bringing on almost immediate deep sleep.

Postop

The *recovery room* is for people regaining feeling from regional anesthesia or waking up from general anesthesia following surgery in the postoperative (postop) phase. Recovery rooms are outfitted with equipment for monitoring the heart, assisting breathing, and intravenously administering fluids, such as blood and painkillers.

It typically takes one to three hours for regional anesthesia to wear off. The time it takes to regain consciousness after general anesthesia varies according to how deep a sleep was induced. Because vision, hearing, and balance may be affected, things often seem hazy; voices appear to be coming from far away; and people may seem to move strangely.

Whether you've had a regional or a general anesthesia, you'll probably receive medication to ease pain once you're out of the recovery room and in your regular hospital bed. Pain medication ranges from analgesics like aspirin and acetaminophen to narcotics such as codeine in pill form, or morphine, which is injected. A nurse may administer these drugs at set intervals, or you may be outfitted with a *patient-controlled analgesia (PCA)* pump device, which allows you to self-administer the drug by pressing a button (see Chapter 24, "Pain Relief"). Medication may also be given by means of an epidural, just like that used for anesthesia. The drug you're given will depend on the type of operation you had and how uncomfortable you are.

Getting Back to Normal

In the hours and days following surgery, pain relief is only one concern. Another is regaining the full function of other body organs such as those of the gastrointestinal and urinary tract and the return of muscular activity and strength. There are ways to cope with the common aftereffects of surgery so that your body recovers as quickly and completely as possible.

Mobility. Discomfort in the area of the incision can make walking difficult, but it's important to get moving as soon as is safely possible, because movement stimulates circulation and prevents blood clots. Turning from side to side, getting out of bed into a chair, and walking also encourage deep breathing, which helps restore the lungs to full capacity and prevents pneumonia (see Chapter 27, "Activity Counts"). You may be given a special device to blow into to encourage deep breathing.

Intestinal Function. Walking also is an antidote to stomach gas, a frequent side effect of surgery to the abdominal region. Gas pains may persist for up to three days. If they don't subside naturally, a tube can be inserted through the nose and the esophagus into the stomach or into the lower intestine through the rectum to help expel the gas.

Similarly, nausea and vomiting are common after surgery but can usually be relieved with medication given by injection or in a suppository. Frequently, eating and drinking are prohibited for 24 hours to allow the digestive tract to regain its ability to digest food.

Urination. Some people find it difficult to empty their bladder after an operation if a catheter is not in place. In that case, medication to stimulate urination may be prescribed, or a catheter may be inserted into the bladder to empty it.

Caring for the Wound

The actual wound or incision usually is covered by a dressing. *Drains*—very thin, soft, rubbery tubes, which may or may not be attached to a collecting device—may be placed into the wound to allow fluid to drain. Hospital personnel trained in sterile technique will care for the wound until healing is ensured. This may mean simply changing the bandage periodically. Some stitches gradually dissolve as the wound heals; other types of stitches and staples are taken out by a doctor. As long as the wound heals normally and is not complicated by infection, little specialized care is needed after you leave the hospital.

In some cases, wound care is not so simple, and healing is not uneventful. When specialized care is needed after you return home, nurses provide instruction before you leave the hospital, and visiting nurse appointments may be arranged to monitor your, or your family's, ability to care for the incision site and to avoid complications such as infection.

Permanent Changes

Sometimes the surgery to treat cancer makes it necessary to change how the body works. For instance, after radical surgery for bladder or bowel cancer, it may be necessary to redirect urine or solid wastes. Typically, an opening, or *stoma*, is created on the surface of the body through which waste flows into a discreetly positioned bag. Women who undergo a mastectomy are faced with living without a breast or, if they choose, with a prosthesis or reconstructed breast. Similarly, someone who loses an arm or leg must adjust to functioning without that limb or learn to use an artificial one (see Chapters 28, "Managing Disabilities and Limitations," and 29, "Body Image and Self-Esteem.")

Complications

Although many side effects of cancer surgery are predictable, unexpected problems sometimes arise. The most common complication is impairment of

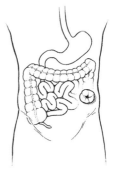

A colostomy is removal of a portion of the colon and creation of an opening through which waste material is excreted. A bag with an opening that fits over the ostomy collects the waste.

lung function, and it usually results from previous lung disease, a smoking habit, or failure to move about adequately after surgery. The ultimate risk, *operative mortality*, refers to a death occurring within 30 days of an operation. This may be due to complications of the surgery, or it may be directly related to the cancer.

The Emotional Impact of Surgery

Although surgery offers hope of substantial relief, in the short term it is a stressful experience. Apprehension about being in the hospital and being operated on, plus the fear of pain, side effects, and temporary or permanent changes in how the body functions, can exacerbate the fear associated with having cancer. However, alleviating as much of that anxiety as possible before surgery will help you achieve peace of mind and improve your chances of a smooth recovery. Research shows that people who are extremely fearful and anxious before an operation tend to experience more complications afterward.

The best way to quell fear is to voice your concerns about the operation and its aftermath to your doctor and other medical personnel. Try to get specific answers to your questions. If you ask when you can go back to work following surgery and are told, "As soon as you feel comfortable," press for a time frame. Likewise, if your doctor prescribes "plenty of bedrest" after you go home, get him or her to explain what "plenty" means. Does it mean that you will need to spend several hours a day in bed or that after a day or so, you will just curtail your normal activities for a while? Details such as these will give you a clear picture of what your life immediately following surgery will be like, and you'll be better able to prepare for it.

If your operation involves changes in how you look or how your body works, again, get as many details as you can. If you are having a mastectomy, discuss with your doctor the pros and cons of a prosthetic device versus breast reconstruction, and if you opt for reconstruction, find out when you can undergo that procedure. Ostomies can be especially traumatic if you don't know what to expect afterward. Find out what the stoma (opening) will look like, and get specific information about caring for it before you leave the hospital. You will be assured that the ostomy will not be noticeable to other people and will not limit the amount of time you can spend away from home, which are two of the biggest fears of people with ostomies.

Often your physician can arrange a visit with a person who has undergone similar surgery.

Equally important are the support of others and learning to relax. A support network of family, friends, and medical personnel can help relieve your fear and anxiety. You may also find it helpful to join an established support group of people who also are cancer surgery patients. They can share with you some of the coping strategies that they've found useful. See Chapter 25, "Coping with Stress, Fear, Anxiety, and Depression," for mind-body techniques to relieve pre- and postsurgery anxiety and manage pain and discomfort. These techniques can prove just as important to you as making the necessary physical preparations.

Surgery is an essential element of cancer treatment, and in many cases it is a positive step toward cure. Even so, the prospect of staying in the hospital, undergoing anesthesia, being "opened up," and facing possible postsurgical consequences such as pain or disfigurement is distressing. Asking questions and carefully weighing the benefits and risks of surgery should lessen your apprehension and give you a more positive outlook.

16

C H A P T E R

RADIATION

More than half of all people who have cancer receive *radiation therapy*, a treatment that uses x-ray waves or a stream of energy particles to destroy cancer cells or damage them so much that they cannot multiply. Radiation therapy is used in a variety of ways, alone or combined with other therapies such as surgery and chemotherapy.

Since radiation kills cancer cells and causes only minimal damage to normal cells, it's a primary treatment for cancer. Vulnerable areas of the body can also be shielded during treatment so they are not exposed to radiation. Radiation is used for palliation, that is, to relieve pain and symptoms or to prevent further complications. For example, palliative radiation therapy can shrink a tumor that is causing pressure and pain because it is impinging on nerves and nearby organs.

This chapter explains how radiation therapy treats cancer, the different methods of targeting cancer cells with radiation, and how the body responds to the treatment. We describe how to cope with side effects and suggest questions to ask when considering whether to have the treatment.

Harnessing Energy to Fight Cancer

Waves of radiation energy, from short to long waves, permeate the atmosphere. This *background radiation* is, for the most part, quite harmless. For example, radiation may be emitted from rocks and soil and even food. In the form of x-rays, radiation is used to diagnose broken bones and visualize internal organs.

Radiation therapy, also called *radiotherapy*, relies on high-energy x-rays, electron beams, or *radioactive isotopes* (from naturally occurring radioactive material such as radium or from artificially produced isotopes such as cesium) to shrink or destroy malignant growths. Radiation does this through a process called *ionization*. Ionizing means removing electrons from atoms, by

Informed Consent for Radiation Therapy

INFORM

YOURSELF

Informed consent is your written permission to receive radiotherapy and the tests that may be necessary to plan the treatment and assess its results. Although the specifics of the form may vary from one state to another, an informed consent form usually attests to the fact that your doctor has explained your condition to you and how radiation therapy will affect it.

Before signing the informed consent form, you should have discussed with your doctor the potential benefits, side effects, and complications of radiation therapy in general and those associated with the particular type of therapy being recommended to you specifically. You should understand how the treatment will be administered. You should also be informed of the pros and cons of the alternative therapies, if there are other options. Finally, when you sign the form, you are acknowledging that you understand there is no guarantee that the treatment will achieve its purpose.

means of a process that breaks up molecules and causes reactions that damage living cells. Sometimes the cells are destroyed immediately; more often, however, certain components of cells, such as DNA, are damaged. Because this injury interferes with the cells' ability to reproduce, they eventually die.

What Radiation Does to Malignant Cells

The life cycle of any cell, malignant or healthy, has four phases, one of which is the dividing or *mitotic* stage. This is the point at which radiation is most effective. Tumors that characteristically grow very rapidly and therefore pass through the mitotic stage frequently are said to be very radiosensitive and so are good candidates for radiation treatment (see the box "Words You Will Hear," page 158). Two examples of highly radiosensitive cancers are leukemia (cancer of the blood cells) and lymphoma (cancer of the lymph nodes). Cancers that are quite radiosensitive include those of the pharynx, bladder, skin, cervix, testicles, and prostate.

When radiation hits a dividing cancerous cell, one of two things may happen: The cell dies or sustains an injury that prevents it from dividing, or if the cell divides, the two new cells cannot divide further.

Cells' sensitivity to radiation also depends on the amount of oxygen in their environment: The more oxygenated the cells are, the more susceptible they are to radiation. Conversely, cells that are *hypoxic* (that is, exist in an environment that contains little, if any, oxygen) are not very radiosensitive. It takes two to three times more radiation to kill hypoxic cells than well-oxygenated ones.

Tumors become hypoxic when they grow very large and their blood supply is diminished. In that case, radiation may first shrink the tumor, which brings the hypoxic cells closer to blood vessels. As the oxygen supply to the cancer cells increases, so does their vulnerability to additional radiation treatments.

Effects on Healthy Tissue

Normal tissues vary in their degree of radiosensitivity. Bone marrow, reproductive glands, skin, mucous membranes, and the organs of the lymph system, such as the tonsils and the axillary nodes (located in the armpit), are all highly radiosensitive. Mature bone and cartilage, the brain, and the spinal cord are not very radiosensitive.

Radiation does not distinguish between tumor cells and healthy tissue, but normal tissue usually is able to recover with little or no permanent damage. Nevertheless, great care is taken to shield healthy body parts during treatment, although certain predictable side effects may occur, as discussed later in this chapter.

Radiation as Cancer Therapy

Radiation is the primary treatment for certain types of cancer, which are especially vulnerable to it. These include certain head and neck malignancies (such as early-stage cancer of the larynx), early-stage Hodgkin's disease and non-Hodgkin's lymphomas, and certain cancers of the lung, breast, cervix, prostate, testes, bladder, thyroid, and brain. Radiation therapy is also used to damage cancer cells that have spread to other parts of the body.

Radiation Therapy Alone

Unlike chemotherapy, which requires exposing the entire body to cancer-fighting chemicals, radiation therapy and surgery affect only the tumor and

CANCER

BASICS

Words You Will Hear

The following are terms often used in discussing radiation therapy:

- *Radiosensitivity* refers to how susceptible a cell, cancerous or healthy, is to radiation. Cells that frequently divide, such as those in the mucous membrane lining the mouth and the gastrointestinal tract, are especially radiosensitive and are affected, though usually only temporarily, by radiation. Remember that cancer cells are more radiosensitive than normal cells because they tend to divide at a faster rate and that well-oxygenated cells are highly radiosensitive.

- *Radioresistance* describes cells that do not respond easily to radiation. The cells of slow-growing tumors, for example, are radioresistant, as are those that are *hypoxic*, or have a poor oxygen supply.

- *Fractionation* is the practice of dividing the total dose of radiation into smaller doses. Radiotherapy is given in these smaller units, or *fractions*, to give healthy tissue time to repair itself between treatments.

- *Protraction* is the period of time during which a course of radiation is given, usually from five to eight weeks.

- The radiation *port* is the area of the body through which external beam radiation is directed in order to reach a tumor.

the area surrounding it. Radiation and surgery have similar cure rates for some types of cancer, but radiation therapy may be preferred to surgery if you have a preexisting condition that makes surgery impossible or if surgery would require removing part or all of a limb or organ. Radiation therapy, therefore, is often chosen to preserve normal organs and/or to keep the body functioning fully. For example, radiation therapy may be used to treat cancer of the larynx in order to preserve the voice.

Combined Treatment

Radiation therapy is frequently combined with other treatments to enhance the chances of curing the cancer. For instance, radiation may be administered before the tumor is removed, in order to kill the outermost cancer cells, which could dislodge and spread during the operation. Or, as in the case of rectal cancer, radiation may be used to shrink the tumor so that it can be surgically removed more easily or to make the operation less radical, thereby preserving more normal tissue.

Radiation therapy also is recommended after surgery to kill cells that can't be easily removed or when cancer cells may remain. For example, radiation may be used after removal of a malignant breast tumor (*lumpectomy*). How soon the radiation therapy begins after an operation depends on the extent of the surgery and how well you are recuperating. In some cases, radiation therapy begins only a few days after surgery; other times, it's best to

---

What Will Radiation Do for Me?

QUESTIONS TO ASK

Part of deciding on a particular treatment is determining whether the benefits of the treatment are worth its costs, side effects, and risks. Therefore, you should understand the goals of the treatment and what your doctor predicts the benefits will be.

The following are some questions to ask:

- What is the purpose of radiation treatment for my cancer? For example, will my therapy obliterate the tumor or shrink it? Will it prevent or curtail the spread of cancer?

- If radiation therapy is to follow surgery, its purpose may be slightly different, and you might ask, "Is this treatment designed to destroy any remaining cancer cells? Could radiation alone be used instead of surgery?"

- If the cancer has recurred or spread to other organs and radiation is being suggested, you might ask, "Why is radiation therapy being suggested? Will it destroy the spreading cancer cells? Will it control further spread? Is it being recommended primarily to relieve symptoms such as pain or bleeding?"

- Whatever the purpose is, what are the chances that the radiation therapy will work?

- Are there other ways to achieve the same goals?

wait about six weeks until the surgical wound has healed.

Chemotherapy can be a helpful addition to radiation therapy; often these two modes of treatment follow surgery to rid the body of any remaining malignant cells. Chemicals may work by rendering cancer cells more radiosensitive, by independently killing cells, or by enhancing the effects of radiation therapy (see Chapter 20, "Combination Treatments").

Types of Radiation Therapy

There are two main types of radiation treatment: *external beam radiation*, or *teletherapy*, which directs radiation from an outside source into the body; and

INFORM

YOURSELF

Team Members

It takes a number of medical professionals to plan and administer radiation therapy, as well as to care for you during the treatment. These people must work together, sharing information about your particular illness. They include the following:

- The *radiation oncologist*, a physician who specializes in treating cancer with radiation. He or she will make many of the decisions affecting your radiation therapy, starting with the recommendation that you should receive radiation in the first place and deciding what kind and approximately how much radiation you should get. The radiation oncologist will evaluate you frequently during the course of treatment and at intervals afterward.

- The *medical* or *radiation physicist*, an expert in medical physics who is trained in planning radiation treatment. He or she helps determine the treatment plan and makes sure the equipment is working properly to deliver the appropriate dose of radiation.

- The *dosimetrist*, a technician who assists the physicist in planning and calculating the dosage of radiation and in deciding how long each treatment will last, often using a computer.

- The *radiation technologist* or *therapist*, a specially trained technician who operates the radiation equipment and positions the patient for treatment.

- The *radiation therapy nurse*, a registered nurse who has trained extensively in oncology and the care of people receiving radiation therapy. For instance, he or she is familiar with the side effects of radiation therapy and will be able to give you information about coping with fatigue, appetite loss, and skin reactions.

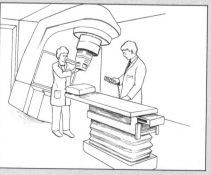

A radiation therapy machine

internal therapy, or *brachytherapy*, in which a radioactive source is placed inside the body, near the cancerous growth.

External Beam Radiation Therapy

External beam radiation therapy is prescribed for many different tumors, including cancers in the head and neck area, breast, lung, colon, and prostate. A machine positioned several feet from the person being treated strikes the target area with radiation.

Low-energy, or *orthovoltage*, radiation does not penetrate very deeply into the body and is used mainly to treat surface tumors, such as skin cancer.

High-energy, or *megavoltage*, radiation is used to treat most other cancers. It is strong enough to penetrate most internal organs and structures and to strike deep tumors. Equally important, megavoltage radiation doesn't attain its full strength until it has reached some depth in the body. This means that the skin and tissues close to the skin receive only mild radiation, which usually causes only minor and temporary side effects. Moreover, the radiation beam is often directed from more than one location so that the radiation is focused on the tumor, sparing all but a small margin of surrounding normal tissue.

Typically, external beam radiation is given daily, Monday through Friday.

Planning External Beam Radiation Treatment. Before the therapy begins, a team of specialists plans how the treatment will be carried out. This treatment planning procedure uses a simulator and treatment planning computer to create images of the areas to be treated and to plan the procedure.

A special diagnostic x-ray machine, called a *radiation simulator*, maps the treatment area. In fact, the simulator does everything the treatment machine does except deliver the radiation beam. Ultrasound or a computerized tomography (CT) scan may also be used to help pinpoint the location of the tumor.

While undergoing radiation simulation, you must lie very still on a table or special chair in the position you will assume for the treatment. For the next 30 minutes to two hours, the simulator and/or other devices are used to make careful measurements, locate the tumor, and delineate the areas on your body through which the radiation will be directed.

Finally, using the images that precisely locate the tumor, the planning team—which includes a radiologist, a physicist, and a dosimetrist—determines, with the aid of a treatment-planning computer, the best plan for treating the tumor.

Marking the Skin. To ensure that the radiation beam is aimed correctly each day, a technician outlines the radiation port with tiny, freckle-sized dots of semipermanent ink. Although the marks will eventually fade away, they need to remain until treatment is completed, so soap and scrubbing on the area must be avoided during the treatment period.

Body Supports and Shields. Before the treatment begins, foam, plaster, or plastic devices may be custom-made to conform to the body. During the treatment, these will help you remain comfortably in the proper position.

Customized lead "blocks" are designed to protect normal tissues and organs. During treatment, these are attached to a transparent plate located between you and the radiation source. During radiation therapy for Hodgkin's disease, for instance, the blocks may be arranged to protect the lungs and larynx.

How Much Radiation? One of the most important elements of the treatment plan is deciding the radiation dosage, which varies with the size, type, and stage of the tumor.

The radiation oncologist prescribes the total amount of radiation necessary to destroy the tumor and then, using a computer in conjunction with a medical physicist, calculates how this total dose should be divided—how much radiation should be administered each day of the treatment, from how many different directions, and for how long. Each daily dose is called a fraction, and the plan for delivering the doses is a fractionation schedule.

The ultimate success of treatment depends in part on whether the cells continue to multiply between fractions. Allowing too much time to pass between fractions gives cells an opportunity to double; and the more cells there are, the less likely it is that a dose of radiation will destroy them all. Therefore, the interval between treatments must be reasonably short for the radiation to kill the greatest number of cancer cells.

Treatment Intervals. External beam radiation therapy is usually given five days a week for five to eight weeks or more, though this may vary. (This schedule prevents the skin and normal tissue from receiving too much radiation at one time.) For instance, radiotherapy may last for two to three weeks when given mainly to alleviate symptoms. For a slow-growing skin cancer, radiation may be administered only two to three times a week for three to five weeks. *Split-course* therapy allows several weeks off in the middle of a radiation treatment to allow the body time to recover from minor side effects while the tumor regresses.

Intraoperative Radiation Therapy (IORT). Radiation is sometimes used to treat the tumor site during surgery. This technique, which utilizes external radiation beam equipment and a special adapter, makes it possible to deliver a large dose of radiation to the tumor without harming healthy tissue in the path of the beam. IORT is often used as a preventive measure, to destroy stray cancer cells that may proliferate, even though the initial tumor has just been removed.

Stereotactic Radiation Therapy. Currently, this type of radiotherapy is used to treat brain cancers, but as the technology evolves, this technique may one day be used to treat tumors in other sites. Stereotactic radiation therapy involves targeting a tumor from many different directions so the beams of radiation converge on the tumor. In that way, the amount of radiation needed to destroy tumor cells is delivered directly to the growth, but the amount of exposure to the area surrounding the tumor is minimal.

During the procedure, your head is held perfectly still by a temporary frame surgically attached to the skull. Then, using a map based on images of the tumor and the brain obtained from computerized tomography (CT) scans,

What to Expect During External Beam Therapy

Typically, external beam therapy is given on an outpatient basis, although sometimes it is begun in the hospital and completed at a clinic. In any case, you may have to undress at least partly, depending on what part of your body is being treated. So it is wise to wear loose-fitting, easily removed clothing.

The actual treatment takes only a few minutes, though you may spend as many as 15 to 30 minutes in the treatment room, "setting up." First, you are asked to lie on a cushioned table, which is then positioned beneath the radiation machine. The technicians focus the machine according to the parameters determined during the simulation. Any pads, casts, or other immobilizing devices designed for you are put in place to ensure that you are in precisely the right position. Lead blocks or shields may be suspended from the machine to protect areas of your body further. These blocks shape the beam so that it is exactly on target.

Once you are positioned correctly, the technicians go into an adjacent room where they can monitor you on closed-circuit TV and talk to you over an intercom.

The machine is then turned on. Radiation equipment is large and often noisy. The machines may whir, click, or sound something like a vacuum cleaner as they move around to aim at the cancer from different angles.

Radiation therapy does not hurt; some people have a sensation of warmth or mild tingling, which is normal. Once the machine delivers the prescribed dose to your body, usually in less than a minute, it is turned off, and the therapist returns to help you out of the immobilization devices. You can then dress and leave. Most people in good physical condition do not need to be accompanied to their radiation treatment and are able to drive themselves home. In fact, many continue to work and engage in their normal activities.

magnetic resonance imaging (MRI), and/or arteriography, a movable, robot-like arm of the x-ray machine is guided by a computer around your head, delivering hundreds of beams of radiation to the brain during a typical 40-minute session.

Special immobilization devices that allow stereotactic treatment without requiring surgery are now available at a number of institutions.

Internal Radiation Therapy

Internal radiation therapy places radioactive material inside the body to deliver radiation to the tumor at point-blank range. Sometimes the radioactive material is inserted into a body cavity, or it may be injected or swallowed in a special solution. Most often, however, internal therapy involves implanting a radioactive substance in or near the tumor.

The most common radiation sources are iridium, cesium, iodine, phosphorus, and gold, all of which give off low-energy radiation, which makes it easier to spare healthy tissue. The advantage of this method is that more radiation can be delivered to the target within a shorter time than with external radiation. Also, the source of radiation is so close to the cancer cells that less healthy tissue is exposed.

Internal radiation therapy is often used as an adjunct to external treatment. For instance, it may "boost" the external radiation therapy directed to a breast following a lumpectomy.

There are several ways of placing radiation inside the body. These procedures usually require hospitalization.

Interstitial Radiation Therapy. Using local or general anesthesia, a radiation oncologist places an implant directly into the tumor and the surrounding tissues. Later it is filled with ribbons of radioactive *seeds*, which are smaller than grains of rice.

When the ribbons are added after the tubes are in place, the procedure is known as *afterloading*. Afterloading takes place in the person's hospital room following surgery.

Implants typically remain in place for three to five days while the radioactive source *decays*, giving off radiation that the tumor absorbs. Like the batteries in a flashlight that gradually lose their power, the radioactive material inside the body gives off less and less energy over time. Most interstitial implants are removed once the prescribed dose has been delivered, but some are left in the body permanently.

Interstitial radiation is a common treatment for cancers of the mouth, tongue, lip, neck, thyroid, and breast.

Intracavitary Radiation Therapy. A radiation oncologist places a hollow applicator into a body space, most commonly the vagina or uterus, to treat a tumor. Usually the radioactive source is afterloaded into the applicator. When the specified dose of radiation has been delivered to the tumor (over 48 to 72 hours), the physician removes the applicator containing the isotope.

Intraluminal Radiation Therapy. Intraluminal radiation therapy delivers radiation to hollow organs. In esophageal cancer, for instance, a surgeon or a radiation oncologist inserts a specially designed tube or applicator into the *lumen*, or opening, of the esophagus. A special imaging technique allows insertion of small radioactive sources into the tube near the tumor so it receives a specified dose of radiation.

High-Dose Rate Remote Afterloading. This method of brachytherapy uses applicators similar to those used for intracavitary or intraluminal radiation therapy but does not require manual loading of a radioactive source. Instead the radiation is delivered remotely from a machine into the applicator through a special conduit. The same radiation dose that may take days to deliver using other implant methods can be given as an outpatient treatment.

Experimental Therapies

Besides these fairly conventional methods of radiation therapy, a few other promising techniques are currently being studied.

What to Expect During Implant Radiation Therapy

Most implants are done in a hospital, where you will need to stay for several days. As a rule, you will undergo minor surgery—with either local or general anesthesia—to place an empty container called an applicator into your body. You will then be taken to your room so that the radioactive material can be afterloaded, or placed inside the applicator.

While the radioactive source is in place, you will remain in your room. Often you must sit or lie very still in bed so that the implant does not shift. Depending on where in your body the implant is placed, you may undergo certain procedures to ensure that you're comfortable and that the treatment will be as effective as possible. For instance, for implants in the vagina or uterus, an enema is given the night before surgery, and a catheter is inserted into the bladder so that you won't have to deal with a bedpan. And the bladder and rectum may be packed with gauze to protect them from the radioactive implant. These procedures are generally done at the same time the applicator is put in place.

Likewise, if implants are placed in your head or neck, a tube may be inserted in your nose so you can receive liquid nourishment in case you have difficulty chewing or swallowing.

During the days that the radiation is active, you will be cared for by nurses trained to deal with radiation. They will be able to provide everything you need, but to protect themselves they will work quickly and may often speak to you from the door of your room. You may be able to have visitors for short periods of time, although some hospitals do not allow them.

Once the treatment is over, the implants are usually removed (although some are left in permanently). You will then be able to check out of the hospital.

High Linear-Energy Transfer Radiation (LET). High LET radiation uses what physicists refer to as large, heavy particles, such as protons, helium atoms, and neutrons, all of which are, of course, invisible. The particles originate in a linear accelerator or one of two other special machines, either a synchrotron or cyclotron. This equipment sends the particles out in a beam, just as other radioactive particles are emitted, but at a superhigh speed.

High LET particles appear to kill poorly oxygenated cells more effectively than does standard radiation (usually referred to as low LET radiation), and tumor cells treated with high LET are less able to repair themselves. The method has been particularly successful in treating sarcomas of the bone and soft tissue, salivary gland tumors, some head and neck tumors, melanomas of the eye, and prostate cancer.

Cell Sensitizers. Drugs called *chemical* or *clinical sensitizers* enhance the effects of radiation. For instance, some drugs take the place of oxygen in hypoxic cells; others transport oxygen to hypoxic cells; and still others are

Will I Be Radioactive?

Because of the powerful effects of radiation, people often are afraid that even when it is used therapeutically, they will become radioactive. They won't. In fact, with external radiation therapy, even the cells targeted by the high-energy waves are affected only for a moment.

When radioactive particles are injected into the body or swallowed, a very small and harmless amount of radiation may be emitted from the body. If the source of radiation is contained in a closed implant, the radioactive material cannot escape, although precautions are taken nevertheless. For these reasons, you are hospitalized, and your visitors are limited. A pregnant woman, whose fetus is vulnerable to even small doses of radiation, is not allowed to visit. Being touched and cared for poses no risk to anyone, provided the exposure time is limited. The health professionals assigned to your care will be able to tell you and your visitors what a safe exposure time is. (Some hospitals do not allow visitors at all.)

If you are given a permanent implant, such as that sometimes used to treat prostate cancer, and discharged from the hospital, the amount of radiation you receive and others are exposed to is safe.

People who receive radioactive iodine are kept in isolation until their bodies no longer contain enough radioactivity to be a radiation hazard.

taken up by the DNA in a cell, inhibiting its ability to repair itself after being damaged by radiation.

Hyperthermia. It has been known for some time that tumor cells are sensitive to heat. Heating body tissues to more than 43 degrees centigrade (105 to 110 degrees Fahrenheit) kills cancer cells directly and enhances the effects of radiation.

Tumors are exposed to heat either before or after radiation therapy. Hyperthermia has become an increasingly refined technique, so that now it is possible to heat the whole body, specific areas, or just the tumor with ultrasound, microwaves, immersion in a heated bath, or a heat probe inserted into the tumor.

Side Effects

Although enormous efforts are made to prevent the radiation beam from striking normal tissue, some contact is unavoidable and side effects often occur. Some of these affect the area being treated; others are more general. But most of them are temporary and there are ways to cope with them.

Fatigue

Tiredness and lethargy are among the most common reactions to radiation therapy, especially among people who are receiving radiation to large areas,

Coping with Fatigue

As your radiation therapy progresses, you may feel tired and sluggish. Generally, by the end of your treatment, your fatigue will have peaked. You may, however, continue to feel tired for a few weeks after the treatment ends.

If you become temporarily fatigued, try to curtail your daily activities and spend your free time doing something restful. Figure out what times of day you feel most energetic, and use that time to do more physically demanding chores and engage in physical activity. Go to bed earlier at night, and if possible, schedule a nap or some quiet time during the day. (It sometimes helps if you plan your rest time for just before or immediately after your treatment sessions.) Turn to family and friends as well: Ask them to help out with housework, grocery shopping, cooking, and child care.

Despite fatigue, diminished appetite, and other side effects of radiation therapy, many people are able to continue working. For some, continuing to live as normally as possible helps them get through the treatment.

If your job makes this difficult, consider taking some time off, or if you can, at least reduce the number of hours you work.

such as the abdomen. Fatigue is likely to begin early and increase during the course of treatment, peaking between the third and fifth weeks.

Why the body reacts to radiation in this way isn't exactly understood, although there are a number of plausible explanations. It may be that the healing process drains the body's energy. Another reason may be the buildup of toxic wastes resulting from cell destruction. An increase in the body's metabolism may play a role, too. Furthermore, daily trips to a radiation center disrupt the normal activities of life and may cut into rest time.

Poor Appetite

Many people receiving radiation lose their appetite. This may happen because changes in the body's cells affect hunger signals or because the perception of taste is altered. The stress of being sick also takes a toll on the desire to eat. It is important not to give in, however, because the energy that food provides is vital to the damaged tissues that are trying to repair themselves. It's important to communicate appetite and nutrition problems to the physician as soon as they occur so that they can be attended to promptly.

Skin Problems

The skin surrounding the area receiving radiation therapy undergoes some temporary changes, reacting much as it would to a long day at the beach without sunscreen. About two weeks after the therapy begins, the skin begins to redden and becomes very dry and itchy. Occasionally, it may peel as the cells in the top layer of skin shed. Rarely, a reaction called *moist desquama-*

Perking Up Your Appetite

While you're receiving radiation, you may not feel like eating, but it is very important to overcome this temporary loss of appetite. Your body is being bombarded with radiation, is using extra energy, and therefore needs more than the usual amount of calories and nutrients. The trick is to note when during the day you feel most like eating and then to take advantage of that time.

Eat when you're hungry, even if it's not a regular mealtime and even if it means eating several small meals each day, rather than three big ones. Be sure to have healthy snacks, such as low-fat frozen yogurt, fruits, and fruit juices. If you are losing weight, you may need to choose high-calorie snacks or nutritional supplements. Take the time to make your meals as pleasant as possible: Play your favorite music, watch TV, read, or dine with friends—whatever makes eating enjoyable for you. (See also Chapter 26, "Food and Nutrition.")

tion may occur, in which skin folds (under the breasts and buttocks, for example) become wet and often very sore. Most skin reactions start to go away within a week or two of completing treatment.

Local Reactions

Some symptoms are responses of the organ or structure receiving radiation. They usually are temporary and are experienced differently by different people. For instance, when the radiation is directed to the head and neck, the mucous membranes of the mouth may become red. You may have difficulty swallowing and suffer from *xerostomia*, extreme dryness of the mouth and lips. Your sense of taste may be impaired, particularly if your tongue is in range of the radiation beam, and your salivary glands may be unable to produce a normal amount of saliva, thereby contributing to the dryness. Drinking a lot of fluids and sucking on hard candy should provide some relief. *Do not use alcohol-containing mouthwash*; it can intensify the radiation reaction. Do not smoke or drink alcohol during your treatment.

Radiation therapy directed to the abdominal or pelvic area may cause nausea and vomiting. Antinausea drugs taken before therapy and as needed afterward may alleviate these reactions. Diarrhea, along with cramping, gassiness, and bloating, also occurs because the radiation affects the function of the bowel, and food slips through the body without being properly absorbed. Over-the-counter preparations for diarrhea, such as Kaopectate, Immodium, or prescription medications such as Lomotil help.

Long-Term Effects

Whereas physical responses such as fatigue and tissue damage become apparent during the course of treatment, some side effects, ranging from mild to severe, do not appear until after the treatment has been completed. Chronic

Caring for Your Skin

Technical improvements have greatly reduced the amount of radiation absorbed by the skin, but local, temporary reactions do occur. You may continue your usual bathing routine. The only skin that will be affected is in the area receiving the radiation. Here are some ways to minimize and treat these problems:

- Wash the skin in the treatment area gently with warm water, and pat it dry; don't rub it. If you must use soap, use a mild, unscented one. Take care not to wash away the skin markings.

- Do not use lotions, creams, perfumes, deodorant, powder, makeup, or other scented or alcohol-containing skin preparations on the affected area unless prescribed by your physician.

- You may be able to relieve dryness with moisturizing creams and lotions such as Eucerin, Aquaphor, lanolin, or gels containing aloe vera (check with your doctor or nurse). Avoid petroleum jelly, since it is insoluble and hard to remove.

- Wear loose-fitting, cotton clothing over the skin exposed to radiation.

- Do not use hot water bottles, heating pads, heat lamps, or cold packs on the area.

- Wear protective clothing in cold weather, and avoid sunlight on the treatment area, particularly while you are receiving treatment. Apply a sunblock or sunscreen with a high SPF if you cannot otherwise cover the area. After the radiotherapy has been completed, the treated area will likely remain more sensitive to sunlight and cold, so you may need to take similar precautions in the future.

side effects or reactions occurring months or years later are specific to the body part being treated.

Infertility. For some people receiving radiation treatment in the pelvic area, the most feared irreversible side effect is diminished fertility. Women may have difficulty becoming pregnant, sometimes stop menstruating, and experience symptoms of menopause. The infertility may be permanent in some cases; however, it's sometimes possible to prevent sterility by shielding the ovaries during treatment so they are not damaged. Nevertheless, women of childbearing age are urged to take precautions that they do not conceive while receiving radiation therapy, since it may be harmful to a developing fetus.

For men, radiation to the testicles can reduce both the number of sperm and their ability to fertilize an egg. Many men have their sperm stored in a sperm bank before beginning radiation therapy. Some men may become impotent after radiation to the prostate gland, and men who have had radiation to the pelvis may have erection problems (see Chapter 30, "Sexuality").

Cancer Risk. Ironically, radiation therapy may infrequently cause the very disease it is treating: Solid evidence suggests that low doses of radiation increase cancer incidence. The most common radiation-induced cancer is leukemia, which usually shows up from five to 10 years after therapy. Thyroid cancer, breast cancer, and sarcomas can appear 15 years or more after treatment.

The incidence of radiation-induced cancer is quite low, however, and depends on several factors. The younger a person is when he or she receives radiation treatment, the greater the risk will be of developing cancer later. Also, the risk is greater with certain types of cancer, namely, Hodgkin's disease and non-Hodgkin's lymphoma. Experts believe that not treating a cancer with radiation is a greater risk than the chance that a secondary cancer will occur as a result of the treatment.

Emotional Risk

Having a life-threatening illness is enough to evoke fear, anger, depression, anxiety, a sense of helplessness, and other strong feelings, and the inevitable fatigue that accompanies radiation therapy only makes these feelings worse. Having to schedule daily radiation appointments—and get to them—also adds to the emotional mix, as does coping with uncomfortable side effects.

It is important to keep in mind that most of the unpleasantness that may develop with radiation therapy will, in all likelihood, last only as long as the treatment continues or for only a limited time afterward. Once the course of therapy is over, a significant step will have been taken in treating the cancer. A support group or therapy group can be helpful in easing emotional symptoms and even some physical ones (see Chapters 13, "Your Support Network"; 25, "Coping with Stress, Fear, Anxiety, and Depression"; and 31, "Coping Strategies").

Follow-up Care

Sometimes the tumor shows measurable changes in size during treatment, but more likely it will take weeks or months after therapy for a tumor to shrink significantly. Some people return to their primary oncologist for follow-up care immediately after their radiation therapy is completed, and others continue to see their radiation oncologist frequently for a while after treatment. During the follow-up visits, blood tests and x-rays are taken to determine the response to treatment and whether further therapy is needed. If it proves necessary, these tests help in the decision about the type of treatment to use next.

The lingering effects of radiation therapy may require some additional care. For instance, some skin reactions take a while to heal, and fatigue continues as tissues regenerate. If you experience these persistent symptoms, continue caring for yourself as you did during treatment—being gentle with the skin and taking naps. As energy levels increase, you can ease back into a normal daily routine, including work, exercise, and sexual activity.

Know the Risks

The side effects and risks of radiation vary according to the area being treated, the type of radiation, and its dose and frequency. Some people never have any side effects, and a very small percentage have severe ones. For the most part, side effects are mild and temporary, subsiding completely within days or weeks after treatment ends. Some cases, however—particularly when large doses of radiation are necessary—produce chronic problems and permanent interruption of body functions.

Considering the range of possibilities, it's important to ask your doctor about all the risks and weigh them against the hoped-for benefits. The following questions are general ones, regardless of the type of radiation recommended. (You may have more specific concerns after reading about your particular cancer in the Encyclopedia section of this book.)

- How will the radiation directly affect the cancer and the area surrounding it?

- What problems typically result from these effects? (For example, radiation to the head and neck may affect swallowing.)

- Which, if any, of these effects will interfere with my functioning? My ability to eat or drink? My physical activity? My ability to work? My sexual activity? My reproductive capability?

- Will any of the effects temporarily or permanently change my appearance?

- How long will the side effect(s) last? Is it likely that any will become chronic?

- What is the probability that the cancer will worsen, spread, and/or recur if I don't receive radiation therapy?

- Is there an alternative treatment that could spare me the risk of a particular side effect? If so, what are the risks and benefits of altering the treatment you have recommended?

CHEMOTHERAPY

At some point in their treatment, most people with cancer receive one or more of some 50 anticancer drugs. These drugs are among the most effective agents available to destroy cancer and often represent the only method capable of treating widespread disease. Whereas surgery and radiation therapy are local therapies, treating a malignant tumor and the area directly surrounding it, chemotherapy can destroy cancer cells that have spread, or metastasized, to parts of the body far from the primary tumor. Chemotherapy has this bodywide, or *systemic*, capability because the drugs enter the bloodstream and are distributed throughout the body.

Because the whole body is involved, chemotherapy can also produce generalized side effects. Although they are not always as bad as expected, their reputation makes chemotherapy the most anxiety-provoking treatment. Fortunately, managing the anxiety helps people tolerate the treatments much more easily than cancer patients did in the past (see Chapter 25, "Coping with Stress, Fear, Anxiety, and Depression").

All the tissues and organs of the body are subject to an anticancer drug's action, which is to destroy rapidly dividing cells or prevent them from reproducing. Cancer cells, which continuously and quickly replace themselves, are obvious targets. But some healthy cells that also divide rapidly, such as those in the hair follicles and lining the intestinal tract, are vulnerable to the drugs as well. Consequently, temporary hair loss and nausea are common side effects.

The challenge, then, for the oncologist is to balance the cancer-destroying benefits of a particular drug or combination of drugs against their toxic effects. It is sometimes quite a delicate balance, but with good emotional and physical care and support the side effects can be managed in most cases and, if not fully controlled, at least made tolerable.

This chapter explains how anticancer drugs destroy malignant cells and how the body responds to the treatment. It includes information on the various ways the drugs are administered and on practical advice for coping with side effects. There also are suggested questions to ask when your oncologist recommends chemotherapy.

How Chemotherapy Destroys Cancer Cells

Chemotherapy—the use of drugs to treat cancer—dates back to World War I, when nitrogen mustard gas was found to inhibit the reproduction of white blood cells, prompting studies of its usefulness in treating diseases such as leukemia. By 1954 the U.S. Congress had invested $3 million in chemotherapy research, and science was well on the way to developing one of the most effective cancer-fighting strategies we have today.

Chemotherapy may either cure the cancer or lead to its remission, meaning that all signs and symptoms disappear temporarily. It also may be used for palliation, to relieve symptoms and improve quality of life. It may slow the tumor's growth or shrink it so that it can be removed more easily with surgery or treated with radiation therapy.

All cells, healthy and malignant, pass through distinct phases in their life cycle: the stage during which the cell produces genetic material (DNA); the mitotic stage, during which the cell is dividing; and the resting stage. Chemotherapy drugs are designed to disrupt a cell's function at one or all of these stages. Cell cycle dependent agents kill only cells actively undergoing division; cell cycle dependent drugs kill both resting and dividing cells. Combinations of these drugs are often used.

Types of Drugs

Five classes of drugs are used in chemotherapy:

- *Alkylating* agents are cell cycle nonspecific. They bind with DNA, preventing the cell from dividing. These were the first anticancer drugs. Examples are cyclophosphamide (Cytoxan), melphalan (Alkeran), and busulfan (Myleran). Cisplatin (Platinol) is usually considered an alkylating agent, even though it inhibits DNA by a mechanism that is different from most other drugs in this catagory.

- *Antimetabolites* are cell cycle specific. They mimic nutrients the cell needs, tricking the cell into consuming them, so it eventually starves to death. Examples are fluorouracil (5-FU) and methotrexate.

- *Plant alkaloids*, also called *vinca alkaloids*, are cell cycle specific. They interfere with those parts of chromosomes necessary for cell division. Examples are vincristine (Oncovin), vinblastine (Velban), VP-16, and VM-26.

Taxol, a drug derived from the bark and needles of the Pacific yew tree (*Taxus brevifolia*), has been studied in clinical trials since 1983. Results have been promising, particularly when used to treat ovarian cancer. Taxol destroys a cancer cell's ability to function and divide by preventing the cell from disassembling its fibrous skeleton of microtubules. When this natural process is inhibited, the cell becomes choked with fibrous structures and dies.

- *Antitumor antibiotics* are cell cycle nonspecific. They are not the same as antibiotics used to treat bacterial infections. Rather, these drugs cause the strands of genetic material that make up DNA to uncoil, thereby preventing the cell from reproducing. Examples are doxorubicin (Adriamycin), mitomycin-C (Mutamycin), and bleomycin (Blenoxane).

- *Hormones* occur naturally in the body and affect certain organs and cells, such as the breast and prostate. Tumors in these organs often depend on hormones to grow, so when the action of one hormone is blocked, the growth of the cancer cells is disrupted. For example, the antiestrogen drug tamoxifen (Nolvadex) is given to women with breast cancer when estrogen receptors are present in tumor cells; it is also being evaluated for use in melanoma, since some cells may depend on estrogen for growth (see "Breast" and "Melanoma" in the Encyclopedia). Examples of hormonal therapy are estrogens, progestins, androgens, and steroids.

What Chemotherapy Can Do

Chemotherapy may be used alone or in combination with other treatments. Whether it precedes or follows another approach depends on such factors as the type of cancer and how advanced the disease is.

Primary Chemotherapy

Chemotherapy may be appropriate before surgery or radiation therapy for a number of reasons. It can reduce the size of the tumor, so it can be more easily removed or targeted by radiation. One advantage of primary chemotherapy, also known as *neoadjuvant* chemotherapy, is that because the cancer cells have not yet been exposed to anticancer drugs, they are especially vulnerable.

On the other hand, a disadvantage of primary chemotherapy is that the drugs must destroy a larger target, since none of the cells were removed with surgery or diminished with radiation. Also, when chemotherapy is the first line of attack, its toxic effects may weaken the body's resistance to the side effects of other treatments that follow, such as radiation therapy.

Adjuvant Chemotherapy

The most common use for chemotherapy is *adjuvant therapy*, which is given to enhance the effectiveness of another treatment. For example, after a tumor has been surgically removed, chemotherapy is administered to destroy cells that may remain near the tumor or have spread to other parts of the body. Such cancer cells are especially vulnerable to chemotherapy because they usu-

QUESTIONS
TO ASK

What Will Chemotherapy Do for Me?

Before you elect to have chemotherapy, you should understand the expected benefits, side effects, and risks. You can get this information from your doctor. Answers to the following questions will give you important facts about your treatment and will help you make a decision about treatment and have realistic expectations about its outcome.

- What is the purpose of chemotherapy for my cancer? Is it expected to kill all the malignant cells in my body so that my disease will be cured or brought to remission? Or is it designed to relieve the symptoms I'm experiencing, without necessarily stopping the disease?

- If the chemotherapy is to follow surgery and/or radiation, you might ask: Is this treatment designed to destroy stray cancer cells that may have been missed by the initial treatment? What are the chances that my cancer will recur if I don't have chemotherapy? Will it improve my chances of cure?

- When chemotherapy is suggested before surgery or radiation, you might ask: Why is this approach being recommended? Will it make it easier to remove or irradiate the tumor? What are the chances that the tumor will respond to the drugs?

- What are the potential risks and side effects of the anticancer drug(s) I will be taking? How do they compare with other treatments or with not receiving any treatment at all?

- How will I be taking my medication, how often, and for how long? Will I be given the drugs in the hospital or my doctor's office?

- Are there ways you will help me prepare for the treatment and to lessen the side effects?

- Will my diet be restricted? My activity? Will I have to take a leave of absence from work or curtail my hours? Will I feel like exercising or pursuing hobbies?

- How much will my therapy cost? Will this cost be covered by my insurance or health plan?

ally are well connected to the body's blood supply where the drugs are circulating. But since chemotherapy subjects the body to side effects, the decision to have adjuvant chemotherapy involves weighing the chances that the drug(s) will destroy cancer cells that have spread against their potential side effects.

Designing a Treatment Plan

Every cancer is unique, and therefore every chemotherapy plan must be individually tailored by an oncologist. He or she must choose the drug or combination of drugs and determine the dosage, how to administer the drugs, how often to give them, and how long the treatment should last.

One of the most important decisions is how much drug to prescribe. Large doses kill more cells. But the more drug that is given, the more likely that it will produce side effects. Still, lowering the dosage to minimize side effects also reduces the chances of success. That is why the usual practice is to use the maximum safe dose for effectiveness, even at the cost of temporary side effects.

Before the Treatment Begins

Because many anticancer drugs are harmful to certain organs, a number of preliminary tests are necessary. For instance, because the bone marrow, where blood cells are formed, is especially susceptible to cytotoxic drugs, a blood sample is obtained to determine that you have a healthy number of red and white blood cells and platelets.

Other important tests include an assessment of the health of certain organs, such as the liver, kidney, and heart. All these tests help determine dosages and whether you will be able to tolerate the chemotherapy. For example, a lower-than-normal white blood cell count can indicate a lowered resistance to infection; therefore, drugs known to suppress the immune system will be too risky until the number of white blood cells returns to normal.

Testing also provides baseline information that the treatment team uses throughout chemotherapy to determine how well the drugs are working or if they are causing damage.

Combination Chemotherapy

Although a single drug can be used to treat cancer, the current practice is generally to combine two to five or more. This strategy serves several purposes. Anticancer drugs often are more powerful when used in combination. Also, if each drug causes different side effects, then a combination that allows a higher dose of drugs can be given without a subsequent increase in any single side effect. And because malignant cells that are exposed to a particular drug eventually develop a resistance to it, mixing several drugs lowers the chances that a cancer will become "immune" to chemotherapy.

Treatment Cycles

Chemotherapy is often given in several phases, called cycles. Each cycle consists of administering the drugs, waiting for them to work, and then allowing the body to recover before beginning the next cycle.

During a cycle of therapy, a percentage of cancer cells throughout the body dies. Between cycles, the remaining cancer cells continue to divide, but before they can reach the original number, the next onslaught of anticancer drugs begins. These cycles continue until there are sufficiently few cancer cells that the body can handle them on its own. Theoretically, for instance, if one cycle kills 75 out of 100 cancer cells, 25 cells will be left. During the rest interval, these cells might multiply to 27, but then the next cycle of treatment will

Informed Consent for Chemotherapy

Informed consent is your written permission to receive chemotherapy, based on your understanding of the drugs the oncologist recommends, how they will be administered, how often and for how long, what their side effects are, and how likely it is that the therapy will be successful. Although many people think of having to sign an informed consent form only before surgery or an invasive test, it is mandatory before chemotherapy. Usually you sign a form that spells out the details of your treatment.

Understanding these details should make chemotherapy less daunting, so make sure you and your immediate support team read the informed consent form carefully and understand what you are agreeing to. If you know what to expect, you can prepare for the side effects. Knowing that the treatment may help you get better should also make it easier to take pills on schedule and keep chemotherapy appointments.

INFORM

YOURSELF

kill 75 percent of these remaining cells, and so on, until the cells are virtually or completely eliminated. The time between treatments is just long enough to allow healthy body tissues that are sensitive to chemotherapy to recover but not so long that the remaining cancer cells have time to regain their original numbers.

Scientists are also experimenting with timing chemotherapy treatment with the body's internal, or *circadian*, rhythms (the biological cycles that occur in about a 24-hour day). The release of hormones, the fluctuation of blood cell production, and the activity of various organs, for example, vary at different times of the day.

Drug Resistance

Sometimes cancer cells do not respond at all to chemotherapy, or the drugs work well for some time but then the cancer cells begin to flourish again despite continued treatment. Some cells do not respond because they are in areas of the body that anticancer drugs cannot easily reach, such as the central nervous system. Other types of cells are inherently resistant to drugs, and some cells develop resistance in ways that are not entirely clear.

Cancer cells that are easily destroyed with chemotherapy at the start of treatment can develop *multidrug resistance*, meaning that the cell is resistant not only to the drugs it has been exposed to but also new ones. It seems that when cells are bombarded with anticancer drugs, a defense mechanism is activated that is effective against many anticancer drugs.

How Chemotherapy Is Administered

Chemotherapy drugs are administered orally or injected into a muscle, under the skin, or into a vein (*intravenous* or *IV*). The method depends on the type of cancer and the particular drug or drug combination. For example, drugs that are not well absorbed by the gastrointestinal tract are injected directly into the bloodstream. Drugs that are in pill, capsule, or liquid form can be taken at home, with regular visits to the doctor's office to evaluate how well the treatment is working. Injections usually are given in a hospital or doctor's office. Sometimes drugs given intravenously require a short hospital stay.

Systemic Delivery

When the goal of treatment is to attack metastatic cells, the drugs must enter the bloodstream for delivery throughout the body.

Oral Chemotherapy. Taking anticancer drugs by mouth is more convenient and less costly than other methods, in large part because you take them at home. In addition, drugs taken orally are often less toxic and cause fewer serious side effects. The disadvantage is that there usually are a lot of instructions to follow: Some drugs require drinking lots of water. Some must be taken on an empty stomach; others should be swallowed with food. Therefore, for oral chemotherapy to be successful, you must keep careful records of which drugs are taken and when. Since accidental overdosing could cause serious problems, doctors often prescribe just enough medication for one treatment at a time.

Intramuscular or Subcutaneous Injection. Rarely are chemotherapy drugs injected into the muscle or under the skin. Although this method does allow for slow absorption, it is not often used because some drugs can damage tissues.

Intravenous (IV) Chemotherapy. The quickest way to get the medication into the bloodstream is by injecting it directly into a vein where cancer cells may be circulating. There are several ways this can be done.

Push or *continuous infusion* is one method. A tiny plastic tube, or catheter, is inserted into a vein in the forearm or hand. The oncologist or nurse then either "pushes" the drugs from a syringe directly into the catheter or mixes the drug in a solution and allows it to flow slowly into the tube from a bag containing the mixture. This "drip" may take up to an hour. Afterward, the IV catheter is removed.

A drawback to this method is that some people have very small veins and thus it becomes difficult to insert an IV needle or catheter repeatedly for subsequent treatments. Although veins in the hand are easier to see, those in the lower arm have more protective tissue surrounding them and may better withstand repeated needle sticks. Even so, veins can become scarred or collapse after several chemotherapy sessions. Also, some chemotherapy drugs, known as *vesicants*, can leak out of veins and seriously damage nearby tissue.

An alternative to a catheter or needle is a *vascular access device* (VAD). This is a catheter that can remain painlessly in place in the skin to provide access to a large vein. Chemotherapy drugs can be injected directly into a VAD or can be administered through an IV connected to the VAD.

There are several types of VADs, including *nontunneled* and *tunneled catheters*. Nontunneled catheters are inserted directly into a vein near the collarbone. The thin catheter has several openings through which the solution flows. Tunneled catheters are inserted into the skin and then tunneled for several inches before "hooking up" to a vein. Insertion of a tunneled catheter requires minor surgery. Both types of catheters need special care.

Another type of VAD is the *port* or *shunt*. This is a small metal or plastic port that is surgically implanted beneath the skin, usually on the chest for access to the vein just below the collarbone or in the upper arm. Drugs are injected into the port via a needle through the skin. The advantage of an implanted port is that it requires no special care, since it is completely under the skin. On the other hand, there is a slight risk that the drug can leak or that the port can shift out of position.

Vascular Access Systems

A port through which medication can be infused directly into the bloodstream can be implanted beneath the skin. It's usually placed in an inconspicuous place such as just below the collarbone. Medication is injected through a needle into a round chamber about an inch in diameter. The person usually feels a mild prick as the needle enters the covering over the chamber, which is a major advantage over having to have repeated intravenous injections. Once in the chamber, the medication will flow through a flexible tube into the bloodstream. The port can also be used to obtain blood samples.

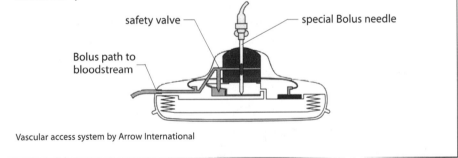

Vascular access system by Arrow International

Regional Chemotherapy

Although chemotherapy is almost always a systemic treatment, sometimes an anticancer drug is delivered directly to a tumor, bathing it in larger than usual doses of the drug without affecting healthy cells. This increases the chances of destroying localized cancer cells while at the same time lowering the risks of the treatment.

Intra-arterial Chemotherapy. Administering the drug to a tumor via the artery supplying blood to the area where the cancer is located is called *intra-arterial chemotherapy.* This is done in a hospital, using a special pump that

Caring for a Catheter

In many ways, having a catheter in place makes the chemotherapy easier, mainly because it avoids multiple injections. But the catheter and the skin around it need special attention. To prevent infection, you must clean the area where the catheter enters the skin and regularly change the bandages covering it. Then a nurse must periodically inject *heparin*, a drug that prevents blood from clotting and blocking the tube. A nurse will instruct you on how to care for the catheter and practice with you until you feel comfortable doing it yourself.

If an infection does develop around the catheter, you may receive antibiotics, or your doctor may decide to remove the catheter.

can override the pressure of the blood flow in the artery and allow the drug to travel to the targeted spot. Some of the areas that might be treated with intra-arterial chemotherapy are the head, neck, and liver.

Intraperitoneal Chemotherapy. Delivering drugs into the abdominal cavity, or *peritoneum*, is called intraperitoneal chemotherapy. A catheter is placed in the abdomen and attached to a special chamberlike device worn on the chest or abdomen. A doctor or nurse fills the chamber with the drugs, which flow through the catheter into the abdominal cavity. Intraperitoneal chemotherapy is often used to treat ovarian cancer and is administered in the hospital.

Intravesical Chemotherapy. Administration of chemotherapy directly into the bladder, or *intravesical* therapy, is designed to treat bladder cancer. The drugs flow through a catheter inserted into the bladder for one to three hours. The person being treated shifts position every 15 minutes so that the drug reaches all areas of the bladder. This therapy is usually done by a urologist on an outpatient basis.

Extravasation Signs and Symptoms

One small risk of chemotherapy is the leakage of drugs from a vein into nearby healthy tissue. Some drugs that are capable of causing serious damage are doxorubicin (Adriamycin), mitomycin (Mutamycin), and vinblastine (Velban). The early signs of leakage may be subtle. Later you may feel pain, stinging, burning, or swelling around the area where the drug was injected. After three to five days, the area may become inflamed and painful to the touch, and within about two weeks, ulceration and other damage can develop that affects the function of tendons and nerves in the area.

Fortunately, serious injury is rare, but any unusual symptoms should be reported to your doctor promptly. Usually only a small amount of drug leaks out, and applying ice to the area and changing the injection site are all the treatment necessary.

How to Choose a VAD

If you are going to receive intravenous chemotherapy, your physician may suggest administration through a vascular access device. There are advantages and disadvantages to each type of VAD. You should discuss them with your doctor. There may be little choice of the type of device you can use, but it's always helpful to know the options and express your preferences.

Device	Pros	Cons
Nontunneled catheter	Does not require surgery; is easy to access; inexpensive.	Cannot be used for more than a month; the catheter is visible and requires regular maintenance—cleaning, dressing changed, flushing with heparin.
Tunneled catheter	Can be used as long as necessary; has a lower risk of infection.	Requires minor surgery; catheter is visible and must be cleaned and flushed regularly with heparin; more costly than nontunneled catheters.
Implanted ports or shunts	Can be used indefinitely; port is visible; no special skin care is needed.	Minor surgery needed to implant and remove port, which may create a small scar; a needle stick is necessary to access the port; must be flushed once a month to prevent blood clotting.

Intraventricular and Intrathecal Chemotherapy. Placing drugs directly into the spinal fluid is most often the method used to treat metastatic cancer of the brain and spinal cord. The drugs are either injected directly into the spinal cord, intrathecal chemotherapy, or are placed in a small rubber bulb called an Ommaya reservoir, which allows the drug to flow directly into the brain for intraventricular chemotherapy. A surgeon implants the bulb under the scalp and threads a small catheter into a ventricle of the brain. Chemotherapy drugs can then be injected directly into the reservoir, avoiding the repeated injections that would be necessary to deliver the drug to the spinal fluid that continuously flows over the brain.

Side Effects

Healthy cells that reproduce rapidly and often—such as those in the mouth, stomach, intestines, and hair follicles—are especially susceptible to temporary damage from chemotherapy. Since chemotherapy also may cause more serious toxic effects—such as damage to the bone marrow—that can be life threatening, anyone undergoing treatment must be monitored carefully and the treatment plan changed if the problems become severe. Some examples of toxic effects are a lowered resistance to infection or damage to vital organs.

No two people experience chemotherapy and its side effects in the same way. This is partly because people have inherent differences and responses and partly because their health varies. In addition, each chemotherapy drug

CANCER

BASICS

Defining Remission

Cancers are often described as being in "remission," a good sign that the chemotherapy is working. *Partial remission* means that the tumor has diminished to less than half its original size and that continued treatment may eventually lead to *complete remission*, the total disappearance of the tumor. Because stray cancer cells are difficult to detect, however, doctors may continue chemotherapy for some time even after they remove the tumor and/or they believe complete remission has been achieved.

differs in its side effects. Many are notorious for inducing nausea, others for causing hair loss, and still others for affecting bone marrow. Most have more than one potential side effect. The side effects also may change as the treatment progresses; some get worse as more and more normal cells succumb to the constant bombardment of drugs. In any case, most are temporary, and there are ways of alleviating them.

Nausea and Vomiting

Nausea and vomiting are two of the most common, and most dreaded, side effects of chemotherapy. Some drugs cause queasiness or are only mildly nauseating; and sometimes a drug induces nausea only when given in large doses. In any case, nausea and vomiting occur when certain drugs stimulate an area of the brain called the *chemoreceptor trigger zone*. Overeating, motion sickness, or nervousness can also activate this zone.

Usually nausea and vomiting start a few hours after treatment and last a very short time. Less often, severe nausea and vomiting can last from 12 to 24 hours and sometimes a day or two, or you'll have a vague, sick feeling that never lets up. For some people, even the thought of chemotherapy

SPECIAL

CONCERNS

Should an Elderly Person Choose Chemotherapy?

It was once assumed that the elderly could not tolerate chemotherapy simply because their organs do not function as well as a younger person's, and therefore they are more vulnerable to side effects. As a result, even though cancer is more common in older people, treatment was often withheld or not provided aggressively enough to do much good.

Scientists now know that older people are usually just as able to tolerate chemotherapy as the young, and treatment can be just as successful for the elderly. For instance, one study of women who had been treated for breast cancer found that those over age 70 live just as long after treatment as younger women do. Therefore, a person's health is a better criterion than age when deciding if chemotherapy is an option.

Coping with Nausea and Vomiting

Besides taking antinausea medications and practicing relaxation techniques, there are some simple steps you can take to curb queasiness and curtail vomiting:

- Eat small meals throughout the day. Avoid sweet, fried, or fatty foods. Foods that are cold or at room temperature are less likely to have strong aromas that may trigger nausea.

- Eat and drink slowly, chewing the food thoroughly so that you can digest it easily.

- Drink liquids at least an hour before and after meals. Clear, unsweetened fruit juices, and "flat" ginger ale or other light-colored sodas are often best.

- Don't eat for at least a few hours before treatment if you tend to become nauseated during chemotherapy.

- If morning nausea is a problem, have some dry cereal, toast, or crackers by the bed to eat before you get up.

- Rest in a chair after eating, but do not lie down for at least two hours (see Chapter 26, "Food and Nutrition").

causes nausea and vomiting (*anticipatory nausea*, as discussed shortly).

Persistent vomiting can cause dehydration and loss of appetite. Both nausea and vomiting must be overcome with medication and/or other measures so that the body gets the fuel it needs to recover from the drugs' effects.

Nausea-Curbing Drugs. Antinausea medications are often given in combinations of two, three, or even four at a time. They are administered intravenously or in pill or suppository form. Drugs to control nausea and vomiting have side effects of their own, however, including sleepiness and fatigue, but for most people the relief is worth it. Some of the most commonly prescribed medications are dexamethasone (Decadron) and metoclopramide. A relatively new drug, ondansetron (Zofran), is administered intravenously or orally and has been found to relieve nausea in up to 85 percent of people using it. It does not cause drowsiness, restlessness, or muscle stiffness, but it is expensive and is therefore often used only for severe nausea and relentless vomiting.

Anticipatory Nausea. According to one survey, about half the people receiving chemotherapy feel queasy even before a treatment session begins, and about a third vomit before receiving any drugs at all. No one knows why this phenomenon, known as anticipatory nausea, occurs. One theory is that after you have undergone a chemotherapy session that made you sick, you associate the treatment room, the smell of the hospital or clinic, or even the sight of the hospital with nausea. The worse your experience with these side effects, the more likely you will develop anticipatory nausea. Those who are prone to motion sickness or are generally anxious or nervous may be more apt to have this problem.

The best way to handle anticipatory nausea is through simple relaxation techniques. For instance, imagining a very pleasant scene can be helpful. You might picture yourself on a beach, feeling the sun on your back and hearing the crash of the waves. Focusing on the detail of this image can distract you from the treatment. (See Chapter 25, "Coping with Stress, Fear, Anxiety, and Depression.")

Diarrhea

Diarrhea can occur when chemotherapy drugs affect the lining of the intestines. It can last briefly or for some time. Your physician may recommend medication for relief. At one time, doctors thought that only prescription medicines could treat chemotherapy-induced diarrhea, but for many people, over-the-counter antidiarrhea drugs work just as well. Call your doctor if diarrhea persists for more than 24 hours.

Mouth Sores

If the inside of your mouth becomes dry and irritated, the mucous membranes may bleed, and sores may develop, making the mouth susceptible to infection. Good oral hygiene is the key to protecting your mouth from the adverse effects of chemotherapy.

Hair Loss

Nausea may be one of the most dreaded chemotherapy side effects, but hair loss, or *alopecia*, can be the most devastating one because it seems like such a gross violation of a healthy appearance. Not all chemotherapy drugs cause hair loss, however, and some people experience only mild thinning that is

TIPS &

ADVICE

Soothing a Sore Mouth

A sore mouth can make eating difficult and is, of course, just plain uncomfortable. Here are some ideas for easing the pain:

- Use a cotton swab to apply Maalox or milk of magnesia to soothe and dry out sores in the mouth.
- Eat foods cold or at room temperature, and choose soft foods such as ice cream, mashed potatoes, cooked cereals, macaroni and cheese, custards, and gelatin.
- Avoid acidic foods, such as tomatoes and citrus fruits and juices, and spicy or salty foods.
- If all else fails, ask your doctor to prescribe a pain-easing medication.

obvious only to them. Others are spared every strand. Some people lose only the hair from their heads, but others also lose eyebrows, eyelashes, and pubic, leg, and underarm hair.

Hair loss doesn't happen immediately. Your scalp may feel tingly and tender for a few weeks after treatment. Your hair may begin to fall out from the roots gradually at first and then in large clumps. Distressing as this is, there are many ways to cope with it.

Remember that hair almost always grows back once the chemotherapy is completed; it may even start growing again before treatment is over. The good news for some people whose hair is naturally straight is that their "new" hair often is thicker and even curly and stays that way for as long as two years (see Chapter 29, "Body Image and Self-Esteem").

Weight Gain

Some people (usually women undergoing adjuvant chemotherapy for breast cancer) put on weight during chemotherapy. It is unclear why this happens. It may have to do with the intense food cravings that develop, despite the nausea. These cravings may be for foods that you used to dislike. Generally, you

TIPS & ADVICE

Strategies for Coping with Hair Loss

If you know that the drugs you will be taking typically cause hair loss, the following are some useful steps for making the transition easier:

- Before beginning chemotherapy, get a stylish, short haircut. This change will prepare you for the effect that the hair loss will have on your appearance. It will also cut down on the amount of hair you find on your pillow or in the shower.

- Once your treatment has begun, handle your hair gently: Wash it with a mild shampoo, pat it dry, and comb it through carefully without pulling or tugging. Use low heat if you must use a dryer. Don't use harsh chemicals such as hair dyes or permanent waving products. Temporary hair rinses are not thought to cause problems, but beauticians are often hesitant to take the chance.

- Sleep on a satin pillowcase to reduce the friction between hair and scalp.

- Some people find the daily handfuls of hair falling out difficult to deal with and so feel more in control if they shave their heads.

- Once all your hair has come out, you may either bare your bald head (many people do) or cover it with a hat, scarf, or wig.

- If you plan to wear a wig, buy it *before* you begin losing your hair. That way you can match your natural hair color and style more exactly. Some shops specialize in wigs for people undergoing chemotherapy; for recommendations look in the yellow pages or ask your doctor, local chapter of the American Cancer Society, or support group. (See Chapter 29, "Body Image and Self-Esteem.")

should eat whatever you want as long as your diet contains enough nutritious foods to fuel your body's energy and repair processes. The average weight gain for women is six to eight pounds, although greater gains are not unusual. Most people prefer to wait until their chemotherapy is completed before dieting to shed the extra pounds. (See Chapters 26, "Food and Nutrition," and 29, "Body Image and Self-Esteem.")

Fatigue

Tiredness is one of the most common side effects of chemotherapy. It can range from mild lethargy to feeling completely wiped out. It may occur because the body is working especially hard to recover from the effects of the drugs and is using lots of energy to dispose of dead cells and build new ones. Tiredness also results from *anemia*, a dearth of the red blood cells that carry oxygen to body tissues.

Fatigue tends to be most severe at the beginning of a treatment cycle, tapering off toward the end, but it may get progressively worse after a number of cycles. When the chemotherapy is completed, the fatigue will gradually disappear.

Should you push yourself? The key to coping with fatigue is listening to your body: If you don't feel like doing something, don't do it. Of course, this advice isn't always practical. Enlist the help of friends and family for the unavoidable tasks of day-to-day life, and pace yourself in regard to other activities. Note when you feel most energetic, and schedule exercise or work for that time. Take rest breaks and naps throughout the day if you can. (See Chapter 27, "Activity Counts.")

You can also plan your treatment session with fatigue in mind. For example, you may feel especially tired the day after intravenous chemotherapy. If so, try to schedule the treatment sessions for a Friday so that you will have the weekend to rest. This way, you may feel more energetic for work by Monday morning.

Effects on Bone Marrow

The bone marrow produces several types of blood cells essential to health. Because these cells are constantly dividing, they are vulnerable to the effects of chemotherapy. The term used to describe impaired bone marrow function is *myelosuppression*.

The bone marrow produces three important blood components: *red blood cells*, which carry oxygen to cells throughout the body; *white blood cells*, which fight infection; and *platelets*, which help blood clot and stop bleeding. A drop in the levels of any of these cells results in specific side effects. Some can be serious, so they are monitored carefully throughout the chemotherapy.

The treatment team performs a blood test to count the blood cells at the beginning of each treatment cycle and again a week to 10 days later. This phase of the cycle, known as the *nadir*, is when white blood cells and platelets reach their lowest levels, leaving the body most vulnerable to infection.

Various drugs have different nadirs; not all of them arrive in seven to 10 days.

Anemia. Anemia is an insufficient number of red blood cells. The symptoms of anemia are fatigue, dizziness, paleness of the skin, and a tendency to feel cold. Usually it is not serious and can be handled with plenty of rest. But sometimes when anemia interferes with daily living, a transfusion of red blood cells or treatment with red cell growth factor may be necessary.

Leukopenia. Leukopenia refers to a lowered number of white blood cells. This condition can make it difficult for the body to fight infection in the mouth, skin, lungs, and urinary tract.

If a blood count shows a drop in the blood cells known as *neutrophils*, the risk of infection is much greater. In this case, some doctors prescribe antibiotics to prevent illness.

Some common signs of infection are fever, sore throat, coughing, chills or sweating, discomfort during urination, wounds that do not heal or become inflamed, and vaginal discharge or itching. Always tell your doctor about these symptoms if they develop.

Thrombocytopenia. Thrombocytopenia is an inadequate number of platelets, which are the cells necessary for blood clotting. A deficiency can cause nose bleeds and bleeding gums, blood in the urine or stool, unusually heavy menstrual flow, or bleeding under the skin, which shows up as bruises. These symptoms can be relieved with platelet transfusions.

Effects on Sex and Fertility

Chemotherapy has direct and indirect effects on sexual function and fertility. Fatigue and nausea can lower libido, and changes in appearance (particularly hair loss) make some people feel they are less attractive to their partners. In addition, the rapidly dividing cells of the reproductive tract are prime targets for anticancer drugs, resulting in a number of side effects for both men and women (see Chapter 30, "Sexuality").

Men. Chemotherapy does not cause erection problems or inhibit sexual intercourse, but the drugs may reduce and/or damage sperm cells, resulting in infertility. Men undergoing combination chemotherapy that includes alkylating drugs are particularly at risk. Once treatment is complete, fertility may be restored, but perhaps not for two to four years. Some men never regain their fertility, and if they do, there may be genetic damage to sperm that could result in birth defects. Consequently, genetic counseling is advisable for a man who wants to have children after chemotherapy. Since it is impossible to predict the extent of damage to sperm production that will result from chemotherapy, it makes sense for men who know they want to become fathers to bank healthy sperm before undergoing treatment.

Women. The ovaries are highly sensitive to chemotherapy drugs, especially alkylating agents. Menstrual periods may come sooner or later than usual and/or last for a longer or shorter time than is normal. Or menstruation may stop altogether during therapy, accompanied by menopause-like symptoms, such as hot flashes, night sweats, and vaginal dryness. Usually, menstruation starts up again after the chemotherapy is completed, although the periods may be irregular for a while. The periods of women who are close to menopause may not resume. Damage to the ovaries can result in either temporary or permanent infertility (see also Chapter 30, "Sexuality").

Effects on Emotions, Mood, and Thinking

The strain of being sick, coupled with the side effects and disruptions brought about by chemotherapy, can take a toll on mental well-being. Chemotherapy can make you feel angry, depressed, anxious, and afraid. It can be emotionally wearing to feel queasy all the time, to have to reschedule work around treatment appointments, or to miss out on enjoyable activities because of fatigue. Many people experience mood swings during treatment because of the drugs, a change in their own biology, or a psychological reaction to therapy. Chemotherapy has also been known to cause confusion, memory loss, agitation, and even periods of unconsciousness. Older people are particularly vulnerable to these side effects, especially if they are taking tranquilizers or painkillers.

It helps to remember that the emotional and cognitive side effects of chemotherapy are temporary and that once the treatment is over, the mood swings will probably end, your thinking will become clearer, and recovery will begin. Meanwhile, talking about your fears, anxiety, anger, and confusion with doctors, friends, family, or support group members can help ease the emotional burden (see Chapters 13, "Your Support Network," and 25, "Coping with Stress, Fear, Anxiety, and Depression").

SPECIAL

CONCERNS

Pregnancy and Chemotherapy

Although chemotherapy often makes both men and women infertile, it is possible to become pregnant during treatment, which may be risky for both the woman and the fetus. Furthermore, the physical changes of pregnancy only compound the unpleasant side effects of chemotherapy. More seriously, the drugs can cause severe birth defects, although current studies are finding that many women who had chemotherapy have healthy babies afterward, even if they were exposed to the drugs early in their pregnancy, when the fetus was most susceptible to damage.

If a woman is already pregnant when she is diagnosed with cancer, it is sometimes possible to postpone chemotherapy until after the baby is born. If not, doctors may recommend delaying treatment until after at least the twelfth week of pregnancy, when the fetus is at less risk of being affected by the drugs. Sometimes, however, the only safe approach is to terminate the pregnancy. Obviously, you must discuss these issues with your treatment team, family, and others who provide your emotional support.

When to Call the Doctor

Even when chemotherapy side effects are fleeting and minor, they may not feel so inconsequential at the time, and some symptoms do signal potentially serious problems. Phone your doctor immediately if you experience any of the following:

- a fever of more than 100 degrees;
- bleeding or unexplained bruising;
- a rash or allergic reaction such as swelling of the hands or feet;
- violent chills;
- pain or soreness at the chemotherapy injection site;
- unusual pain, including intense headaches;
- shortness of breath;
- diarrhea or prolonged vomiting;
- bloody urine.

Nerve and Muscle Side Effects

When chemotherapy drugs affect the nervous system, a condition called *peripheral neuropathy* results. The symptoms include tingling, burning, weakness, or numbness in the hands or feet or both. When the nerves are affected, you may experience a loss of balance and clumsiness, jaw pain, hearing loss, stomach pain, constipation, and difficulty walking or picking things up. Your muscles may be affected as well, and you may feel weak, tired, and sore. Even when such symptoms are mild, you should always report them to your doctor.

Life After Chemotherapy

Once the chemotherapy has ended, the body usually returns to normal, often bouncing back from most side effects in a relatively short time: Lost hair grows in and energy levels rise. But some consequences may linger, such as infertility, menstrual changes, damage to organs, and a low white blood cell count. Similarly, anxiety and fear may continue, especially regarding the possible recurrence of your cancer. Many cancer survivors are helped greatly by joining support groups, where they can share their feelings with others who are going through a similar experience. After treatment ends, family members may not understand why you are not acting like everything is all right again. But cancer survivors know full well about the emotional course of the illness (see Chapters 31, "Coping Strategies," and 32, "Issues for Families and Friends").

BIOLOGICAL THERAPIES

For many years the three main methods of treating cancer have been surgery, chemotherapy, and radiation. Recently, excitement has grown about a fourth approach, one that stimulates the body's own immune system to recognize, attack, and destroy cancer cells. It's called *biological therapy* or *biotherapy*, because the agents are made from living body cells.

Biological therapy began with the discovery of immunization more than 200 years ago. In modern times, research has centered on isolating specific cells of the immune system and their chemical products and manipulating them in the laboratory to target their activity and control their effects.

Research in humans is under way throughout the world in hopes of identifying which biological approaches work best for which types of cancer, and in which kinds of people. Also, because the side effects can be serious, even life threatening, and can significantly alter the person's quality of life, studies to determine how the agents can be used safely is an active area of scientific endeavor.

With few exceptions, biological therapy is not considered a frontline approach. In other words, although it can be used in conjunction with surgery or chemotherapy, it does not replace these other methods, nor is it usually the first treatment tried. In fact, according to one estimate, only about one or two out of 100 people with cancer will be offered this option. Also, in most instances, biological therapy is considered an experimental treatment (see Chapter 21, "Investigational Treatments").

Some biological agents may be given at home, but therapy usually requires hospitalization. With the exception of interferon and some growth factors, treatment is administered or prescribed by an experienced health care team at a major cancer care center. It is unlikely that experimental biological therapies will be offered at a community hospital.

Currently, a few biological agents have been approved by the U.S. Food and Drug Administration (FDA) for use in particular types of cancer. Alpha-interferon, for example, is approved for a rare type of cancer called hairy-cell leukemia, the more common chronic myelogenous leukemia, and Kaposi's sarcoma. Interleukin 2 is approved for treating kidney cancer. However, clinical trials—a step toward FDA approval—of these agents for other uses as well as other agents are being conducted in medical centers nationwide.

Biological therapy is not an option for everyone with cancer, however, so you may wish to skip this chapter or merely skim it to get a general sense of the direction in which cancer therapy is going. If you read on, you will learn a little about the immune system, the principles of biological therapy, and the benefits and side effects of some promising treatments. Since this is a rapidly developing field, it is impossible to describe every biological therapy currently being investigated, so we will talk about only some of the most promising ones.

Defending the Body

To understand biological therapy, it helps to know a few basics about the immune system, the network of organs and cells in the bloodstream and the

What to Ask the Doctor About Biological Therapy

QUESTIONS TO ASK

Weighing the physical, emotional, and financial costs of biological therapies and the serious nature of their side effects against the potential benefit is difficult. One reason is that the risks and benefits are hard to pin down, since experience with biological therapy is so limited. Therefore, try to discuss the state of the research with more than one physician. It may also help to talk about the option being suggested to you with a person who has undergone the treatment.

The following are some suggested questions to ask your physician:

- Is biological treatment an option for my kind of cancer?
- What agent will be used and why?
- Has the agent been proved effective?
- If not, why do you believe it will help me?
- At what point in my illness will biological treatment be used?
- What experience do you have with this particular agent?
- What are the chances of success?
- What are the risks? The complications?
- How much will it cost? Is this treatment covered by my insurance or health plan?
- Will I be part of a research protocol?
- What are the immediate side effects? Long-term effects?
- Will I have to be in the hospital during my treatment?
- Will I be in an intensive care unit?
- What will happen if I stop the treatment?

lymph system that recognizes foreign materials and attempts to rid the body of them.

There are two basic types of immune defense. The first involves the skin, mucous membranes, lining of the respiratory tract, and so on. Like the wall surrounding a castle, this first line of defense is a physical barrier. It produces a *nonspecific response* because it works regardless of the invader.

If that defense fails, the *specific response* (also called *acquired immunity*) is set in motion. First the body must recognize the invaders, such as bacteria, viruses, or cancer cells, as being foreign. Then it must develop the specific weapons needed to fight the particular invader and send those weapons to the site of the battle. After achieving victory, it must be able to remember what the invader looked like so that next time its response will be even swifter.

This military imagery—invaders, weapons, battles—is appropriate, since the immune cells circulating throughout the body are very much like a well-organized, well-trained army. As in any army, success in the battle against the cancer, or any foreign invader, depends on the ability to communicate.

Understanding how cells exchange messages and finding ways to make these messages clearer and stronger are the goals of research in biological therapy. The following section briefly describes the key components of the immune system. The main point to keep in mind is that each of these components, indeed each step in the immune response, represents a potential avenue for the development of a cancer therapy.

Cells of the Immune System

The most important cells of the immune system are the white blood cells, known as *lymphocytes*. Lymphocytes come in two main varieties, T cells and B cells.

Killer T cell

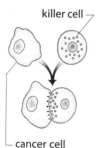

Natural killer cells in the bloodstream release potent chemicals into cancer cells on contact.

T Cells. T cells get their name from the fact that they multiply and mature inside the *thymus*, a gland high in the chest. The job of the T cells is to link up with a foreign invader. What happens then depends on which of the five kinds of T cells is called into action.

- *Killer* T cells destroy the invader directly.

- *Lymphokine-producing* T cells release proteins called *lymphokines*, such as the interferons and interleukin 2, which in turn speed up the activity of the immune system.

- *Helper* T cells boost the activity of the B cells.

- *Suppressor* T cells slow down the immune response to keep the system from going too far and attacking normal cells.

- *Memory* T cells keep a record of the type of invader encountered, so that the next time the body is exposed to it there will be an efficient response.

B Cells. B cells are named for the fact that they develop within the bone marrow. Attracted by signals from helper T cells, B cells circulate to the invasion site and link up with foreign cells. The B cells quickly mature and become factories for producing a specific kind of *antibody* against the invader. Millions

A Brief History of Biological Therapy

In 1798 Edward Jenner discovered the benefits of injecting humans with fluid taken from sores on cattle infected with cowpox, a disease also known as *vaccinia* (from *vacca*, the Latin word for "cows"). This fluid contains the organisms that produce the disease. Although Jenner did not know it, his inoculation—for which he coined the term *vaccine*—worked because the cells of the immune system developed antibodies against the cowpox organism. Jenner applied the same technique to inoculate people against smallpox, and so the age of biological therapy began.

After Jenner's work, the existence of circulating antibodies was suspected, but it wasn't until 1890 that they were discovered. William Coley, a New York surgeon, noticed that people with some kinds of cancer appeared to enter remission after developing certain bacterial infections. He reasoned that the body's response to the infection must be exerting some effect on the cancer.

Coley injected cancer patients with live bacteria, and later with filtered toxins, to induce an infectious response that sometimes led to a remission of their cancer. The so-called Coley's toxins were a treatment option for decades and produced remission in many people with soft-tissue sarcomas and lymphomas. But the use of Coley's toxins dwindled when the focus shifted to treatment with radiation and chemotherapy. Lately, though, researchers have realized that Coley was practicing a kind of biological therapy. It is now known that immune cells respond to bacterial infection by releasing powerful proteins that stimulate the T cells and NK cells. Once in circulation, these cells may also work against cancer cells, which accounts for the remissions that Coley noticed.

Paul Ehrlich, a European contemporary of Coley, theorized that the surfaces of cells carried receptor molecules, which he called side chains. His theory that antibodies attached to these side chains and triggered the release of antitoxins earned him the Nobel Prize in 1908. Ehrlich believed that antibodies might be developed that could home in on invaders, like guided missiles. Were he alive today, Ehrlich would recognize that *monoclonal antibodies*, compounds developed in the lab from immune cells for use against specific targets, were the direct result of his work.

In 1957, two researchers, Alick Isaacs and Jean Lindeman, discovered a lymphokine released by T cells. They named the substance *interferon* because it interfered with viruses' ability to reproduce. But another 30 years passed before researchers realized that interferon had anticancer potential. Unfortunately, the biological treatments developed before 1980 proved to have serious drawbacks. They were generally complicated and expensive, and worse, they didn't usually work, at least not very well. By the late 1970s, many frustrated clinicians had virtually given up on the biological approach. But a good part of the problem lay not in the concept but in the failure to understand the complexity of the immune system and its intricate network of chemical messengers.

The pace of research picked up again in the mid-1980s. Encouraging results were seen in the use of interferon to treat a rare blood disorder called hairy-cell leukemia. Before the decade had ended, the FDA had approved interferon for this disease, chronic myelogenous leukemia, AIDS-related Kaposi's sarcoma, and genital warts.

At the National Cancer Institute in the early to middle 1980s, researcher Steven Rosenberg and his colleagues experimented with doses of a lymphokine called interleukin 2 (IL-2) in people with severe kidney cancer. About 20 percent of those given the treatment experienced at least a partial remission; some even had a complete remission. By 1985 Rosenberg had proved that the human immune system could be directed to discriminate between healthy cells and cancerous ones. Handled properly, immunotherapy could indeed stimulate the body's defenses. In 1992 genetically engineered IL-2 received the FDA's approval for treating advanced kidney cancer. In 1994 clinical trials were started to determine whether yet another interleukin, IL-12, might have some benefit against metastatic cancer and AIDS.

of antibody molecules released from the B cells then circulate in the blood and lymphatic system to seek out other invaders of the exact same type.

Other Immune Cells. Null cells are a kind of lymphocyte only recently identified, and their function is not entirely known. It appears, however, that the cells known as *natural killer (NK)* cells and *lymphokine-activated killer (LAK)* cells evolve from these null cells. NK cells get their name because they function naturally; that is, they can attack invaders without having to be "switched on" by messages from other immune cells. LAK cells, in contrast, need a jump start from a lymphokine such as interleukin.

Monocytes are cells that circulate in the bloodstream, but when they settle in tissue, they develop into *macrophages*, which means "big eaters." The macrophages engulf the invaders and actually digest them.

Therapy from Within

There are two basic categories of biological therapy. The first and most advanced is *immunotherapy*, which generally works by triggering an immune response or by using immune cells to create a hostile environment for the cancer. Immunotherapy can be either active or passive.

The second main category of biological therapy is sometimes called *cytotoxic* (cell-killing) therapy. This approach uses proteins called *cytotoxins* that are produced by the body's cells to attack the cancer either by destroying the cancer cells or by making it difficult for them to grow and reproduce. Another term for this approach is *tumor cell modulation*.

Active Immunotherapy

Every cell in your body contains an identical copy of your unique DNA, the molecule that serves as a blueprint for making more cells. In a sense, DNA is

Biological Therapies

Classification	Examples
Active Immunotherapy	Nonspecific; Immune-boosting substances such as bacille Calmette-Guérin (BCG)
	Interferon
	Interleukin 2
Passive Immunotherapy	Specific; Immunization with tumor cell vaccines
	Antibodies
	Monoclonal antibodies
	LAK cells
	Tumor-infiltrating lymphocytes (TIL)
Cytotoxic (Tumor Cell Modulation)	Inhibition of tumor growth factors or angiogenic (blood vessel) factors

CANCER
BASICS

like a cellular identity card proving that a particular cell belongs to you. Accordingly, cells that do not carry the same DNA look foreign to your immune system. The surfaces of these cells are studded with molecules called antigens that reveal the invader to be "nonself."

Certain cancer cells contain antigens that appear foreign to your immune system. In some cases, it is possible to remove cancer cells, analyze them in the lab, and identify their antigens. Theoretically, once the antigens are known, a treatment can be designed that stimulates a specific immune response against them. This is called *specific active immunotherapy*. Results of this approach have been disappointing, however, and clinicians have generally abandoned it.

In contrast, a *nonspecific active* approach uses agents that set in motion a general immune response, activating a wide range of immune cells. The agents used in this method include interferons and IL-2, as well as bacillus (or bacille) Calmette-Guérin (BCG), the organism that causes tuberculosis. As William Coley (see the box entitled "A Brief History of Biological Therapy") discovered more than 100 years ago, the immune response to tuberculosis can also cause certain cancers to regress.

Researchers have achieved some success by injecting nonspecific agents directly into body cavities where tumors are growing. In two studies, for example, the use of BCG led to the complete remission of recurrent bladder tumors in about 70 percent of the patients.

Passive Immunotherapy

Passive immunotherapy may prove to be the key to biological therapy. In this strategy, antibodies and other agents that have been activated in the lab are given to the person with cancer. This approach is sometimes called *adoptive immunotherapy* because the person adopts an immune response that has been developed in a test tube. This technique, a result of genetic engineering technology, is expensive and requires long hospitalizations and close monitoring during and for some time after treatment.

As with active immunotherapy, the passive approach can be specific (aimed at certain targets) or nonspecific (aimed at a range of targets). Specific treatments include monoclonal antibodies (MABs), the so-called magic bullets, which can be designed to target certain cancer cells.

One nonspecific technique involves removing some of the person's T cells, culturing the cells in the lab, and reinfusing them into the bloodstream in larger numbers. Using interleukin 2 (IL-2) to stimulate these T cells can make them even more powerful. Additional doses of IL-2 may follow. An alternative approach is to activate lymphocytes taken from a person's tumor to create yet another agent, called *tumor-infiltrating lymphocytes* (TILs) and returning these "stranger" cells to the patient where they can fight the cancer cells.

Cytotoxic Therapy (Tumor Cell Modulation)

Tumor cell modulation changes the cancer cells' biology so that they become weak and die. Some of the agents used in this approach are called *cytotoxins*. Perhaps the best-known cytotoxin in this category is *tumor necrosis factor* (TNF), a toxin secreted by activated macrophages to selectively kill tumor cells, principally by interfering with their blood supply.

Certain agents make the antigens on cancer cells more recognizable to antibodies or make them stickier so that antibodies bind to them more easily. Other compounds interfere with cells' ability to metastasize.

The Agents of Biological Therapy

This section describes some of the most common approaches to biological therapy and their side effects.

Interferons

Interferons are proteins secreted by immune cells that interfere with a virus's ability to reproduce and proliferate. This action is how interferons got their name, but it does not account for how they work against cancer.

In the laboratory, low concentrations of interferon help boost the killing power of natural killer (NK) cells, T cells, and macrophages. At higher concentrations, interferons kill cells directly or keep certain cells from reproducing. It is not yet clear whether these effects translate into antitumor activity in the body. One of the more remarkable recent discoveries is the fact that interferons can inhibit the development of the blood vessels that tumors need in order to grow, a phenomenon called *angiogenesis* (see Chapter 33, "Metastasis and Recurrence").

There are three main types (and 17 subtypes) of interferon, and it is possible that more will be discovered. So far, only alpha-interferon has been approved as a cancer treatment, but beta- and gamma-interferon are being studied as well.

Interferons have been licensed in more than 40 countries for more than a dozen therapeutic indications. Given their many functions, the interferons may one day prove useful as treatments for a wide range of benign and malignant tumors.

Approved Uses. The first approved indication for alpha-interferon in this country was for the treatment of hairy-cell leukemia. It has produced at least some benefit in 60 to 90 percent of people with the disease, but complete remission is rare.

The FDA has also approved interferon for the treatment of chronic myelogenous leukemia, or CML, which is more common than hairy-cell leukemia. The use of alpha-interferon in the stable or chronic phases of CML can produce complete remission in as many as seven out of 10 people. In the advanced stages of CML, however, the treatment has little effect.

The FDA has also approved interferon for use in AIDS-related Kaposi's sarcoma, a cancer of the skin and connective tissue. A good response to the treatment means that the lesions flatten or disappear. The response is usually dose related; in other words, the higher the dose is, the greater the response will be. Up to 35 percent of responses occur at high doses. Although treatment does not correct the immune deficiencies seen in AIDS, those people who respond experience a lower incidence of infections.

Interferon is also indicated for the treatment of genital warts known as condylomata acuminata, which have been linked to cervical cancer.

Investigational Uses. The evidence suggests that the interferons may have wide application in a number of different forms of cancer, including low-grade lymphoma, cutaneous T-cell lymphoma, melanoma, myeloma, ovarian cancer, colon cancer, and glioma (a cancer of the brain and spinal cord). Alpha-interferon causes tumors to shrink in about 15 to 20 percent of cases of kidney cancer. So far it appears that the response in these cases is partial and continues only as long as the interferon is administered. Studies have also noted responses to interferon in cases of superficial bladder cancer, Hodgkin's disease, aggressive forms of non-Hodgkin's lymphoma, and cancer of the soft palate. As a rule, interferon appears to be most active when used in cancers of the blood and is not as effective against solid tumors. In some instances, as with colorectal carcinoma, alpha-interferon appears to enhance the effectiveness of other treatments, such as the chemotherapy drug fluorouracil (5-FU).

In laboratory studies, beta-interferon seems to enhance the effects of radiation therapy; whether similar results will be seen in humans is not yet clear. This approach may have particular value in treating cancer of the bronchial tubes of the lung. Beta-interferon also suppresses cell growth and differentiation, especially when used in combination with other interferons, tumor necrosis factor, or interleukins.

How Interferon Is Given. Interferon can be adminstered in the hospital or on an outpatient basis. Initially, close monitoring of side effects is essential. Often, though, injections can be provided at home if the people responsible have been given careful guidance.

A typical course of treatment involves three to seven doses of interferon each week for a period of time from a month to a year.

Side Effects. The injection site can become red and sore. When the agent is given intravenously, possibly serious *phlebitis* (vein inflammation) can result. The most typical problem, affecting nine out of 10 people taking interferon, is flulike symptoms: fever, chills, and aches. The chills usually begin between two and six hours after administration and are marked by teeth chattering, shivers, and a pale complexion. The shivers cause the body temperature to rise, along with the pulse rate and the blood pressure.

The day after the interferon is administered, the fever usually abates, but it is often replaced by a washed-out feeling. The muscles ache, and an oppressive sense of fatigue sets in. Some people are so affected that they can barely drag themselves out of bed; they may neglect their diet and their personal hygiene. Sometimes just knowing what to expect will lessen the impact of these side effects. Also, a kind of tolerance develops that helps in enduring the treatment.

Long-term side effects may be distressing and can have a serious impact on a person's quality of life. For instance, the fatigue can become chronic. About 70 percent of people taking interferon experience confusion, disorientation, and depression. They may have trouble concentrating, performing simple calculations, or remembering appointments. Not surprisingly, these difficulties may interfere with their ability to work.

Many people stop taking interferon because of the chronic fatigue and/or the cognitive problems, feeling that the benefits are not worth the costs. But others find effective ways to manage the problems.

Some side effects stem from high doses of interferon. These reactions, which are usually temporary and reversible, include nausea, vomiting, diarrhea, low blood pressure, burning or prickling sensations, sleepiness, and a general "slowing down" of the body. Tests of liver and kidney functions may be abnormal, indicating that these organs are temporarily compromised. Heart function can also be affected, and in rare cases, there is danger of an irregular heartbeat, loss of blood flow to the heart, and acute cardiac failure.

Monoclonal Antibodies (MABs)

The idea of a magic bullet, a single agent that could pass harmlessly through the body to target and destroy cancer cells, seemed close to reality when monoclonal antibodies were developed in 1978. These laboratory-made antibodies are manufactured or cloned from the same living parent cell (hence the word monoclonal) and are designed to link up with matching antigens on the surface of particular cancer cells.

Designed to Destroy. These designer antibodies can be made to react directly against cancer cells or to carry radioactive molecules or anticancer drugs to them. Monoclonal antibodies have been used by pathologists in the laboratory to test blood and tissue samples and experimentally by radiologists to highlight sites of metastasis so they will be noticeable on x-rays.

MABs can play a key role in bone marrow transplantation. For example, cells harvested from donated marrow are mixed with antibodies in the lab and prepared to seek out and disable T-lymphocytes that would normally lead to rejection of the marrow. The marrow, now free of the T cells, can then be infused into the host.

The greatest potential for MABs is for cancer treatment, but using them to attack cancer cells is still largely experimental, with several difficulties to surmount.

Managing the Side Effects of Interferon Therapy

The severity of the flulike symptoms in interferon therapy often depends on the dose. Unfortunately, at this time, high doses appear to be most effective. However, there are ways to manage the side effects.

Acetaminophen alleviates the aches and fever. (Aspirin can interfere with immune function.) Ask your nurse or physician about how much acetaminophen you should take and how often. Your doctor may offer to prescribe acetaminophen with codeine if the over-the-counter medication doesn't adequately control your pain.

Commonsense remedies such as blankets and warm beverages can provide relief for the chills and shaking, which occur for up to six hours after an interferon injection. In severe cases, morphine may be needed to reduce muscle contractions.

Ask your doctor about taking the interferon injection in the evening, so that you might sleep through the worst of the adverse reactions.

You may experience a change in your taste for food. Old favorites may lose their appeal, or you may have no appetite at all. A dietitian can help with planning meals so you get the most nutritive value from the foods you do eat and you don't lose too much weight. Sometimes sipping high-protein, high-calorie liquid meals can get you through days when you just don't feel like eating anything (see Chapter 26, "Food and Nutrition").

Inflammation at the site of injection is common. Alternating sites minimizes the risk of serious infection, and corticosteroid medication can help relieve inflammation, redness, and pain.

Low blood pressure often can be managed with increased fluid intake and by avoiding sudden changes in position, such as quickly standing up from a chair or a bed. If you are taking a medication for high blood pressure, your doctor may lower the dosage or take you off the medication for a while.

Since interferon can lead to trouble concentrating, you may want to ask your family or a close friend to check with you often during therapy about the medicines you're taking and to be certain you keep your doctor's appointments. Time off from work may be necessary, and it may help to delegate such responsibilities as paying bills to someone else for a while.

Fatigue is the most distressing side effect and one that can dramatically affect your quality of life. You might need to cut back on activities, allow plenty of time for rest, and take naps frequently. Don't hesitate to ask others for help, even for small things like getting dressed or helping you wash your hair. You need to conserve your strength so the treatment has the best chance of working.

Obstacles to Therapy. Success with MABs has been elusive, for several reasons. Some cancers, such as small-cell lung cancer, may produce cells whose surfaces are studded with not just one type of antigen but a variety of them. In such cases, the very specificity of the antibodies works against the therapeutic process, since a whole fleet of different MABs would be needed to destroy this kind of cancer cell.

Another problem is that once MABs bearing anticancer drugs are injected, they must hold onto their cargo long enough to reach the target site. If released too soon, toxic or radioactive molecules can enter the circulation and destroy healthy cells or tissues. On the other hand, the antibody may successfully bind to the antigen but then fail to release its toxic payload.

Cancer cells are wily opponents, defending themselves in a variety of ways against attack by MABs. They sometimes shed their antigens, thereby leaving the MABs without a docking site. Or the cancer cells may secrete a blocking factor that coats their antigens, disguising their appearance.

Finally, as with other biological therapies, there are side effects.

Side Effects of MABs. Often there is pain or inflammation at the injection site. Many people experience flulike symptoms of fever, fatigue, chills, headache, nausea, and vomiting. There may be a decrease in blood pressure, weight gain, and shifts in body fluids, resulting in mild swelling. To some extent, the side effects depend on the target of the antibodies. For example, MABs aimed at colon cancer may cause diarrhea, and those used against a blood disorder may cause the number of white blood cells to decrease.

Some people experience allergic reactions, including cough, wheezing, and skin rash. In severe cases, there is an extreme, potentially fatal allergic reaction, called *anaphylaxis*, which produces a drop in blood pressure, swelling, severe rash, and difficulty in breathing. The risk of allergic reactions increases with each injection because the body eventually forms antibodies against the monoclonal antibody itself.

People receiving monoclonal treatments need to be in a facility equipped with resuscitation equipment in case of an allergic reaction. Close observation for at least an hour after the injection is crucial. Heart and lung functions are checked frequently, and various blood tests, scans, and tumor measurements routinely monitor the body's response to treatment.

The Prospects. The problems and side effects associated with MAB therapy are the subject of several areas of research. For example, many MABs used today are produced from mouse cells because monoclonals from human cells, though reducing the risk of allergic reaction, are less reliable as antibody factories. More efficient human MABs may be developed in the future. Also, figuring out ways to prevent tumor cells from changing their antigens would facilitate the MABs' ability to bind to their targets. It is likely that combinations of treatments using MABs and other biological agents, such as IL-2 or interferon, will increase the success of this approach. The greatest potential for MAB therapy lies in treatment for cancers in which tumor-specific antigens can be identified, such as B-cell lymphomas and certain forms of leukemia.

Interleukins

Lymphocytes produce interleukins, hormone-like substances that activate several components of the immune system. Individual interleukins are identified by number, such as interleukin 2 (IL-2). Several different ones are under study, but IL-2 which can be mass-produced using genetic technology, is the first and so far the only approved biological treatment for kidney cancer. Studies show that IL-2 reduced the size of tumors in 15 percent of those taking the drug, and in 4 percent of the patients, the tumors disappeared completely. IL-2 has had some success in correcting T-lymphocyte abnormalities in people with AIDS.

Treatment with IL-2 is complicated, toxic, and expensive. In a typical protocol for renal cell cancer, for example, IL-2 is given intravenously four times a day for four or five days. Then, a week later, a second IL-2 cycle begins.

Combined Therapy. Much of the current interest in IL-2 focuses on its use with *lymphokine-activated killer cells*, or LAK cells. In one procedure, T cells are removed from the blood and grown in the laboratory along with IL-2. The interleukin "primes the pump" by stimulating the T cells to release cytokines such as tumor necrosis factor (TNF) and gamma-interferon. These stimulated cells, now called LAK cells, are then reinjected intravenously. Once inside the body, the LAK cells can destroy a variety of tumor cells. Often an additional dose of IL-2 is given at the same time to enhance the LAK cells' activity.

Administering IL-2 in low doses as quickly as possible and then giving IL-2 for long periods after the infusion of LAK cells help reduce the risk of life-threatening toxic reactions.

Studies indicate that IL-2 and LAK cells produce at least some response in 15 to 30 percent of people with renal-cell carcinoma and in up to 40 percent in those with melanoma. Positive results have also been reported when LAK cells are used to treat people with gliomas.

Side Effects from IL-2. Treatment with IL-2 carries considerable risk of serious side effects; therefore, it is typically given in intensive care units (ICUs) or at least in hospitals that have an ICU and emergency physicians available. Blood pressure, urine output, and breathing must be monitored closely for a few days.

Of great concern is *capillary leak syndrome*, in which fluids escape from small blood vessels, resulting in swollen tissues. Symptoms include rapid weight gain, a drop in blood pressure, and difficulty breathing. Left untreated, the syndrome can cause kidney failure or respiratory arrest.

Other potentially life-threatening reactions include cardiac arrhythmias, angina, myocardial infarction, infections, neurologic problems, and gastrointestinal bleeding. People whose kidneys fail require dialysis for a period of time. About 2 to 4 percent of people given IL-2 for kidney cancer die as a result of therapy. However, most people do recover from the treatment, and even though these problems are serious, they can be reversed within two or three days.

Less serious consequences, such as skin rashes and the flulike symptoms of chills and fever and nausea and vomiting are common. Sometimes even more distressing is the profound malaise and fatigue that affects almost everyone who undergoes IL-2 therapy.

People receiving this treatment, therefore, need nursing care. They may also want to avail themselves of support services, such as counseling, to help them deal with apprehension and to enable them to continue the treatment.

Growth Factors and Hormones

These substances help normal cells to grow. Growth factors are also known as *colony stimulating factors* or *hematopoietic growth factors*. There are two types used in cancer treatment that are FDA approved: ones that stimulate bone marrow to make normal cells and others that act as anticancer agents. These include the following:

Erythropoietin. Called *epo* for short, erythropoietin is one of the first growth factors to be synthesized and is perhaps the best known. It was approved in 1989 for use in chronic kidney disease. This hormone, partially produced by the kidneys, causes immature red blood cells to develop and stimulates their release from the bone marrow.

People with advanced kidney failure often cannot make enough epo, and so in addition to dialysis, they may require many blood transfusions. Injections of epo, however, maintain a healthy level of red blood cells and can eliminate the need for dialysis and transfusions altogether.

This treatment does not address the cause of kidney failure directly, but it does offer a valuable form of support that enhances the quality of life. Epo replacement also helps reverse the anemia that often results from chemotherapy with cisplatin, a drug used in the treatment of metastatic testicular and ovarian cancers and advanced bladder cancer. People receiving epo report a sense of well-being and higher levels of energy that allow them to live more normally.

Granulocyte-Macrophage–Colony-Stimulating Factor (GM–CSF) and Granulocyte–CSF (G–CSF). *Granulocytes* are cells containing tiny granules, or particles, essential to various immune functions. CSFs (colony-stimulating factors) are proteins that induce granulocyte cells to multiply.

Given intravenously to people with small-cell lung cancer, for example, G–CSF increases the number of certain granulocytes that destroy microorganisms. It can be given before chemotherapy to reduce side effects. Both G–CSF and GM–CSF help increase the number of white blood cells following chemotherapy and after bone marrow transplantation.

The ideal dosage and treatment regimen with growth factors are not yet known. These agents usually cause few serious side effects, although some people experience mild fever, muscle aches, headaches, and nausea; less common reactions include bone pain and difficulty breathing.

Transforming Growth Factor-Beta. Like other growth factors, transforming growth factor-beta regulates immune cell activity. It also directly affects the ability of cancer tumors to develop their supportive structure and the blood vessels necessary for growth.

Tumor Necrosis Factor (TNF). TNF, secreted by macrophages and other cells, kills tumor cells directly. It appears to enhance the effectiveness of some anticancer drugs and gives a boost to the interleukins and interferons. There is some evidence that injecting TNF directly into AIDS-related Kaposi's sarcoma lesions provides some benefit. Many researchers believe the role of this growth factor will be to shrink tumors, enabling other treatments that activate the immune system to destroy malignant cells more effectively.

The side effects with TNF resemble those of other biological treatments: flulike symptoms of shivers, fever, and headache and inflammation at the injection site. People with abdominal disease may experience nausea and vomiting. Less common side effects include a change in blood pressure, rapid heartbeat, mild chest discomfort, and fatigue.

The route of administration is determined by the type and severity of adverse reactions. Intravenous infusion produces longer-lasting and more severe shivering and fevers, but after injection under the skin, fatigue is more common and severe, and skin rash more likely. Fortunately, people who are given daily doses of TNF often find they become able to tolerate the side effects fairly well.

Thymic Hormones. Because the thymus is in many ways the master control center of the body's immune response, some researchers believe that supportive treatment using hormones to regulate the gland may be of value, especially in preventing infections.

Clinical trials have explored the role of two compounds, *thymosin fraction 5* and *thymosin-alpha-1*, in children and adults undergoing cancer therapy or in people with HIV infection before the development of AIDS or other autoimmune diseases.

The side effects associated with thymic hormone treatment are very mild, usually nothing more than inflammation at the injection site. Toxic reactions are rare. People taking these hormones often say that their sense of well-being has improved and that they are better able to function in their daily lives. Their infection rate drops, and they often regain lost weight. Some people even notice an improvement in chronic conditions such as arthritis.

Vaccines. Vaccines are appealing to scientists because they have proved to be so effective in preventing infectious diseases, from smallpox to polio. For cancer, the idea is to design a vaccine that can immunize people against their own tumors. Cancer vaccine development and testing is in its infancy, and although results have been mixed, they are improving and nationwide trials are being planned. One of the most active areas of research involves melanoma vaccines. A few early, small studies indicate that some combination treatments employing a vaccine prolong survival time, and several larger trials are being planned to evaluate melanoma vaccines developed by different groups of scientists. In one study, a vaccine will be combined with interferon treatment. Attempts are also being made to identify people who have been treated for melanoma but are at high risk of recurrence and, therefore, are likely candidates for vaccine treatment.

The Future

Each day, the immune system gives up more of its secrets. Researchers are learning more about how cells multiply and mature and how they exchange messages. Just as important, they are learning about the relationship between the host and the disease, how tumor cells and immune cells interact and how they try to outwit each other in the battle for survival.

Data from worldwide studies of the human gene structure will provide countless opportunities for gene therapy aimed at improving the body's ability to fend off disease. For example, clinical trials show that tumor cells removed from the body can be inserted into genes programmed to make extra quantities of TNF and then reinjected into the body.

For researchers, health care providers, and people with cancer, the promise of biological therapy has been a roller coaster ride. The hope that biological therapy would produce a cure or at least a vaccine has been scaled back to a more reasonable understanding that biological treatments have clear value in certain cancers when given in certain ways. There is no doubt that the role of biological treatment will continue to grow in the years ahead.

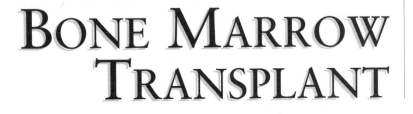

Bone Marrow Transplant

A *bone marrow transplant (BMT)* is the removal of bone marrow from one person and the return of its blood-forming cells later to the same person or the transfer of the blood-forming cells to someone else. Although BMT was developed for people whose defective marrow caused conditions such as aplastic anemia, today about 90 percent of transplants are performed to help treat cancer.

Bone marrow is tissue within the cavities of bones that contains fat (yellow bone marrow) and blood-forming tissue (red bone marrow). Healthy bone marrow tissue constantly replenishes the blood supply and is essential to life. Unfortunately, the amount of drugs or radiation needed to kill cancer cells also destroys bone marrow. Replacing the bone marrow with healthy cells (which find their way from the blood to the marrow) counteracts this adverse effect. BMT, therefore, is not always a treatment in itself, as many people think, but it allows those with cancer to undergo very aggressive therapy.

Exciting Developments

In the 1950s, scientists discovered that red bone marrow drawn from one person could be infused into someone else and that the immature cells (*stem cells*) it contained would shortly begin to produce normal blood cells. In this way, stem cells in the bone marrow that had been destroyed could be replaced and begin turning out oxygen-bearing red blood cells; infection-fighting white blood cells; and platelets, which assist blood clotting.

In the 1960s, when techniques were developed that allowed precise genetic matching of bone marrow recipients and donors, BMT became a viable tool in the treatment of leukemia, a form of cancer that affects blood-manufacturing cells in the bone marrow, lymph nodes, and spleen. By the 1980s, BMT had been used as part of the treatment of other cancers, and today it is considered one of the most exciting and rapidly evolving developments in cancer therapy. Techniques that enhance the recovery process—for example, using new drugs to boost cell production—are making BMT safer and shortening hospital stays. Studies are under way that allow for outpatient care for part of the procedure. More than 500 specialized transplant centers throughout the world perform BMT on a daily basis.

Still, BMT is a very demanding treatment, and the decision to have it is not an easy one to make. BMT requires a tremendous investment of time, energy, and patience. It also demands bravery, because of the risks of rejection, death, and the long-term consequences.

BMT is more successful in some people than in others. Younger people usually do better than older ones. And researchers are discovering that the treatment works best in the earlier stages of disease.

When Is BMT an Option

In some cancers, particularly those involving the blood cells, BMT is used to attack the malignancy directly; acute leukemia, for example, was the first cancer to be treated with BMT. Most often, however, BMT is a *rescue procedure*, replacing destroyed bone marrow tissue when extremely high doses of chemotherapy drugs or radiation have been used. BMT is now used for the following:

- several types of leukemia: acute myelogenous, acute lymphocytic, chronic myelogenous, and chronic lymphocytic leukemias;

- myelodysplastic syndromes;

- multiple myeloma;

- non-Hodgkin's lymphoma and Hodgkin's disease;

- solid tumors, including cancers of the brain, testes, breast, and lung.

Some of these uses—such as those for breast cancer and chronic lymphocytic leukemias—are considered experimental.

Recovery and Cure

About 60 to 70 percent of BMT procedures are successful; the recipients have a smooth recovery and are discharged promptly from the hospital. The long-term response rate varies greatly, however, depending on the type of cancer. For example, the expected cure rate when BMT is performed in the early stages of acute myeloblastic leukemia is about 50 percent; when BMT is done late in the disease, the rate may drop to 10 percent. For brain cancer, the cure rate with BMT is around 30 percent. It is considered too early to predict cure rates for other cancers, such as breast cancer.

Finding a Donor

As more people learn about the success of BMT, more are volunteering to become donors. In one recent year, about 1.5 million volunteers were regis-

Finding a Bone Marrow Transplant Center

Your doctor will refer you to a bone marrow transplant center, but you may prefer to evaluate others as well. Choosing one nearby will help lower the cost and be easier on family members and friends. However, there are some important points to consider besides location. Some centers have more experience with specific cancers. It's helpful to visit the center(s) you are considering. (Most of them will request a "transplant interview" before accepting you.) Speak with the physicians and other staff members. Take along your donor if possible so that both of you will understand the process better. Ask the following questions:

- Does the center have extensive experience in treating the type of cancer I have?

- Has the physician likely to treat me had experience with similar cases?

- Does the center meet the minimal criteria set up by the American Society of Clinical Oncology and the American Society of Hematology, which have jointly recommended standards for BMT centers? (There is no accreditation of BMT units, although the hospitals that house them or are associated with them must meet the general accreditation standards of the Joint Commission on Accreditation of Health Care Organizations.)

- Does the center sponsor support or discussion groups for BMT patients and their families? If not is there a referral service to connect me to such groups or help?

- Is there a waiting list?

tered. Nevertheless, because finding an unrelated donor whose bone marrow is genetically similar is extremely difficult, most people begin their search among family members, particularly their siblings, whose bone marrow is much more likely to be a good match.

Although this solution is the simplest one, it still can be difficult. Family members from around the country or even abroad must be contacted and their blood tested. If a good match is found, it may be necessary to arrange and pay for travel.

Sometimes the family member whose bone marrow matches is not the BMT candidate's favorite person, which can create other problems. For example, you might feel guilty asking a sibling that you have not talked to for years to provide bone marrow. Or a relative may decide not to be a donor, which can create resentment and anger. And if the BMT candidate was adopted, it can be even more difficult to find relatives who are potential donors.

In the early years of BMT, a person without a relative who could be a donor would have to search on his or her own for a volunteer whose bone marrow closely matched. It was like looking for a needle in a haystack and, at best, a haphazard process. Now, with computers and large marrow banks such as the National Bone Marrow Donor Program (see Appendix I,

"Resources"), it is increasingly possible to find that needle. Some communities even host "matching" parties, inviting people to come to a barbecue or pancake breakfast for testing to see whether they might be potential donors.

Testing the Donor

The technique that has improved the matching process is *HLA* (*human leukocyte antigens*) tissue typing. HLAs are produced by HLA genes; they are proteins on cell surfaces that help the cell recognize foreign substances. They thus play a key role in the immune response and in the acceptance of the transplant. The better the match of the donor's and recipient's antigens, the less likely the marrow will be rejected and the fewer complications there will be. Once a match is made, the donor is tested for human immunodeficiency virus (HIV), hepatitis infection, and other diseases that might be spread by the transplanted cells.

The Donor's Responsibility

The donor's job is not easy. He or she must fully understand the scope of the undertaking before agreeing to it. Aside from the actual discomfort of the procedure—which has been described as a toothache-like pain—the donor must be "on call," waiting for the best time to have his or her marrow removed (a procedure called *extraction*), depending on the recipient's blood count and general health.

Most donors are happy that they can help, but some worry that their marrow won't be "good enough" to cure the recipient. Some people also feel responsible for the success or failure of the treatment, as if it were under their control. Although some donors are hesitant to mention it, they may feel ignored, as most of the concern and attention are focused on the recipient.

Types of Transplants

Transplants are categorized according to the source of the bone marrow, which indicates how close a match it is.

Syngeneic Transplant

The most compatible bone marrow is that of an identical twin. There is no risk of rejection of this syngeneic transplant because the twins' HLA genes are the same; the match, therefore, is perfect.

Allogeneic Transplant

An allogeneic transplant is donated by a person chosen through the HLA-typing process. The better the match is, the less the risk of rejection will be. Siblings are always a closer match than parents and are more likely to be compatible than other family members. The best matches also come from someone of the same ancestry. That is, it is more difficult to find a match for people belonging to minority populations, such as those of African or Asian descent, because fewer minorities are in the donor pool at this time. An effort is being made to recruit minorities and encourage them to become donors, so this scarcity may be overcome in the future.

Autologous Transplant

An autologous transplant is the removal of bone marrow from the person with cancer before treatment and its return to him or her after treatment with high doses of chemotherapy or radiation therapy or both. During the weeks that the therapy is under way, the bone marrow cells are frozen.

Although there is no risk of rejection, because the marrow is the person's own, there is a chance of reintroducing cancer cells that remain in the marrow. To minimize this risk, some laboratories treat the marrow with chemotherapy, special antibodies, or other substances before reinfusing it (a procedure called *purging*).

Autologous transplants are still considered experimental but are being used for solid tumors such as cancers of the breast.

A recent development is banking of umbilical cord blood, obtained when a baby is born, for use at a later time, should the child need high-dose chemotherapy or radiation therapy. Eventually, allogeneic transplant of these immature blood cells may be possible.

A variation of BMT is *blood stem cell harvesting*, now being studied. Immature blood cells are withdrawn from the recipient's blood and later, in the laboratory, are stimulated with natural chemicals called growth factors to produce enough stem cells for a transfusion.

Candidates for BMT

Since you have absolutely no bone marrow for some time during the BMT and the number of circulating blood cells takes a while to return to normal after the marrow is transplanted, you must be strong enough to withstand a variety of potential complications as well as endure the aggressive treatment. With this in mind, physicians at BMT centers carefully screen each candidate.

Age

The risk of complications generally increases with age. BMT is commonly performed in people up to age 50, provided they meet certain health criteria. In some cases, BMT is approved for people age 55 or even 60. The maximum age has been increasing, and it is not unreasonable to expect the age limit to climb as techniques become better and success rates improve. Children often tolerate the procedure better than adults do.

Sex

For unexplained reasons, women tend to tolerate BMT somewhat better than men do.

General Health

People who undergo BMT must be in reasonably good health aside from their cancer and not have had infections recently that may have weakened them.

How Much Does BMT Cost?

Typically, a BMT procedure requires about four to six weeks in the hospital and costs $75,000 to $200,000. Whether or not a transplant will be covered, especially for cancers in which its use is considered "experimental," varies widely from one health care plan to another. And even when the cost of the transplant is reimbursed by insurance, there still can be staggering out-of-pocket, uncovered expenses such as return visits to the transplant center and travel and housing for family members who want to be nearby during the procedure.

Fungal infections, such as thrush in the mouth, can be especially dangerous and usually rule out BMT or are a good reason to postpone it.

Intestinal difficulties are another reason that a person may not be accepted for BMT, because the high doses of anticancer drugs or radiation can damage tissue in the intestinal tract, making existing intestinal problems worse.

Pneumonia usually rules out or postpones BMT, even if the patient is under age 30, because the lungs are especially vulnerable to complications after BMT.

Therapy Trial

Chemotherapy or radiation precedes BMT. A course of treatment with regular doses of either therapy will reveal whether a person's cancer is responsive to that therapy.

Emotional Resilience

BMT centers differ in how they evaluate a potential recipient's ability to cope with the psychological stress of the procedure. Some insist on psychiatric interviews. Some ask potential recipients to complete a questionnaire that assesses whether they are emotionally capable of enduring the BMT procedure and can cope with the uncertainty of the outcome. At many centers a social worker evaluates every candidate and decides whether a consultation with a psychiatrist would be helpful.

The Procedure

Allogeneic BMT begins with a pretreatment or *conditioning treatment*. Very-high-dose chemotherapy or radiation therapy or both are given to kill the cancer cells, which destroys the bone marrow. This treatment also suppresses the immune system temporarily, which allows your body to accept the transplanted cells.

In the case of autologous BMT, the preconditioning treatment will be preceded by *harvesting* or retrieving bone marrow from you. This step may be accomplished on an outpatient basis.

QUESTIONS

TO ASK

What to Ask the Doctor About BMT

When considering a bone marrow transplant, ask your doctor the following questions:

- Is BMT the best option for me? Why?
- What are the chances of success in my case?
- Is BMT considered experimental for my disease or my type of cancer? Why?
- What are the risks of the BMT?
- What type of pretreatment conditioning will I receive?
- What is the estimated cost? What costs, if any, will be covered by my insurance or health plan?
- What side effects might I expect? How severe are they likely to be? How long will they last? Can they be controlled by medicine or other means?
- When will I be able to visit with people? Participate in social functions? Return to work?
- What type of monitoring will be required after BMT? How often?
- What are the chances that my cancer will recur even after BMT?

Chemotherapy

Most commonly, cyclophosphamide is the anticancer drug used for the conditioning treatment. Other options include dimethylbusulfan, cytosine arabinoside, toposide, melphalan, carmustine, and nitrosourea (see Chapter 17, "Chemotherapy").

The conditioning treatment usually takes three to five days, during which time you will be hospitalized. Such side effects as nausea, vomiting, and diarrhea are nearly universal, and drugs called *antiemetics* are given to ease the distress. Because large doses are prescribed, you will feel heavily sedated. Intravenous fluids are often given to prevent dehydration and to provide nutrients. Bladder inflammation and bleeding may occur. Because cyclophosphamide can be toxic to the heart, electrocardiograms may be taken periodically. Temporary hair loss, which may affect all body hair—including that on the head, eyebrows, legs, armpits, and pubic areas—is common. (For a more detailed explanation of the side effects of chemotherapy and ways of coping with them, see Chapter 17, "Chemotherapy.")

Radiation Therapy

Total body radiation (TBI)—the use of high-energy x-rays to kill cancer cells throughout the body—may be given alone or in combination with chemotherapy in one session or over several days. Although the side effects are less severe than those following chemotherapy, nausea and vomiting are not unusual. (For more information on the side effects of radiation and ways of coping with them, see Chapter 16, "Radiation.")

QUESTIONS

TO   ASK

Treatment Decisions

Deciding whether to undergo BMT can seem like an overwhelming decision. Here are some questions to consider:

- Can my cancer be treated by any other method besides high-dose radiation or chemotherapy?
- Is a good donor match likely?
- Am I strong enough, or can I get strong enough, for the procedure?
- Does my family understand the length of time, the expense, and the effort of this treatment?
- Do I have a strong support system in place to help with the physical and emotional side effects?

Donor Preparation and Procedures

The timing of getting the marrow from the donor to the recipient is critical. If marrow transfer is delayed for even 24 to 48 hours, the recipient could die. Therefore, when the recipient is nearing the end of the pretreatment, the donor is admitted to the hospital.

To extract the marrow, the donor is taken to the operating room and given a general or spinal anesthesia. The surgeon then inserts a large needle into the pelvic bones, which are rich in red marrow. As many as 200 punctures may be needed to gather the one to two pints of marrow needed.

The procedure takes about an hour and a half. Afterward the donor may receive a blood transfusion and, after the effects of the anesthesia have worn off, pain medication. He or she is usually discharged from the hospital a day or so after the extraction and can return to normal activity within a few days. Antibiotics may be prescribed to prevent infection. There are few risks to the donor, other than those related to the anesthesia.

The Transplant

Marrow harvested from the patient or a donor contains some undesirable materials like fat, which can enter the lungs and cause problems, so the marrow must be carefully filtered before being given to the recipient. The best transplant samples contain many stem cells, which reproduce, and few adult cells, which do not reproduce.

When the marrow sample is ready, a tiny tube is inserted through a needle into the recipient's vein, through which the cells are transfused over about an hour and a half, much like a blood transfusion. No anesthesia is needed. The transplanted cells gradually make their way into your marrow. The new marrow usually begins to produce new cells in a week or so, but it takes several weeks for the number of red and white blood cells and platelets in the bloodstream to return to normal and resume their functions. It is during this three- or four-week period that the most life-threatening complications are likely to occur.

After the Transplant

For several weeks following the transfusion, the focus of health care is on maintaining your health until the transplant begins to function. The following are common short-term complications and a brief discussion of how the health care team works to prevent or treat these problems. Although most people survive them, no one should consider BMT without recognizing that complications may occur.

Infection. The most serious early danger is infection, so recipients often stay for three to six weeks in a *laminar airflow room*, a special sealed-off hospital room in which an air filter continuously removes bacteria and other impurities. Because of the risk of infection, visitors are limited, and those who are permitted must wear sterile gowns and masks. You are closely monitored for fever and other signs of infection and receive antibiotics as well as red blood cells and platelets.

Nausea and Vomiting. Almost everyone who undergoes BMT experiences lethargy, nausea, and vomiting because of the high doses of chemotherapy and/or radiation that precede the transplant. Mucositis, an inflammation of the membranes lining the mouth, causes intense pain and is a common side effect. Nurses often help you rinse your mouth with a saline solution every few hours and administer pain medications.

Veno-occlusive Disease. According to some studies, a third of all transplant recipients with a malignancy develop *veno-occlusive disease*, a very serious disease of the liver. Although it can be fatal, two-thirds of those who get it survive. It is most common during the first three weeks after BMT. Symptoms include weight gain and pain in the upper right side. To cope with this disease, for which there is no treatment, doctors immediately decrease the stress on the liver, which may mean discontinuing certain drugs designed to prevent other complications, such as infection.

Rejection. One of the major risks of allogeneic BMT is that the recipient's immune system will reject the transplanted, "foreign" marrow. If the donors are unrelated, which is increasingly common, the likelihood is greater that the new marrow will be rejected. Initially, the marrow appears to function, but then it fails. Blood counts may not return to normal, or if they do, the number of blood cells suddenly drops. In about half the cases, an immediate second transplant is successful.

To avoid rejection, your ability to fight the donor cells is decreased with immunity-suppressing drugs.

Graft Versus Host Disease (GVHD). In about half the BMT recipients, rejection occurs in reverse; that is, the white blood cells (T-lymphocytes) in the newly transplanted marrow (the *graft*) recognize you, the BMT recipient (*host*), as foreign and launch an attack against your own cells.

Often the skin, liver, and gastrointestinal tract are affected, and symptoms range from a mild skin rash to severe diarrhea to life-threatening liver damage and hemorrhage. Initially, GVHD may be difficult to diagnose, because the symptoms so closely resemble other complications or side effects of the chemotherapy and radiation therapy. Most people survive acute GVHD and the disease disappears. However, severe symptoms are associated with a poor prognosis and about 16 percent of recipients die of GVHD.

The risk increases in those over the age of 30. Generally, the older both the recipient and the donor are, the greater the risk. It is also higher among those whose donors are of the opposite sex. For unexplained reasons, female recipients whose female donors previously were pregnant have a higher risk. The less well matched the donor and recipient are, the greater the risk of GVHD.

Pneumonia. A grave danger for BMT recipients is *adult respiratory distress syndrome (ARDS)*, a kind of pneumonia. The symptoms are similar to other types of pneumonia, but ARDS usually comes on more rapidly, with such symptoms as a dry cough and difficult and rapid breathing. It occurs about two months after the transplant, after you have been discharged from the hospital and appear to be doing well. It is usually treated with steroid drugs. ARDS is the most common cause of death in the all-important 100-day window after a transplant.

The most frequent cause of pneumonia is infection by the *cytomegalovirus (CMV)*. Since it is such a grave danger, some physicians suggest screening potential marrow donors to make sure they do not have the virus.

Long-Term Complications

For about 70 percent of recipients, everything goes smoothly and they return home promptly, but the long-term response rate varies greatly.

Months or years after an apparently successful transplant, complications can occur. After a year, the complication rate drops to about 5 to 10 percent, and after two years, it declines even more, to less than 5 percent. The following are common long-term complications:

Chronic Graft Versus Host Disease. About one-quarter to one-half of people who survive longer than 100 days develop chronic GVHD, and about 5 to 10 percent of them have it severely. Skin symptoms (temporary hardening and darkening, a kind of mottled appearance), dry mouth and eyes, infections, and weight loss are typical. Problems also may arise in the intestinal tract, including the esophagus and liver. Lung problems can be serious, even life threatening.

There is no convincingly effective therapy for the chronic form of GVHD. Treatment with drugs that suppress the immune system may be given for as long as two years, but their use is a delicate balancing act between the benefits of the drugs and their side effects.

Some experts believe the key to preventing chronic GVHD is in effective pretreatment, which involves removing or inactivating the T-lymphocytes, a component of the immune system, so that they won't attack the transplanted marrow.

Cataracts. Very high doses of radiation can cause cataracts, a clouding of the eye's natural lens, as long as five years after treatment. This condition can usually be corrected surgically.

Fertility Problems. Because high doses of radiation and chemotherapy make people sterile, some men about to undergo BMT should consider banking their sperm before the pretreatment. For women the issue is more difficult. Retrieving eggs requires surgery and is not generally recommended for female BMT candidates. And even if a woman successfully stored her eggs, it would be questionable whether her uterus could later support a pregnancy after such aggressive cancer treatment. Women under age 25, however, often maintain their fertility if they do not receive high doses of radiation to the pelvis. In children, BMT may delay or arrest puberty.

Learning Problems. Experts notice a tendency among children to develop permanent learning disabilities, especially if they have received high doses of radiation to the brain or if they have taken high doses of the drug methotrexate. Therefore, it is becoming common practice to test for learning disabilities as soon as is feasible in children who have undergone BMT.

Emotional Problems. Isolation is an immediate obstacle in the hospital and afterward, and it can be six months or more before the recipient is free to go out into public where germs proliferate. But it's the longer-term problems that can hamper your quality of life. Studies of BMT recipients have concluded that sexual problems, occupational disability, and mood disturbances are not unusual. In general, older people have a harder time returning to a normal life.

Memory Lapses. Memory problems, poor concentration, and shortened attention span may follow BMT. Although such problems as slowed reaction time and difficulties in problem solving and reasoning are rarely severe, they can last for several years.

Recurrence

The main reason for BMT failure is recurrence of the original cancer. The relapse rate has been reported to be as high as 70 percent for acute leukemia if the recipient was in relapse at the time of BMT. But relapse has dipped as low as 10 to 12 percent among recipients who have undergone BMT when their leukemia was in its first remission.

New cancers at other sites also can occur after BMT. Of some 9,700 BMT recipients in the International Bone Marrow Transplant Registry, about 100 developed a new malignancy during the five to 10 years of follow up.

Some experts believe that the treatments designed to destroy the original cancer—radiation, chemotherapy, and immunosuppression—may predispose a person to develop another cancer. To put this risk in perspective, remember that the initial treatments were often the only hope for eradicating the original cancer.

Nutrition and BMT

Because of appetite loss, nausea, vomiting, diarrhea, and other side effects of aggressive treatment, nutritional monitoring and counseling are vital before, during, and after BMT. Taking into account individual differences, experts offer the following suggestions:

- Meal replacement products are not well tolerated immediately after BMT. Within a few weeks, though, such supplements may be helpful (see Chapter 26, "Food and Nutrition").

- Total parenteral nutrition (TPN) or intravenous feeding may be necessary to ensure an adequate intake of fluid and nutrients.

- Because nausea and vomiting can make eating difficult, try clear liquids, salty foods, and fruits such as watermelon, and avoid very sweet and greasy foods. Drink and eat slowly and avoid sudden movements, which can precipitate vomiting.

- A dry mouth can make it difficult to chew and swallow foods such as meat and bread. Gravies, broths, or sauces make these foods easier to swallow. Citric acid from lemonade or sugarless lemon drops increase saliva production. Also try eating crackers, plain meat, and bananas.

- Thick saliva makes swallowing difficult. Try an all-liquid diet. Hot tea with lemon or sour lemon drops can help break up the thick saliva.

- Changes in the way foods taste are widespread and may last as long as two months after BMT, but it's the first 25 days when it interferes most with eating. (Adults suffer changes in taste perception more often than children do.) Interestingly, smell perception isn't affected, so foods with an attractive aroma may stimulate your appetite. As long as there is no inflammation in your mouth, strongly flavored foods are the most appealing. Avoid bland, unsalted, and overcooked foods. Eventually, taste perception returns to normal. Sweet taste comes back first, followed by bitter, sour, and salty.

- If possible, work with a dietitian to ensure an adequate intake of food and liquids.

Coping with the Treatment and Its Aftermath

After BMT, many of the recipients who are placed in laminar airflow rooms feel especially isolated. There, in the sterile calm, you may realize, perhaps for the first time, the seriousness of your condition and the demands of the treatment.

Feelings of isolation can be extremely stressful for even the most emotionally stable person, but the combination of isolation and physical discomfort is particularly distressing. Most BMT centers have a social worker available to help you and your family and friends cope during the hospital stay. In addition, the center's staff members are usually trained to deal with the unique issues surrounding BMT.

Although a few bone marrow recipients sail through with few psychological repercussions, many become quite depressed and anxious. Some experts believe that being informed beforehand about the entire process and what emotional upheaval to expect will help you cope better. Then you won't be surprised by your physical and emotional reactions, and you'll be able to accept feelings that you otherwise might construe as abnormal.

Getting and Giving Support

The recovery period following BMT is quite prolonged. Recovery takes six months to a year, and even then, the return to work may be delayed another six months or longer. During this time, joining a support group can be extremely valuable. In a group, you'll discover that most of your feelings are universal, or at least not uncommon. You also can share your feelings in a safe environment and learn ways that others have used to cope with their disease successfully (see Chapter 13, "Your Support Network").

Today experts in BMT recognize that the family members or friends involved in a recipient's care are under enormous pressure and have serious emotional needs as well. They often feel exhausted in their roles as supporters and caregivers and, sometimes, as stand-in breadwinners. And frequently they believe they must keep a stiff upper lip. This kind of forbearance can take a toll on their health and emotional well-being (see Chapter 32, "Issues for Family and Friends").

Support groups can give family and friends, too, an opportunity to talk about their experiences and learn how others have dealt with similar issues. A good transplant center is likely to offer support groups for BMT recipients and to provide outreach programs for family members or be able to refer them to counseling services, which many BMT recipients take advantage of for many months.

It is important to remember, though, that ongoing support groups are not helpful for everyone. Some BMT recipients remain friends with fellow recipients, drawing strength from them. But others want to cut off such relationships once they leave the hospital, feeling that being around others who have undergone BMT only reminds them of all the unpleasant possibilities.

Others draw strength from each other. Frequently, people who "graduate" from BMT centers volunteer to help other BMT recipients. They enjoy the feeling of repaying the center that saved their lives.

Quality of Life

Because the side effects of BMT can be seriously debilitating for some people, the difficulties raise questions about the quality of life after BMT. It is especially important for those contemplating the procedure to be aware that their life may not return to normal following their recovery from the actual procedure. Nausea, vomiting, poor appetite, and changes in taste may be nagging side effects, as can the skin itching and mottling that even makeup can't conceal, sleep problems, diarrhea or constipation, mouth sores, and

CASE HISTORIES

TRUE STORIES

How One Woman Coped

Jean was 25 when she was diagnosed with leukemia. When her doctor suggested aggressive chemotherapy followed by BMT, she set to work finding a donor. Fortunately, her sister was a good match.

Jean's goal was to survive so that she could care for her four-year-old twins, one of whom had undergone heart surgery the year before. She decided to "go for the cure" as soon as possible, so other complications wouldn't weaken her.

She asked question after question, including how to best help her husband care for their sons when she had to be hospitalized. Jean made good use of the social worker at the BMT unit at her hospital, conferring with her frequently.

A combination of humor and grit helped Jean get through the ordeal. She joked about windy days, because her wig wouldn't stay on. She had to learn to deal with adults who made cruel comments about her mottled skin. Nonetheless, everything went well for about eight months after the transplant, and then she developed chronic GVHD. She was fatigued and unable to do things for her children, such as drive them to kindergarten and take part in social functions. She felt she was not contributing to the family, even though she spent many hours with them. The goal then became how to control the GVHD. Jean now accepts the fact that she often cannot do everything she could before BMT. But she hopes that her strength will return or at least improve.

She credits her very close-knit family, especially her husband, with helping her keep a grip on reality. He has taken over many of the child care tasks and keeps the atmosphere as upbeat and cooperative as possible.

Her bottom line: Even though she has a chronic disease, Jean firmly believes the BMT was worth doing. She can still take part in many aspects of her family's life together. And she values being with them, every day.

dizzy spells. Joints can be stiff. Headaches, blurred vision, and shortness of breath may be a problem.

But not everyone has these experiences, and many BMT recipients do report a return to normal. In one survey, about 93 percent of recipients for whom BMT was successful said they could perform normal activities within six months. Eighty percent said their social activities were not impaired or just slightly affected. Severe or even moderate pain was uncommon. Sixty-five percent had returned to work full or part time.

To improve the outlook even more, researchers say they are focusing on clarifying areas of unresolved psychological needs. Then, social workers and others can concentrate on those needs and improve the overall quality of life for more and more people who choose this often life-saving procedure.

COMBINATION TREATMENTS

Today it is uncommon for cancer to be treated by only one method. Combining two or more types of treatments—such as surgery, radiation, and chemotherapy—may be more effective than a single therapy alone. Under certain conditions combination or *multimodal* therapy not only can achieve a greater likelihood of cure than a single approach, but can do it with less damage to vital organs and tissues.

A dramatic example of the success of combining therapies is the treatment of osteosarcoma, a cancer of the bone found most often in young people. Not long ago, amputation of the affected limb was the only treatment. Today radiation therapy directed to the tumor and chemotherapy delivered through the bloodstream may destroy the cancer without loss of the limb containing the tumor. Another example is the change in treatment of early-stage breast cancer from mastectomy (removal of the entire breast) to lumpectomy (excision of the lump) followed by radiation therapy. This has allowed many women to retain their natural contour without compromising the possibility of cure.

Why Treatments Are Combined

Doctors often combine two or three standard treatments—and in some cases, experimental therapies—in situations where

- one treatment may be more effective at a certain stage than another;

- one may enhance the effectiveness of another;

- one may reduce the extent or intensity of another;

- one alone may not affect the tumor.

Multimodal therapy requires a well-planned strategy designed to exploit the unique qualities of each of the component treatments. It should balance their strengths and weaknesses, thereby increasing the likelihood of success.

The first questions physicians must answer when planning multimodal therapy are

- What kind of cancer is it?

- How big is the tumor?

- How far has it spread locally?

- How likely is it to spread to distant organs?

This process is called *staging* the tumor. (See Chapter 2, "The Language of Cancer.") Depending on the stage, the oncologist chooses a *primary* or *definitive* therapy, the one that might have the greatest impact on the cancer. Then one or more other therapies may be selected to increase the possibility of cure. The *secondary* treatments may come before, after, or at the same time as the primary one.

Often the therapies are equally important, so it is hard to say which one should be called primary. In certain breast cancers, for example, both surgery and radiation are essential; omitting either one could lead to failure.

Multimodal approaches can be designed to work in various ways. One treatment can fill in the gaps of another. For example, radiation therapy is generally most effective at the edges, or margins, of a tumor, where the bulk of the tumor is small and the cells are well supplied with blood vessels. (Blood brings in the oxygen required for radiation to work.) However, radiation therapy may not be as effective in the center, or *core*, of a tumor, where there is a dense collection of cells with a poor oxygen supply (see Chapter 16, "Radiation"). Surgery, on the other hand, can remove the tumor, but in some cases it may be unable to eliminate all cancer cells surrounding it without cutting out too much normal tissue. Therefore, the two treatments can cover for each other's weaknesses.

Combining therapies may enhance the immediate and long-term effects of both. For example, the chemotherapy drugs fluorouracil (5-FU) and mitomycin C (Mutamycin) can make certain kinds of cancer cells more susceptible to radiation and are often given along with radiation therapy.

Combining two therapies may also allow for a less intense treatment than would be required if one were given alone.

The mixture and sequence of therapies depend chiefly on the risk of spread and on whether the cancer cells are dividing rapidly or slowly—along with such factors as your age, general health, and ability to tolerate the therapy. The various modalities may interact in ways that vary with the kind of cancer and its stage. Because there are so many aspects to consider, physicians caution patients against comparing their treatment plan with that of another person, even if he or she has the same kind of cancer.

Of greatest importance is that the doctor discuss the whole treatment plan and any options with you in advance. Of course, some changes may be necessary during treatment. For example, if a you seem to be responding unusually well to a certain drug, your doctor may alter the dose and schedule

Terms You May Hear

The following terms are used to describe how several therapies may be used together.

- The words *combination* and *multimodal* are often used interchangeably, although they may have somewhat different meanings. *Combination* sometimes describes a single treatment that incorporates more than one variety of the same therapy. For example, chemotherapy may include two or more different drugs, or radiation may be delivered from an external source and an implant. *Multimodal* refers only to the use of two or more kinds of therapy (for example, surgery and chemotherapy). It may consist of a sequence of treatments, such as surgery followed by radiation therapy; *simultaneous* treatments, such as radiation and chemotherapy given during the same time period; and various combinations of type and timing, such as alternating courses of radiation therapy and chemotherapy.

- *Adjuvant therapy* refers to giving a secondary treatment after the primary treatment, such as radiation after surgery.

- *Neoadjuvant therapy* is sometimes referred to as *up-front treatment* because it is given before the primary therapy. Sometimes both neoadjuvant and adjuvant therapies are used. One recent approach for treating advanced lung cancer is surgery "surrounded" or "sandwiched" by chemotherapy.

to take advantage of it. Of course, the regimen will change as well if you experience excessive or unexpected toxicity. For these reasons your primary physician or oncologist must carefully monitor your response and adjust the treatment strategy as needed.

Combination therapy calls for a team approach using the expertise of several doctors to ensure the most effective type and timing of treatments with the least risk. The primary physician, radiologist, pathologist, surgeon, oncologist, and other specialists confer to tailor therapy for each patient. Among the issues they discuss is how to integrate conflicting treatments. For example, radiation therapy before surgery may help to shrink a tumor and thereby make it easier to remove surgically, but it also can permanently affect other vital organs or slow the healing process or both. The surgeon and the radiologist work together to assess these possibilities.

In the ideal situation members of the team don't simply manage their part and then turn the treatment over to the next specialist in line. Nor do they administer one therapy and then try to decide what to do next. Preferably, all the specialists will express their views and recommendations at the beginning, reach agreement with you on the treatment plan and its details, and continue to consult with each other and you throughout the administration of therapy. This is why assessing a physician's willingness to work with others is important when choosing the primary doctor (see Chapter 11, "Getting Help: Who, What, Where, and How").

How Combinations Evolved

It was once believed that cancer started in a local site, spread throughout the region by following a direct path to nearby lymph nodes (where its progress was at least partly blocked), and only much later extended in an orderly way out into other parts of the body. For many years surgery was the only accepted treatment for cancer, on the assumption that the disease could be cured if the local tumor was removed.

When scientists discovered that x-rays and radium could kill growing cells, physicians attempted to treat cancer with external radiation or implanted radium instead of surgery. The results were no better than those of surgery alone. However, researchers soon learned that adding radiation therapy to surgery for breast cancer, for example, produced better results than either treatment alone. Later, the same combination proved helpful for lung and colorectal cancers.

These results led to the revised view that cancer does not always move directly and progressively outward from its primary site (see Chapter 33, "Metastasis and Recurrence"). Instead, cancer cells may travel from the local site to a distant area through the blood and lymphatic systems. And they may do so before the primary tumor is discovered or produces symptoms. It has been estimated that as many as 70 percent of people with certain solid tumors may have such microscopic metastases when they are first diagnosed. These distant colonies may be so tiny they cannot be detected by available tests. (Fortunately, all these tumor cells do not develop into invasive cancer.)

Thus, the reason for recurrences—and the need for another kind of treatment—became clear. Surgery and radiation therapy both act locally; neither addresses the problem of tumor cells that escape surgery or that have already established themselves elsewhere. Something more is needed.

That something was found in the 1960s. Research showed that certain drugs could kill cancer cells throughout the body. Doctors began combining chemotherapy with surgery for advanced stages of breast cancer, and the outlook for people with this disease improved.

These results quickly led to combining surgery and chemotherapy for many cancers, beginning with those of the head and neck. Such tumors had continued to have a high relapse rate even after doctors began treating them aggressively with surgery and radiation. A combination of chemotherapy with surgery, however, achieved startling results. The size of more than three-fourths of tumors so treated was reduced by at least 50 percent when chemotherapy was given berfore surgery, and one tumor in every five was eradicated.

Although multimodal treatment is now the most common approach, some cancers and certain circumstances call for a single type of treatment. For example, early-stage skin cancer is curable with surgery alone. Similarly, certain types of leukemia and lymphoma can be cured using chemotherapy or radiation therapy alone. In these situations multimodal therapy would be unnecessary and could be detrimental.

What Lies Ahead?

Cancer specialists are constantly adjusting, refining, and investigating ways to improve treatment planning, primarily through the use of clinical research tri-

Questions to Ask

Multimodal therapy is not a standard recipe for treatment but a strategy that must be tailored to your unique situation. The answers to the following questions will help you understand your treatment plan. You will also want assurance that you are getting the teamwork that combination treatments require. Your primary physician or oncologist can answer these questions.

- Why is multimodal therapy being recommended for me? Does this mean my cancer has spread or is likely to recur?

- What is the evidence that multimodal treatment is best for my kind of cancer?

- What are the major side effects? How long will they last? Are any permanent?

- Who are the people on my treatment team? Did they agree on the details of the proposed plan? Will they all be involved throughout? Who will monitor the different types of treatment?

- If I get better after the first kind of treatment, can I skip the next one?

- Will the first treatment have side effects that may affect the second treatment? If I get radiation or chemotherapy first, will I have to delay surgery? For how long? How will it affect my recovery?

- What if I choose not to have additional treatment?

- What is the timetable for treatments? How long do I wait in between? How long will the whole plan take? Will I have to be hospitalized? Can any of the treatment be done on an outpatient basis? Will I be able to continue working? Will I be able to travel?

- How much will it cost? Is my treatment plan covered by my health care plan?

- Is there a clinical research trial available for my type of cancer?

als (see Chapter 21, "Investigational Treatments"). One of the newest developments is to add biological therapy—drugs that bolster the body's natural immune defenses—to the mix (see Chapter 18, "Biological Therapies").

Hormones or hormone suppressants are being added to enhance chemotherapy in some multimodal plans for cancers that are influenced by their hormonal environment, such as cancers of the breast, uterus, prostate, thyroid, and kidney. Another treatment being used increasingly is bone marrow transplantation to replace vital stem cells that are destroyed by high doses of chemotherapy (see Chapter 19, "Bone Marrow Transplant").

Neoadjuvant Therapy

Because surgery was for so long the only treatment for cancer, most people still assume that it is always the physician's first and most important weapon. This is not always the case. Surgery is not the first in a sequence of therapies with certain cancers and specific treatment circumstances.

If there is a suspicion that your cancer has spread, your physician may attempt to eliminate distant colonies of cancer cells by ordering radiation therapy or chemotherapy before surgery. Radiation therapy or chemotherapy may also be used before surgery to reduce the size of a very large tumor so that less drastic surgery is required. Doctors sometimes call this *debulking* surgery.

Radiation Therapy

Doctors may prescribe neoadjuvant radiation therapy when they are concerned about cancer cells becoming dislodged during surgery and spreading elsewhere in the body. The radiation not only prevents these cells from reproducing if they are displaced, but also can shrink tumors so they are easier to remove.

Chemotherapy

Chemotherapy before surgery or radiation is infrequent, but it can be useful in shrinking cancers that would otherwise require drastic or extensive surgery. Neoadjuvant chemotherapy is also being evaluated in cancers that are not expected to respond well to other therapies.

Timing Treatments

Treatment schedules vary widely, depending on the type of cancer, the extent of spread, and your physical condition. The timing of any combination depends on how each therapy works and how it relates to the others. Radiation treatment may precede surgery by only a few days or even hours. On the other hand, several months of chemotherapy may precede radiation therapy (in certain head and neck cancers) or surgery (particularly for brain tumors).

Neoadjuvant radiation is usually given in the smallest possible doses over the shortest time period, to destroy cancer cells with minimal side effects and the least delay before surgery. A typical schedule might consist of radiation therapy five days a week for two weeks, followed by a two-week recovery period before surgery.

Advantages

Neoadjuvant therapy has several advantages:

- People may tolerate radiation therapy or chemotherapy better before surgery because they are usually stronger and in a better nutritional state.

- The blood supply hasn't been interrupted by surgery, so chemotherapy can reach the tumor in high concentrations. A good oxygen supply via the bloodstream also makes cancer cells more susceptible to radiation.

- Large numbers of rapidly growing cells can be destroyed.

- Neoadjuvant therapy provides a guide for later treatment. For example, a good response to chemotherapy before surgery usually means a good response to chemotherapy afterward.

Disadvantages

Neoadjuvant therapy does have disadvantages:

- It can mask the true extent of the disease. Reduction of the tumor makes it harder for the surgeon and the pathologist to determine where its original margins were; thus, the operation may not be extensive enough.

- When radiation therapy is provided first, it may make proper staging impossible.

- Other treatment may be delayed or limited, sometimes seriously. This is a minor disadvantage if the first treatment produces no complications, and the second treatment is postponed only for the normal time needed to administer the first.

- Immune defenses may be weakened just when they are especially needed to promote recovery from surgery.

Risks and Complications

All cancer therapies have some side effects and can cause complications, but combining them doesn't necessarily pose greater risks. However, where a certain therapy is more toxic when used with another, the physician chooses it only if the benefits outweigh the added burden of side effects.

Radiation therapy or chemotherapy given first in the treatment plan may exaggerate some of the potential long-term and permanent side effects of surgery. These include such complications as adhesions of tissues, fibrosis, abscesses, and fistulas.

Radiation therapy may trigger side effects from subsequent chemotherapy. Doxorubicin (Adriamycin), for example, given weeks after radiation therapy may be followed by a sunburnlike reaction of the more sensitive skin in the area treated with radiation.

One of the greatest risks of neoadjuvant therapy is that it will be ineffective or produce intolerable side effects. Both possibilities should be part of the treatment planning decision.

Knowledgeable physicians, careful monitoring during treatment, use of the safest and most effective doses, and continuous teamwork are the keys to preventing or managing most complications.

Adjuvant Therapy

Adjuvant therapy is a kind of one-two punch. First, definitive primary treatment removes the tumor. Then either a supplemental local treatment kills any cancer cells remaining in the immediate area or a systemic treatment destroys cancer cells in other parts of the body. A common sequence is surgery followed by radiation, chemotherapy, or both. The choices depend on the type of tumor, whether there is a danger of recurrence, if it is largely local or systemic, and how rapidly the cancer cells are growing.

Timing

Chemotherapy usually begins as soon as possible after surgery, allowing time for a necessary degree of recovery. Postsurgical radiation therapy, however, must be delayed until the wound has healed. (Chemotherapy may sometimes follow radiation therapy.) However, a long delay may lower the chances of cure.

Advantages and Disadvantages

Performing surgery first allows the surgeon, pathologist, and radiologist to review the results of surgery, looking at the size and type of the tumor that was removed and examining cells from the surrounding area. This direct analysis helps them to determine whether postoperative radiation therapy will be helpful and to define the precise target area. The team can also identify those who won't benefit from radiation therapy and who should therefore be spared the exposure.

A disadvantage to surgery first is that it may reduce the oxygen supply to tumor cells, making them resistant to radiation therapy. In specific cases it has other disadvantages; for example, certain kinds of abdominal surgery may make the small intestine more susceptible to damage from radiation therapy.

Risks and Complications

Adjunctive chemotherapy and radiation therapy may have the same side effects as either treatment given alone, but they don't necessarily have any additional ones when combined. Nor do they aggravate the consequences of previous surgery, as long as adequate time is allowed for postoperative recovery. Conversely, the acute and long-term effects of surgery don't seem to increase or change the side effects of chemotherapy or radiation therapy.

Intraoperative Radiation Therapy

Radiation is sometimes used during an operation to treat the tumor and the surrounding area directly (see Chapter 16, "Radiation"). After the tumor has been exposed or removed but before the surgical wound is closed, the radiologist may direct a single high dose of radiation directly to the tumor site while holding normal skin, tissues, and organs aside or otherwise shielding them. Sometimes this *intraoperative therapy* is given in addition to postoperative external radiation therapy. Intraoperative radiation therapy is being used in cancers of the breast, colon, rectum, stomach, brain, pancreas, and female reproductive organs.

Radiation Therapy and Chemotherapy

When there is a known likelihood of recurrence or clear evidence that cancer has spread, doctors may combine radiation and chemotherapy to treat both the primary cancer and any potential disease. Depending on the extent of the cancer, these treatments may even be used without surgery.

In some cancers both radiation therapy and chemotherapy are advantageous because each attacks different "volumes" of cells—that is, large tumor masses versus microscopic scattered cells. Chemotherapy given first can shrink a tumor to make it more susceptible to radiation therapy, which tends to work best against smaller tumors.

The effects of chemotherapy and radiation therapy also supplement each other, depending on the cancer cells' rate of growth. Radiation therapy works better against older and slower-growing cells; chemotherapy is best against the younger, more rapidly growing ones.

In some cases the two therapies are used because one makes the other possible. In head and neck cancer, for example, chemotherapy may be given for a few months before radiation therapy begins. Or chemotherapy may be given simultaneously with radiation therapy to make the cells more vulnerable to the radiation. For instance, rectal cancer is often treated simultaneously with fluorouracil (5-FU), mitomycin C (Mutamycin), and radiation. Here chemotherapy and radiation are combined because the total effect seems to be greater than the sum of the parts.

Staying with the Plan

Occasionally, people stop their cancer treatment or fail to keep their medical appointments. Those undergoing multimodal therapy are especially vulnerable to this kind of noncompliance, because the treatments are often long term, inconvenient, and expensive—not just in medical costs but in out-of-pocket costs, such as transportation to the doctor's office.

Unfortunately, some people who respond dramatically to the first part of a treatment plan may think that they are cured and don't need to proceed with adjuvant therapy, especially if the next treatment is expected to have unpleasant side effects. Multimodal therapy, however, is an overall strategy that must include all its interlocking parts to be successful.

CHAPTER

INVESTIGATIONAL TREATMENTS

Scientific studies involving humans are crucial to conquering cancer. Over the last 40 years, such investigations, called *clinical trials*, have led to a greater understanding of how cancer progresses, the development of more precise methods of detecting and diagnosing it, and the planning of highly effective prevention and treatment strategies.

Clinical trials are designed to follow the tenets of ethical medical practice and to provide nothing less than the current *standard of treatment*—that is, the therapy that oncologists, the National Cancer Institute, the Food and Drug Administration, and the American Cancer Society agree is the most effective and safe. In fact, since new drugs are approved and regimens are altered continuously, many people enter a trial to ensure they will receive the most current therapy available.

The potential benefit to a person volunteering for a clinical trial varies considerably, depending on the stage of the research. In the earliest phases, direct benefits are limited, because the purpose of these trials is to establish whether the treatment or drug should be evaluated at all. In the last phase, where the prospects of the treatment or drug's usefulness are good, the potential for benefit is much greater. Some people enter clinical trials in the last phase, because they want to be among the first to benefit if the new treatment being studied does prove superior to the current standard of care available.

Some people also volunteer for altruistic reasons. They have the satisfaction of knowing they are helping to solve the mysteries of the disease. And even if the treatment fails to cure their illness, they have contributed to future, more successful therapies.

Fewer than 3 percent of adults with cancer now participate in clinical trials, yet many experts believe that if more people volunteered, cancer treatment would be improved significantly. About half of those with cancer today are cured, but that rate could climb considerably if more would join research studies. Considering that the large number of children in trials has been accompanied by steadily higher survival rates for some childhood cancers, this prediction seems plausible (see Chapter 35, "Cancer in Children"). More than 50 percent of the children with Wilms' tumor, neuroblastoma, acute lymphocytic leukemia, and Ewing's sarcoma are enrolled in clinical trials today.

Thousands of research studies are currently under way in the United States. Researchers are investigating basic biology to learn what causes cancer, testing current diagnostic methods, and evaluating new ones to determine how best to detect and define the disease. Epidemiologists are studying the impact of suspected risk factors such as diet on the incidence of cancer, and other researchers are conducting prevention trials to learn what might help people avoid developing cancer. Some studies focus on rehabilitation methods after treatment, and some aim to devise better ways of controlling some of cancer's most devastating effects, such as pain. But most clinical trials are designed to test potentially improved treatments. These may include new chemotherapy drugs or different combinations of standard ones, innovative types of radiation therapy and ways of combining standard radiation therapy techniques with surgery and/or chemotherapy, different surgical approaches, and various biological therapies—either alone or in combination with standard treatments.

Besides looking at how a particular treatment may improve chances for cure, researchers often examine how it may enhance a person's quality of life—perhaps by relieving pain, psychological stress, or other symptoms—thus allowing more people to continue working and enjoying life as long as possible.

This chapter explains how clinical trials are conducted, and defines the different types of studies. It describes what's involved in a trial and how to find a treatment study that may be beneficial to you.

From the Laboratory to Real Life

Currently, the National Cancer Institute alone sponsors research on more than 250 anticancer agents. The main thrust of these studies is to see if a new drug or combination of drugs or therapies is ultimately more effective than the interventions currently in use. Clinical trials are part of the long, slow, and often expensive process that improves standard treatments. Typically, it takes up to 14 years and $70 million for a new drug to become established as a standard treatment.

Before human testing of a drug begins, researchers conduct rigorous preliminary experiments in the test tube (*in vitro*) and in animals (*in vivo*) to determine which drugs are most likely to affect the cancer and make educated guesses about how best to administer them. Finally, if the laboratory research is promising and the Food and Drug Administration (FDA) approves the drug for investigation, scientists begin human studies in three phases.

INFORM YOURSELF

Informed Consent for Clinical Trials

An informed consent agreement that details the potential benefits and risks is essential for many treatments (see Chapter 14, "Principles of Treatment"). But it is especially important in the case of clinical trials, since the outcome of the proposed intervention is unknown to some degree or may have some risk.

The details of an informed consent form for clinical trials include the expected benefits of the study, other treatment options, assurance that your personal records will be kept confidential, provisions for compensation for injury, and a statement that your participation is voluntary and that you are free to withdraw without penalty at any time.

To cover all this information, consent forms are often lengthy and riddled with medical terminology with which you may not be familiar. For that reason you should ask your physician, nurse, or other medical personnel to go over the form with you before you sign it and to help you fully understand every aspect of the study you are considering. In fact, most people are given informed consent forms to read on their own, and then make appointments soon after to discuss their questions and concerns with the doctors and nurses involved with the trial.

Even though you sign the form, you are not legally bound to complete the trial. The informed consent form will state that you will be regularly updated regarding any new results coming from the trial, including unexpected risks or toxicity. Similarly, you or your physician may determine that problems you are experiencing do not warrant your staying in the trial. In either case, you can leave the trial at any time if you or others determine it is wise to do so.

Phase I Trials

During a phase I trial—the initial investigation of a treatment's safety and effectiveness in humans—a promising new therapy is tested to learn if it is worthy of further investigation. In the case of a new drug, this is when researchers learn about its effects by gradually increasing the dosage in a stepwise fashion and carefully analyzing the responses among the participants.

These are preliminary trials in which the researchers learn, for example, how well the drug is absorbed by the body, how much of it reaches the bloodstream, and how it is metabolized and eliminated from the body. The results let the scientists know if a larger study is possible that will reveal the drug's potential effectiveness.

Because participants in phase I studies can experience toxic and other undesirable side effects, only a few people are recruited. Usually a person will not be considered for a phase I study unless the cancer is advanced and conventional therapies have been employed and are no longer of any benefit. Typically, the person who enters this early phase of a clinical trial has no other treatment possibilities, and the study offers some hope of a response.

Compassionate Need

In some instances a promising anticancer drug may receive considerable favorable publicity before all the trials have been completed and it is approved for use by the FDA. In this case, an argument can be made for compassionate need, which is a process that has been developed allowing cancer patients who have exhausted most available standard therapies to receive the experimental drug. The use of the drug is called *off protocol*, meaning that even if the person is eligible, he or she is not part of a clinical trial.

Phase II

Once researchers confirm the possible value of a drug (or other treatment) and determine the safe dosage and other specifics of administering it, they focus on how effective it is on people with one or more types of cancer. Phase II studies often are slightly larger than phase I studies.

In some ways, a phase II trial is a preview of a new treatment. The results may not indicate for certain that a treatment is an improvement on current therapy; instead they may show whether it has the potential to be better.

Participants in a phase II trial often have been treated with a standard therapy before but have had a relapse or recurrence of their cancer. Although they are no longer responding to the standard treatment, their doctors believe the new approach being evaluated may be of benefit.

To gather information about how well people are responding, researchers may measure the size of tumors for shrinkage or, in the case of a systemic blood disease such as leukemia, they may analyze blood samples for changes in the circulating blood cells. The study may also involve monitoring the patient's blood for substances called tumor markers that often indicate whether their cancers are growing or shrinking. Subjective experiences, such as relief of certain symptoms, are noted, but objective measures allow for accurate analysis and comparison of treatment results.

Phase III

Phase III is the final and definitive round. Often many hundreds of people who have the same type of cancer at the same stage are involved in these studies. Phase III trials require a large number of participants for several reasons. For one, the levels of improvement may be small, and so many subjects are needed to determine by reliable statistical methods if the benefit is truly better than that achieved with standard treatment.

Phase III trials are designed to help physicians determine if the new experimental intervention is better than, as good as, or inferior to the accepted standard treatment. As a general rule, participants in a phase III trial are receiving the drug or therapy being studied as their initial treatment—that is, they have not received any prior interventions for their cancer. In this way, the researchers know that any changes in the subjects' condition are due to the treatment they receive in the study and not to the delayed effects of any other therapy. Depending on the approach being evaluated, other factors may influence the outcome and confuse the results of the study, making some patients ineligible for entry into the trial. For example, a person who has another disease with the potential to affect his or her health is likely to be ineligible for a clinical trial.

The study design usually provides one group of people with the treatment currently thought to be the best available. Another group receives the new treatment being studied, which is often a modification of the standard one. For example, in the case of a chemotherapy trial, the promising treatment may be an entirely different medication, or it may be the standard drug plus a second one that scientists believe may boost the effectiveness of the first.

If at some point during the study the new treatment is found to be more effective than the standard one, the trial is stopped, and all the participants receive the more successful intervention. If there is any evidence that the new intervention is inferior, unduly toxic, or otherwise harmful, the trial is also stopped to protect the participants.

The trial may be completed, or closed, when enough people have been treated to satisfy the statistical requirements for answering the experimental question, but the final answer is likely to take more time as the researchers continue their observations. The ultimate answer may be that the new treatment offers better results in terms of preventing a recurrence or of lengthening survival time. Or it may have other advantages, such as improved function and fewer undesirable effects.

Once a drug has been through the final stages of testing in such a trial and is found to be safe and effective, the FDA is likely to approve it for commercial use. At this point it is available to anyone who might benefit. However, even when a new drug becomes "standard," scientists may continue to study it for long-term side effects.

From Phase I to Phase III

Although most experimental cancer treatments go through all three trial phases, there are exceptions, such as studies designed to assess a prevention strategy. Usually, evidence from population studies has already indicated that the intervention, such as a dietary change, may be beneficial, so a phase II trial to determine the potential efficacy of a particular change is unnecessary. What remains to be tested is whether the new intervention or strategy can be implemented and whether it is truly beneficial. For example, a phase I trial, which is sometimes referred to as a *pilot study*, may determine that it's possible to get people to modify their diets in a particular way. It will then be compared to other prevention strategies or to no specific preventive measures in a phase III trial to establish the effectiveness of the intervention.

Myths and Misunderstandings

You may be hesitant to participate in clinical trials because you have heard that there's no guarantee you will receive appropriate treatment, or that you

Terms You Will Hear

These are terms commonly used in discussing clinical trials:

- *Protocol* is the written outline of a clinical study. You are not likely to receive a copy of the protocol, which spells out, among other things, the objectives of the trial, how it will be carried out, and a list of scientists involved in the study. However, you will receive an abbreviated form that is written in language you can understand, called the *informed consent* document. If you request it, you can review the actual protocol.

- *Standard treatment* refers to the therapy for a particular cancer that is accepted by the medical community and has FDA approval, if it is a drug. This standard treatment for cancer is promoted by both the National Cancer Institute and the American Cancer Society in most instances and is used for comparison with the "new" treatment. (The experimental treatment is usually a variation of the "standard" treatment. The researchers hope the variation will yield better results, but it may not.)

- A *placebo* is a harmless inactive substance given to members of the control group when the study is attempting to evaluate the benefits of adding a new drug to current treatment. A placebo is necessary as a standard of comparison. It is usually a pill, capsule, or injection resembling the active drug being tested.

- *Control group* refers to those people in a clinical trial not receiving the experimental treatment but undergoing the standard treatment approach.

- *Randomization* is a distribution process. The participants are randomly assigned to a control group or to one or more other groups receiving the new or modified treatment. Chance determines who goes into which group.

- *Double blind* describes a randomized trial in which neither physicians nor participants know which treatments are being administered to whom until the study is over.

- *Study arm* is the group in a study to which a participant is assigned: Each arm receives a different treatment.

CANCER

BASICS

will be lost in some scientific shuffle. If you are considering joining a clinical trial, it's important to know what's myth and what's reality.

Fear of Being Treated Like a "Guinea Pig"

A common worry of trial participants is that they will no longer be treated as individuals, that they will become just a "face in the crowd" and their care will be compromised in the name of science. In fact, study participants typically receive the best care available. Rather than being treated by only one or two doctors, they are monitored carefully by a number of specialists who are aware of privacy concerns and care about the subjects' well-being. If anything, clinical study participants in phase III trials have a better chance of gaining from treatment than nonparticipants, because they will receive either the best standard treatment known or an experimental therapy with the potential to be even more effective. (The likelihood for benefit with phase I and phase II trials is considerably less than that with phase III trials.) Most physicians in clinical trials are very sensitive to patients' experiences, the demands of participating in a clinical trial, and the need for individualized care. It is a general rule among physicians working with experimental therapies that these needs are considered and supersede those of the trial. The patient comes first.

Fear of Side Effects

It is true that, depending on which phase a trial is in, an experimental treatment may have unknown side effects. Most side effects in drug trials are similar to those brought about by standard drug therapies, such as hair loss, diminished blood counts (increasing the chance of infection), and nausea, and they are usually temporary. Although there is considerable information about side effects from animal studies that precede phase I trials, as a general rule more is known about how people will tolerate a drug during a phase III trial than in a phase I trial.

Of course, it is always possible that a treatment under investigation will cause serious, even life-threatening problems. These may be permanent, or they may not appear for a long time after the treatment is completed (for example, problems affecting the kidney or heart, or the later appearance of a second cancer). (Some of these problems are associated with standard treatments also.) Consequently, all possible risks are carefully discussed with potential participants during the informed consent process described earlier in this chapter.

You and your physician together should weigh the risks of side effects of a particular treatment plan on the type and stage of the cancer you have and your general health. Then you can discuss the potential benefits of the experimental treatment. Your decision to participate should not be made impulsively; it may require several discussions with your physician and other members of the treatment team. You may also want a family member or close friend to meet with the doctor responsible for the trial and help you weigh the risks and benefits of volunteering.

Fear of Receiving a Placebo

The use of the term placebo is often misleading. Clinical trials of anticancer drugs are never designed so that any participant will receive a placebo as the sole treatment unless, of course, the current standard is no treatment (see the box "Terms You Will Hear"). For instance, in a clinical trial evaluating the effects of a new drug given with radiation therapy on a particular type and stage of cancer, radiation therapy alone may be the recommended treatment. Therefore, all study participants will receive radiation therapy; but some will also receive the drug being tested. Those in the control group will take a placebo in addition to the radiation therapy. No one in such a study will go without treatment. If during the course of the research the new drug is found to boost the effectiveness of the radiation therapy, all participants will immediately get the additional drug and the trial will end.

Fear of Missing Out on a Promising Treatment

Some experimental treatments are available outside of the clinical trial arena, and some doctors, encouraged by reports of promising results early in the investigation phase, may offer unapproved treatments as standard care. You may be tempted to seek treatment in this way rather than via a trial. Some people do this because they fear that if they enter a study, they will be part of the control group that does not receive the new and potentially beneficial experimental treatment. This perception is unfortunate on two counts: If a treatment is still being investigated, it has not been proven to be better than standard care; also, its risks and side effects may not be clear.

Despite these cautions there are circumstances when some physicians are convinced that an unproven new treatment is the preferable approach. A recent example of this situation is high-dose chemotherapy facilitated by bone marrow transplantation in women with breast cancer who have extensive spread to the lymph nodes, which is a poor prognostic sign. The majority of oncologists recognize the need to determine whether bone marrow transplant (BMT) for this stage of disease is beneficial (see Chapter 19, "Bone Marrow Transplant"). However, the somewhat misleading publicity generated by those who consider BMT "the only hope" is confusing to the public.

Whatever you choose to do about an investigational treatment, it's important to understand that there is no proof that it is superior to any other option. The physicians conducting the trial are not biased in favor of either the new or the standard therapy. If they were, the study would be jeopardized.

Financial Fears

Extra follow-up office visits and frequent monitoring with laboratory tests are part of participating in a clinical trial. The extent to which insurance and health plans cover these additional costs varies. Some do pay for the cost of phase III trial treatments. Indeed, there is much pressure being put on managed care organizations to include clinical trials as treatment options. However, if your plan doesn't cover the costs of experimental treatments, be sure the researchers in charge of the study you are considering are aware of it. Most physicians who plan clinical trials know the status of coverage and are careful to keep the number of office visits, laboratory tests, hospital stays, and other potentially costly conditions of clinical investigations to a minimum. In fact, clinical trials are sometimes less expensive to patients than receiving standard treatment, since many of the charges may be borne by those funding the study.

As for travel costs, as more and more trials are conducted in community hospitals rather than in major cancer centers, participants travel no farther for treatment and checkups than if they were receiving standard care.

Safeguards

Although there are no guarantees about the outcome of a clinical trial, safeguards are built in. One of the most important is the *Institutional Review Board (IRB)*, a group of doctors, knowledgeable lay people, and other experts such as nurses, scientists, and clergy based at the facility where trials are carried out. IRBs are specifically responsible for protecting the welfare of trial participants in their institution. Members examine all aspects of each study before it is initiated to make sure that the risks are reasonable compared to the potential benefits to the patients. These groups also periodically monitor the data from the trial at their institution while it is under way. Studies funded by the federal government and under its jurisdiction also are reviewed by the National Cancer Institute.

How to Find a Clinical Trial

Most cancer studies are funded by the National Cancer Institute through cancer centers or cooperative networks made up of research institutions, university and community hospitals, and clinics associated with them.

Currently, the NCI is sponsoring hundreds of experimental treatment programs. Many of these studies take place at community hospitals as part of the *Community Clinical Oncology Program (CCOP)*. This links community oncologists and primary physicians with NCI-funded researchers at medical centers, so that people can participate in cancer treatment trials without having to leave their area (see Appendix I, "Resources").

Most pilot or exploratory studies (phases I and II) are carried out by single institutions such as universities and/or cancer centers. Even pharmaceutical companies that have a vested interest in proving that a medication works must adhere strictly to the scientific rules of research outlined earlier. Often they join forces with university medical centers to conduct the necessary studies of drug efficacy, and any reputable company will scrupulously avoid potential conflict of interest.

There are many ways to go about finding out about a clinical study that may benefit you. The most obvious place to start is the office of your own oncologist. You can also contact an NCI-designated clinical cancer center. The Cancer Information Service (CIS), a program supported by the National Cancer Institute, can provide you with the names and numbers of centers near you (800-4-CANCER). (See Appendix I, "Resources.")

When contacting the CIS you can also request a Physician's Data Query (PDQ) search. PDQ is a computerized database system supported by the NCI. It contains information about the latest nationwide cancer treatments for each type and stage of cancer. It lists more than 1,500 ongoing clinical trials and is updated monthly.

You can also access the PDQ on line with your own computer. In addition, the NCI has begun to collaborate with patient advocacy groups (starting with NABCO, the National Alliance of Breast Cancer Organizations) to offer information about relevant clinical trials through their own Web sites. Patient advocacy organizations can be excellent sources of information about

Questions to Ask

If you are considering entering a clinical trial, you will want to gather as much information about the study as you can before you make a decision to participate. The following questions are a good start:

- What is the study trying to find out? Is the purpose to determine the safest dosage of a new drug or to determine the most effective treatment for my type of cancer?

- Who is sponsoring the study? Has it been reviewed by a bona fide national group, such as the National Cancer Institute? Has it been approved by an institutional review board?

- How is my cancer most likely to progress or change if I join this study? What will happen regarding treatment if I don't?

- What are the other alternatives to the treatment proposed in this study? Are there standard options that may be just as beneficial as those in the study? What are the risks and advantages of these alternatives?

- What kinds of additional tests, such as blood tests or biopsies, will I undergo for the specific purpose of the study? Do any of these have side effects or risks that are of particular concern to me?

- How will being in the study affect my daily life? Will I be able to continue work? Will I feel like pursuing social activities?

- Will I have to be hospitalized? How often and for how long?

- How long will my active participation in the study last?

- Where will I be treated and evaluated? Will I have to travel? How frequently? Will much of my time be taken up by visits to the doctor or place where the trial is being coordinated, or can much of the treatment be given at my local cancer treatment center?

- What are the potential short-term and long-term side effects of the treatment alternatives? Are any of them likely to be permanent or life threatening? Will I be allowed to take medications to alleviate side effects such as nausea? Will I be able to continue other medicines?

- How will I know if the treatment is working properly or if I am responding? How will I know whether I should receive a different treatment plan from the one being studied?

- What if I seem to be harmed during the research program? Will I be entitled to care for problems related to the treatment?

- Will the treatment involve additional expense? Will any or all of the costs be covered? If not, are there other sources I can turn to for financial help? Do you know of any organizations that can help me convince my insurance company or health plan to cover the costs?

- What type of follow-up care will I receive after the study is completed?

- How much will my personal physician be involved?

- Who will be professionally responsible for my health care while I am in the trial?

experimental treatments generally. See Appendix I ("Resources") and Appendix II ("Cancer Information On Line").

Another valuable source of cancer research information is the American Cancer Society (800-ACS-2345).

ALTERNATIVE AND COMPLEMENTARY THERAPIES

In recent years, there has been a tremendous resurgence of interest in *alternative* methods, those approaches to treating cancer that differ from the conventional medical treatments and are currently under study or otherwise unproven. According to a study published in 1993 in the *New England Journal of Medicine*, 34 percent of the 1,500 people surveyed in 1990 had used at least one unconventional therapy in the previous year. Interestingly, fewer than three in 10 users of such unconventional therapies had told their physicians about the treatments.

Today the widespread curiosity about some of these alternatives—also known as *unconventional, unproven, nontraditional, holistic,* or *questionable* methods—is very different from earlier peaks of interest in nontraditional medicine in the 1920s and at the turn of the century. That is, the current resurgence has been fueled by some positive reports from the medical community itself. In addition, disparaging terms like *quackery* can no longer be applied to all alternatives, when some of them, such as mental imagery or visualization and meditation, are being taught to patients in some of the most prestigious cancer centers in this country.

Although many bogus treatments are still being sold to the public, and charlatans continue to promote their "cures," there are some nontraditional practices that well-respected scientists and the U.S. government believe are worthy of serious study. The key word here is *study*. Just because a treatment is initially promising or some people claim to benefit from it does not mean that it will be safe, effective, and promote enough of an improvement in a large number of people to be considered a valid therapy (see Chapter 21, "Investigational Treatments").

This chapter describes some of the better-known alternatives, pointing out which methods are being evaluated for their usefulness as adjuncts to tra-

What Does *Alternative* Mean?

The meaning of the words sometimes used interchangeably with *alternative* varies according to who is using them. The following are the American Cancer Society's definitions:

- *Questionable methods* are lifestyle practices, clinical tests, or treatment methods that are promoted for general use for the prevention, diagnosis, or treatment of cancer and that, on the basis of careful review by scientists and/or clinicians, are deemed to lack real evidence of value.

- *Alternative treatments* are remedies in popular use that are under study or are otherwise unproven.

- *Complementary treatments* are those approaches used as a supplement to or in conjunction with conventional cancer treatments.

ditional treatments, which approaches may help relieve symptoms and promote recovery, and which ones have *not* been proved effective or have proved ineffective and perhaps even dangerous. It will also help you ask the right questions of your doctor or proponent of an alternative therapy if you are considering one.

A New Look at Alternatives

Researchers are finding that some techniques, such as acupuncture, appear to relieve some symptoms. And positive preliminary studies of the benefits of stress reduction and support groups conducted in clinical research settings have stimulated funding for more investigations of the mind-body connection. In fact, in 1992, the National Institutes of Health established a special department for this, called the Office of Alternative Medicine (OAM). The purpose of the OAM is to put the most promising practices through the same thorough testing processes used to determine whether conventional treatments should be made available to the public.

One of the OAM's objectives is to establish clinical research centers at leading medical institutions where unproven treatment methods can be studied in a scientific environment. When the OAM was established in 1992, two of the first three therapies evaluated for further study were cancer therapies.

More than two dozen highly respected medical schools and hospitals such as Harvard University's Beth Israel in Boston, Georgetown University in Washington, D.C., and Columbia University in New York City have established departments or centers for the study of complementary medicine and at least 27 medical schools offer alternative medicine courses. *Complementary* is a recent term for those therapies that are used along with mainstream medical care. For the most part, these methods are thought to help improve the quality of life, including relieving symptoms of the disease, alleviating side effects of treatment, and/or providing psychological benefits. They are not curative, however.

The Appeal of Alternatives

There are several reasons for the growing appeal of alternative medicine, but for many people with cancer, there is one overriding attraction: Unless their disease is discovered at an early stage, most mainstream treatments cannot promise cure. Often, alternative therapies do.

Furthermore, many conventional treatments may be accompanied by unpleasant, even toxic, side effects. And for people with very advanced disease, no therapy can ensure long-term survival. Naturally, a treatment that *claims* to cure or prolong survival time and has no objectionable side effects is enormously tempting.

Unconventional therapies not only cannot cure, they have not been held to the same standards of proof of safety and effectiveness as have the drugs and treatments prescribed by physicians. Nevertheless, vulnerable people—already leery of or frustrated by standard treatments—may find that anecdotal evidence and testimonials provide more hope than do the statistics of conventional treatment. Whether incorporating certain complementary therapies into a treatment plan can actually boost the chance of recovery has not yet been established.

Another reason for the appeal of alternative medicine is disillusionment with technological advances, the hospital environment, and the modern health care system. To many, caregivers seem to place a particular treatment and what it may accomplish ahead of what the person with cancer considers to be an acceptable quality of life. Although the medical community is finally recognizing the importance of maintaining a person's psychological and emotional well-being during treatment and recovery, those with cancer still are sometimes disappointed with the attention given to these needs. In contrast, alternative practitioners often appear more sympathetic to these feelings, listening and talking to their patients more than do overscheduled physicians in busy managed-care or oncology settings. Not surprisingly, being cared for and listened to is enormously appealing.

What Can It Hurt?

Although many alternative treatments are harmless and inexpensive and can renew a person's feelings of hopefulness, not all are benign. Some treatments may interfere with the effectiveness of a conventional medical therapy. Some may cause injury or infection or other kinds of problems. For example, certain diet therapies actually cause nutritional deficiencies that interfere with the body's ability to heal and withstand the side effects of conventional treatment. Others may involve procedures that can lead to serious injury or infection. At the very least, the promises made by the proponents of these treatments create false hope and can represent a significant waste of money. What often causes so much dismay among traditional practitioners is that unproven therapies sometimes steer people away from treatment that would have been effective if they had not delayed it. In sum, *trying an unproven approach may mean losing the best opportunity to control the cancer and prolong life.*

It also is unfortunate when those with very advanced disease turn to an unconventional therapy simply because they believe they have "nothing to lose." This decision to pursue a treatment as a last resort, without careful consideration of what the real costs are, may lead to unnecessary grief and pain. People have been known to spend their remaining weeks receiving ineffective and expensive treatments overseas, for instance, rather than enjoying the company of loved ones, receiving care that keeps them comfortable, and seeing to their financial affairs. Even when an alternative therapy is less costly than conventional medicine, the fees paid for it may still be wasted.

It is extremely difficult to determine which of the many proliferating alternatives are safe or provide any benefits at all. Just because a practice is legal does not mean it is benign. Laws and regulations protecting people from unsafe practices are sometimes vague, and few attempts are made to enforce those that do exist. In general, the U.S. Food and Drug Administration (FDA) requires proof of safety and efficacy before a medication can be sold. But there is a lot of leeway between the FDA's regulations and a person's freedom of choice, particularly when the option is not a drug. Certainly, there is no law against traveling to another country for a treatment that is illegal or not available in the United States. Indeed, several treatments that are not considered effective by American physicians are used in mainstream practice in European countries, which only increases the confusion for someone with cancer.

Complementary Methods

Some unconventional therapies, however, are beginning to take their place alongside conventional treatments. Called complementary treatments because they supplement conventional cancer treatments or are used in conjunction with them, these methods often improve the quality of life during treatment. For example, because stress is thought to play a part in how well a person handles the rigors of a treatment such as radiation therapy, some type of relaxation therapy may be helpful (see Chapter 25, "Coping with Stress, Fear, Anxiety, and Depression"). Likewise, a carefully constructed diet may make it easier to eat well and maintain a healthy weight even when experiencing appetite loss and vomiting caused by chemotherapy (see Chapter 26, "Food and Nutrition").

A number of complementary methods have been found to relieve symptoms such as nausea and pain from either the treatment or the cancer itself. Some can also alleviate anxiety and stress. Prayer, massage, meditation, nutritional counseling, and yoga are considered complementary methods. Some experts and organizations also refer to these as *lifestyle* approaches.

Nutritional Therapy

Cancer affects your nutritional needs in a variety of ways (see Chapter 26, "Food and Nutrition"). Ideally, a registered dietitian or other credentialed nutrition professional will design an eating plan for you, taking into account your special needs as well as likes and dislikes. Foods are chosen to help improve well-being, tolerance of treatment, and quality of life. Typically, considerable attention is paid to variety, balance, and moderation, and calories are calibrated to keep body weight from dipping dangerously low. Some experts feel that eating a low-fat, high-fiber diet may improve your chances of avoiding a recurrence of a cancer that has been treated effectively, and studies to test this belief are under way. There is no evidence, however, that any diet, food—such as wheat grass or barley juice—or specially grown, organic food can cure cancer.

Support Groups

Research shows that social support can be an invaluable part of cancer treatment and can have a positive effect on your quality of life and overall attitude (see Chapter 13, "Your Support Network"). Meeting with people who are having similar physical and emotional experiences can help diminish your feelings of isolation.

If you feel you must put up a positive front for your family, friends, and others, support groups provide a place where you can let down your guard and express your emotions among sympathetic people. Many self-help groups are run by health professionals who can contribute important information about dealing with both the physical and the emotional effects of cancer, such as diet advice and stress-reducing strategies.

Preliminary research indicates that people who join structured support groups during or following treatment not only feel better but also may live longer. For instance, in a Stanford University study, those women with advanced breast cancer who went regularly to therapist-led support group meetings lived an average of 18 months longer than did those women who did not join a structured support group. Another study was conducted at UCLA among people with malignant melanoma, all of whom had undergone surgery for this deadly form of skin cancer. Half went on to meet once a week for six weeks to learn about the disease and prevention of recurrence, deal with stress, cope with problems, and seek emotional support from one another. Six years later their death rate was reduced by 60 percent compared with the men and women who did not participate in the groups. Also fewer of the group participants experienced a recurrence of the cancer. Other studies have shown that carefully structured support and coping programs seem to improve the immune functioning of those who take part, at least in the short term. Still, while these studies are promising, none has been conducted with a sufficiently large number of subjects to draw definitive conclusions.

Several theories explain why social support is beneficial. First, people who feel that others care about them are more likely to eat well, get enough sleep, take their medication as directed, and otherwise care for themselves. Some evidence also suggests that social support may affect the immune system positively.

Meditation

Meditation is a way to relax, counter stress, even relieve pain by freeing the mind so that mundane matters and negative emotions are set aside while concentrating only on the moment. Reports have suggested that meditation can reduce anxiety, depression, discomfort, and pain in people with cancer, but no evidence confirms that stress reduction through meditation or other psychological means such as mental or guided imagery and visualization can alter the course of cancer (see Chapter 25, "Coping with Stress, Fear, Anxiety, and Depression").

There are many ways to practice meditation, such as sitting quietly and concentrating on breathing in a regulated way, focusing on a repeated word, or concentrating on an object such as a lighted candle. Similarly, a form of yoga called *hatha yoga* also can relieve stress and anxiety. Rather than focusing on a word or object, you concentrate on breathing while assuming various physical postures.

Acupuncture

Acupuncture originated in China some 2,000 years ago. It is based on the ancient belief that energy—*qi* or *chi*—flows through the body along specific pathways called *meridians*. Acupuncture, inserting extremely fine needles into points along these meridians, called *acupoints*, or pressing on them (*acupressure*) is believed to enhance the flow of energy to corresponding organs or systems.

In the United States, an estimated 5,000 physicians practice acupuncture, carrying out as many as 9 to 12 million treatments each year. In many states many more nonphysician practitioners are allowed to practice acupuncture.

Although acupuncture is used throughout the world to treat a variety of ailments, including asthma and cancer, most people only know about its use as an anesthetic and pain reliever. Studies suggest that it works at least as well as a placebo for relief of certain types of nausea and vomiting and treating drug addiction.

No one knows for certain how acupuncture works, but theories abound. Some research maintains that the acupoints lie near areas where major nerves and nerve endings join muscle or bone and that any interference in those places can relieve pain. Other studies have found that acupuncture can trigger the release of *endorphins*, natural painkillers produced in the brain.

If you are considering acupuncture as an adjunct to cancer treatment, check with your state medical board to find out whether and how practitioners are regulated in your area. (Also make sure when you have a treatment that the acupuncturist uses disposable needles, to avoid contracting any blood-borne diseases.)

Unproven Therapies

The American Cancer Society defines unproven cancer therapies as "those diagnostic tests or therapeutic modalities which are promoted for general use in cancer prevention, diagnosis, or treatment and which are, on the basis of careful review by scientists and/or clinicians, not deemed proven nor recommended for current use." (These are sometimes referred to as *questionable* or

Asking About Alternatives

You should ask the same questions about an alternative treatment that you would ask about a conventional one, such as surgery, chemotherapy, or radiation therapy (see the lists of questions to ask in those chapters). Then ask the following questions as well:

- How thoroughly has this treatment been evaluated?
- Have any clinical trials been done, or are any under way?
- Have articles or studies of the treatment been published in peer-reviewed medical journals?
- What are the qualifications of those responsible for providing the treatment? What about those actually administering it? Do they have medical degrees from accredited schools?
- Is the treatment or method provided at a hospital or other medical setting?
- How long has the treatment been available? How long has the clinic or center offering it been in business?
- Will I be able to see my doctor and continue my regular treatments while trying the unproven method?
- How much will the treatment cost? Would I be willing to pay that amount if I knew for certain that the treatment was unlikely to work?
- Will I have to travel outside the United States for the treatment?
- Why isn't it offered here?
- Does the treatment promise what no one else is willing to tell me—that it can cure my cancer or add years to my expected life span?

unorthodox treatments.) Because such therapies lack proof of effectiveness or, in some cases, proof of their ineffectiveness, the ACS does not endorse their use. The following are some of the best-known unproven treatments. With the exception of shark cartilage, all have been evaluated by the ACS and have been found to have no objective benefit in the treatment of cancer.

Nutritional and Metabolic Therapies

The underlying theory of metabolic therapy is that cancer results when toxins and waste materials in the body interfere with its metabolism and healing. Although specific methods to "detoxify" the body and eliminate these wastes vary among practitioners of metabolic therapy, most involve a combination of diet, very large doses of vitamins and minerals, "internal cleansing" (in other words, enemas), and spiritual and emotional restoration.

Gerson Diet. For a number of years, the Gerson diet, also known as the Gerson treatment, has been a popular metabolic therapy. It was developed by Max Gerson, M.D., a German-born physician who emigrated to the United

States in 1938. While still in Germany, Gerson designed a dietary regimen to treat his own disabling migraine headaches. He developed similar therapies for disorders such as arthritis. In 1928, Gerson treated his first patient with cancer, and by the time he had settled in the United States and passed his state boards in New York in 1939, he was concentrating on treating cancer.

Gerson theorized that cancer was a degenerative disease caused by a failure of the immune system and the inability of the body to produce an "allergic inflammation," which, he believed, was a healing reaction. He thought cancer was caused in part by eating foods grown in poor soil that was contaminated by insecticides and herbicides. The goals of Gerson's regimen—a special low-sodium, high-potassium diet; juices; supplements such as iodine; and coffee enemas—were to eliminate "toxins" from the body and improve the cancer patient's general condition. He published the case histories of some of the patients he treated in *A Cancer Therapy: Results of Fifty Cases*.

Today the Gerson treatment, provided in Tijuana, Mexico, relies on a diet of fruits and vegetables and as many as 13 glasses of fresh juices a day. Heavy animal fats are avoided. The Gerson Institute literature says that metabolism is stimulated with liver extract injections; pancreatic enzymes; and thyroid, potassium, and other supplements. Coffee or chamomile tea enemas may be used. Adjuvant treatments such as laetrile, hyperbaric oxygen therapy, and shark cartilage may be recommended also.

Although Gerson submitted 10 case histories to the National Cancer Institute in 1947 to prove that his program was successful, an NCI statement says their review did not find the treatment to be effective. After Gerson died in 1959, the NCI reviewed his book and concluded that many of the case reports it contained did not meet the basic criteria for evaluating the benefits of therapy. The NCI found no demonstration of benefit. According to the U.S. Office of Technology Assessment (OTA) report, *Unconventional Cancer Treatment*, members of the Gerson Institute argue that some evidence was dismissed on the basis of technicalities.

Serious illnesses and deaths have occurred as a result of some of the treatments, such as coffee enemas, which can affect the body's electrolyte balance and may cause infection. Accordingly, the ACS warns against using the Gerson method for any medical condition.

Kelley Metabolic Therapy. Thirty years ago the Kelley metabolic therapy, also known as the Kelley Ecology Therapy, was one of the most popular alternative treatments for cancer. Since then, several variations have evolved, including, according to the OTA, the method currently being practiced by Nicholas Gonzalez, M.D., in New York City.

William Donald Kelley, an orthodontist who had been diagnosed with pancreatic cancer, developed biochemical tests, one of which he called the "Protein Metabolism Evaluation Index," which was intended to diagnose cancer months or years before it became apparent. Believing that cancer indicated a deficiency "particularly of a pancreatic enzyme" and inadequate protein metabolism, Kelley developed a one- to two-year, five-part program that included a special diet, some 25 nutritional supplements (among them pancreatic enzymes said to destroy defective cells) that could amount to about

300 pills a day; detoxifying treatments such as coffee enemas; moderate exercise; fasting and purging; neurological stimulation such as chiropractic and osteopathic treatments; a spiritual component to "purify the emotions and spirits"; and, of course, a diet. Kelley recommended avoiding meat, milk (except as yogurt and buttermilk), and peanuts. Almonds and vegetables supply the protein. Fresh vegetable juice (at least a quart of carrot and a pint of celery juice a day), and salads, fruits, and fruit juices are advised. Whole grains are encouraged, but white flour, tea, coffee, chocolate, liquor, and white rice, among other foods, should be avoided.

According to the OTA report, in 1970 Dr. Kelley was ordered not to practice medicine and to stop distributing the booklet about his treatment, *One Answer to Cancer*. An OTA review of 50 patients' case histories selected from Kelley's files and written by Gonzalez had mixed results: unconventional reviewers found some positive effects; mainstream reviewers found most cases unconvincing.

Today, according to the OTA report, the Gonzalez regimen is similar to Kelley's. It consists of nutritional supplements, including digestive enzymes such as pancreatic enzymes, pepsin, hydrochloric acid, and bile; coffee enemas; and a diet designed especially for each patient. For some people an entirely vegetarian diet may be prescribed, whereas others may be told to eat a lot of meat—sometimes red meat three or four times a day. Neurological stimulation and spirituality are not part of the Gonzalez regimen.

Manner Metabolic Cancer Therapy. Biologist Harold W. Manner, Ph.D., described cancer as resulting from a weak immune system, which his metabolic therapy was designed to restore to its normal, healthy condition. Underlying causes include inadequate nutrition and the inability of glands such as the pancreas to produce enzymes.

While studying the development of fish, frogs, salamanders, and mice at Loyola University in Chicago in the 1970s, Manner became interested in the purported anticancer drug laetrile. He published a paper reporting that his injections of vitamin A, laetrile (see below), and enzymes into tumors in mice caused the tumors to regress completely in more than 89.3 percent of the animals tested.

According to Manner's book *The Death of Cancer*, the various components of metabolic therapy are a pretreatment-phase hair and blood test to detect mineral imbalances, a special diet, and detoxification with a daily coffee enema. Next, he prescribed enzymes (some of which are injected directly into the tumor), and various combinations of laetrile and large doses of vitamins A, B15, C, and E; RNA and DNA; and minerals. Maintaining a positive attitude is also a component of the program.

Several risks are involved with this treatment. Laetrile has been shown to cause serious side effects, and deaths from cyanide poisoning have been reported following its ingestion. Large doses of vitamin A can cause drying, cracking, and peeling of the skin, and megadoses of vitamin C may lead to nausea, diarrhea, and kidney stones.

Manner died in 1988, but the Clinica Manner continues to operate in Tijuana, Mexico.

Macrobiotic Diet. The macrobiotic diet was developed in the 1950s by a Japanese teacher, George Ohsawa, and was described a decade later in *Zen Macrobiotics and The Philosophy of Oriental Medicine*. In the late 1960s and early 1970s, several deaths as a result of the diet were reported, and the American Medical Association's Council on Foods and Nutrition issued a statement describing the nutritional shortcomings of one form of the diet consisting of 100 percent cereals and the problems associated with it.

A resurgence of interest in macrobiotics began in the late 1970s when a well-known proponent and teacher of the diet, Michio Kushi—who founded the Kushi Institute for One Peaceful World and wrote *The Cancer Prevention Diet*—modified the diet. According to the OTA report, Kushi no longer advises people not to combine a macrobiotic diet and traditional cancer treatments, such as radiation therapy or chemotherapy. However, some people with cancer refuse conventional therapy in the hope that the macrobiotic diet, a primarily vegetarian diet, will help them. Today it is one of the most popular unconventional approaches to cancer treatment.

Macrobiotics is frequently defined as a way of life rather than as an approach to eating, combining elements of Zen Buddhism with dietary principles based on simplicity and the avoidance of toxins that come from eating too many dairy products, meats, and oily foods.

The modified macrobiotic diet consists of unprocessed, organically grown grains, vegetables, fruits, beans, and seafood. Liquids are restricted to soy-based miso or tamari broths, nonstimulating teas, cereal grain coffee, and tepid water.

The guidelines for combining and preparing these foods are very specific and complicated, based on Eastern principles of restoring balance to the body. The amount of each food is described as a percentage. For instance, 50 to 60 percent of the macrobiotic diet is made up of cooked, organically grown whole grains; 25 to 30 percent, of vegetables; 5 to 10 percent, of beans and seaweeds (nori, wakame, kombu, dulse); and 5 to 10 percent, of specific types of soups. Fish and fruit are occasionally permitted. Meat, poultry, animal fat, eggs, dairy products, citrus fruits, bananas, potatoes, tomatoes, spinach, coffee, canned and frozen foods, refined sugars and honey, and vitamin supplements are not allowed. Other "rules" of the macrobiotic diet include exercising regularly, maintaining a good mental attitude, and avoiding synthetic fabrics and chemical fumes.

There have been no controlled studies of the effects of such a diet on cancer, although the OTA has reviewed a number of case studies of people with pancreatic and prostate cancers who had adopted a macrobiotic lifestyle. The results were inconclusive. The Office of Alternative Medicine (OAM) has funded a pilot study to determine if a macrobiotic diet may prevent cancer.

What is known about this diet, or any strict vegetarian diet, is that it can lead to nutritional deficiencies, especially of vitamins B12 and D, particularly when followed by seriously ill people and/or those undergoing cancer treatments, who need more of certain nutrients and more calories than healthy people do. Macrobiotic practitioners have adjusted the diet somewhat to avoid deficiencies. In some ways, a modified macrobiotic diet is better for a well person than the typical American diet is, because it is lower in fat and cholesterol and higher in fiber, complex carbohydrates, vitamins A and C, and beta carotene.

After reviewing the Kushi Institute's literature, 11 major scientific databases, and reports in the medical literature, the ACS finds "that the usefulness of macrobiotic diets in cancer treatment is undocumented and that if not properly planned to be nutritionally adequate, such diets could provide insufficient nutrition for cancer patients."

Hoxsey Herbal Treatment. The Hoxsey treatment originally consisted of a paste applied to external cancers, then a tonic for intestinal cancers made up mostly of herbs, and finally a combination of various tonics and a diet that avoids pork, vinegar, tomatoes, pickles, carbonated drinks, alcohol, bleached flour, sugar, and salt. In *You Don't Have to Die*, Harry Hoxsey describes the formulas.

Today the Hoxsey treatment—including the brown tonic, which is presumed to contain potassium iodide, licorice, red clover, buckthorn bark, burdock, pokeweed roots, other herbs, and the pink tonic of potassium iodide and elixir lactate of pepsin—is available only in their Tijuana, Mexico, clinic. The tonics are said to stimulate "the elimination of toxins which are poisoning the system, thereby correcting the abnormal blood chemistry and normalizing cell metabolism."

Hoxsey died in 1974, but his nurse Mildred Nelson continues to administer the Hoxsey treatment at the Bio-Medical Center in Tijuana, Mexico. She is said to have added the dietary component and the emphasis on the importance of having the "right attitude." The center also offers vaccine therapies. According to Nelson, the therapy restores to normal "impaired metabolism and immune dysfunction" and "deals with the DNA."

The FDA banned the distribution of the tonics across state lines in 1960. During the many legal battles over the internal tonics, various experts testified about the effects of their ingredients. The licorice and pepsin, for example, are primarily flavorings; the buckthorn bark is a laxative, but large doses of it can cause severe nausea, vomiting, and diarrhea; red clover has no proven therapeutic value; burdock root is believed to boost appetite; berberis root has some antibacterial effects; and pokeroot has been used for everything from an emetic to a narcotic, but one expert in medicinal plants reported that it is not useful for anything.

When the FDA evaluated the case histories of some 400 cancer patients treated by Hoxsey, it found not a single documented cure. The American Cancer Society does not recommend the use of Hoxsey medicines by cancer patients and considers the internal treatments to be useless and the external ones archaic.

Special Preparations

From time to time, tonics, teas, vaccines, vitamins, folk remedies, and new chemical combinations make headlines. Some also fall from favor just as quickly, but several continue to attract proponents.

Laetrile. Laetrile is one of the best-known alternative cancer treatments. Laetrile, derived from a substance called amygdalin, found in the pits of apricots and other fruits, has been called vitamin B17, although scientists do not recognize it as a nutrient.

Laetrile was first used by Ernst Krebs Sr., M.D., in the 1950s. By the mid-1970s it had become a popular, though unproven, cancer treatment. Proponents claim that it selectively destroys cancer cells and relieves pain in advanced disease. Political pressure resulted in clinical trials at three prestigious institutions, which found laetrile ineffective. Although it has been proved that the drug is not beneficial, it continues to be available at some cancer clinics in Mexico, and many Americans continue to take it in the hope of a cure.

Because laetrile breaks down in the body to form cyanide, a deadly poison, it causes many problems, such as nausea, vomiting, headache, and dizziness. A few cases of death have been linked to the substance. Studies sponsored by the National Cancer Institute found that the drug produced no substantial benefit in terms of cure, improvement or stabilization of cancer.

Vitamin C (Ascorbic Acid). In the early 1970s Ewan Cameron, a Scottish surgeon, and Linus Pauling, an American Nobel Prize laureate, paved the way for using large doses of vitamin C to treat cancer. They believed that vitamin C would help slow the progression of the disease by increasing the amount of a substance in the blood known to inhibit tumor growth and by strengthening the tissue around the tumor to make it more resistant to the cancer cells.

Cameron and Pauling proposed using megadoses of vitamin C—from 2 to 10 grams (2,000 to 10,000 milligrams) of vitamin C daily (the Recommended Daily Allowance is 60 milligrams)—as an adjunct to conventional treatment. Pauling and Cameron reported that megadoses of vitamin C given by mouth or intravenously provided many benefits for cancer patients, such as improved appetite, increased mental alertness, and diminished need for pain medication. The researchers published the effects of their treatment in *Cancer and Vitamin C* in 1979.

Three studies funded by the National Cancer Institute and conducted by researchers at the Mayo Clinic in Rochester, Minnesota, did not find any significant improvements in people who took large amounts of vitamin C, compared with those who took a placebo. The studies did show, however, that such large quantities of vitamin C can cause side effects like nausea, vomiting, leg swelling, heartburn, and diarrhea. Excessive amounts of vitamin C are also known to inflame the stomach lining and to break down red blood cells. Furthermore, excess vitamin C may actually promote tumor growth.

Supporters of vitamin C therapy argue that the Mayo Clinic's studies were flawed and that the patients selected for them had already received chemotherapy. Cameron believed that such patients would be less able to respond to the vitamin C treatment.

Immuno-augmentative Therapy. Lawrence Burton, Ph.D., an American biologist, developed immuno-augmentative therapy (IAT) in the early 1970s. In 1977 Burton moved to the Bahamas and opened the Immunology Research Centre, Ltd. Later, clinics were also opened in Germany and Mexico.

Burton believed that cancer develops because of a breakdown in the immune system. IAT is a series of biological products that strive to correct that imbalance. They include the "tumor complement" taken from the blood of cancer patients and "tumor antibodies" and "deblocking protein" derived from the blood of healthy people. Cancer patients receive injections of these products according to a prescribed regimen. Burton endorsed surgery to remove a tumor before IAT treatment, but he discouraged other treatments such as chemotherapy. Burton died in 1993, but the Bahamian Clinic remains in operation under the direction of R. John Clement, M.D.

Studies have not found IAT to be effective, and attempts to conduct a well-designed clinical trial have fallen through. Moreover, samples of the IAT serum were found to be contaminated with hepatitis and the HIV virus that causes AIDS. For this reason, the Bahamian government closed the Immunology Research Centre for a time, and, in 1986, the FDA prohibited bringing IAT into the United States, but according to the OTA report, "There has, however, been no report that the ban has been enforced."

Antineoplaston Therapy. One of the best-known and most controversial alternative therapies today is antineoplaston therapy, which was developed in the late 1960s by Stanislaw R. Burzynski, M.D., Ph.D., a Polish physician and biochemist who came to the United States in 1970. He believes the body contains substances, *antineoplastons*, that are part of a biomedical defense system. Unlike the immune system, which destroys defective cells, the peptides and amino acid derivatives that form antineoplastons correct the defects, he claims, restoring the cells to normal.

Originally, these peptides were retrieved from the blood and urine of healthy people, but now they are synthesized. According to Burzynski, research indicates people with cancer have fewer antineoplastons.

Patients receive antineoplaston therapy intravenously, often through an implanted catheter, or orally at the Burzynski Clinic in Houston. A small percentage of people experience side effects, according to the clinic literature, which includes "excessive gas in the stomach, slight skin rash, slightly increased blood pressure, chills and fever."

Animal studies have shown that antineoplastons are retained in brain tissue and have a low toxicity.

In 1991, the National Cancer Institute reviewed a series of Burzynski's "best cases" and visited his clinic. The NCI concluded that antitumor activity by antineoplastons may have been demonstrated in seven cases of incurable brain cancer, and the agency agreed that trials to confirm these effects would be worthwhile. (It is noted, however, that several patients received the treatment shortly after taking radiation therapy.) However, for various reasons, the joint effort by the OAM and NCI to study the therapy in children with brain tumors failed, and antineoplaston therapy remains very controversial.

Oxygen Therapy. Oxygen therapy is also known as *hyperoxygenation therapy, oxymedicine, oxidative* or *bio-oxidative therapy*, or *oxidology*. It is based on the premise that cancer is caused by a deficiency of oxygen, a theory developed by a German chemist and two-time Nobel Prize winner, Otto Warburg, M.D. The way to counter cancer, he believed, is to expose cancer cells to high levels of oxygen. Since then, many have advocated this therapy and several have written books about it. Indeed, hyperoxygenation is claimed to be effective against countless diseases besides cancer. The most common types of oxygen therapy use ozone (a gas) and hydrogen peroxide (a liquid). Enzymes such as superoxide dismutase also are used in oxygenation therapy. Supplements, such as germanium sesquioxide, which is sold in health food stores, are promoted as "oxygenators." Diluted hydrogen peroxide may be given orally, rectally, intravenously, or vaginally. It may even be used directly on the skin, in a bath. According to the OTA, ozone enemas are given at the Gerson clinic.

Ozone is usually administered in a process called *blood infusion*, in which blood is removed, treated with ozone, and returned intravenously to the person. One company has applied to the FDA to study the antiviral effects of ozone, but animal studies must be submitted before Phase I studies are permitted.

Thus far, no studies have shown that oxygen therapy is a viable treatment for cancer. In fact, although oxymedicinal therapies are often touted as natural and nontoxic, ozone, hydrogen peroxide, and other oxidizing agents can have serious side effects, including damage to healthy organs. At some doses these substances can even be lethal. Nevertheless, oxygen therapy is available at cancer centers outside the United States, especially in Mexico and Germany.

Shark Cartilage. Some scientists—led by William Lane, Ph.D., author of *Sharks Don't Get Cancer* and, more recently, *Sharks Still Don't Get Cancer*—believe that sharks have amazingly strong immune systems powered by a substance found in the cartilage of their skeletons. This substance appears to prevent *angiogenesis*, the growth of new blood vessels, which are essential to tumor growth.

In recent years there has been a growing interest in powdered shark cartilage as a cancer treatment. It is available in health food stores and some drugstores in capsule form. Some mainstream scientists say that the active ingredient of these supplements is not absorbed by the body and is excreted.

There have been no clinical trials to prove its effectiveness. The FDA has granted permission to Lane Labs–USA, a pharmaceutical company, to test BeneFin, a drug derived from shark cartilage, to treat prostate cancer and AIDS patients with Kaposi's sarcoma. Bovine cartilage (Catrix) is being evaluated for use against cancer, and some positive effects have been reported. Some scientists report that bovine cartilage has far more angiogenic activity than shark cartilage.

Herbal Treatments. More than 3,000 different plants have reportedly been used to treat cancer all over the world. Many herbal treatments are based on folk remedies and traditional Chinese medicine. Some herbs are used alone, such as mistletoe or chaparral, which is usually prepared as a tea. Others are combined. For example, a tea called *essiac*, developed by a Native Canadian and popularized in the 1920s by Rene Caisse (which spelled backward is essi-ac), consists of Turkey rhubarb, sorrel, slippery elm, and burdock. Caisse never revealed the formula, so the health food store varieties are different versions of the herbal combination.

So far, there has been scant evidence that any of the most popular herbal treatments provide any benefit for people with cancer. In fact, some herbs are harmful. Chaparral, for example, may cause liver damage. But the interest in herbal remedies is increasing, and many studies evaluating herbs for medicinal use are under way.

Iscador. In 1920 Rudolf Steiner, Ph.D., founder of the privately funded Society for Cancer Research in Arlesheim, Switzerland, proposed using iscador, a preparation made from mistletoe found in apple, fir, pine, oak, and elm trees, to treat cancer. It is available in many European clinics, and several countries are funding studies of iscador's effects on cancer.

A few studies have been done in the United States. One indicated that iscador simulates the thymus gland and speeds blood-forming cell regeneration after exposure to x-rays. Another showed that cytotoxic alkaloids (see Chapter 17, "Chemotherapy") could be extracted from the preparation, and studies of mouse and human leukemia cells showed that their growth could be inhibited. But in another animal study, tumor growth rates were not significantly reduced. The FDA has not tested Iscador, and it is not approved for use.

Dimethyl Sulfoxide (DMSO). DMSO, an industrial solvent, has been touted as a treatment for various diseases and conditions, including cancer. (In the United States it has been approved by the FDA only for the treatment of interstitial cystitis, a bladder condition.) DMSO has been used in conjunction with other alternative treatments and preparations, such as Harold Manner's metabolic therapy, laetrile, and the well-known "youth drug" of the Romanian physician Anna Aslan, M.D., procaine hydrochloride, which is also known as *GH3, Gerovital,* or *KH3.* In the late 1980s several studies were done to evaluate DMSO's activity in the test tube and in humans with bladder cancer. DMSO did not increase the activity of standard chemotherapy drugs, nor was it helpful in treating patients.

In 1971 the National Academy of Sciences' National Research Council evaluated data on the use of DMSO in humans and found that it did not warrant approval and, moreover, caused side effects in the skin and eyes.

Cancell. Cancell (also known as *Entelev*) is a solution containing 12 different compounds, including inositol, nitric acid, sodium sulfite, potassium hydroxide, sulfuric acid, and catechol. It has been known by several names: *Jim's juice, crocinic acid, Sheridan's formula, JS-114, JS-101,* and *126-F.* Cancer is just one of several diseases and conditions that it is said to cure when taken internally or applied externally to an area pretreated with DMSO.

Both James V. Sheridan, a columnist, and Edward J. Sopcak manufactured some form of Cancell/Entelev, and each describes its purported anti-cancer activity in a slightly different way. Their claimed end result, however, is similar: The cancer cells return to a primitive state that allows them to be digested.

In 1978 and 1980, the National Cancer Institute, using Sheridan's preparation, did tests on animals and found no anticancer activity. In 1990 and 1991, the preparation was examined again by the NCI, which "determined that no further action will be taken on this compound."

Revici Method. The Revici method of "biologically guided" chemotherapy is based on a complex theory of cancer developed by Emanuel Revici, M.D., a Romanian-born physician who came to the United States in 1946 and practiced for many years in New York City. At one time he maintained his own hospital, Trafalgar Hospital, where he was chief of oncology. Although some academics have described Revici as an "innovative medical genius," his hospital was suspended from the Medicaid program because of fraud and in 1982, his license to practice medicine was temporarily suspended. He was allowed to continue to practice, albeit with several restrictions. In 1993 the New York Board of Regents found Revici guilty of violating probation on a charge of professional misconduct and his license was revoked..

Revici determined what treatment a patient should receive based on urine and blood tests that revealed whether his or her cancer was "anabolic" or "catabolic." His form of "biologically guided chemotherapy" would, Revici believed, correct the "offbalance": Lipid alcohols, lithium, zinc, iron, and caffeine are considered anabolic agents, and fatty acids, sulfur, selenium, and magnesium are catabolic.

The National Cancer Institute, the Committee of Cancer Diagnosis and Therapy of the National Research Council, and the University of Wisconsin have made several attempts to objectively evaluate Revici's methods and claims. Unfortunately, Revici's Institute of Applied Biology could never agree on the procedure to be followed. In the 1960s, a study by a Clinical Appraisal Group of New York City researchers found "no instance of objective tumor regression" in some 30 patients they studied. Revici objected to the group's findings.

Fresh Cell Therapy. The Swiss physician Paul Niehans, M.D., developed fresh cell therapy (also known as live cell therapy or cellular therapy) in 1931 based on the theory that intramuscular injections of cells from cancer-resistant animal embryos could repair and regenerate human cells and organs. Cellular therapy, proponents claim, also stimulates the immune system. Cancer, Niehans believed, resulted from the degeneration of epithelial cells, but the disease was not the primary indication for his treatment. According to the OTA report, injected cells are said to travel to an organ similar to the one from which they were taken and stimulate the organ's function.

Niehans died in 1971, but his fresh cell therapy is still administered in several clinics in Tijuana and Switzerland. The Swiss Clinic La Prairie is probably the best known, because so many celebrities have gone there for cellular therapy to combat aging. However, the chief physician of the clinic says it is not a cancer clinic, and injections of sheep fetus cells are used only when all other standard treatments have failed.

The dangers of the treatment, according to the FDA, are infections and allergic reactions, including anaphylactic shock and death. In 1985, the FDA asked the U.S. Customs and Postal Service to bar from entry all cellular therapy powders and extracts intended for injection. In addition, the German Medical Association has warned against fresh cell therapy because of fatal immune reactions.

The Greek Cancer Cure. Hariton-Tzannis Alivizatos, M.D., a Greek microbiologist, claimed to have successfully treated skin, bone, uterine, stomach, and lymphatic system cancers with intravenous injections of his "secret" serum. It is said to contain sugars, vitamins, and amino acids, among other things, though an American laboratory that analyzed the ingredients of some syringes used to deliver the treatment found nicotinic acid, one of the B vitamins.

A series of serum injections over six to 30 days is said to boost the immune system. The patient also eats a diet low in salt and acids, limits physical activity, and avoids some drugs such as aspirin and laxatives.

Alivizatos was investigated for medical malpractice and had his license suspended for two years. Although Alivizatos died in 1994, some physicians in Poland and Greece are said to be using the Greek Cancer Cure.

Livingston-Wheeler Therapy. According to physician Virginia Livingston-Wheeler, the cause of cancer is a weak immune system that allows proliferation of a bacteria she named *Progenitor cryptocides*. (The possibility of a bacterial link is not new, though most scientists abandoned the idea 50 years ago. Furthermore, researchers have never discovered a *P. cryptocides* organism.) In *The Conquest of Cancer*, Livingston-Wheeler claimed an 82 percent success rate in those cases described in the book.

The treatment is a combination of a vaccine made from each patient's own strain of bacteria obtained from his or her own urine, blood, or tumor tissue (an *autologous* vaccine) and other vaccines such as Bacille Clamette-Guérin (BCG) (a tuberculosis vaccine). Injections of gamma globulin, sheep spleen extract, crude liver extract, and vitamin B12 are also used. Injectable or oral preparations of spleen and liver extracts, Levamisole, and whole blood transfusions are sometimes administered.

And there is more: castor oil, Epsom salts, and enemas are used to cleanse the bowels, followed by daily coffee, lemon juice, or hot water enemas. Lactic acid bacilli are used to maintain the intestinal flora and remove toxins and digestive enzymes are prescribed. Megadoses of vitamin and mineral supplements in pill or injectable form provide extra vitamins A, C, D, E, and individual Bs; calcium; magnesium; selenium; and iodine. A vitamin A derivative, abscic acid (Dormin), is said to inhibit tumor growth.

Finally, Livingston-Wheeler prescribes a strict vegetarian diet that is 75 percent raw fruits and vegetables and is supposed to boost immunity. No poultry, meat, eggs, milk, sugar, processed foods, food additives, alcohol, caffeine, and fluoridated water are allowed. But once the patient graduates to a "maintenance diet," fish (not shellfish), lamb, and more grains are permitted.

Even though vaccines are currently being actively investigated to treat cancer, Livingston-Wheeler's autologous vaccine—like other aspects of her treatment—is not considered effective against the disease. The ACS has found no evidence that the therapy offered at the Livingston-Wheeler Clinic in San Diego, California, is of any benefit to people with cancer.

Psychological Approaches

Meditation, relaxation therapy, mental imagery, and visualization techniques have proved helpful to cancer patients coping with certain symptoms and stress, although no psychological therapy has been found to cure cancer.

Guided Imagery

Guided imagery is a psychological approach to cancer treatment that was developed in the 1970s by O. Carl Simonton, a radiation oncologist, and Stephanie Simonton-Atchley, a psychotherapist, and is taught in Simonton's Center in Santa Barbara, California. The Simontons devised a technique that they claim empowers the mind to relieve cancer-related stress, anxiety, and fear and make the immune system work more effectively. According to the OTA report, the regimen is presented as an adjunct to conventional treatment.

The procedure the Simontons recommend three times a day is to first become totally relaxed. Then the person pictures his or her tumor as a mass of disorganized cells and visualizes that they are being overwhelmed by white blood cells. Conventional treatment is seen as powerful. Dead cancer cells are visualized as being eliminated. Then the person imagines being healthy and full of energy.

The method was published in *Getting Well Again*, in which the Simontons claimed that over four years, their patients who used guided imagery along with conventional treatments lived significantly longer than those who did not use imagery. They reported that imagery could enhance the immune system and "alter the course of a malignancy," although these claims were not based on a controlled study and are not conclusive.

The terms *guided* or *mental imagery* or *visualization* are used in complementary medical settings to define certain techniques that help cancer patients relax, deal with the stress of procedures, and relieve symptoms (see Chapter 25, "Coping with Stress, Fear, Anxiety, and Depression"). In these situations, though, imagery is *not* being promoted for any antitumor effect.

Where the American Cancer Society Stands

The ACS examines questionable therapies and attempts to answer fundamental questions typically asked of any treatment that claims to be of value in diagnosing or treating cancer. The following are questions that physicians and other health care professionals and researchers use when evaluating a treatment and its claims. You too can use them when a treatment seems questionable.

Warning Signs That a Treatment Is Questionable

There are several indicators that a treatment is truly bogus. You can save yourself time, money, and disappointment by avoiding any practitioner and/or therapist who causes you to answer yes to any of the following:

- The practitioner claims that the treatment is based on a "secret" ingredient or method.
- The proof that the treatment works and is safe is based only on testimonials.
- The therapist refuses to speak to your physician.
- The treatment claims to cure your cancer or prevent its recurrence.
- The treatment is described as a "scientific breakthrough" or "miraculous."

- Has the method been objectively demonstrated in peer-reviewed scientific literature to be more effective than doing nothing?

- Has the method shown a potential for benefit that clearly exceeds the potential for harm?

- Have objective studies been conducted properly, appropriately evaluated by other qualified scientists, and approved by responsible human studies committees to answer these questions?

The ACS, through its Medical Affairs Subcommittee on Alternative and Complementary Methods of Cancer Management, provides information on unproven therapies to health professionals and the lay public. You can receive information from your local ACS or by calling 1-800-ACS-2345.

Making Choices

It is sometimes difficult to be objective when you so much want a treatment to deliver the hoped-for cure. Nevertheless, it is important to try not to let fear or desperation affect your judgment. One of the criticisms you most often hear of alternatives is that they have not been proved safe and effective according to standard scientific methods (see Chapter 21, "Investigational Treatments"). For example, before the FDA approves a drug, it is studied in a large number of people. These studies are then published in peer-reviewed medical journals that your doctor can read, and he or she can search the literature for the opinions of qualified specialists. In this way, both you and your doctor can get some idea of the success of a particular treatment, its side effects, and any toxicity. Little of this important information is available about alternatives, however.

Therefore, it is important to discuss with your oncologist the treatment you are considering. Some studies indicate that people are unwilling to tell their doctors that they are seeking an alternative therapy. They may fear being criticized or that their doctor will stop treating them. Whatever the concern, it clearly stands in the way of the open, trusting communication that is so important when dealing with a life-threatening disease. For some people, openness to alternative therapies is not an issue, but if it is for you, a discussion with your oncologist is in order. Just as he or she should respect your right to make choices, you need to feel confident of your doctor's judgment and trust his or her opinion. Today many doctors do not object to complementary treatments, and some have no problem with some alternative ones, provided they are not dangerous and do not delay or interfere with medical treatment. Likewise, you can best help yourself by understanding that wishing or hoping a treatment will work is one thing but that true, measurable improvement is another.

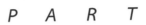

LIVING THE BEST YOU CAN WITH CANCER

THE PAIN CHALLENGE

Each day, more than 1 million Americans and 9 million people around the world experience cancer-related pain. But a more important statistic is that nine out of 10 of these people can find some degree of relief through treatment. If you experience pain caused by cancer or its therapies, you have the right to demand—and receive—relief.

For far too long, the importance of managing cancer pain was overlooked. Pain was seen as something to be endured, an inevitable consequence of the disease process. Now research is providing growing evidence that in the great majority of cases, pain can be controlled.

Pain control (or pain management) means treating pain aggressively to provide the maximum degree of relief possible. Usually this means treatment with drugs and other methods, such as surgery. But it also includes techniques that improve the quality of life and the ability to work, enjoy recreation, and function as normally as possible. It may involve psychological therapy, training in relaxation techniques, and a number of other strategies that do not require medications.

Current studies are determining what approaches work best for people with different forms of cancer. New federal guidelines for relieving cancer pain have been published, and nearly every state has launched a cancer pain relief initiative to promote awareness of pain-control strategies. Education is helping overcome myths and misunderstandings that doctors and nurses as well as patients have maintained in regard to pain treatment. In addition, the importance of mind-body approaches to pain, such as certain relaxation techniques, is being recognized by doctors and caregivers in traditional hospital settings.

This chapter explores the causes and effects of cancer pain and shows how you can communicate with others about your discomfort and how you and your care providers can work together to ease the burden of pain and achieve the highest possible quality of life. Although some reference is made to pain relief techniques, Chapter 24 is devoted to how pain is treated.

What Is Pain?

On one level, pain is simply any feeling that hurts. Throughout the body are thousands of nerve endings that react when something is wrong. (These nerve sites are technically known as *nociceptors*, a word that means "harm receptor.") The signals travel along nerves to the brain, which then processes the sensory information.

Cancer causes pain when the disease invades bones, muscles, or blood vessels. It also occurs if the cancer presses on nerves, blocks hollow organs such as the bowel, pinches blood vessels, or produces inflammation. In addition, the treatments aimed at the cancer sometimes are painful.

But pain has many dimensions beyond the merely physical. The longer the pain persists, the greater the suffering it causes in virtually all aspects of life. Unrelieved pain makes it hard to carry out many of the basic activities of life: dressing, eating, walking. It can cause you to feel anxious, angry, or depressed. It strips away personal dignity, shatters relationships with friends and family, and leads to mistrust of doctors and other care providers. In a vicious cycle, pain may make it impossible for some people to comply with the treatment for their cancer—the very treatment that holds some promise for relieving their pain.

Pain is a unique experience for each person. Some can tolerate it more easily than others. Tolerance is partly the result of cultural conditioning. For example, many people who live in Western cultures prize the stiff upper lip philosophy of enduring hardship. And athletes might believe in the motto "No pain, no gain." There is nothing to be gained, however, from enduring the pain associated with cancer.

Myths and Misconceptions

Fear gives rise to myths about the meaning of pain. For example, when you first learned you had cancer, perhaps you automatically assumed you would have pain. Although pain is indeed a common complication of certain kinds of cancer, it is not inevitable. In fact, most early cancers do not cause pain.

Even if pain does develop in the early stages, it is by no means certain that it will get worse. Often the treatment that removes or shrinks tumors also relieves pain.

Nor is pain a sign that the cancer is incurable. About 15 percent of people with nonmetastatic cancer have pain. In cases of metastatic cancer, about one in three people report pain severe enough to disrupt their activities and that requires the use of pain-relieving medications. Between 50 and 90 percent of those with advanced metastatic disease do have substantial pain.

TIPS & ADVICE

Pain Control Strategies

Stay on top of the pain. Anticipate it if possible, and respond to it quickly. The more you can prevent pain from developing or becoming severe, the more effective the treatment will be and your doses of medication may be lower.

Don't try to tough it out or wait until the pain becomes unbearable before seeking relief. Generally, the worse the pain is, the longer it takes to get relief.

Don't be afraid to admit you have pain. Only you know how you feel. Communicating to family members and caregivers about your pain is essential. Don't worry about being seen as a complainer or a difficult patient. Pain relief is vital to managing cancer, and unless others know about your situation, they can't help you as much as you may need.

Resist comparing your situation with someone else's. Your pain, like your cancer, is unique, and so is the treatment you require.

Try to follow your doctor's orders. You may need to take a medication at certain intervals, even if you're not in much pain at the time, to get the most benefit.

Let people know if you're not getting the relief you expected. The effects of cancer on your body can change from day to day, and sometimes a medication that worked in the past may not work in the future. Don't wait for your next appointment before letting your doctor know if the pain therapy isn't working.

Take note of and immediately report any side effects of the pain treatment.

A New Awareness

According to a 1992 survey of 1,200 cancer physicians, only 50 percent believed that pain control in their hospitals was adequate, and 85 percent believed that patients were undermedicated for pain. Many steps were immediately taken to remedy this situation. Programs now exist in most states to educate health care professionals (and also people with cancer) about undertreated pain. These programs alert people to the problem, describe options for pain control, and work to make cancer pain relief a high priority. In 1992 the National Cancer Institute began giving grants to support projects whose goal is to raise awareness of the need for better pain management.

Some states are working to remove legislative barriers. For example, California and Texas each adopted a so-called Intractable Pain Act that reduces the red tape and protects doctors who prescribe narcotic analgesics (painkillers) from the legal risks of using these controlled substances.

Many hospitals are revising patient charts to track the severity of pain and the results of pain control strategies. Pain is now considered a vital sign, and monitoring it is as significant as checking body temperature and heartbeat.

On an even more basic level, medical schools are making pain treatment part of the training program for oncologists. Such training is essential to change attitudes and to bring new pain control strategies into the mainstream.

Today, depending on the circumstances, the professionals involved in pain assessment and treatment may include oncologists, nurses, anesthesiologists, home health care providers, psychiatrists, psychologists, social workers, and therapists versed in complementary techniques ranging from hypnosis to biofeedback.

The Experience of Pain

The most important person on the team, of course, is you. The more involved you are, the more you will understand your perceptions, which will make you better able to communicate your feelings and bring your pain under control.

It's Personal

A number of factors make the experience of pain a highly individual one. For example, some people with cancer may feel they should downplay the extent of their pain. Others may not want to distract their caregivers from the task at hand, namely, addressing the cancer itself. And some people may fear that pain treatment may cause further suffering or complications, such as addiction to narcotics. Some people want to put up a brave front, to protect loved ones from knowing how much they are suffering. The best thing to do, though, is to speak up: Tell others what is happening to you so that you can get the help you need.

Psychological factors play a key part. Fears and worries about the disease and about death can influence your perception of pain. If you worry a lot, you may be tense, anxious, and unable to sleep, and insomnia and fatigue can make the pain worse. On the other hand, if you believe that you have good control over your situation, that you know your limits of tolerance and what steps to take to feel better, you may experience less pain than does a person who doesn't have such confidence.

Life experience also plays a part. Your ability to cope with challenge, level of emotional maturity, attitudes toward doctors and medications, and the impact of the illness on your life goals all influence your perception of pain. And clearly, social support—love and understanding from family and friends—makes a big difference.

Emotional or psychological problems may contribute to the experience of pain. For example, chronic pain tends to cause a depression-like syndrome. People with cancer may feel highly anxious about the treatment they must endure or the outcome of their illness. Thus, even though emotional symptoms and difficulties may not cause pain directly, they can increase the awareness of and vulnerability to discomfort.

Beliefs and Meanings

Most people react to pain in one of three ways: as a punishment, as an enemy, or as a challenge. Those who see it as a punishment wonder what they did wrong in life to have earned such grief. Those who see it as an enemy feel they are being attacked or robbed and often feel hopeless. But those who see it as a challenge believe they can do something to overcome the pain and feel they have more control over their situation. These people have lower levels of depression, more and stronger strategies for coping, and—most important— less pain.

Being aware of the meaning you ascribe to pain can translate directly into better pain management. In some cases, counseling can help uncover troublesome beliefs about pain. Someone who sees pain as a punishment or a lesson from God may benefit from talking with a member of the clergy or other spiritual counselor. Open, honest communication about such feelings is essential.

Why It Hurts

The pain associated with cancer comes from the tumor itself, the cancer treatments, complications of the disease, or a combination of all three. The pain relief choices are determined by what is causing the discomfort and whether or not that cause is transient. Over the course of the illness, the quality of the pain—as well as what is causing it—may change.

Most complaints are a direct reflection of the tumor's growth and spread. When cancer cells invade bones or vital organs or press on nerves or blood vessels, pain can result. Pain can also result from the effects of the various hormones and other chemicals the body produces in response to cancer.

Cancer treatments may cause a variety of uncomfortable sensations. Surgery, of course, is a major trauma to the body, and strong medications are temporarily needed. But as the body begins to heal, the discomfort usually diminishes, and medications are given less often and in lower doses. However, some types of pain related to surgery persist long after the wounds have healed and may require long-term pain relief.

Less well known are the side effects of certain chemotherapy drugs, such as a burning sensation in the hands or feet. (Tricyclic antidepressants and anticonvulsant medications have been shown to be helpful for this type of pain.) And depending on the treatment site, radiation therapy may produce uncomfortable sensory changes that last for several months. Cancer can suppress the immune system too, increasing the chances of infection, a symptom of which may be local irritation and soreness in the area affected.

Simply being confined to bed may lead to various complications, from bedsores to constipation, all of which are uncomfortable. Finally, the emotional stress of coping with such confinement can lead to muscle tension, which causes pain. Precautions can be taken to prevent these complications, but when they do occur, each symptom must be addressed individually and promptly.

A small percentage of people sometimes have another illness or disorder in addition to cancer that produces pain, such as migraine headaches, osteoporosis, or degenerative disk disease. Although these conditions may complicate the cancer treatment, the discomfort must be attended to.

Communicating Your Pain

An essential element in effective pain management, at all steps in the process, is communication. The person who feels pain is the best source of information about it: how bad it is, where it is located, what works, and what doesn't. All too often, though, there is a wide gap between the way a person experiences pain and the way others perceive that pain. One study found that doctors and nurses consistently rated patients' pain as less intense than did the patients themselves. In fact, nurses and the people in their care agreed on the level of severity only about 7 percent of the time. No one knows where and how you hurt better than you do. If you can communicate clearly, there's a better chance that your care providers can determine what is causing the problem. That, in turn, improves the odds of obtaining the relief you need.

Pain can be described in a number of ways. The type of cancer involved, the part of the body affected, the combination of treatments you receive—even your work life and support network—have some bearing on the extent and impact of pain and its management.

How Long Does It Last?

One of the chief characteristics of pain is how long it lasts. *Acute pain* appears suddenly and recedes fairly quickly. Besides the painful feelings, people in acute pain may experience rapid heartbeat and an increase in blood pressure. They may wince and rub the affected area. Such pain may come from the cancer itself, usually from the swelling of a tumor. When the tumor is removed or made to shrink, most people experience dramatic pain relief. The use of analgesic medications, taken as needed, can provide relief. Acute pain can also be a response to cancer therapy. Many people find it easier to bear such pain when they learn that it comes and goes in a predictable way and that the benefits of treatment—a successful outcome—are well worth the drawbacks.

In contrast to acute pain, *chronic pain* lasts more or less continuously for several months. Like acute pain, it can be caused by the disease itself or may be a consequence of the treatment. The pain may grow more severe as time passes, or it may persist at a constant level. Of course, the longer it lasts, the greater its impact on your quality of life.

Over time, the body's nervous system adapts to chronic pain by becoming less physically responsive to pain signals. For example, the heart may no longer beat as rapidly as it did during an episode of acute pain. Although the painful sensations may become less intense, they can give rise to emotional difficulties. Like depression, chronic pain can produce mood changes, irritability, disturbed sleep, reduced appetite, and difficulty concentrating. Such pain can lead to changes in personality, lifestyle, and ability to function. Robbed of the ability to enjoy even simple daily activities, a person may lose hope of recovering. But the resulting fear of death only increases the overall level of pain and suffering.

Fortunately, cancer pain is more readily treated than is the pain from other long-term illnesses such as sickle-cell disease. Morphine and related drugs are very effective, even over long periods of time, and the risk of becoming addicted to narcotics for the treatment of cancer pain is extremely low.

Acute pain is often obvious to an observer because it produces symptoms such as rapid heartbeat. But chronic pain can become invisible over time. By letting people know how you feel, you can get the help you need.

Where Is It?

Pain can originate from a particular place, such as when a tumor affects nerves in a specific area. This is known as *focal* pain. Pain sensations can also spread out along the length of a nerve, causing what is known as *radiating* (or *radicular*) pain. But some parts of the body, including some of the internal organs and tissues, do not have pain receptors. When something goes wrong in these areas, the brain reacts by responding as though the pain were occurring somewhere else along the same nerve network. For example, gallbladder disease often produces pain in the right shoulder area. This is known as *referred* pain. Knowing that pain sensations may not actually arise at the site of the problem helps in deciding the type of treatment needed. For example, anesthetic or surgical approaches may be more appropriate for focal pain, whereas medications may be more effective for referred pain.

What Type Is It?

Another way to characterize pain is by the changes it produces in the body. Most cancer-related pain is physical or *organic* in nature. (So-called psychosomatic pain, originating in the mind, is rare in people with cancer, although psychological distress certainly contributes to the severity of pain.)

There are three types of organic pain. *Somatic* pain affects the pain receptors and typically causes you to feel a constant dull or aching sensation in a specific area. Examples are metastatic bone pain, pain felt along a surgical incision, and musculoskeletal pain.

Sometimes the pain arises from the stretching and enlarging of tissues or organ structures in the abdominal cavity. This is known as *visceral* pain. Such pain is usually less focused and tends to be referred to distant locations. People often describe visceral pain as a deep squeezing or pressured feeling. If it comes on suddenly, it may lead to nausea, vomiting, and sweating.

A third type of organic pain, *neuropathic* pain, arises from damage to nerves, from either the cancer or its treatment. People often describe this type of pain as severe burning, stabbing, viselike, or shocklike sensations. Neuropathic pain does not usually respond to narcotics but may improve after certain kinds of surgery or the use of regional anesthetics. Antidepressant and anticonvulsant drugs may also be helpful.

A Picture of Pain

A complete assessment of pain is much like a diagnostic procedure. There is a discussion during which you describe your situation and undergo an examination to evaluate your physical condition.

How Do You Feel?

The caregiver (usually a nurse or a physician) asks questions about the history of your pain, as well as other pertinent details about your illness. Typical questions include

- How bad is your pain?

- Where do you feel it?

- When did it begin?

- What does it feel like?

- Is it constant? Does it vary? Is it worse at some times of day than others?

- How long does it last?

- How does it affect your ability to carry out your activities?

- What have you done to relieve the pain?

- What does or does not work?

- What has worked in the past to relieve pain?

Some physicians show you a picture of the body and ask you to point out where you feel the pain.

There are a number of ways in which caregivers assess the intensity of pain. One of the easiest is to ask you to describe the level of the pain on a scale of 0 to 10. As a measure of severity, for instance, 0 might represent no pain at all and 10 might indicate the worst pain you can imagine. Such numbers are highly subjective—one person's 7 might be another person's 4. What is important, though, is the *consistency* of your responses over time.

The *pattern* of pain also is relevant. It helps to know, for example, if the pain is constant or if it comes and goes; if it changes throughout the day or is usually the same in intensity and location; if certain activities (such as moving your arms, breathing, swallowing, standing up, or lying down) trigger painful feelings. Especially valuable is a verbal description of the pain. Such descriptions provide clues to what is happening inside the body (see box on page 269).

To arrive at a true measure of your pain, your caregivers should also ask about its psychological and social impact. They will want to know about the degree of suffering, about its effect on your mood, the extent of physical disability it causes, how you function with your family or on the job, and what concerns you may have about money or death. Sometimes these questions are best answered by a spouse or other close relative or friend. It helps enormously if someone who knows you well, who can talk about the impact the pain is having, can be present for the assessment. If you are incapacitated or otherwise unable to speak, the presence of such an ally is essential.

The Physical Exam

A doctor or nurse may look for signs of inflammation or tenderness and check vital signs, since heart rate (pulse) and blood pressure may increase during pain. These signs are not useful, however, when attempting to measure the amount of pain, nor will pain show up on an x-ray or under a microscope. Even so, certain imaging procedures can help pinpoint the cause of pain or reveal the extent of tissue injury or damage. Computerized tomography (CT) scans, for example, can reveal changes in bones and certain soft tissues. Magnetic resonance imaging (MRI) helps evaluate damage to the vertebrae, spinal cord compression, or the metastasis of cancer cells to the brain. In many cases, these procedures may not be necessary to obtain the information needed to carry out treatment.

To the greatest extent possible, caregivers should provide relief for people in pain at the time of the assessment, before proceeding. Pain is not an excuse for not doing a careful work-up, particularly since the results of the assessment will determine a course of action that might alleviate it.

Words for Describing Pain

Flickering	Jumping	Pricking	Sharp
Quivering	Flashing	Boring	Cutting
Pulsing	Shooting	Drilling	Lacerating
Throbbing		Stabbing	
Beating		Lancinating	
Pounding			
Pinching	Tugging	Hot	Tingling
Pressing	Pulling	Burning	Itchy
Gnawing	Wrenching	Scalding	Smarting
Cramping		Searing	Stinging
Crushing			
Dull	Tender	Tiring	Sickening
Sore	Taut	Exhausting	Suffocating
Hurting	Rasping		
Aching	Splitting		
Heavy			
Fearful	Punishing	Wretched	Annoying
Frightful	Grueling	Blinding	Troublesome
Terrifying	Cruel		Miserable
	Vicious		Intense
	Killing		Unbearable
Spreading	Tight	Cool	Nagging
Radiating	Numb	Cold	Nauseating
Penetrating	Drawing	Freezing	Agonizing
Piercing	Squeezing		Dreadful
	Tearing		Torturing

INFORM

YOURSELF

TIPS &
ADVICE

Keep a Pain Diary

It's hard to remember when you experience the pain, the nature of it at any particular time, what you did for it, what you were doing when it occurred. Keeping a daily pain diary can help you communicate to your caregivers and track which pain relief methods work best. Here is a sample page for one day.

Time	Severity from 1 (very mild) to 10 (never worse)	Description (choose from list on page 269)	What you were doing when it began (such as walking, sleeping)	Name and amount of medication taken	Nondrug techniques you tried (such as meditation, heat)
Midnight					
1 a.m.					
2 a.m.					
3 a.m.					
4 a.m.					
5 a.m.					
6 a.m.					
7 a.m.					
8 a.m.					
9 a.m.					
10 a.m.					
11 a.m.					
Noon					
1 p.m.					
2 p.m.					
3 p.m.					
4 p.m.					
5 p.m.					
6 p.m.					
7 p.m.					
8 p.m.					
9 p.m.					
10 p.m.					
11 p.m.					

PAIN RELIEF

Decisions about pain relief always are subject to reevaluation. If one approach does not bring comfort, other options almost always exist. However, to ensure an active role in the decision making, it's important that you or a close family member learn as much about pain relief strategies as possible. Education is also critical to overcoming the myths and misunderstandings surrounding cancer pain and its management.

This chapter describes the basic approaches to pain relief: the pharmacologic, surgical, anesthetic, neurologic, and mind-body methods typically incorporated in a treatment plan. As you consider the possibilities and discuss them with your caregivers, remember that you have a right to accept or reject any treatment that is proposed. And if the therapy is inadequate, you need to say so.

Whatever the plan, continuity of care is crucial to its success. Oncologists, nurse clinicians, and primary physicians must work with social workers, therapists, and any other caregivers on the team to provide consistent and aggressive pain relief in the hospital and at home. If care is fragmented (for cxample, if the primary physician has no idea what approaches have been recommended by the hospital staff or if a home care worker has no idea what treatments or dosages are known to work best) confusion will result.

Getting Control

In many instances, cancer therapy removes or shrinks the tumor and thus eliminates the source of the pain. The basic cancer treatments can also be palliative, that is, prescribed for pain relief. Radiation eases pain in more than half the cases and is usually the fastest and most effective strategy, especially for pain caused by bone metastases. Surgery, such as tumor resection, drainage of abscesses, or treatment of bowel obstruction, also can ease pain.

Chemotherapy has some palliative value, but it is unpredictable; its effects are often delayed; and it carries the risk of toxicity.

Drug Options

At least 70 percent of people with cancer who have pain find relief through the use of *analgesics*, agents that alleviate pain without causing a loss of consciousness. The other strategies, used alone or in combination with analgesics, can help most of the remaining 30 percent.

A few years ago the World Health Organization (WHO) became concerned that not enough was being done to treat pain in people with cancer. After studying the problem, the WHO devised a "ladder" approach to pain management. As shown in the box, the ladder image conveys the basic plan for using pain-relieving drugs: Start with the simplest and gradually proceed to the most powerful narcotics until a satisfactory level of relief is reached.

Nonnarcotic Analgesics

In many cases of mild to moderate pain, nonnarcotic drugs, several of which are available without a prescription, provide good relief. This is especially true if the person is able to "stay on top of the pain," that is, is able to anticipate the need for medication and take it as directed before the pain becomes severe.

INFORM
YOURSELF

Ladder of Pain Treatment

The first step on the ladder is the use of a nonnarcotic, such as aspirin or acetaminophen, and nonsteroidal anti-inflammatory drugs (NSAIDs), such as ibuprofen and naproxen. These are used alone or with *adjuvant* medications, that is, additional drugs directed at specific complaints. If none of the nonnarcotic analgesics or NSAIDs works, the second step is to try a weak narcotic in addition as needed. (A *narcotic* is an agent that has a numbing effect. It usually means an *opioid*, that is, a natural or synthetic drug that has a morphinelike action.) If high doses of this regimen are not adequate, the third step is to use a potent opioid, usually morphine, with or without NSAIDs or other adjuvants.

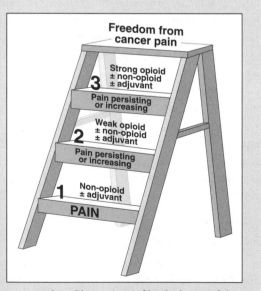

Freedom from cancer pain

3 Strong opioid ± non-opioid ± adjuvant

Pain persisting or increasing

2 Weak opioid ± non-opioid ± adjuvant

Pain persisting or increasing

1 Non-opioid ± adjuvant

PAIN

Like other pain relievers, nonnarcotic analgesics work by affecting the nervous system. However, unlike narcotics, which dull the central nervous system, these painkillers as a rule do not cause euphoria, drowsiness, or loss of consciousness. They have few serious side effects (although they can have some; see below) and do not lead to tolerance or dependence. Rather, they provide temporary relief, usually for about three or four hours, although some may be longer lasting. The choice of nonnarcotic analgesics boils down to acetaminophen (Tylenol is a well-known brand) and the nonsteroidal anti-inflammatory drugs (NSAIDs) such as ibuprofen (Motrin, Advil, Rufen, Nuprin) and naproxen (Naprosyn, Anaprox, Aleve). Some people cannot tolerate the NSAIDs because of gastrointestinal side effects. Numerous kinds of NSAIDs are available, some over-the-counter, some by prescription only. One NSAID may effectively relieve pain for one person, whereas another type may not, so switching drugs can be helpful.

Treatment with nonnarcotic analgesics generally begins with low doses, which may be increased over two or three weeks. These drugs have what is known as a *ceiling dose*, beyond which additional doses do not do any good. In this way, they differ from narcotics, which do provide more relief at higher doses. Always drink plenty of water when taking nonnarcotic analgesics, and even if you purchase them over the counter, take them only as your doctor suggests.

Side Effects. The risk of side effects increases with the dose of nonnarcotic analgesics and with the length of time the medication is taken. Although aspirin is generally a very safe drug, it can cause bleeding in the stomach, usually noticed as blood in the stools or unexplained bruising. For that reason people should not take it who are also using anticancer drugs that may cause bleeding. Others who should avoid aspirin include those taking steroids, such as prednisone or blood thinners such as Coumadin, and those who are allergic to aspirin or have a history of ulcers or gout. In children, aspirin may cause Reye's syndrome, a serious illness that can lead to respiratory arrest, mental confusion, coma, and death.

Other side effects of aspirin are ringing in the ears, hearing loss, unusual sweating, rapid breathing and heartbeat, nausea, vomiting, and diarrhea.

Comparison of Some Nonnarcotic Analgesics

	Reduce pain, fever	Reduce inflammation, pain of swollen joints	Can irritate stomach	Can affect blood clotting	Can cause Reye's syndrome	Can worsen kidney problems
Aspirin	Yes	Yes	Yes	Yes	Yes	No
Acetaminophen	Yes	No	No	No	No	No
Ibuprofen	Yes	Yes	Yes	Yes	No	Yes
Naproxen	Yes	Yes	Yes	Yes	No	Yes

INFORM

YOURSELF

Side effects associated with acetaminophen are rare, which accounts for its popularity. Liver or kidney damage, however, may result from large doses taken daily for a long period of time.

NSAIDs are generally safe but can cause nausea, vomiting, indigestion, and constipation. The drugs interfere with blood clotting, so people with low platelet counts should not take them. Other potential side effects of NSAIDs are dizziness, headache, ringing in the ears, fluid retention, dry mouth, and increased heart rate.

Narcotic Analgesics

If a trial with nonnarcotic analgesics does not bring sufficient pain relief, the next step on the ladder is the use of narcotics, or *opioids*. Unfortunately, narcotics have become associated with drug addicts and traffic in illegal "street" drugs. Furthermore, myths and misunderstandings about narcotics have led to the underuse of these drugs, which are exceedingly valuable in relieving cancer pain. Recently, though—in large part because of the experience gained from the hospice movement in England—care providers have come to recognize the benefits of long-term use of narcotic analgesics.

Narcotics (the word comes from the Greek term for numbness) range in strength from mild to strong. Some, such as codeine, can be either mild or strong, depending on their dosages and how they are used. As a rule, the low-strength products work only about as well and for as long as aspirin does.

Narcotics can be given alone, but some are used in combination with nonnarcotic analgesics. These drugs are usually given by mouth, but some are given as IV injections or as rectal suppositories if you have difficulty swallowing. A long-lasting (12-hour) form of morphine also is available.

There is no best choice of drugs, nor is there any such thing as a standard dose of narcotics. Each person in treatment has different needs, a different level of pain, and a different threshold for tolerating medication and its adverse effects.

Morphine is considered the gold standard of narcotic pain relief. Morphine (MS Contin, Oramorph), or a related drug called hydromorphone (Dilaudid), is frequently the first choice for treating pain, especially among the elderly with severe cancer-related pain. Other narcotics frequently used are levorphanol (Levo-Dromoran), methadone (Dolophine), or oxycodone (an ingredient in Percodan and Percocet), and meperidine (Demerol).

Narcotic Analgesics

Mild	Strong	
Codeine	Fentanyl	Morphine
Hydrocodone	Hydromorphone	Methadone
Oxycodone	Levorphanol	Oxymorphone
Propoxyphene	Meperidine	

INFORM

YOURSELF

Generally, physicians start with low doses of narcotics and increase the dose until pain is relieved or unpleasant side effects begin. If at that point the pain has not been relieved, the doctor may prescribe another kind of narcotic or add a nonnarcotic analgesic plus some other adjuvant medication.

Research has shown that usually the best treatment plan is giving a fixed dose of narcotic every four hours around the clock, plus additional "rescue doses" if the pain breaks through. This strategy has several advantages. Most important, of course, is that it effectively controls pain. It also provides additional relief should something happen—a change in the cancer or a treatment procedure—that suddenly increases the level of pain. Furthermore, it means that you can get relief without having to request it. This eases the feelings of guilt, awkwardness, hesitation, and responsibility that can accompany constant requests for more relief.

Side Effects and Other Concerns. One problem in using narcotics is that different drugs produce pain relief at different dosages. For instance, 10 units of one drug might have the same effect as 100 units of another. The method of delivery can also make a difference: A drug given by mouth may have a vastly enhanced effect if injected directly into the vein. Morphine taken orally, for example, must pass through the stomach before it can enter the bloodstream and find its way to the pain receptors.

Sometimes, however, caregivers are unaware of the differences in changing the route of administration or the type of narcotic, which in practice usually results in a tragic undermedication for pain. Today, however, cancer care providers are becoming more aware of the need to provide *equianalgesia*, in other words, to adjust for the differences in the type of drug or the route of administration to achieve the same results.

Gastrointestinal Side Effects. Although side effects are a less serious problem than the underuse of analgesics, they are fairly common, especially as the doses increase. Virtually everyone taking narcotics can expect to become constipated. These medications reduce the intestines' motility, which makes it harder to move the bowels and results in dry, stubborn stools. Other problems associated with cancer and its treatment, such as reduced activity, poor appetite, and weakness, only make the problem worse. Constipation can be alleviated by eating foods with lots of fiber (fruits, vegetables, oatmeal, stewed prunes, prune juice, bran cereal, or added bran) and by drinking eight to 10 glasses of water a day. Exercise helps too. Caregivers may suggest the use of a stool softener combined with a laxative, such as milk of magnesia. Before taking steps to deal with constipation, check with the physician, nurse, or nutritionist.

Low-grade nausea can be a problem, especially when appetite is already affected by cancer or its treatment. The incidence of nausea and vomiting is higher among ambulatory people. Accordingly, staying in bed for an hour or so after receiving the pain medication reduces the risk of nausea. Depending on the symptoms, antivomiting medications may be prescribed. Sometimes people taking narcotics feel as though their stomachs are always full, but a drug called metaclopramide makes the stomach empty faster and thus reduces this symptom. Switching to another narcotic can help as well.

Sedation. Narcotics can produce undesirable levels of drowsiness and sedation, depending on the drug and the dose. (Sometimes, though, the sleepiness is a direct result of the pain relief; freed from torment, you are at last able to catch up on much-needed rest.) In many cases, therefore, the drowsiness disappears after a few days. If not, taking lower doses more often or switching to another kind of opioid drug may help. Sometimes mild stimulants such as caffeine or amphetamines relieve the problem.

Respiratory Depression. Respiratory depression is the slowing down of breathing, and it can be the most serious consequence of using narcotics. Although this is seldom a problem in medical treatment, especially with oral morphine and when the dosage is tailored to your individual needs, respiratory depression can sometimes occur after the short-term use of high doses of a narcotic or after an overdose. Usually, the risk of this side effect diminishes over time. Should it occur, respiratory depression can be reversed through the administration of naloxone, a drug that blocks the action of narcotics.

Other Problems. At high doses over long periods of time, narcotics such as meperidine can cause muscle twitching or seizures, especially in people whose kidneys are not functioning fully. Reducing the dosage or using another medication can help. Other side effects include dry mouth and itching. Urinary retention can develop, especially in people with prostate or pelvic cancers. Changing the drug or discontinuing any adjuvant medications that can contribute to such problems, such as antidepressants, can minimize these side effects. Narcotics such as methadone and levorphanol have a long half-life (the time it takes for the dose to break down in the body). For that reason the dose can build up in the bloodstream while you are waiting for the benefits, which poses some risk of damage to certain organs in the body.

Fear of Addiction

Perhaps the most important point to be made in this chapter is that *people who take narcotics to relieve pain caused by a medical disease are not addicts, nor are they at serious risk of becoming addicts, no matter how much of the drug they take or how often they take it.*

The irrational fear of addiction causes many care providers to resist administering narcotics, many people with cancer pain to fear taking them, and many well-meaning friends and family members to pressure their loved ones not to comply with the treatment when narcotics are prescribed. One survey found that nearly half of people with cancer-related pain were reluctant to report their suffering, apparently out of concern that they would be given narcotics. Half were also afraid to take pain medications as prescribed. This fear of addiction, which is almost totally unfounded, prevents many people with cancer from achieving the degree of pain relief to which they are entitled.

A big part of the problem is confusion over the meaning of the terms *tolerance*, *dependency*, and *addiction*.

Tolerance. Narcotic drugs commonly produce tolerance, which means that you may need to take higher and higher doses to achieve the same effects as before. Although many people remain comfortable on stable doses of narcotics for long periods of time, one sign that you are becoming tolerant is that the pain relief from your usual dose does not last as long as it used to. This might happen because the disease is progressing or you are under greater psychological distress. In any case, for people who have become tolerant of narcotic painkillers, the medically correct strategy is to increase the dose or the frequency with which the medication is given. Unlike the nonnarcotic analgesics, narcotics have no ceiling dose, and sometimes large amounts of the drug are needed to achieve adequate pain relief. Another approach is to switch to a different type of narcotic.

When so-called recreational narcotics users become tolerant of a drug's effects, they too increase their use. But tolerance by itself does not mean that you are becoming addicted.

Although the situation is improving, many physicians and nurses still do not understand that tolerance differs from addiction. Therefore, if they see a patient becoming tolerant of a narcotic, they may reduce its use. These caregivers may have the mistaken notion that if "too much" of the drug is used now, the medication will not work later when the person "really needs it." The flaw in this argument is the assumption that people with cancer "really need" a narcotic only when their pain is not relieved by other strategies.

Dependence. Dependence, on the other hand, is a different issue. Dependence comes in two varieties: physical and psychological.

Physical dependence is a normal, predictable, and not very serious result of using narcotics. People who take high enough doses of a drug for a long enough time will likely become physically dependent on it. The most salient sign of dependency is that when they suddenly stop taking the drug, they experience withdrawal symptoms: agitation, fear, chills, sweating, shaking, sleeplessness, and worsening of pain. As bad as it sounds, the withdrawal syndrome can be easily avoided and well managed if the use of narcotics is reduced slowly over time. Note that even though narcotics addicts may become physically dependent on a drug, *physical dependence is not addiction.*

Psychological dependence is what most experts today mean when they speak of addiction. Addicts take drugs to satisfy physical, emotional, and psychological needs, not to solve a medical problem. Their lives become centered on obtaining and taking drugs. And they keep taking narcotics despite serious financial, legal, or health consequences.

The use of a narcotic is only one factor in developing a psychological dependence; a person's social, economic, and psychiatric background also plays a critical role. Unless he or she has a history of drug abuse, there is little risk that a patient being treated for a painful medical illness like cancer is at risk of developing a psychological addiction to a narcotic drug. Indeed, the incidence of psychological dependence among cancer patients is "vanishingly rare." According to a report in the *New England Journal of Medicine*, for which researchers reviewed the records of nearly 12,000 hospital patients with pain who had no history of drug addiction and who were treated with narcotics, the scientists found that only four out of these many thousands developed a psychological dependence—a risk of about three hundredths of 1 percent.

The Myths About Narcotics

- "Narcotics pose a strong risk of addiction." False. The risk is less than one in 3,000. Unfortunately, the misplaced fear of addiction often means that these drugs are not used as frequently as they should be, or in the right doses, to provide adequate pain relief.

- "Narcotics produce euphoria, which inevitably leads to being hooked." Not true. People taking narcotics for pain relief seldom report feeling euphoric. Even if they do, it is unlikely that they will continue to seek drugs for their euphoric effects after the pain has abated.

- "People are given morphine only when they're at death's door." No. In good cancer management, narcotics are administered as soon as pain becomes moderately severe. As the ladder strategy suggests, narcotics are appropriate treatment when nonnarcotics alone fail to provide the amount and duration of relief the person needs.

- "Morphine doesn't work when taken by mouth." False. This belief originated from some faulty studies done some years ago. In fact, oral morphine is very effective. (Injected narcotics may work faster at lower doses, however.)

- "Heroin is a better narcotic than morphine." Untrue. Anyway, the body converts heroin to morphine.

- "People always need high doses of narcotics." Wrong. Every person is different. Effective doses of morphine can range from 5 to 180 mg every four hours. Most people require only moderate doses; in fact, many people with advanced cancer and chronic severe pain need no more than 20 mg every four hours, no matter how long the therapy lasts.

- "I'll die of an overdose." Not likely. Many people fear narcotics because of news reports about drug users who die of overdoses. Even though the doses required for adequate pain relief are sometimes high, they are rarely, if ever, large enough to cause death. Among substance abusers, death usually results when they take outrageously high doses or consume dangerous combinations of substances, like a heroin-and-cocaine "cocktail." And addicts often take illegal narcotics manufactured by amateur scientists, compounds that contain impurities or are "cut" with adulterating substances such as talcum powder.

- "There's a limit to the effective dose of a narcotic." Not so. The stronger the pain is, the more is required for relief. Again, NSAIDs do have a ceiling dose, but narcotics can be used in increasing amounts until they bring the pain under control. Furthermore, increasing the dose (often a necessary step in managing the pain of progressive cancer) does not increase the already minimal risk of addiction.

- "People taking narcotics always need to take antivomiting drugs." Some do, especially in the beginning. Women are more prone to experience vomiting. But in most cases, the antivomiting therapy can be stopped after a few days.

- "People should take morphine only when they feel the need." No. The best strategy is to take regular doses around the clock, rather than on an as needed, or p.r.n., basis.

Adjuvant Medications

In many instances, drugs that treat a variety of complaints other than pain can enhance the effectiveness of analgesic therapy. Scientists are not sure why this is true, and they lack solid evidence showing which adjuvant drugs work best for people with various kinds of cancer. Still, adjuvant medications often do more than nonnarcotic or narcotic analgesics alone.

Tricyclic Antidepressants. Tricyclic antidepressants enhance the activity of various *neurotransmitters* in the brain and can be very useful drugs for managing pain. Tricyclics such as amitryptyline (Elavil, Endep), doxepin (Adapin, Sinequan), and imipramine (Tofranil) are especially effective for relieving the dull, burning pain due to nerve infiltration by cancer cells. The doses needed for pain relief are lower than those used in treating depression.

Anticonvulsants. Carbamazepine (Tegretol) and other anticonvulsants relieve the sharp stabbing or burning pains of tumors pressing on nerves, especially those in the head and neck. Such pain is notoriously resistant to narcotics. These drugs also are used to manage pain following surgical injury and for people with stump pain or pain in the lower extremities.

Corticosteroids. For many people, dexamethasone (Decadron), used in treating back pain due to compression of the spinal cord, produces significant relief and lowers the need for analgesic drugs. Prednisone (Deltasone) relieves

Adjuvant Medications for Cancer Pain

Type of Drug	Example(s)	Uses
Tricyclic antidepressants	Amitriptyline, doxepin, imipramine	Dull, burning pain due to nerve infiltration
Anticonvulsants	Carbamazepine, phenytoin, clonazepam	Stabbing pain due to nerve infiltration or compression, surgical injury, stump pain
Corticosteroids	Prednisone	Advanced cancer
	Dexamethasone	Back pain due to spinal cord compression
	Others	Diffuse bony metastases, nerve infiltration
Neuroleptics	Methotrimeprazine	Terminal stages, people tolerant of narcotics
Butyrophenones	Haloperidol	Reduce narcotic doses, psychosis, or delirium
Antibiotics	Various	Reduce pain secondary to infections
Miscellaneous	Hydroxyzine (minor tranquilizer)	Residual pain, nausea, or anxiety
	Dextroamphetamine	Post-op pain, counter sedation

INFORM
YOURSELF

pain in people with advanced cancer. Other steroids may help people with bony metastases or nerve infiltration. Steroids also can have positive effects on appetite and mood, and there is some evidence that they may work directly against certain kinds of tumors. Accordingly, people with advanced cancer who receive steroids often need lower doses of narcotics to control pain.

Getting the Drugs into the Body

Over the course of their illness, most people need to take pain medications via a number of different routes. Most need two routes. This is important, because the way that the drugs are administered can make a big difference in the way they work against pain. For example, drugs given orally or rectally may take longer to take effect, but they may last longer than when the drugs are given intravenously. However, many people become anxious and distressed while waiting for the medication to work. This becomes a concern when making decisions about medications, particularly when the individual is transferred home from the hospital or to a hospice. Caregivers and family members should therefore be aware that the way in which drugs are given can change the degree of pain relief.

As a rule, chronic pain is best treated orally. This route is easier, cheaper, and safer and generally provides longer relief. People who do not have to be attached to tubes and poles are more mobile and can participate more fully in life. Drugs taken orally are generally given in higher doses than those given by other means, because the drug must pass through the stomach's acidic environment before it can be absorbed into the bloodstream. Morphine is available in an elixir form, which can be swallowed or absorbed through the mucous membrane of the mouth. This may be the route of choice for people who have difficulty swallowing.

Other routes can be used if drugs cannot be taken by mouth. For example, an intestinal obstruction or nausea and vomiting following chemothera-

INFORM
YOURSELF

Routes of Administration

- Oral (swallowed)
- Sublingual (under the tongue)
- Continuous infusion
- Subcutaneous (under the skin)
- Intravenous (through a vein)
- Epidural (injected into a space along the spinal cord)
- Intrathecal (injected into the spinal canal)
- Rectal (suppositories)
- Intranasal (into the nose)
- Transdermal (skin patch)

py may temporarily rule out oral drugs. *Intranasal* drugs, which are absorbed through the nasal membranes, or *transdermal* drugs, which are absorbed through the skin, sometimes are an option for people who have difficulty receiving injections.

Injection directly into the spinal canal (*epidural* or *intrathecal* administration) puts the drug closer to its target, the nervous system. As a result, less drug circulates to the brain, which reduces the risk of side effects.

Morphine and other narcotics are available as suppositories so that they can be administered through the rectum.

Do-It-Yourself Pain Therapy

One of the most promising approaches to cancer pain management allows you to administer drugs to yourself at the rate and dosage you choose. *Patient-controlled analgesia,* or *PCA,* is becoming more common in many cancer care facilities. In fact, some experts predict that PCA will soon become a mainstay of treatment.

PCA (sometimes called *demand* or *self-administered analgesia*) uses an electronic pump attached to a drug reservoir and a timing device. A tube is connected to a small needle inserted under the skin or into a vein. When you feel pain, you press a button on the pump and receive a preset dose of medication. The timer is adjustable, so that no more than a certain amount of drug can be taken over a given time. (For example, no more than four doses of a drug may be released in an hour, no matter how many times you press the button.) PCA is often used after surgery or for anyone with severe pain.

Although some experts question whether this approach will prove cost effective in the long run, studies have found that people who self-medicate tend to be discharged earlier and may suffer fewer chronic pain problems later. People who can control their pain themselves may use lower total doses of drug than would have been prescribed by their caregivers. And most people prefer this arrangement to being stuck with a needle every few hours. If nothing else, PCA provides a psychological edge, because pain is easier to bear if you know it can be relieved instantly whenever you want.

Thanks to advances in technology, many people today can use miniature pumps that fit into a fanny pack, backpack, or purse and that deliver a continuous infusion of analgesic medication. One device even straps to the wrist like a watch. You can thus enjoy the benefits of pain relief while living a more normal life.

Nerve Surgery

Nerve surgery is performed when pain relief from a cancer treatment or from the use of analgesics is inadequate. The goal is to isolate the painful part by interrupting the pathway along which pain signals travel to the brain. The process (sometimes called *neuroablation*) cuts or destroys part of the pain nerve fibers. Such procedures are expensive because they are usually performed by highly skilled experts at special treatment centers. Only those with clearly localized pain are likely to benefit; moreover, serious risks are involved, including the temporary or permanent loss of feeling or motor control in some parts of the body.

Cordotomy is a neuroablative procedure often used to relieve pain in the leg or hip on one side of the body. The technique is usually not helpful if you have pain in the upper body or on both sides of the trunk. A miniature electrode is inserted into a spinal cord nerve; then heat from the electrode creates a lesion that disrupts the nerve signal. You must be awake during the procedure in order to help the surgeon place the needle and to report what you are feeling. Nine out of 10 people experience significant pain relief following a cordotomy, but in about half, the pain returns within a year.

Cordotomy can involve complications, including mild paralysis, loss of coordination, and, most seriously, respiratory dysfunction. Loss of bladder control and pain on the side opposite the cordotomy site may result.

Hypophysectomy, removal of the pituitary gland, is a technique for relieving generalized pain that does not respond to other strategies. In most cases, this procedure can reduce pain from metastatic cancer. The benefits, however, last for only a few months.

Other neuroablative strategies target different sites in the body. For example, *neurectomy* affects the nerves on the surface of the body; and *thalamotomy*, the thalamus, which is a part of the brain through which sensory and pain impulses pass to reach another part of the brain where pain is recognized, the cerebral cortex. Thalamotomy prevents pain impulses from getting to the cerebral cortex.

Anesthetics

Anesthetic techniques may help people with well-defined local pain caused by a tumor that is infiltrating surrounding tissue. Some anesthetic methods work for short periods of time; others, such as *cryoanalgesia*, or freezing, can cause permanent nerve blockage. From two to eight out of 10 people whose pain does not respond to other approaches may benefit from these techniques.

A drawback of this strategy is that many nerves may need to be blocked to achieve adequate relief. Up to 13 percent of people may suffer permanent side effects such as urinary or rectal incontinence, motor weakness, or abnormal tingling or burning sensations (*paresthesias*).

Most anesthesia techniques block nerves. For example, pain in the chest wall and abdominal wall can be relieved by interrupting the nerves that exit from the spinal cord to supply these sites. Pain in the legs, groin, and low back can be helped by infusing drugs into the epidural or intrathecal spaces to numb the nerves that receive pain signals from these sites. Patients with upper abdominal pain from pancreatic cancer can get good relief from interruption of the nerves near the pancreas.

Continuous epidural infusion is used when the pain is difficult to treat, as in cases of advanced metastatic disease involving the pelvis and lower body. An infusion pump delivers the drug to the spinal column through a catheter, or a small reservoir is surgically implanted in the body to dispense the drug in small doses over time. The advantage of this method is that it provides effective relief without disrupting the function of the muscles and nerves.

Stimulating Nerves

Blocking the nerves is one way to reduce pain. Another is to stimulate the nerves with signals that are *not* painful, such as gentle vibrations. This technique is believed to crowd out the painful feelings and keep them from traveling along the spinal cord to the brain. In a way, it's like flooding a switchboard with telephone calls to prevent other calls from getting through. Nerve stimulation is very safe, but it seems to work best only in the short term; long-lasting analgesia is rare.

Common techniques include stimulating the skin with pressure, friction, temperature change, or chemicals. The simplest and most widely used method is *counterirritation*, for example, brisk rubbing of the painful part, often following the use of a cooling spray.

Another method is *transcutaneous electrical nerve stimulation (TENS)*, which requires placing a small electrical device over the painful region to activate the nerves. The resulting relief can be substantial, but the effect usually lasts only as long as the machine is turned on. After a few months, or even days, many people no longer get relief. A variation on TENS is the surgical implantation of a small electrode to produce stimulation.

Acupuncture is a method of using needles to stimulate specific nerves. Many people report that it brings relief. Recently, the World Health Organization conducted a careful study of the technique as it is performed in China. Although acupuncture alone does not appear to provide adequate pain relief, it may help when used to supplement other techniques (see Chapter 22, "Alternative and Complementary Therapies").

Physical Approaches

The value of physical therapy techniques is often overlooked in the treatment of cancer pain. For example, a surgical corset can relieve back pain in people with progressive vertebral disease. Arm or shoulder splints ease pain due to nerve infiltration in those regions. Physical therapy can prevent or delay muscle contractions or frozen joints in people who are partly immobilized. Massage, muscle stretching, or the use of hot or cold compresses can prevent muscle pain. Apart from their physical benefits, these techniques offer some degree of self-control over pain, which can lead to psychological benefits and more independence.

Pain and the Mind

The strategies discussed so far focus on the physical aspects of pain relief. Psychological methods also provide important benefits, because the way that you think and act affects the way you feel. In a very real sense, your attitude toward pain is an important part of your experience of pain. It stands to reason that if you can change the way you think about pain, you can change your susceptibility to it and your feelings and reactions. Psychological techniques restore the sense of personal control and allow you to participate more actively in your own care. The sooner these methods are attempted, the more likely they are to succeed. This in turn makes you more likely to continue using them and enhances their benefits.

Mind-body strategies, such as imagery, hypnosis, and relaxation, increase your sense of personal control over pain, a benefit not found in many analgesic treatments in which the drug is responsible for controlling pain. These mind strategies reduce feelings of hopelessness and helplessness and offer a calming diversion of attention. As yet, few studies have explored the role of such techniques in managing cancer-related pain, although recent research has found that hypnosis can be very effective. Experience suggests that for many people these methods can be an important adjunct to an overall program of pain therapy. Most likely to benefit are those with

- intermittent, predictable pain such as that associated with treatment procedures;

- incidental pain associated with metastatic bone disease that flares up during movement;

- chronic pain accompanied by anxiety.

Because many of these techniques are helpful in managing a number of cancer symptoms in addition to pain, they are discussed in greater detail in Chapter 25, "Coping with Stress, Fear, Anxiety, and Depression."

Cognitive and Behavioral Techniques

Cognitive and behavioral strategies help you learn to divert your attention from your pain, improve your ability to tolerate it, and increase your feelings of control over your situation. Cognitive techniques include learning about the disease, discovering distraction techniques, and focusing your mind through controlled mental imagery. In cognitive therapy you learn healthier ways to think about your illness and interpret its meaning in your life.

A word about imagery: This cognitive method can help you fill your mind with beautiful or soothing pictures, allowing you to disconnect temporarily from pain. Such a strategy may have tremendous value. Despite the message of certain popular books and articles, however, imagery is *not* a treatment for the cancer itself. It has not proved effective in shrinking tumors or eliminating metastatic cells.

Behavioral methods help eliminate behaviors such as the tensing of muscles that may contribute to the severity of pain. Some behavioral strategies teach skills to help you cope with pain and modify your reactions to it. These techniques are especially effective in managing acute pain arising from cancer procedures and as adjuncts to an overall program of chronic pain therapy.

Perhaps the most important and basic cognitive-behavioral techniques are relaxation and distraction. As mentioned, muscular tension—which can arise directly from the pain or from the fear of anticipating future pain—makes the experience of pain worse. The ability to relax, then, is an essential survival skill. When you relax, you break the vicious cycle of pain-anxiety-tension-pain. You waste less energy, are able to sleep better, feel less anxious, and can benefit more from other methods of pain relief.

Approaches to relaxation include breathing exercises, biofeedback, music therapy, medication, massage, and imagery, all of which are discussed in Chapter 25, "Coping with Stress, Fear, Anxiety, and Depression."

Psychiatric Therapy

Chronic pain can make anyone vulnerable to severe depression. Short-term supportive psychotherapy provides education and emotional support and helps everyone, family members included, adapt to their difficult situation. Therapy can help you identify your strong points, determine what methods of coping work best, and learn new skills. In addition, a therapist may recommend medications to reduce anxiety or feelings of depression. As noted earlier, some antidepressant drugs also relieve pain when used as adjuvants to analgesics.

Insist!

Not everyone with cancer has pain. Of those who do, most can find relief through treatment with medications alone or with a combination of medications, surgical procedures, and psychological strategies. Narcotics, including morphine, are extremely valuable weapons, but because of fear and misunderstandings, they are too often underused in the fight against cancer pain. Fortunately, that picture is changing.

People with cancer, including those in the terminal stages, have the right to insist on the highest possible quality of life when dealing with their disease, and this means they are entitled to request and receive aggressive pain management. Cancer care is not complete until pain is under control.

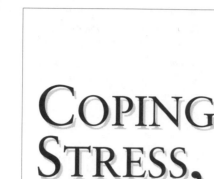

Coping with Stress, Fear, Anxiety, and Depression

Dealing with the emotions triggered by having cancer is as important to your comfort and recovery as managing the physical symptoms. Stress, fear, anxiety, sadness, confusion, and feelings of depression or helplessness are common at all stages of the illness, beginning with your first concern that something might be wrong. At the very least, these reactions can lower your tolerance to pain and make the treatments harder to endure, robbing you of quality of life, the strength or desire to fight the illness, and the ability to make the best decisions.

There is growing evidence, as well, that states of mind can influence the course of cancer. Although claims that negative attitudes cause cancer have not been proved, studies suggest that stress may influence the immune system.

On the other hand, as research has begun to suggest, techniques of psychotherapy and behavioral medicine—such as supportive group psychotherapy, relaxation training, hypnosis, and meditation—not only offer psychological relief but also may enhance the body's ability to respond to cancer. At the very least, although these techniques are not cures, incorporating them into your overall treatment plan offers you a way to ease discomfort and to take an active role in your care.

Normal or Not

It is normal for someone with cancer to experience emotional upheavals for short periods of time, especially around crisis points, such as the time of diagnosis, the beginning or end of treatment, the anniversary of the treatment, or the advanced stages of illness (see also Chapter 31, "Coping Strategies"). When you pass in and out of distressing states of mind, the techniques offered in this chapter can make them easier to tolerate or to control.

But when mental anguish becomes unremitting and severe or leads to despair and/or the desire to die, such feelings are not normal. Having cancer does not mean you should resign yourself to feeling at the end of your rope, and anyone who tells you, "Of course you're depressed—you have cancer!" is at best misinformed. Even among those with advanced illness, extreme mental anguish and the wish to die are closely related to clinical depression, a condition that can be remedied. Painful, continuing psychological states can be alleviated and should always be investigated. For everyone, regaining a sense of mastery is critical to a decent quality of life that can be yours at every stage of illness.

This chapter first explores anxiety and depression, from the types that many people with cancer confront to the more severe kind for which specialized care is needed. The remainder of the chapter presents numerous specific techniques of behavioral medicine—or mind-body medicine—for dealing with the emotional and physical stresses of cancer, its symptoms (including pain), and its treatment (such as the nausea associated with chemotherapy).

All the techniques and advice in this chapter also apply to caregivers and others close to the person who is ill, who experience their own huge share of stress (see Chapter 32, "Issues for Families and Friends").

Anxiety

Anxiety is an emotional response to fear. When you are anxious, your body responds as if it were under physical attack. Your heart beats faster, your blood pressure increases, muscles tense, and stress hormones such as adrenaline are released into the system. Ordinarily, when the perceived danger passes, these systems return to normal. But under chronic stress, your body remains in a state of arousal, and over time, this can affect the immune system. Among anxiety's many mind and body symptoms are muscle tension, sweaty palms, pounding heart, difficulty breathing, racing pulse, headache, jitteriness, upset stomach, excessive worrying, difficulty concentrating, problems making decisions, and panicky feelings.

Action to reduce anxiety is always recommended, to control unpleasant emotions, reduce tension, and provide a sense of direction, control, and hope. Many of the mind-body methods described later in this chapter can ease mild anxiety. But if these feelings last longer than two or three weeks, if they prevent you from taking adequate care of yourself or from participating fully in your treatment, or if you find yourself haunted by undefined or excessive fears, it is advisable to consult a mental health professional who is knowledgeable about cancer care. Medication, counseling, and/or behavioral techniques may be prescribed to help you feel more comfortable, relaxed, and able to cope.

Anxiety that you may have suffered before your cancer diagnosis may increase or recur under the strain of being sick. Anyone with a history of phobias or panic disorders is advised to consult a mental health professional before treatment begins, to plan strategies for managing the situations that trigger these reactions. *Stress inoculation*, as such a preventive approach is called, has been shown to reduce distress and maximize coping.

Psychological Causes

Most people with cancer fear being disabled, disfigured, or dependent; losing income or significant relationships; losing control or experiencing pain; and/or dying. Sometimes the anxiety associated with these fears is mixed with depressed feelings, and it is hard to sort out which is which (see box, "Am I Anxious? Am I Depressed?").

Am I Anxious? Am I Depressed?

QUESTIONS

TO ASK

Ups and downs in mood are expected for anyone who is coping with a life-threatening disease. But if the bad feelings last longer than two or three weeks, are getting worse, or are preventing you from taking an active role in your care, professional help is needed. The following questions can help you identify feelings of anxiety or depression or both:

1. Have you been experiencing insomnia or restless sleep or are you sleeping much more than usual?

2. Does life seem like a constant struggle, as if you're pushing a weight up an increasingly steep hill?

3. Are you feeling overwhelmed by life?

4. Do you think you are having more problems coping than most people would in your situation?

5. Are you having difficulty in your relationships with others?

6. Are you able to stay busy?

7. Are you able to make decisions?

8. Are you able to face your problems?

If you answered yes to questions 1 through 8, you may be experiencing anxiety or depression, or both.

9. Do you constantly feel stressed?

10. Are you sometimes scared or panicky for no particular reason?

11. Do you often feel nervous or edgy?

12. Are you sometimes too nervous to do anything?

If you answered yes to questions 9 through 12, you may be experiencing anxiety.

13. Have you persistently been sad?

14. Have you lost confidence in yourself?

15. Do you feel that you're worthless?

16. Do you ever feel that life is hopeless?

If you answered yes to questions 13 through 16, you may be experiencing depression.

As you can see, the distinction between anxiety and depression is not always clear. More important is the amount of distress you are feeling. Ask for help: See your doctor or a mental health professional for further evaluation.

Anticipatory anxiety refers to the distress and associated physical symptoms that occur before surgery and such procedures as needle biopsies, endoscopies, sigmoidoscopies, radiation, chemotherapy, and scans. Magnetic resonance imaging (MRI) requires that you lie immobilized in a narrow cylinder for a prolonged period, and so people with even mild claustrophobia may become apprehensive in such circumstances. Before chemotherapy, many people experience anticipatory anxiety in the form of nausea and vomiting.

Mild antianxiety medications, such as Valium, and a number of behavioral techniques, including progressive relaxation, systematic desensitization, distraction, guided imagery, and hypnosis, have been used successfully to manage these symptoms.

Physical Causes

Hormone-secreting tumors, found in cancers of the pancreas, lungs, thyroid, and adrenal glands, often produce anxiety and sometimes even panic. Anxiety also is associated with liver cancer and with certain cancer-fighting drugs, including the corticosteroids. In such instances, doctors may prescribe antianxiety medication (a tranquilizer) that is compatible with other aspects of the treatment.

Inadequately controlled pain produces overwhelming anxiety that the suffering will be prolonged. Often simply adjusting the pain medication can help relieve this distress, as can the numerous techniques of behavioral medicine, described later in this chapter, that help you deal with pain (see also Chapters 23, "The Pain Challenge," and 24, "Pain Relief").

Depression

As with intermittent anxiety, occasional depressed feelings are not unusual in people living with cancer. Depression that does not abate, however, can and should be treated. Symptoms include unremitting sadness, feelings of loss, hopelessness, irritability, irregular sleep patterns (insomnia or sleeping too much), difficulty concentrating, a desire to be alone, and diminished interest in sex.

Appetite and weight changes and a lack of vim and vigor are key symptoms of depression as well, but they also are common symptoms of cancer and its treatment. Many people with cancer and sometimes even their caregivers assume that these changes mean the cancer is worsening, but that is not always the case. In fact, depression can be the sole culprit, and with appropriate treatment the depression will lift, taking these alarming symptoms with it and giving you much more hope and satisfaction in your day-to-day life.

Depression and Loss

Learning that you have cancer almost always produces feelings of loss. These emotions may deepen when the treatment ends or if the cancer becomes advanced. Sometimes a depressed mood is triggered by a form of cancer or cancer treatment that strikes at a basic source of your identity or self-esteem.

For example, a woman who has a mastectomy or a hysterectomy may experience a blow to her sense of herself as a woman, just as having his prostate gland removed or irradiated might undermine a man's self-concept, or bone cancer could challenge a professional athlete's meaning in life. Many people become sad or even despondent in response to disfiguring treatments or to hair loss from chemotherapy (see Chapter 29, "Body Image and Self-Esteem").

Physical Factors

A depressed mood may also have a physical origin. For example, depression is a common symptom of pancreatic cancer and certain brain cancers and, like anxiety, is a side effect of inadequately controlled pain. Pain can have a depressing effect, and in turn, a depressed mood makes pain harder to tolerate.

Systemic imbalances, such as thyroid problems or nutritional deficiencies, may cause mood changes. Some cancer medications, such as the chemotherapy drugs vincristine (Oncovin), vinblastine (Velban), procarbazine (Matulane), L-asparaginase (Elspar), amphotericin B, and interferon, have a depressive effect. So do some of the medications used to control the nausea associated with chemotherapy, such as reserpine (Diapres), barbiturates (Nembutal), diazepam (Valium), propranolol (Inderal), and prochlorperazine (Compazine). Prednisone and dexamethasone—key components in many cancer treatments—may cause emotional upsets ranging from minor mood swings to severe depression and suicidal feelings.

Getting Help

It is not always easy to tell whether a down mood is associated with the cancer itself or its treatment, whether it is a temporary emotional reaction that is adaptive under the circumstances, or whether it is a sign of a more serious clinical depression that may have nothing to do with the cancer. A thorough diagnosis by a mental health professional who is knowledgeable about cancer is essential if your symptoms last longer than two or three weeks; if you experience guilt, hopelessness, or plummeting self-esteem; or if you have a prior history of depression. If you are having suicidal thoughts, get help immediately. Any prolonged depression destroys the quality of life that you are entitled to at any stage of illness, even at the end of life. It also robs you of the ability to make reasoned, sensible decisions on your behalf.

Sometimes one or more of the many types of antidepressant medications can relieve the symptoms. Likewise, counseling or psychotherapy alone can be an effective approach for some people. More often, however, persistent, severe depression is best managed through a combination of medication, counseling, mind-body interventions, and/or group support.

Although any medical doctor can prescribe antidepressants, a psychiatrist generally has more experience in administering such medications and monitoring their potential interaction with cancer and cancer treatments. Ask your oncologist or a social worker or psychologist involved in your care for a referral.

Dealing with Depression

Being depressed is different from just being sad. Depression permeates your whole existence and causes an emotional paralysis that can devastate you if you're not prepared. When you're depressed, you become thoroughly convinced that your glass is half empty and draining fast: you are sure there is no hope that you will ever feel better. Attempting to change that attitude can help restore your ability to take pleasure in the life that is yours and in the people who care for you.

Here are some suggestions for developing a positive attitude. Try them as an exercise even if you're convinced they won't help, and remember that when you're depressed, by definition you believe that nothing will be of benefit; that's the depression talking.

- Resist thinking about what you've lost. Concentrate on what you still have left and what you have gained by your experiences. You may find you have a great deal to offer others.

- Keep your mind active. Push yourself to go to movies. Read. Listen to music. Enjoy the company of interesting, stimulating people. Try to spend less time dwelling on your own situation. Distract yourself.

- Exercise to the extent that you can. Aerobic exercise (see Chapter 27, "Activity Counts") and general physical activity are among the best antidotes to depression. Even if your down mood returns later, at least you'll know there's something you can do to make yourself feel better for a while.

- Listen to audiotapes that concentrate on positive images. Even if you're not sure they will help—or that you can get well—listen anyway. At least you'll be spending your time in a positive environment.

- Don't expect too much of yourself. Reward yourself for positive thoughts and activities. But don't be too hard on yourself if you give in to depression now and then. Just gently and persistently draw yourself away from it when you can.

- Know that you're not alone. People who are depressed tend to withdraw from others, which makes them feel even more isolated. Even if you think that you don't have the energy for company or that nobody would want to be with you, stay involved with other people. If there's no one you feel close to or if the people in your life seem unresponsive, join a support group for people with cancer, who will understand how you feel. And always feel free to ask for professional help and guidance from a psychiatrist, social worker, pastoral counselor, or psychologist knowledgeable about cancer. The social work department at the hospital at which you are being treated can be a good source for information, assistance, or referrals. Don't wait until your depression becomes severe.

- See Chapter 31, "Coping Strategies."

TIPS &
ADVICE

Help for Depressed People with Advanced Cancer

People with advanced cancer are particularly vulnerable to depression, and so the risk of suicide is greatest at this point. Supportive psychotherapy combined with spiritual counseling can be beneficial, along with antidepressant or stimulant medications and behavioral techniques such as music therapy. Taking small but significant actions, such as talking with family and friends, taping recollections, or writing a living will (see Chapter 34, "Supportive Care"), can help shake some fears and feelings of futility and restore a sense of living fully in the time remaining.

Mind-Body Medicine

The burgeoning field of mind-body medicine, which focuses on the interplay of thoughts, emotions, and health, offers an array of noninvasive behavioral techniques to deal with the physical effects, side effects, and mental stresses of having cancer. These methods are almost always used in conjunction with medication, counseling, and group support.

Relaxation therapy, meditation, and hypnosis, once considered "alternative" methods, are just a few such approaches now often included in mainstream cancer care (see Chapter 22, "Alternative and Complementary Therapies"). Wherever you are in the disease process, mind-body techniques can help improve your mood and therefore the quality of your life. If you are relaxed and free of distress, you will be better able to focus your attention on important decisions you may have to make concerning your care. There is evidence that people who feel they are actively managing their treatment have less pain.

It also is important to encourage family members and others on your support team to learn these techniques. Not only will they be able to help you in your efforts, but they, too, will benefit.

Setting Goals

Mind-body techniques are safe and, in many cases, are easy to learn to do on your own. But like any interventions, they are most effective as part of a well-supervised comprehensive treatment plan. A social worker, psychiatrist, psychologist, psychiatric nurse, or other mental health care professional with expertise in cancer care and behavioral medicine can help you draw up a program of techniques for relieving stress, emotional symptoms, pain, and unpleasant treatment side effects and can act as your coach in learning to use them. Be sure your oncologist is aware of any techniques you try, particularly self-help methods. If he or she is not supportive, have your counselor call and discuss with the doctor how important these techniques are to you.

The method that will be most beneficial depends on your medical condition, your personality, how active or sedentary you are, and your treatment goals. For example, are you trying to relieve short-term pain? To learn to distract yourself during an uncomfortable test or procedure? To overcome a fear of needles? Or do you have a larger goal—perhaps to use the experience of having cancer as an opportunity to learn positive coping skills and more adaptive mental habits?

Approaches

Mind-body methods fall into three broad categories:

Physical. Body-centered interventions—including deep relaxation, deep breathing, and massage—are excellent for relieving the tension associated with anxiety and stress. Body-centered techniques can decrease muscle tension and lower blood pressure and heart rate and help relieve pain, anxiety, and depressed feelings.

Mental. Mental approaches, many of which draw on the link between positive thoughts and healing action, are useful for changing self-defeating patterns of thinking and for developing skills to alter your perception of pain and to improve your mood. Techniques that let you mentally rehearse uncomfortable or unpleasant encounters until they seem less threatening can aid you in managing everything from claustrophobia to nausea. Hypnosis, imagery, meditation, distraction, thought stopping, cognitive restructuring, graded task assignments, and music therapies are all mental approaches.

Behavioral. Regaining a sense of mastery over feared situations or stimuli through effective action can help you cope with the emotions associated with having cancer. Relaxation training, focused breathing, and systematic desensitization, presented in this chapter, fall into this category, as does exercise.

Help or Self-Help?

Some of the methods outlined in the remainder of this chapter, such as hypnosis and systematic desensitization, require a health professional to serve as your guide, at least initially. In most cases, you will be given audiotapes or other tools so you can continue practicing on your own. Other methods, such as distraction (diverting your mind from tension and discomfort) are easy to learn without professional help.

Relaxation

Being able to relax both body and mind is one of the most useful skills for managing the discomfort associated with cancer and stress. You can use *progressive relaxation*—relaxing the body part by part (see "Body Scan," page 295)—to dispel anxiety while awaiting treatment or surgery, to aid sleep, to relieve pain, or to enter a deeply relaxed state for imagery work or hypnosis.

Studies show that when you are rested and relaxed, you may need less pain medication. Relaxation also helps the body counter the effects of stress by reducing muscle tension and lowering blood pressure and heart rate.

There are dozens of time-tested methods of relaxation. Yet just the simple act of deeper breathing provide direct physiological benefits. Taking long, slow, relaxed breaths is an easy way to calm your emotions during a stressful procedure or a bout of crying.

Commercial relaxation tapes are widely available in bookstores or by mail order (see the end of this chapter), but many people find a familiar voice more soothing. An individualized tape is particularly effective; a therapist or counselor can make one using images and instructions that are especially meaningful to you.

T I P S &

A D V I C E

Basic Relaxation and Imagery for Coping with Cancer

Basic relaxation and imagery is an exercise designed specifically for cancer patients. It helps you reduce muscle tension and feel relaxed, comfortable, safe, and in control. It also teaches you how to narrow your focus and concentrate on a word, idea, or image—a skill that is integral to many other mind-body techniques, including imagery, hypnosis, and meditation.

You can ask another person to lead you through the exercise, or you can record the instructions yourself in advance.

Find a comfortable, relaxed position, sitting or lying. Feel free to shift about at any time during the exercise, to feel more at ease.

You may close your eyes or keep them open. If your eyes are open, fix your gaze on one spot and continue to stare at it throughout the exercise.

Now, allow your attention to shift to your breathing. Breathe in through your nose and out through your mouth. Breathe slowly and deeply from your diaphragm. Feel your abdomen moving out when you inhale and moving in when you exhale. Continue to take deep, comfortable breaths. You do not need to control your breath. Just observe your relaxed, steady breathing.

As you breathe in a relaxed, comfortable way, imagine that you are breathing out any tension, anxiety, confusion, or fear. If you wish, you may repeat silently each time you inhale, "Relaxation in," and each time you exhale, "Tension and confusion out."

At any point, if your mind wanders to a safe, comfortable, pleasant place or if you experience a comfortable feeling, feel free to allow it to continue. If extraneous thoughts drift into your awareness, just let them drift away and bring your attention back to your breathing.

Now let your attention shift to one specific feeling (or word or idea or image). Let yourself feel even more comfortable, relaxed and in control. Experience that feeling (word, idea, image) deep in your muscles, your joints, your bones. Let this special feeling (word, idea, image) absorb you. Now let it carry you to an imaginary, special, safe place, somewhere you feel whole and complete.

Gradually let yourself become aware of the sounds around you, and prepare to come back to the room. Begin counting backward from 10 to 1. Ten, 9, 8—you're becoming more aware of the sounds around you and the sensations in your body, especially your fingertips. Six, 5, 4—you're feeling more alert, awake, and refreshed. Three, 2, 1—now open your eyes.

Body Scan

Body scan is a basic relaxation exercise for everyone. Focusing on each part of your body in turn and relaxing your muscles one by one helps you develop more awareness of how your body feels when it is tense and when it is relaxed so that you can quickly sense and release tension. Until you have learned the exercise, you might have someone read the instructions aloud as you perform them. Or you can tape the instructions in advance. Plan to spend about 15 to 20 minutes on the exercise, but avoid it immediately after meals.

Find a comfortable position. This usually means lying on your back with your legs slightly apart, letting your feet fall outward, and your arms resting at your sides with your palms up or down. You can also sit in a chair or stool if that's more comfortable, with your feet flat on the floor and your hands resting lightly on your thighs or arms of the chair or between your legs. Loosen any tight clothing, particularly your waistband or anything that constricts your breathing.

Close your eyes. Begin to take slow, deep breaths with your mouth closed. When your breathing is relaxed, mentally begin to scan your whole body for tension, as follows: Each time you inhale, focus on a body part (your foot, for example). Think about whether that part of your body is tense or relaxed. What does that feel like? Then as you exhale, release any tension that you locate in that area. What does it feel like now?

Begin with your left foot. Focus on the sole of your foot, then the toes, then move slowly to the instep, the top of your foot, your ankle. Slowly scan upward, to your calf, your knee, your thigh. Then repeat the process on your right leg.

When you reach the top of your right thigh, turn your attention to your torso. Be aware of any tension in your buttocks, the small of your back, your hips, your abdomen, your stomach. Then move upward, scanning your chest, heart area, lungs, and the top of your chest.

Now focus on your left hand, starting at the fingertips and working upward through your fingers, hand, wrist, forearm, elbow, upper arm, shoulder. Slowly shift your attention to your right hand and repeat the process. When you have finished scanning your right shoulder, turn to your neck, your throat, then your face, scanning your mouth, nose, ears, eyes. Slowly move up your forehead to your scalp, and then imagine any remaining tension being released through the top of your head.

Now, keeping your eyes closed, spend a few minutes lying or sitting quietly, letting your body sink deeper and deeper into a relaxed state. Notice what it feels like to have your body and mind deeply relaxed. Then, when you are ready, take a few deep breaths and slowly open your eyes. Repeat this exercise once or twice a day and at bedtime.

TIPS & ADVICE

Choose a relaxation position that is comfortable for you.

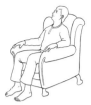

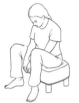

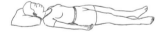

Focused Breathing

Deep, rhythmic breathing can relax the body and focus the mind, helping to relieve anxiety, depressed feelings, pain, and fatigue. The following is a simple exercise based on a yoga technique. Plan to spend about five to 10 minutes on it, once or twice a day and whenever you are feeling stressed.

Sit up straight in a chair with your legs uncrossed and your feet flat on the floor, or, if you prefer, sit cross-legged on a cushion, or lie flat if that is more comfortable for you.

Inhale slowly and deeply, breathing through your nose and keeping your mouth closed.

Imagine your breath filling up your lower abdomen, then your stomach, then your chest. Then slowly release all the air, pausing briefly before beginning the next inhalation.

As you continue breathing, be aware of the breath coming in and out your nose, of your abdomen expanding and contracting, of your diaphragm rising and falling.

You do not need to control your breathing. Just observe it as it becomes steadier and deeper and more relaxed.

Meditation

Although some people think of meditation as primarily a spiritual practice—which is in itself a good way to cope with the stress of serious illness—there is clinical evidence that it also has medical benefits, by inducing relaxation. In studies at Harvard University and at the Menninger Foundation meditators were able to control normally involuntary physiological processes, countering the physical effects of stress by lowering their heart rates and blood pressure.

Meditation is focusing your awareness on one thing to the exclusion of everything else. (In this sense, the focused breathing exercise described in the box above is a form of meditation.) The object of concentration can be a thought, word, sound, image, prayer, or body process (such as breathing). Learning to focus the mind can give you a sense of self-control, as you find that you can shift your attention away from those feelings and thoughts you believed were overwhelming. After consistent practice, meditation can also help you deal with physical pain or painful thoughts.

To provide benefit, meditation should be practiced once or twice daily, for 10 to 20 minutes. Once you're familiar with the technique, you may find it helpful to meditate before you undergo unpleasant procedures or even during them.

Imagery/Visualization

The imagination can be a valuable healing tool, and imagery, also known as visualization, is used in many cancer care settings. Alternative therapies that recommend using active imagery to attack the cancer itself have received a lot

Basic Meditation

Sit or lie still in a quiet place, with your eyes shut. Simple meditation is mentally following your breath in and out, or counting from one to four as you exhale, and then repeating the process over and over. Or you may wish to repeat a word to yourself (called a *mantra*), such as a nonsense word, the number one, or a word that has spiritual meaning for you, perhaps peace or love.

If your mind wanders, just bring it back gently to the breath or the counting. Do not judge, resist, or try to talk yourself out of unwanted thoughts that cross your mind. Just let them go.

Listening Meditation

Instead of counting, watching your breathing, or repeating a mantra, open your ears to the sounds in your environment as they occur. Don't think about what you hear, just let the sounds in. You can practice this listening meditation with music, trying to hear each note as it occurs. Don't hum along or sing, but simply let the sounds, and the silences, happen.

TIPS & ADVICE

of attention (see Chapter 22, "Alternative and Complementary Therapies"). But so far, there is no evidence that imagery alone can alter the course of the disease.

Passive Imagery. In passive imagery, once you are in a relaxed state, you look at the visual images or other sense impressions that spontaneously appear in your mind. When carried out under the guidance of a therapist, this exercise can be helpful in uncovering fears or resistances that might be interfering with your treatment—anything from money worries to a fear of dying.

Active Imagery. A more widely used approach is active imagery, in which you consciously choose the images, conjuring up sensory impressions to quell anxiety, lift depression, induce sleep or deep relaxation, manage physical symptoms, prepare yourself for surgery or treatment, or achieve other goals. Studies show that the body responds physiologically to mental images as if they were real events. Therefore, envisioning yourself lying in a grassy meadow on a warm summer day can have the same beneficial relaxing effect as actually being there.

Guided Imagery. In guided imagery, a therapist leads you through the process, or you can listen to taped instructions. The therapist may make a special tape with instructions and images that are particularly evocative for you, or may recommend ones for you to buy. Generally, in the first part of the exercise you settle into a deeply relaxed state. To do this, you might be asked to envision yourself in a place with peaceful associations: a beach, the woods, a mountaintop, a flower garden, a lake, or perhaps a special spot remembered from childhood. Alternatively, you might simply visualize a color, such as sky blue, or a pleasing aroma—your favorite perfume, perhaps. Then other images will be introduced, related to what you want to achieve.

Let's say your goal is to manage pain. Many people find it useful to transform the pain into a more tolerable sensation, such as heat or cold or tingling. One person might imagine trailing his hands in a cool mountain stream or running them under a sprinkler; another might see herself warming her hands in front of a crackling campfire or burying them in her cat's fur.

Some people prefer to experience their pain as an integral part of their imagined scenario—pretending, for example, that the pain is the sweet agony of running a marathon or of crashing into another player in a hockey game. Others might opt to rise above the pain with an image of floating on a mattress of fluffy white clouds.

Just as athletes use imagery to rehearse successful outcomes—seeing themselves performing all the movements necessary to clearing the high hurdles, for example—you can use it to envision clearing a treatment hurdle, such as enduring a diagnostic test, chemotherapy, or surgery, with a minimum of discomfort and a prompt recovery. To control the nausea associated with chemotherapy, for example, you might envision yourself driving to the hospital, walking confidently down the corridor, being hooked up to the IV, and then having the chemo flow into your arm like beautiful liquid gold.

Guided imagery can also help you rehearse a positive outcome to a difficult emotional scene. Perhaps you want to tell your family that you are frightened about having cancer and need them to be more supportive, or you want to tell your boss that you have cancer and will need time off for treatment. Visualize yourself taking every step necessary to tell them what you need.

Distraction

If you have ever daydreamed in class, counted sheep to get to sleep, worn a Walkman to avoid the boredom of exercise or a bus ride, or kept busy to avoid thinking about something unpleasant, you are an old hand at distrac-

TIPS & ADVICE

Some Hints for Successful Imagery

Don't be afraid to try imagery even if you, like many people, have difficulty creating mental pictures. Even though it is commonly referred to as visualization, imagery involves evoking any and all sense impressions, sounds, smells, tastes, and touch, as well as what you can see in your mind's eye. In fact, the more senses and details you can include in your imagery, the more lifelike and effective it will be. Let your imagination freely embroider on the scene: Add pleasing sounds and smells, and feel the coolness and texture of the objects you envision. And imagine yourself feeling calm and comfortable all the while.

tion. It is one of the easiest and most useful mind-body methods for handling short-term discomfort.

Distraction encompasses a wide range of techniques, from imagery, as just described, to watching funny movies to thought stopping (see page 301). All these methods are aimed at directing your awareness away from the physical or emotional distress at hand. Distraction is particularly useful to

- control anticipatory anxiety before surgery or treatments.

- control the nausea or vomiting associated with chemotherapy.

- handle acute (short-term) pain.

- manage treatment-related phobias, such as a fear of hypodermic or IV needles or claustrophobia during MRI.

- stop repetitive, negative thoughts about the treatment or outcome of your disease.

Are you one of the many people who grows breathless or panicky when confined within an MRI machine? If so, an effective distraction might be to imagine that the tube is a rocket ship and that you can blast off to wherever you want to go or that the top and sides of the tube have fallen away and you're floating through space on a magic carpet. If you have difficulty spontaneously generating such images when you're in a stressful situation, you can make a tape of the exercise in advance and listen to it before or even during any such procedure in which you have to lie still for a long time. Check to see whether there's an audio system through which you can pipe in your tape, since you can't bring in a tape recorder with you. Another way to distract yourself during a scan is to listen to music or a recorded book through a headset attached to an audio-input system (such as on an airplane); check beforehand to see if one is available.

Distraction through visualization (page 296) is an especially useful tool for people who are normally very physically active, especially children and adolescents. To handle tense moments, for example, they can imagine themselves doing those things they typically do to work off stress, such as riding a bicycle or a motorcycle, or playing a sport. For example, a young man undergoing radiation and chemotherapy for Hodgkin's disease envisioned himself skiing, in order to distract himself from his abdominal pains; the distraction also helped control the nausea and vomiting associated with his treatment.

If the mere smell of the hospital's chemotherapy wing makes you ill, you can distract yourself by taking along a small bottle of perfume or a scented oil such as basil or peppermint to sniff when you feel nauseated.

Laughter

Humor is a powerful distraction. The late Norman Cousins, in his classic book *Anatomy of an Illness*, described how reading funny books and watching tapes of the Marx brothers' movies and *Candid Camera* TV episodes helped him manage pain. (To borrow *Candid Camera* videos, contact the Alan Funt Fund, P.O. Box 827, Monterey, CA 93942.)

Desensitization

Systematic desensitization is a tried-and-true technique used by behavioral therapists to help overcome fears. It can be particularly useful in dealing with treatment-related fears and anticipatory anxiety, as well as pain and insomnia. This is not a self-help method; rather, you will need to work with a professional trained in behavioral techniques.

Desensitization entails learning to put yourself into a relaxed state or to distract yourself, as previously described, and then being exposed gradually to the fearful stimulus or situation so that you can learn to control your emotional reactions. Say, for example, you are unable to face chemotherapy because of a fear of needles. While in a state of relaxation or distraction, you might be asked simply to hold the needle and then later to stick it into an orange. Next, you would progress to holding the needle against your skin, gradually building up to the point of even giving yourself a "fake" injection.

This process allows you to rehearse the specific situation until you develop a tolerance for it. And it has another benefit as well: creating a sense of mastery that helps you recognize that you can overcome much that you thought you could not.

Hypnosis

Hypnosis is another effective tool for managing pain (a National Institutes of Health panel recently found "strong evidence" for its effectiveness with cancer-related pain), anxiety, nausea, vomiting, and aversions to certain cancer treatments. It can also be useful in uncovering and dealing with unresolved fears or conflicts related to your disease, such as a fear of dying or sorrow over hopes and plans that you now must revise or abandon.

Hypnosis is a method of putting you in a state of heightened mental concentration so that you can focus on a problem or symptom and be receptive to ideas and images for resolving it. It is not a self-help technique, but in most cases a hypnotherapist will work with you for one or several sessions and then teach you self-hypnosis so that you can control your symptoms on your own.

Hypnosis begins with an induction: While you are sitting or lying quietly, the hypnotherapist repeats a series of verbal suggestions enabling you to become deeply absorbed and focus your awareness. Then the therapist offers suggestions consistent with your goals. If, for example, you have a burning pain in the chest—this is common after a mastectomy—the hypnotherapist might suggest that every time you experience the discomfort, you should imagine pouring cool water over the area. Or the suggestion might be to imagine applying ice to the painful part or to imagine yourself taking a cooling dip in the ocean.

Despite the demonstrated effectiveness of hypnosis, some people mistakenly fear that harmful ideas will be "planted" in their minds while they are in a trance or that they will be made to do things against their will. But hypnosis is not brainwashing. Although it increases receptivity to suggestion, part of the brain always remains alert during the process, acting as an inner censor that prevents you from acting out ideas you find unacceptable.

As in any medical procedure, however, it is important to choose a trained professional. Ask your doctor or social worker for a referral, or contact the Society of Clinical Hypnosis, Des Plaines, Illinois (847-297-3317), or the Society for Clinical and Experimental Hypnosis, Liverpool, New York (315-652-7299).

Cognitive Restructuring

Cognitive methods are based on the theory that it is not what happens to you in life but rather how you interpret it that leads to emotional consequences. Dealing with cancer gives you an opportunity to review your habitual ways of responding to stress and, if necessary, to modify your coping style by thinking through the problem differently.

Cognitive restructuring can help you identify maladaptive thoughts, fears, or fantasies and replace them with more constructive or realistic ones that lead to positive action. For example, a woman with leukemia who was suffering greatly from burning and tingling sensations in her joints believed that her pain was inevitable and beyond her control. With counseling, however, she came to see that even though pain was likely to occur from time to time, she did not have to accept it passively and "suffer in silence." Instead, whenever she felt pain, she interpreted it as a signal to start mobilizing her pain-coping techniques—in her case, active imagery. She imagined the burning pain as red hot and then envisioned painting her entire body a cooling shade of purple. This technique also worked as a distraction.

In addition to managing pain, cognitive restructuring can be useful for coping with morbid thoughts and anticipatory anxiety. If you know what problem you want to handle, you can use the method on your own. If you don't, a therapist can help you identify the problem and decide on a replacement thought or action.

Thought Stopping

Cancer raises no end of fears, it sometimes seems. It is hard not to worry about everything from deteriorating health to medical expenses and family and work pressures. But continual worry can undermine healing efforts. Thought stopping is a classic technique of behavioral therapy that provides a simple self-help tool for interrupting repetitive or unpleasant thoughts.

First, identify the thought you want to stop (for example, "What if I'm dying?" or "How will I ever pay the hospital bill?" or "Poor me"). Then every time you have this thought, visualize a big red stop sign (or another image that means "halt" to you) and say "Stop!" loudly and firmly. Practice the exercise until it is second nature. Then whenever the thought pops up, so will the image, and your inner voice will silently command the thought to stop.

T I P S &

A D V I C E

Music Therapy

Expressive therapies using art, dance, and music provide a way of getting in touch with your feelings and fears about cancer. Music therapy, in particular, can also help you manage pain and other physical discomforts.

Music, whether you are listening to it or playing it, is an almost universally pleasing distraction. It can soothe anxiety, lift depression, reduce tension, and create a general sense of well-being. Making music, even in the most amateurish way, helps restore a sense of mastery and control.

Listening to music through a headset can be a relaxing distraction during scans or chemotherapy. For some people, it can even reduce nausea. And music's power to evoke deep memories and feelings makes it an important tool for therapists to help people reveal fears and sorrows. For example, a middle-aged man struggling stoically with advanced cancer was finally able to express his anguish after listening to spirituals he had loved as a child.

Music not only triggers emotional release but also seems to reduce the actual physical sensation of pain.

Some comprehensive cancer care teams now include a music therapist. If your medical team does not, you can ask for a recommendation from a cancer social worker.

Massage and Touch Therapies

One of the oldest forms of health care is the simple act of touching. Studies show that *therapeutic touch*, a form of the laying on of hands that is practiced by nurses in many hospitals, can reduce pain and increase well-being. Gentle massage therapy can relieve joint stiffness, as well as stimulate circulation and help maintain muscle tone. This is particularly useful if your cancer is limiting your ability to exercise and stay active.

Some people worry, however, that massage might make their cancer spread. Although there is some evidence that deep massage could break off bits of a tumor, gentle stroking that avoids the tumor area is not likely to be harmful. In any case, always check with your oncologist before receiving any kind of body work or massage.

To find someone trained in medical massage, ask a cancer social worker for a referral.

Graded Task Assignments

Graded task assignments constitute a valuable self-help technique for handling the strains that having cancer can cause in your relationships with others.

The method is to identify a goal and then to list small steps to achieve it. Let's say, as frequently happens, the demands of treatment make it hard for you to keep in touch with friends. When your treatment is over, you would like to resume these friendships but feel overwhelmed by the task of trying to rebuild your life. First, identify your goal: to reconnect with your support system. Then give yourself graded task assignments—specific, manageable steps toward that goal. You might make a list of people with whom you've lost touch and then call one friend a day. The next tasks might be to make one lunch date a week, to go on that date, and to talk with a friend about how it feels to pick up the pieces after cancer. Step by step, you can reach your goal without exhausting yourself physically or emotionally.

Coping Resources

Audiotapes, books, and videotapes that may help you cope with cancer are widely available. Use them to help you cope, but always remember that any claims that stress reduction will cure your cancer are groundless (see also Chapter 22, "Alternative and Complementary Therapies").

Although audiotapes that are tailored by a therapist precisely to your needs are best, for general stress reduction, you might try *Mindfulness Meditation Practice Tapes* by Jon Kabat-Zinn, Ph.D. These are a series of four practice tapes developed for participants in the Stress Reduction Clinic at the University of Massachusetts Medical Center. Tape 1: "Guided Body Scan and Guided Yoga." To order them, write Stress Reduction Tapes, P.O. Box 547, Lexington, MA 02173.

Kabat-Zinn is also the author of *Full Catastrophe Living: Using the Wisdom of Your Body and Mind to Face Stress, Pain, and Illness* (Dell), the self-help manual on mindfulness meditation and healing, based on the stress reduction program.

The Relaxation & Stress Reduction Workbook (New Harbinger) is a comprehensive guide with step-by-step instructions for a range of techniques, including progressive relaxation, self-hypnosis, and thought stopping. It is written by Martha Davis, Ph.D., Elizabeth Robbins Eshelman, M.S.W., and Matthew McKay, Ph.D.

FOOD AND NUTRITION

Nutrition plays an increasingly important role in the treatment of cancer. Doctors and dietitians have long urged people with cancer to "eat hearty" to maintain their strength and overall well-being. This is good advice for most people, particularly those whose cancer is in an early stage or whose loss of appetite is caused by depression or chemotherapy. However, the role of nutritional support in advanced cancer is being reconsidered. Research in recent years is raising doubts about exactly what supplementary feedings can accomplish in advanced disease.

This chapter discusses the basics of a healthy diet during and after cancer treatment. It explains the various mechanisms underlying *anorexia*, or loss of appetite, and weight loss in all stages of cancer, to help you understand what is going on in your body. And it describes how the disease affects appetite and the absorption of nutrients and offers practical advice for dealing with nutritional problems.

Nutrition Basics

A healthy diet helps maintain strength and resistance to infection, prevents body tissues from breaking down, and helps rebuild tissues that have been affected by therapy. Those who eat well and maintain their weight are in better shape to withstand the side effects of therapy and may even be able to handle more aggressive treatments and, therefore, increase their chances for survival.

Eating well for people who have cancer means eating the same healthy diet generally recommended for all Americans: one that is high in complex carbohydrates and low in fat while ensuring an adequate intake of protein.

A Nutritional Cure for Cancer?

Eating a balanced, healthy diet during cancer treatment and recovery is important to promote strength and healing. When they learn they have cancer, many people immediately change their diets. For example, according to one survey of women recently diagnosed with breast cancer, 80 percent altered their food intake in some way, and 85 percent started taking vitamins.

But nutrition is no panacea. Despite the increased interest in and research on the relationship of nutrition to health and healing, no unimpeachable evidence yet exists that a particular diet or combination of nutrients can bring remission or cure. The interrelationship of nutrients and cancer is extraordinarily complex and not yet well understood. Thus far, more light has been shed on the role of diet in prevention than in treatment or cure.

When supplementing a conventional cancer treatment with an unconventional nutritional intervention, beware of any practitioner who claims to have a dietary cure for cancer or even asserts that controlled clinical studies strongly support his or her nutritional point of view (see Chapter 22, "Alternative and Complementary Therapies").

SPECIAL **!** CONCERNS

Carbohydrates

The most efficient source of energy in the diet is carbohydrates, which should account for 55 to 60 percent of the calories eaten each day. Most of the calories should come from starches (also called *complex carbohydrates*) rather than sugars.

Starches are found in grains (cereals, pastas, rice, flour, and bran), legumes (beans, lentils, peas), potatoes, and other vegetables. Sugars are found in fruit, milk, honey, table sugar, jams, jellies, syrups, and other sweets.

The body needs the energy from carbohydrates to breathe, move, and handle extra stress posed by cancer and its treatment. If the diet doesn't contain enough carbohydrates, the body will turn to its protein stores for energy, thereby risking the loss of lean body mass.

Fat

Most Americans eat too much fat. Even though numerous health authorities suggest limiting fat calories to 20 to 25 percent of daily intake, the average American's diet is 35 to 40 percent fat.

The links between fat and cardiovascular disease are well known. Less well defined but under careful study are possible links between fat and cancer, especially colon and prostate cancer. Recent research has questioned the link between fat and breast cancer that earlier studies had suggested.

The amount of fat in the diet can be reduced simply by eating only lean meats; removing the skin from chicken and turkey before eating the meat (and preferably before cooking it); avoiding fried foods, spreads like butter and mayonnaise, and fat-filled fast foods and snacks; and substituting skim milk for whole milk. When oils are needed for cooking, monounsaturated fats like canola and olive oil should be used instead of butter or lard. If you need extra calories to maintain your weight, it is wiser to obtain them from starches and sugars than from fats.

Protein

Protein is vital to the life of every cell, as it continuously builds, maintains, and repairs cells. Therefore, during treatment for cancer, protein requirements increase as the body rebuilds damaged tissue.

Protein should account for 15 to 25 percent of the day's total calories, depending on your age and nutritional status. Quality sources of protein are nonfat dairy foods, such as skim milk and cheeses made of skim or low-fat milk, grains, legumes, fish, lean meat, and poultry.

Counting Calories

Most people only think about calories when they want to lose weight, but those with cancer may need to count calories in order to maintain or gain weight.

The easiest way to determine your daily calorie needs is to multiply your current weight in kilograms by the recommended calorie needs for your sex and metabolic needs (see below). For women, this is 20 to 30 calories per kilogram of current body weight, and for men, it is 25 to 35 calories per kilogram. When your body needs extra energy and more calories, such as before and after surgery or when you are running a fever, your intake should be boosted to 40 to 50 calories per kilogram.

INFORM
YOURSELF

Calculating Your Caloric Needs

To determine the range of your daily caloric needs, first weigh yourself and convert your weight in pounds to your metric weight in kilograms, by multiplying the number of pounds by 0.45. Then multiply your current weight in kilograms by 25 and then multiply your weight in kilograms by 35 if you are a man, or by 20 and then 30 if you are a woman.

Let us use as an example a woman weighing 140 pounds, or 63 kilograms. If we multiply her metric weight first by 20 and then again by 30, we will get an estimated daily need of 1,260 to 1,890 calories to maintain weight. For a man of 190 pounds, or 85.5 kilograms, the recommended range for weight maintenance comes to about 2,138 to 2,993 calories.

Vitamin and Mineral Supplements

When cancer or its treatment interferes with the body's absorption of certain nutrients, especially the B vitamins, supplements are sometimes recommended. Further, recent research suggests that certain vitamins—called *antioxidant* vitamins because they help prevent the oxidative destruction of cells—may help lower the risk of cancer. The antioxidants are vitamin C, vitamin E, and beta carotene (which is converted to vitamin A in the body), although recent research has raised some doubts about the value of this last substance. All these vitamins are in plentiful supply in colorful foods: Yellow and orange foods such as cantaloupe, carrots, and sweet potatoes are good sources of beta carotene; citrus and other fruits and dark green vegetables such as broccoli and green peppers are rich in vitamin C; and green leafy vegetables, dried beans, and whole-grain cereals and breads contain vitamin E.

Because cancer and its treatment can affect the body's metabolism in many ways and some vitamins may interfere with the action of certain chemotherapeutic drugs, you should discuss taking supplements with your physician.

What to Eat Every Day

Eating a wide variety of foods is the best way to ensure getting the nutrients you need. The following are recommendations adapted from the U.S. Department of Agriculture's Dietary Guidelines:

INFORM
YOURSELF

Food Group	Minimum Daily	Sample Servings
Breads, cereals, grains	6	1 slice bread; small roll or muffin; 1/2 cup cooked cereal, rice, or pasta; 1 oz. cold breakfast cereal; 3 to 4 small crackers
Vegetables	3 or more, including dark green leafy vegetables and dry beans or peas several times a week	1/2 c. cooked vegetables; 1/2 c. chopped raw vegetables; or 1 c. leafy raw vegetables such as lettuce or spinach several times a week; 1 medium potato
Fruits	2 or more	1 whole medium fresh fruit, such as an orange, apple, or banana; a grapefruit half; a melon wedge, 1/2 c. berries, 3/4 c. fruit juice, 1/2 c. cooked or canned fruit, 1/4 c. dried fruit
Meat, poultry	2	daily intake should total no more than 5 to 7 oz. cooked lean meat, poultry, or fish *alternative protein sources:* 1/2 c. cooked beans, 1 egg, or 2 T reduced-fat peanut butter (equal to 1 oz. meat)
Milk, cheese, yogurt	2	1 c. skim milk, 8 oz. low-fat yogurt, 1.5 oz. low-fat cheese

Planning Daily Meals

It may be useful to schedule an appointment with a registered dietitian who is familiar with the nutritional demands of cancer. You may need help determining, for example, how many calories you need daily and how to select foods that will provide those calories and be healthful.

Understanding Weight Loss

More than half of all people with cancer lose some weight, and about 15 percent lose more than 10 percent of their body weight. As many as two-thirds of people with advanced cancer develop *cachexia*, in which body wasting is accompanied by weakness, hormonal disturbances, and progressive failure of vital functions.

Not surprisingly, the prognosis for those who lose too much weight is not as good as for those who are able to maintain their weight. However, it is still not clear whether survival time is affected directly by weight loss. It may be that weight loss is a symptom of an aggressive form of cancer and that it is the disease—not the body wasting itself—that is responsible for the shortened survival time.

Maintaining body weight requires eating enough calories to replace those being burned and being able to digest food and absorb the nutrients. Any impairment of digestion and metabolism can lead to malnutrition, and in advanced cancer, weight loss may not be preventable.

People who suddenly lose a significant amount of weight often say they feel weak. The reason is that they are losing skeletal muscle as well as fat and that their oxygen-carrying red blood cells are in short supply (a condition known as *anemia*).

Cachexia also compromises the body's immune system. The white blood cells that battle disease are not functioning properly and thus are lowering the person's resistance to even minor infections. Furthermore, once malnutrition is under way, changes occur in the gastrointestinal tract that only worsen the situation. For example, cells lining the small intestine may be shed, thereby reducing the absorption of food. So even though the person may eat, the food's nutrients are not put to use.

In some people, severe weight loss that results from or is aggravated by a treatment's side effects may require stopping the treatment until their nutritional state can be improved.

Secondary Anorexia

In early or localized cancer, poor appetite may be due to emotional upset or depression or may be a side effect of the treatment. This is known as secondary anorexia, and those affected are encouraged to do whatever they can to stimulate their appetite and eat healthy meals—that is, meals low in fat; high in complex carbohydrates such as fruits, vegetables, and grains; and with adequate protein.

Mind, Body, and Appetite

The impact of stress, anxiety, fear, and depression on appetite varies from person to person. Some people eat more when they're stressed, whereas others can't stand the thought of food. Indeed, a change in appetite is one of the diagnostic hallmarks of depression. Because a diagnosis of cancer can be so frightening and its treatment uncomfortable and disruptive to daily life, anxiety and appetite loss are not uncommon. (See Chapter 25, "Coping with Stress, Fear, Anxiety, and Depression.")

Other aspects of the daily life of a person with cancer can also impair appetite. For example, someone who has done most of the cooking at home but is no longer able to do so may miss its appetite-stimulating effects. Or perhaps the food prepared by others is not as appealing because the seasoning is different or because unfamiliar foods may not be appetizing. And the appetite of someone accustomed to sharing meals with others may suffer if he or she is no longer able to socialize.

Pain interferes with appetite, too. When the brain is focused on dealing with discomfort, responses to other stimuli, even pleasant ones such as the aroma and taste of a delicious meal, may diminish.

The Mechanics of Digestion

A malfunction anywhere—from the mouth to the colon—can affect your nutritional status. Obviously, if a tumor is pressing on an area of the digestive tract or affecting one of the digestive organs, it can impair the normal movement of food or nutrient absorption or both. For example, tumors in the mouth or throat can interfere with chewing and swallowing. Tumors in the stomach or intestines can block the passage of food or decrease the flow of fluids, interfering with their absorption. Tumors in the liver or pancreas cause deficiencies in digestive enzymes and hormones.

Mechanical difficulties may also cause early *satiety*, a feeling of fullness that occurs shortly after you begin to eat. This can happen when a tumor decreases the size of the stomach or causes changes that slow the movement of food through the intestinal tract. Early satiety is apt to worsen during the day; that is, it may be absent at breakfast, mild at lunch, and severe at dinner. Reversing the typical order of meals can help; you could eat the main meal for breakfast or have many small meals throughout the day.

Treatment Effects

Many treatments for cancer affect, temporarily and sometimes permanently, your nutritional needs and ability to eat.

Surgery

Immediately after any type of surgery, nutritional needs normally increase as the body heals. Unfortunately, it is at just this time that most people least feel like eating. Furthermore, if the surgery has involved the mouth, throat, or any part of the intestinal tract, eating may be uncomfortable, and the absorption of nutrients from food may be compromised. For example, the surgical removal of all or part of the stomach or small intestine may mean that food moves through the system and reaches the colon too quickly, leading to a condition known as *dumping syndrome*, which can cause nausea, diarrhea, rapid heartbeat, weakness, and dizziness. (See Chapter 15, "Surgery.")

Radiation

When radiation therapy is given to kill tumor cells, a certain number of normal cells surrounding the cancer also are destroyed. Damage to cells anywhere along the intestinal tract affects a person's ability to eat. For example, radiation to the head and neck can inhibit the activity of the salivary glands, leading to dry mouth (*xerostomia*); cause a sore throat and/or mouth; and lead to dental problems that inhibit chewing or change the taste of food. Radiation to the stomach or intestines may cause nausea, vomiting, or diarrhea. (See Chapter 16, "Radiation.")

Chemotherapy

Nausea and vomiting are well-known side effects of chemotherapy and are likely to diminish the desire for food. Many people receiving chemotherapy experience *stomatitis*, an inflammation of the mouth that can cause a sensation of heat, pain, and increased saliva flow. Other side effects may be similar to those of radiation therapy, such as a sore or dry mouth or throat, diarrhea, and a change in the taste of food. Constipation is also common.

Does Chemotherapy Cause Vomiting? Some of the drugs used in chemotherapy are more likely than others to cause nausea and vomiting. The drugs are selected in accordance with their likely effectiveness against the particular cancer, not the side effects they may cause. However, other drugs can be prescribed to help minimize the nausea and vomiting.

In contrast to the appetite and weight loss associated with most cancer treatments, *hormonal therapy* (for instance, using tamoxifen or steroid drugs) can stimulate the appetite and cause weight gain. In this case, you may be advised not to eat too much, particularly high-fat foods, to avoid becoming overweight. (See Chapter 17, "Chemotherapy.")

Biological Therapy

Also known as immunotherapy, biological therapy alters the body's immune function in an attempt to destroy the cancer. Unfortunately, it may have some of the same side effects as those seen in chemotherapy, including nausea and vomiting, diarrhea, sore mouth, dry mouth, and changes in the taste of food. Moreover, anorexia and weight loss may be severe. (See Chapter 18, "Biological Therapies.")

Coping with Appetite Loss and Eating Problems

In most cases, it's not difficult to explain the loss of appetite and to understand the ways of dealing with it.

What's the Cause?

Consider *when* it occurs. If you began to lose weight when your cancer was first diagnosed or in anticipation of a doctor's visit or chemotherapy or radiation therapy, the cause is probably related to depression or anxiety. If you started to lose your appetite after chemotherapy or radiation therapy was initiated, the cause is probably the treatment (that is, it's likely to be secondary anorexia).

Your doctor can help assess your situation. He or she can also help you respond to the anorexia at any stage of your treatment.

If your cancer is advanced and you have no desire to eat, your cancer is probably the cause (*primary anorexia*), discussed later in this chapter.

Drugs to Stimulate Appetite

A variety of drugs have been used to stimulate appetite, including the antihistamine cyproheptadine (Periactin), corticosteroids such as prednisolone and methylprednisolone (Medrol), progestin hormones such as medroxyprogesterone acetate and megestrol acetate (Megace), anabolic steroids such as nandrolone decanoate (Deca-Durabolin), and hydrazine sulfate.

Although some of these drugs have led to reports of improved appetite, little actual increase in caloric intake or weight gain has been observed in con-

Appetite Boosters

Sometimes simple changes in daily habits boost appetite, especially if psychological factors appear to be the underlying problem. Here are some suggestions:

- Ask those preparing your meals to follow your recipes or preferences.
- If you usually cooked your own food and are not feeling nauseated, stay in the kitchen to participate in its preparation even if you are not physically able to do the cooking.
- Ask friends and family to bring food from home to the hospital, if it is permitted.
- Arrange to eat meals with others.
- Disregard the "rules" of specific meal times. Instead, eat when you're hungry.
- Have small, frequent meals—six or more times per day—rather than three large ones.
- Foods that are visually appealing can stimulate the appetite. For example, brightly colored foods can accent pale ones. Fruits could be served over cereal or cottage cheese. Green and yellow vegetables and other garnishes could decorate pale sauces and casseroles. Contrasting texture and temperature also enhance the appeal of food. For example, soups could be seasoned with crunchy croutons; raw vegetable curls could top a soft casserole.

TIPS & ADVICE

trolled clinical trials. In fact, the side effects of some are worse than the problem they were supposed to solve. Others pose specific hazards when used in advanced disease, when the problem is primary anorexia. For example, although anabolic steroids do increase appetite and muscle mass, muscle requires more calories to maintain, and, as we pointed out earlier, even when a person with cachexia eats more, lean body tissue may not increase as expected.

Although drugs may yet be found that will help maintain weight in advanced disease without stimulating the tumor to grow, considerable research is needed before these drugs can be widely recommended.

Coping with Treatment Side Effects at Mealtimes

When treatment side effects cannot be avoided, dietitians offer a variety of techniques to alleviate the problems while still ensuring adequate nutrition.

1. *Mouth inflammation, difficult chewing or swallowing*: Avoid spicy, salty, and acidic foods. Instead of hot food, try eating room-temperature or chilled foods. Also try soft foods such as milkshakes, bananas, applesauce, cottage cheese, mashed potatoes, macaroni and cheese, cooked cereals, pureed vegetables, and scrambled eggs. In addition, ask your doctor about anesthetic lozenges and sprays that temporarily numb your mouth.

2. *Dry mouth*: Eat soups and foods in sauces or gravies. Liquify foods in a blender, or drink liquids between bites. Very sweet or tart foods and beverages may help you produce more saliva.

3. *Altered taste perception*: If sweet foods don't seem sweet enough, add a little extra sugar, such as honey, molasses, marmalade, syrup, apple butter, or jam. If your sour or bitter threshold is decreased, you may find that beef and pork taste bad. The addition of extra herbs and seasonings may remedy the problem. Or simply avoid the offensive foods and choose other sources of protein, such as poultry, fish, beans, peanut butter, nuts, and seeds. In particular, tart foods such as oranges or lemonade, or foods seasoned with citrus, may be appealing.

4. *Diarrhea*: For 12 to 14 hours after the diarrhea subsides have only clear broths and tea and an occasional piece of toast. Then add foods such as bananas and rice dishes, and low-fiber foods such as farina, scrambled eggs, pureed vegetables, canned fruit, and skinned poultry. Eat small amounts frequently, rather than three large meals, and include plenty of fluids. Foods and beverages should be at room temperature. Avoid foods and beverages that produce gas; greasy, fatty, spicy, or fried foods; as well as raw vegetables and fruits and high-fiber vegetables. Medication to stop diarrhea may be needed.

5. *Constipation*: Increase your consumption of fluids and fiber-containing foods, such as salads, colorful vegetables, bran, and other whole grains. If possible, get some exercise, such as walking, every day. If this regimen is not well tolerated, try a daily dose of psyllium seeds in products such as Metamucil. Medication to relieve constipation may be necessary.

6. *Nausea*: If possible, stay out of the kitchen to avoid cooking aromas that may trigger nausea. If you must do the cooking, avoid aromatic foods (such as cabbage) and keep foods covered during cooking to minimize odors. Try to eat slowly in a relaxed atmosphere, avoiding a room that is stuffy or too warm. Eat dry bland foods such as crackers or toast before meals. Eat your largest meal in the morning, when you may be less apt to be nauseated. Or eat small meals throughout the day, stopping when the nausea hits. Avoid any food that seems to trigger or aggravate the nausea, such as fatty, spicy, or other strongly flavored foods. Foods that are chilled or at room temperature may be better tolerated than hot foods. When nausea hits, take deep breaths to relax and sip small quantities of a carbonated beverage or warm tea or chew ice chips until the nausea passes. Rest for a half-hour after eating, preferably sitting in an upright position, as reclining may trigger reflux, nausea, and vomiting.

7. *Vomiting*: Do not try to eat or drink until the vomiting has stopped. Then try drinking a teaspoonful of clear liquid such as tea every 10 minutes. Gradually increase the quantity until you can hold down 2 tablespoonsful every 30 minutes. Other liquids can be gradually introduced. If you know when nausea and vomiting are likely to occur, such as shortly after a treatment, eat a bland, easy-to-digest meal several hours beforehand, making sure to avoid milk products. If home remedies are not sufficient to control nausea and vomiting, ask your doctor about medication.

Primary Anorexia

Primary anorexia and weight loss caused directly by the presence of a tumor in the body continue to mystify researchers. There are two theories to explain

SPECIAL

CONCERNS

What About Marijuana?

One of the best-known side effects of the "recreational" drug marijuana is increased appetite. Marijuana, or the synthetic drug Marinol (delta-9-THC), also helps relieve nausea, among other reported medical effects. However, although efforts are continuing to reverse the prohibition against the medical use of marijuana, in most states all uses of the drug currently are against the law. Therefore, doctors cannot prescribe it under any circumstances. They may, however, prescribe the synthetic form of the active ingredient, called Marinol, which some claim is not as effective as the real thing.

If you are offered marijuana, which though against the law is nonetheless widely available in some places, be aware that it has other effects and side effects that may upset you. For some, it promotes a feeling of well-being, but its psychoactive effects can be unsettling and may produce anxiety and fear, particularly in those inexperienced in its use. Also, as with any "street" drug, its quality, strength, and effects can be unpredictable.

the phenomenon. One is that the tumor secretes a substance that suppresses the appetite or affects the body's use of energy or both. The other theory is that the body secretes substances that have an anorexic effect, which enables it to defend itself against the tumor. Although the research is not conclusive, it may be that the anorexia starves the tumor. Many scientists believe that multiple mechanisms may be at work.

Clues to these phenomena have been found in many research studies. For example, a brain chemical called *tryptophan* is elevated in animals with tumors. Tryptophan is used by the body to make a neurotransmitter called *serotonin*, which plays a key role in controlling the appetite. Although it is not known why or how the tryptophan level rises in people with cancer, the finding supports the theory that the body's chemistry changes and leads to

TIPS & ADVICE

Coping with a Dry Mouth

A dry mouth is a common side effect of cancer therapy. Although you may think of it as merely uncomfortable, the shortage of saliva can have long-term effects, such as increasing the risk of gum disease and tooth decay, especially below the gums. A dry mouth also means that old fillings, caps, and bonding are more likely to become dislodged. Consequently, your oral hygiene should be scrupulous.

Brush your teeth at least twice daily, using a soft toothbrush and an antibacterial toothpaste formulated especially for those with dry mouth. Ask your dentist about home fluoride treatments, with either an additional daily brushing using a prescription fluoride product or a mouth rinse.

Daily flossing also is important to remove debris on and between your teeth. Learn the correct technique from your dentist to avoid damaging your gums. In some cases, a small interdental round brush that slips in the spaces between teeth may be more effective than flossing. It also is less likely to damage gums or dislodge dental fillings, caps, or bonding.

Several methods can help keep your mouth moist during the day, including artificial saliva products in gel or liquid spray form. You can experiment with different brands and flavors to find one that appeals to you. Some people keep at hand a low-calorie, nonsugary fluid, such as water, sodium-free seltzer, water-diluted fruit juice, or no-sugar soda, taking small sips throughout the day. However, make sure not to fill your stomach with fluids that contain calories but no nutrients, especially if your appetite is poor. Filling up on fluids may make you less apt to eat the nutritional foods you need. You can keep your lips moist with petroleum jelly or other lip salves.

Finally, make sure your dentist knows both that you have cancer and the type of treatment you are receiving. Those with dry mouth may need professional dental cleanings every three months or more often because they lack the saliva that normally helps keep the mouth clean. You also need frequent dental evaluations and prompt treatment of gum disease and cavities. Dentures may need refitting if the shape of your gums changes.

anorexia. Also supporting such theories is the discovery that people with cancer may metabolize carbohydrates, fats, and proteins differently.

In addition, certain types of cancer cause specific metabolic abnormalities contributing to anorexia. For instance, a cancer that begins in or spreads to the liver produces high levels of lactic acid, a chemical that can cause both anorexia and nausea.

Beyond overall appetite loss, many people—especially those with metastatic cancer—report changes in their taste and smell sensations and say they develop aversions to certain foods. Meat and meat products, for instance, can become quite distasteful. Such people may have increased tolerance for sweet substances and decrease their tolerance for sour and salty foods. Although such changes may occur as a side effect of treatment, they may also stem from the body's response to the tumor.

Although people with primary anorexia do eat—albeit far less food than is usual for them—they lose weight (both lean body mass and fatty tissue) far out of proportion to their caloric intake. This type of weight loss seems to indicate a wide range of metabolic abnormalities, including aberrations in energy expenditure and in the body's use of sugar, fat, and protein.

Today, cancer experts and nutritionists are rethinking their advice that even people with advanced cancer *must* eat. Now doctors are concluding that loss of appetite and weight in the presence of cancer should not necessarily prompt efforts to force-feed or give supplements. That is, food is not necessarily what the body needs as it does battle with advanced or metastatic cancer.

It is important to remember that tumor cells require nutrients to grow, just as normal cells do. And when a tumor cell uses large quantities of nutrients, healthy cells may be deprived of essential nutrients. Such body wasting is very disturbing, yet the body's response may be the best one.

Extreme Weight Loss

People with primary anorexia should not be urged to eat beyond what they want, which may be an extraordinarily difficult message for family members to hear. The urge to try to feed a person who is losing weight is very difficult to overcome.

Because malnutrition and cachexia are associated with a poor prognosis, it's not surprising that it was long believed that nutritional support might improve the outlook. However, when routine nutritional support (in the form of tube and intravenous feedings) was evaluated in clinical trials, no benefits were consistently found. The survival rates for people with advanced cancer did not improve, and in most cases efforts to reverse cachexia had little if any benefit.

New Attitudes About Intravenous Feeding

Oncologists have become more discriminating in turning to intravenous supplements when a person doesn't want to eat, regardless of the stage of illness. Although there are exceptions (see "When Extra Nutrition Is Necessary," page 316), most experts feel that when therapy is effective, appetite will return and the person will regain some lost weight. It simply doesn't work to try to force weight gain before therapy is successful.

Parenteral, or intravenous, nutrition is not routinely recommended for those receiving chemotherapy either. In fact, the American College of Physicians issued a position statement concerning people receiving this treatment who are *not* malnourished. According to the statement, intravenous feedings "...should be strongly discouraged [because it] was associated with net harm."

When Extra Nutrition Is Necessary

Although oncologists now believe that nutritional support with liquid-food supplements or tube or intravenous feeding should not be routinely implemented, regardless of the stage of cancer, there are some exceptions.

Surgery. Extra energy is needed to cope with the stress of recovery from an operation and to promote healing. Although the American College of Physicians has concluded that for most people, the routine use of intravenous nutrition is not justified, it did find that such nutritional support is useful for certain high-risk patients. For example, a number of studies have shown that seven to 10 days of aggressive pre- and postoperative nutritional support in cancer patients reduces the morbidity and mortality associated with surgery.

Supplementation also is recommended, even for those who are well nourished, for people about to undergo operations (such as removal of the stomach) that will result in a postoperative period of 10 days or more when they will not be able to eat. It is advised as well for those who develop postoperative complications that similarly impair the ability to eat.

Bone Marrow Transplantation (BMT). The stresses on the body from BMT are enormous, and the recovery period is difficult. Studies have shown that well-nourished BMT recipients who receive intravenous feeding before and during transplantation have a significantly higher survival rate, as well as longer disease-free periods than do people who do not receive nutritional support.

Gastrointestinal Tumors. People who have mechanical difficulties that interfere with their ability to eat and digest food may not obtain adequate nutrition from meals. Furthermore, radiation therapy to the gastrointestinal system can cause side effects that damage the ability to eat, digest, and/or absorb food. In such cases, a period of tube or intravenous feeding, depending on the site of gastrointestinal impairment, can help maintain body weight until the person is again able to eat.

Although these are the major exceptions to the general rule of not force-feeding, all treatment must be tailored to the particular patient. Therefore, physicians may have specific reasons for recommending nutritional support in other situations.

Supplementary Nutrition

When nutritional supplements are necessary, three different approaches are available: commercial meal replacements taken orally; *enteral nutrition*, also

SPECIAL

CONCERNS

A Word to Family Members: Food Is Not Necessarily Love

We grew up learning that "food is love" and "food is good medicine," so it's hard to accept that the opposite may be the case in advanced or metastatic cancer.

"He's becoming a skeleton," many a wife has lamented. How can she resist heading to the kitchen to whip up her husband's favorite high-calorie —and probably high-fat—dessert when cooking has been one of the ways she has expressed her love throughout their marriage? How can a partner resist taking his or her cachectic mate to a favorite restaurant to offer cheer and "put a little meat on your bones?" How can one *not* provide the nourishment to a parent that he or she never withheld?

If it is clear that the appetite and weight loss are primary, rather than the result of emotions or treatment side effects, resist the urge. Your desire to see your loved one gain weight is well meaning but ill founded. Don't hound him or her!

known as tube feeding; and *total parenteral nutrition (TPN)*, also known as *hyperalimentation* or intravenous feeding.

Commercial Meal Replacements

In situations when not enough nutrients can be obtained from a normal diet, such as when the effects of chemotherapy or radiation cause the gastrointestinal system to function improperly, commercial meal replacement products may be used instead of food or to supplement real food meals.

Some products are liquids that can be sipped immediately; others are powders that first have to be mixed with water. The products' nutritional contents vary widely: Some are classified as complete mixtures of nutrients; some are *modular*, providing sources of protein, carbohydrates, or fatty acids alone or with a carbohydrate; some are designed specifically for those with liver, kidney, or lung failure; and some address various needs, such as lactose intolerance. The physician's choice of a supplement is based on your specific nutritional needs. Most are available in drugstores and supermarkets.

When a specific commercial meal replacement is recommended, another product should not be substituted, as it may not contain the same nutrients. However, if the taste of a formula is offensive, the doctor or dietitian can suggest ways of flavoring it. Sometimes just a few drops of vanilla, mint, or anise can make it an enjoyable beverage.

Enteral Nutrition

When chewing or swallowing is difficult but the stomach and intestines are working normally, enteral nutrition may be recommended. For example, this may happen if your mouth, throat, or esophagus are severely inflamed because of radiation therapy. Or it may be needed when neurologic or psychiatric disorders, including severe depression, prevent normal eating.

The most common method of enteral nutrition involves a *nasogastric* tube, a flexible plastic tube that is passed through the nose into the stomach. A specific formula is delivered directly to the stomach through the tube, which remains in place continuously. Less commonly, an *orogastric* tube is used, entering through the mouth rather than the nose. If you cannot tolerate a tube in the nose or mouth, a surgical opening can be made in the abdomen, and a *gastrostomy* tube is placed directly into the stomach or, if the stomach must be bypassed, a *jejunostomy* tube is inserted directly into the small intestine.

The nutrients delivered through a tube are usually in a liquid formula such as those provided in commercial meal replacements. With surgically placed tubes to the stomach or intestine, sometimes normal food pureed in a blender can be used. Enteral nutrition may be delivered to the stomach at specified meal times every three or four hours (called *bolus* feeding), intermittently, or continuously by a special pump.

Once the tube is in place, enteral nutrition can be provided in the hospital or by a trained family member or health care worker at home. This has become a relatively common and safe practice that permits you to be sent home earlier, where you may recuperate more rapidly and calmly. In any case, when you are receiving enteral nutrition, you must be monitored for such side effects as nausea, vomiting, diarrhea, and constipation. A change of formula can usually alleviate these problems.

Total Parenteral Nutrition

Total parenteral nutrition (TPN) delivers nutrients directly into the bloodstream. It may be recommended when the intestinal tract is not functioning. For example, intravenous feeding is helpful when there is an absorption problem, such as dumping syndrome (see page 310). It may be most valuable when a very aggressive treatment has caused a temporary but severe gastrointestinal malfunction. TPN also may be prescribed for those whose cancer has been cured but who radiation therapy has left with severe and permanent gastrointestinal tract damage. These people may need TPN indefinitely.

For short-term nutrition of less than ten days, a catheter is inserted into a vein in the arm, delivering a solution of amino acids, simple sugars, electrolytes, and vitamins. This is called *peripheral TPN*. For longer-term nutritional support, a catheter is inserted into a large vein, the *subclavian vein*, in the chest. The catheter extends through the vein into the *superior vena cava*, which is the principal vein draining the upper portion of the body. This is called *central TPN*. It empties directly into the heart, from which the nutrients are pumped throughout the body.

As with tube feeding, once the catheter for central TPN is in place, nutrition can be provided either in the hospital or at home by home health workers or trained family members. *Hyperalimentation*, or intravenous feeding, need not be continuous but can often be done while you sleep at night.

During the day, the catheter can be disconnected from the intravenous tube and discreetly concealed.

Central TPN is the least preferable route for providing nutrition because of the high risk of mechanical difficulties, infection, and other complications. In addition, it is a relatively complicated procedure and requires an open wound in the body. It must be dressed every day using a strict aseptic technique. It also necessitates frequent blood tests for assessment of blood sugar and electrolytes, urine testing, and weighings to ensure adequate nutrition. Moreover, TPN is expensive: The cost for at-home TPN can range from $75,000 to $150,000 a year.

C H A P T E R

ACTIVITY COUNTS

The evidence in favor of the health benefits of physical activity continues to accumulate, even for people with cancer. Research is beginning to show that exercise may help prevent the disease; it also seems to help counter some aspects of cancer and to relieve some of the unpleasant reactions to its treatment. Although the effects of exercise on people with cancer have not yet been studied extensively, one well-proven advantage is that it enhances your sense of autonomy and self-esteem. Men and women who exercise report that they simply feel better.

Of course, the capacity to exercise depends on your physical condition, including the stage and type of cancer you have, your treatment and its side effects, and your general health. For instance, a fitness regimen that might be beneficial to a woman recovering from a mastectomy could be counterproductive for a man in the late stages of lung cancer.

This chapter explains how exercise can help prevent some physical problems and relieve others. There are suggestions too for sedentary people beginning an exercise program as well as ideas for previously active people adjusting their routine.

Why Exercise?

Spotty though the research is, exercise appears to be beneficial. Although no one knows whether it can prevent a recurrence of cancer or slow the progress of metastasis, it is helpful for those with cancer to exercise and reap some of its positive effects.

Physical Benefits

Exercise builds muscle tissue, strengthens the heart, increases the capacity of the lungs to take in oxygen, and improves circulation. It may even help healthy tissue compensate for compromised tissues and organs. For example, walking

Exercise and Cancer Prevention

Scientists have begun to speculate about the role of physical inactivity in the development of cancer, and some intriguing findings have emerged. It's now known, for instance, that physically fit people tend to have a lower incidence of cancer. According to one large study of people at various levels of fitness, the least fit men died from cancer at a rate that was more than four times higher than that of the most fit men, and the least fit women had fully 16 times the cancer death rate of the most fit women. Several studies have shown a correlation between an inactive lifestyle and colon cancer in men, and in women there appears to be a link between inactivity and endometrial cancer.

Unfortunately, finding a correlation is not the same as identifying a cause, but researchers are exploring several theories that may explain the link between inactivity and cancer. People who exercise tend to be leaner than those who do not, and excessive body fat is a risk factor for cancer, specifically endometrial, colon, and possibly breast cancers (see Chapter 10, "Cancer Causes and Risks").

Another theory is that because exercise such as walking or running speeds food through the digestive tract, carcinogens (including certain bile acids that help digest fat) interact with the intestinal wall for a shorter time. Girls who exercise vigorously begin menstruating later, which appears to reduce their chances of getting breast or reproductive cancers in the future. This finding has led some scientists to speculate that by affecting hormone levels, exercise might help prevent certain forms of cancer.

CANCER BASICS

or swimming twice a day for 15 minutes may increase the efficiency of the healthy areas of the lungs and enable a person with lung cancer who has no distant metastasis to breathe more easily.

Stimulating Appetite. Moderate activity stimulates appetite when worry and the physical effects of the disease or the side effects of treatment interfere with the desire for food.

Boosting Energy. Men and women who have survived cancer and exercise regularly say the main reason that they keep active is that they feel more energetic. This probably occurs for two reasons: First, exercise increases stamina that has been diminished by bed rest or depression; second, activity increases muscle strength, so movement requires less effort.

Improving Immunity. Aerobic exercise is any activity that increases the blood flow to the heart and the amount of oxygen the lungs take in. Fast walking or running are common examples. Aerobic exercise is believed to improve the immune function by enhancing the production of interferon and interleukin 2, normal body proteins that also are being used to treat cancer (see Chapter 18, "Biological Therapies"). This may explain why physical activity seems to help the body fight infection.

Remember, though, that moderation is the key, for some evidence suggests that overtraining—that is, repeatedly working out to the point of exhaustion—can depress immunity.

Preventing Complications. Poor physical condition invites a worsening of problems that arise from confinement to bed or restricted movement. These can range from minor annoyances, such as generalized aches or localized muscle spasms, to serious health problems such as pneumonia and poor circulation. Regular movement of the entire body will help avoid these effects of immobility.

If you've been very active, you may find that you have to start at a much lower level of activity after surgery or chemotherapy, for instance, and then gradually build up your stamina again. You may or may not achieve your pretreatment level of conditioning, but by working with a physician who can help monitor your progress and physical capability, a program can be designed that works for you. If your lifestyle hasn't included much physical activity until now, begin slowly and gradually increase your level of exertion so that it challenges but does not exhaust you.

Fighting Fatigue. Traditionally, the only medical treatment for fatigue has been rest, yet this can create a dangerous *fatigue spiral*: The more you rest, the weaker your muscles become and the more your circulation is compromised, which increases your tiredness. In fact, to regain the lean muscle mass lost during one week of bedrest, it's necessary to exercise regularly for two to three weeks.

A program of moderate exercise combats the fatigue syndrome by keeping muscles in good condition and elevating your mood. The best kinds of exercise to combat fatigue are stretching, yoga, walking, and swimming, because they stimulate the muscles and circulatory system without putting stress on the joints. In one study of women with breast cancer, those who exercised experienced less fatigue than nonexercising patients, whose fatigue actually increased.

One note of caution when exercising to counteract fatigue: Be sure to get enough rest between periods of physical exertion. Muscles require at least a day to recover from strenuous exercise. And what you may have done as part of your normal routine before your cancer treatment may be too strenuous after it.

Also, if you cannot relax and continually worry about your condition, your skeletal muscles will be tense and unable to recover adequately from exercise. Don't be tempted to push too hard to prove you are still strong. A person who attempts strenuous exercises too frequently can actually perpetuate fatigue.

Maintaining a Range of Motion. Studies show that increasing physical activity improves the range of motion of the body's joints, which often diminishes as the cancer progresses or whenever bed rest or general inactivity is prolonged. (Range of motion is the degree to which a joint can be moved in a circle.) Maintaining and restoring flexibility and range of motion are essential to preserving general strength. See "Exercises to Do in Bed" on pages 336–37 in Chapter 28.

Countering Nausea. Whether activity affects the cause of nausea or simply distracts you from it is unknown, but aerobic exercise has been shown to diminish this unpleasant side effect of chemotherapy. Unfortunately, nausea also can interfere with the ability to tolerate physical exertion and can cause balance problems, so it is not always possible to exercise.

Preserving Lean Tissue. Muscle fibers, which give your body strength and allow you to move freely, consist of lean tissue. If you lose too much weight or lose weight too quickly, you usually lose lean tissue. Activity, however, can help counter that loss. As you build strength and endurance through exercise, you increase the amount of lean tissue. This is sometimes referred to as *lean body mass* or *lean muscle tissue.* However, when exercising, if you burn more calories than you consume, you risk losing muscle.

If your prognosis is good and you can tolerate a 1,500-calorie diet, it's usually safe to do some form of aerobic exercise four or five times a week, along with some strength training to build muscle.

Weight Gain. Exercise can also prevent or reduce some of the weight gain associated with hormones and certain anticancer drugs, by flushing excess fluid from the body and raising the body's metabolic rate so that calories burn faster.

Weight Loss. The interrelationship between your disease and how you exercise and how much you eat is complicated when the cancer is advanced. Since exercise helps preserve lean muscle tissue, it may slow the wasting process that accompanies advanced disease. However, this benefit has not been confirmed by research, so most physicians believe that if you feel up to it, moderate exercise is probably not harmful.

Emotional Benefits

Exercise enhances emotional well-being in a variety of ways. Immediately after their cancer is diagnosed, people often feel depressed, lethargic, hopeless, anxious, or angry, or a combination of all these emotions. Exercise can go a long way to counteract these feelings, by inducing feelings of relaxation and optimism (see Chapter 25, "Coping with Stress, Fear, Anxiety, and Depression").

Depression. Activities that are pleasurable and constructive appear to decrease feelings of apathy, inadequacy, and helplessness. The relief may come because exercise provides a sense of accomplishment, control, and independence. Or as some scientists speculate, aerobic exercise may have a direct effect on the brain's chemistry, increasing those natural agents that enhance pleasurable sensations and reducing those associated with stress.

Anxiety. Exercise also has a temporary calming effect on angry or anxious people. Muscle tension is especially troublesome, because when the muscles are tense, their blood supply is constricted, which contributes to a generalized weakness. Fatigue may follow, which often contributes to depression.

Self-Esteem. Exercise can give you a feeling of control in a situation in which constant tests, visits to the doctor, and treatments make it easy to feel helpless. Therefore, exercise is a worthwhile activity, if only to regain a sense of autonomy and personal power. It also provides goals to work toward and accomplish, which can be quite satisfying.

An Exercise Prescription

Exercise falls into two categories: aerobic and anaerobic. Walking, jogging, cycling, and swimming are examples of aerobic exercise. Any of these activities can increase the heart rate and, as a result, increase the lungs' capacity to take in oxygen. Thus, more oxygen is delivered to the muscles. Aerobic exercise also increases metabolism, which may help control the weight that some people gain during chemotherapy. Regular aerobic exercise lowers the amount of blood cholesterol, strengthens bones, and increases endurance.

Anaerobic exercise is characterized by short bursts of intense activity. Weight lifting or sprinting, for example, helps develop muscles and strength, speed, and power.

- *Walking.* Walking is an excellent exercise for people with cancer, because it increases lung function, stimulates bone growth, and strengthens leg and back muscles. Although a metastasis to the leg, back, or pelvic bone rules out running, it may not rule out walking, because walking does not jar the joints. (If you have metastatic disease in your bones, consult your physician before starting any exercise program.) Walking in a swimming pool is especially gentle yet stimulates the heart and lungs, building endurance.

- *Swimming.* When walking is painful because of metastasis in the spine, hip, or pelvis, swimming can be a good substitute. It is not stressful to any body part, and if you swim far and fast enough, you will increase your aerobic capacity. Swimming's major advantage is that it stretches the muscles, including those of the rib cage, which increases the amount of air you can inhale and exhale. Swimming also strengthens your muscles as your body moves against the water's resistance without jarring.

- *Strength training.* Lifting weights or working out with weight resistance machines is sometimes recommended for people with cancer because the repetitive movements against resistance help build muscle. However, because the more lean muscle mass you have, the more calories you will burn, close supervision and weight monitoring are important to make sure your increased calorie needs don't exceed the number of calories you are able to eat.

  Some experts feel that weight resistance machines are safer than free weights because they are more easily controlled. If you have never done strength training before, work with an experienced trainer who understands the needs and limitations of a person with cancer.

- *Stretching and yoga.* Stretching and yoga promote flexibility and relieve muscle tension. Well-stretched muscles also are less vulnerable to injury than tight muscles are, and they require less energy and effort to move. Stretching and yoga are gentle movements designed to extend and tone muscles that have become shortened as a result of lengthy periods of inactivity, such as prolonged bed rest after surgery. Stretching also produces a feeling of well-being and increases blood circulation.

  In addition, yoga and the deep breathing it requires can help you relax and gain a feeling of serenity. Some experts say it helps restore emotional equilibrium.

Getting Started, Keeping Going

There are no rules in regard to maintaining your current level of activity, but if you have been sidelined for a while or want to begin an exercise program for the first time, it's important to consult a physician first. Some tests of heart and lung function may be needed to make a safe recommendation. For example, a runner or a person with a previously diagnosed heart condition may need to have an exercise stress test to be certain that his or her heart can handle the increased workload. A physical exam that includes an evaluation of joint and muscle function is important to forestall such problems as stiffness of the hips or unstable knees. If the cancer has metastasized, x-rays of the legs, pelvis, spine, and other areas may be needed.

People who have never exercised before or active people who have been confined to bed for a while need to start slowly, perhaps walking only 5 to 10 minutes several times a day initially. With daily effort, endurance will increase. The key is to have a willing, positive attitude; to set reasonable goals; and to stick to a program. Avoid competitive activities, if they make you feel tense; exercise should promote relaxation.

The Right Combination

If you enjoyed exercising before your diagnosis, you will probably be able to continue the activities that gave you pleasure. Much depends on where your cancer is and the treatment you have received. If you are a runner or a golfer, for example, you should still be able to run and play after a prostatectomy, a mastectomy, partial removal of the large bowel, or even removal of one kidney. Many who have had a portion of a lung removed return to their original level of activity. But you must avoid intense exertion that produces exhaustion and muscle strain and that lowers the body's resistance to infection. People with cancer also frequently have anemia, which makes them tired and susceptible to cold. Never exercise so vigorously that you are feel unable to do your normal activities. For instance, don't walk so long in the afternoon that you are too tired to eat dinner that evening.

An ideal exercise program combines aerobic and anaerobic exercises such as strength training with stretching components as part of the warm-up and cool-down. It's a good idea to alternate aerobic and strength-training exercises. Or if you enjoy a half-hour walk every day, you might add a strength-training session two or three times a week.

Warming up for five to 10 minutes before exercising avoids injuries. To warm up, start the activity slowly; then briefly limber up muscles in the arms, legs, and trunk through stretching movements. As circulation to the muscle increases, pick up the pace. Finally, do the last few minutes of the activity at a slower pace. This cooling down is necessary to allow the muscles to relax and to prevent subsequent cramping. Each episode of exercise should begin and end with some gentle stretches.

Where to Get the Right Supervision and Help

Your doctor or the physical therapy department at the hospital where you're being treated should be able to recommend an exercise professional to you. For help with all types of exercise, you can check with your local American Heart Association for cardiac rehabilitation classes, which are designed for people who need to be careful about how much they stress their system. The YMCA and YWCA may have programs for people with cancer, and the American Lung Association offers special programs in some areas. Road runner clubs, local hiking groups, and cycling groups also may have programs for people with chronic diseases and/or cancer.

Yoga and stretching classes are offered at health clubs throughout the country. It is important to speak to the teacher beforehand, to make sure he or she understands your limitations. There are several excellent books and videos on yoga and stretching.

In any class or program, stop if you feel pressured to push yourself to the point of discomfort or if you feel any discomfort.

TIPS & ADVICE

Why Walk?

Walking is the perfect exercise. It can be done in nearly any type of weather and is not jarring to the joints. Moreover, a five-year longitudinal study showed no significant difference in the improvement of aerobic capacity between joggers and walkers who kept to a brisk pace. In addition, walking provides a feeling of well-being, relaxation, and emotional uplift.

Begin by walking for 10 minutes three times a week, and then build to 20 minutes four times a week. Ultimately, your goal should be to walk four to seven times a week for 30 minutes.

If you are over age 35, walking at least four times weekly for 30 minutes will maintain or improve your aerobic capacity. This is particularly important when cancer has phases of exacerbation. During the acute stage, you may be unable to walk, but you can build up your aerobic reserve by walking when your disease is not active.

Limitations on Physical Activity

Despite the obvious benefits of exercise, people with cancer need to take into account their special circumstances. Each person is the best judge of how much activity is tolerable. There is nothing to be gained from attempting to "work through" symptoms or the side effects of treatment with excessive exercise. Also, even if physical activity was your way of coping with stress and tension before you became ill, pushing yourself too hard now may be discouraging and end up making you feel worse.

Be aware, too, that some chemotherapy drugs may affect specific organs in ways that limit physical activity (see Chapter 17, "Chemotherapy"). Adriamycin, for example, can be quite toxic to the heart. Bleomycin can affect the lungs. And sometimes drugs given to relieve side effects have side effects of their own. For example, the antinausea drug compazine can cause dizziness.

Chemotherapy can adversely affect the capacity to exercise by inducing nausea and decreasing the number of red and white blood cells and platelets, which not only reduces the body's ability to deliver oxygen to the muscles but raises the risk of infection and bleeding. However, during chemotherapy, walking and yoga, which are gentle and incorporate deep breathing, can be helpful.

Conditions That Exercise Can Aggravate

Although it is important to resist the impulse to stop exercising altogether when you're not feeling energetic, there are times when it's wise to give yourself a break. Some of the following situations or conditions may alter your ability to exercise:

- *Dehydration.* Some cancers can cause electrolyte imbalances and deplete the body of fluids. Dehydration in these cases can have severe consequences. Never exercise in extreme heat, and always drink plenty of fluids. If you perspire a lot, you may feel better drinking a sport drink that is fortified with electrolytes such as salt and potassium.

- *Bone stress.* Many people with cancer are at risk for bone fractures, especially in the long bones, spine, pelvis, and ribs. If the cancer has spread to the bone, strength training is not recommended. Activities such as basketball or tennis that involve jumping or twisting the hips are not advised if there is bone loss or metastatic disease in the bones.

- *Anemia.* If the cancer has metastasized to the bones or treatment has affected the bone marrow, anemia and a low platelet count—which causes bruising or bleeding into the joints and elsewhere—can make you vulnerable to injury. Accordingly, activities that exert a force on the bones, such as running or step classes, may be restricted. Until the condition is corrected, your activities may be limited to walking and gentle yoga or stretching.

- *Hypercalcemia.* Too much calcium in the blood, or hypercalcemia, may occur in women with breast cancer because of hormonal changes that accompany the disease as well as some types of treatment, such as the use

CASE HISTORIES

TRUE STORIES

My Life as a Runner with Cancer, by Fred Lebow

Fred Lebow, a member of the national Track Hall of Fame and founder of the New York City Marathon, died of brain cancer, a recurrence of lymphoma, four years after his condition was diagnosed, longer than his doctor had expected. In 1992, while his cancer was in remission, Lebow completed the 26-mile marathon he created—in five hours, 32 minutes, and 34 seconds. In the introduction to *The New York Road Runners Club Complete Book of Running*, Lebow described how important exercise was during his illness:

My physical fitness was critical. I used it to make sure I didn't stagnate. You can be sick in bed, unable to do almost anything, but you can still wiggle your fingers and toes. I found this out through experience. Over the months in and out of hospitals, I believed that if I let myself be ruled by the disease, I could succumb to my own laziness. I fought that tendency with exercise.

On the journey to save my life, I started chemotherapy, a horrible odyssey of nausea, weakness, weight and hair loss. I felt like Methuselah in his nine hundredth year—yet I continued to proclaim myself the healthiest cancer patient on earth.

The first day back in my own apartment, I decided to walk in Central Park. I was tired before I started. But I was spurred on by greetings from the doorman I used to pass on my daily runs during my pre-disease days. Every day I went walking, starting with one mile, and by the third day I walked 2 3/4 miles in one hour. After about three weeks of walking, I was able to insert short bursts of running, 10- to 15-yard jogs, into my walking routine. I never thought running could be so difficult! I was amazed how I could be jogging and every walker in the park could still pass me. But with each day I improved, inserting more and longer intervals of jogging. One minute of running became ten, and eventually, I worked my way up to past levels of training.

Then I began a 31-day cycle of radiation at Memorial Sloan-Kettering Cancer Center. Because the hospital is within blocks of my apartment, it was convenient to walk there for treatments. This was the only convenience, however.

With chemotherapy, I lost my hair. With radiation, I lost my trademark beard. Initially, I became bloated, then I lost weight. Eventually I was down to 124 pounds from my running weight of 144. I had no hair, and very little meat on my bones. But I had made great progress in my recovery. One day I managed an entire lower loop of the park running. It took me 30 minutes to cover the 1.7 miles. Pills, operations, doctor's guidance, and the love of family and friends all aid recovery. But there is something more, something crucial to overcoming the failure of the body, and that is physical fitness.

When I look back over my experience with cancer, I am struck by how little other patients exercise. At Mount Sinai [Hospital], younger, fitter patients than I didn't move a muscle. Only one other patient—a 2:48 marathoner—ever seemed to join me in activity.

> *When I became ill, I got the best doctors, treatment, and advice. And then I did more. I moved my hands, my legs. I made my blood pump. Other patients at Mount Sinai would ask me, "Why do you do this?" I'd respond, "The question isn't why I'm doing this, but why you aren't."*
>
> *I know it's sometimes hard to get motivated to run even in the best of health and under the best conditions. Part of my desire to run is to stay in shape to race. Even after cancer therapy, I walked, then ran, with the goal of getting back into racing. However, I was no longer racing to break a 7-minute per mile pace. I'm delighted now to break 10 minutes per mile.*
>
> *Since my illness, I have been taking my life back, slowly but confidently. My body has changed. I'm not as strong as I was before, but I can manage more and more each day. I'm thinner, but I've always been fairly "runner thin." But the real change is inside me, a change I understand best through my running. I'm glad to be alive and I live with that feeling every day. It's like being a beginner again, in love with the idea of my body moving along, content with the weather, the seasons, and the sound of each footfall.*

of tamoxifen. This condition causes muscle weakness and leaches calcium out of bones, making them vulnerable to fractures. Acute hypercalcemia can even cause cardiac arrhythmia and kidney failure, and so aerobic exercise that stresses the heart is not recommended until the condition is corrected.

- *Nerve damage.* If your brain or nerves are affected and you are unsteady, exercising by yourself is not advised. Plan walks with a friend. You could also consult with a *physiatrist*, a specialist in rehabilitation medicine, to learn compensatory training methods to help you overcome some problems such as unsteadiness in walking (see Chapter 28, "Managing Disabilities and Limitations").

Exercise in Advanced Illness

Exercise counteracts feelings of listlessness and can slow the fatigue spiral and tissue loss, so some form of physical activity is beneficial at an advanced stage of cancer, even when generalized weakness is present.

Activity for those confined to bed may consist of passive (someone else moves your extremities for you) range-of-motion exercises and general stretching. A physical therapist can show you and a friend or family member a passive exercise routine. What's most important is listening to your body. If it hurts, stop. Although it may be impossible to stem the loss of muscle, the physical activity will help you maintain some mobility and relieve muscle tension, providing a temporary psychological boost. In fact, pain medication combined with stretching exercises is one of the best solutions for keeping comfortable when confined to bed.

The Gift of Exercise

Besides all the good reasons for exercising, remember that physical activity also can be pleasurable. It can add to your quality of life by making you feel better mentally and physically. The bonus can be a sense of pure joy, which improves your quality of life.

Many with cancer who exercise revel in meeting personal challenges. Some run marathons, ride in bikeathons, or just walk the length of their street. They thrill to see their own capabilities increase and take pride in their successive accomplishments. Some of them are champions.

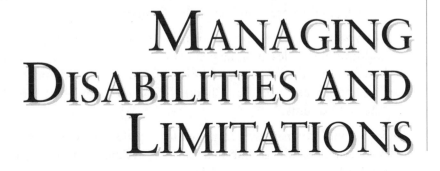

MANAGING
DISABILITIES AND
LIMITATIONS

Cancer treatment causes almost everyone to experience some change in their physical being and ability to care for themselves. The effects may range from the trivial to the overwhelming, from temporary inconvenience to lifelong disability. Therapy can alter a body function, appearance, or both, possibly affecting the way you speak, walk, eat, eliminate, or perform an activity that you once took for granted.

How these changes affect any individual varies enormously. A young woman with breast cancer, for example, may not face the same problems as does a postmenopausal woman with the same disease, and neither of them has the same needs as a man with a colostomy or a child whose leg must be amputated. This is why one of the basic principles of *rehabilitation medicine*, a specialty concerned with enabling people to attain their full functioning potential, is that you must help plan your therapy. The main purpose of rehabilitation is to regain independence, but the circumstances of your illness, ongoing changes in physical ability, the type and site of the cancer, and age are always viewed as part of the process.

Ideally, rehabilitation begins at the time of diagnosis, in the form of psychological support. It continues through treatment and is an essential aspect of follow-up care. The goal is to help you return to a life as close as possible to the one you lived before you learned you had cancer. This chapter tells you the options and helps you learn how to get what you need.

Unfortunately, many people don't benefit from all that rehabilitation medicine can offer simply because they don't know that it exists and, even when they do, they often don't know how to gain access to it.

What Rehabilitation Can Do for You

The objectives of rehabilitation were summed up by the National Cancer

Institute as part of a broad effort to improve the quality of life for people with cancer:

- *Psychological adjustment:* overcoming anger and fear, developing a positive attitude, learning how to relax, and becoming secure enough to express yourself sexually. (See Chapters 25, "Coping with Stress, Fear, Anxiety, and Depression," and 30, "Sexuality.")

- *Physical functioning:* coping with side effects; recognizing your strengths and limitations; learning new skills in daily functioning; adapting to the loss of limbs, organs, or capabilities; maintaining good nutrition; and getting enough exercise. (See Chapters 26, "Food and Nutrition," and 27, "Activity Counts.")

- *Vocational counseling:* arranging for productive work and recreation, recovering socially, getting your support system in place, and renewing or establishing contacts with friends. (See Chapter 13, "Your Support Network.")

- An effective rehabilitation plan always recognizes challenges to self-esteem and personal relationships. (See Chapters 29, "Body Image and Self-Esteem," and 31, "Coping Strategies.")

When Rehabilitation Begins

When you first learn you have cancer is a crucial time for obtaining psychological support, learning about your illness, developing coping skills, and doing preventive work. Learning about your potential for recovery early on can help alleviate some of the fear and anxiety about your treatment and your future. Knowing what to expect, what you can do to recover as rapidly and fully as possible, and how to make the best of your situation can greatly diminish your fear of the unknown and the tendency to imagine the worst. Information and early preparation can be enormously helpful.

Many people find that accepting the diagnosis, becoming comfortable with the changes to their bodies, and learning the self-care that might be necessary are easier when they are shown that living with a disability need not be as terrible as they may fear. For example, a clear explanation of what happens when you have an *ostomy* (a surgically created opening in the abdomen for waste elimination) offers some sense of control in a situation in which the loss of control over body functions is a central concern. For this reason surgeons typically invite an ostomy specialist, called an *enterostomal* or *stoma therapist*, to talk with their patients before such surgery.

Who Needs Rehabilitation?

Nearly everyone who has been treated for cancer needs some rehabilitation, even if it's only help in regaining strength after bed rest.

The following are some examples of specific difficulties that extensive, focused rehabilitation can address:

- *Head and neck cancer:* swallowing, eating, drinking, maintaining adequate food and water intake, talking, and appearance.

- *Cancer of the uterus, ovary, vulva, or vagina:* hormonal changes from treatment-induced menopause, changes in internal or external anatomy, fear of the loss of femininity and of one's partner's reaction, compromised sexual function, and loss of childbearing ability.

- *Cancer of the bowel or bladder:* loss of voluntary control, adequate food and water intake, dietary changes, feelings of social isolation or stigma, sexual difficulties because of anatomic changes, difficulty in traveling, and interference with hobbies, work, and recreation.

People with advanced cancer of any type are usually better able to cope with its emotional demands when they can care for themselves as much as possible. Rehabilitation goals can include relieving symptoms that diminish well-being, making the environment safe and workable, and ensuring physical and emotional support.

Getting the Help You Need

Although rehabilitation is a widely accepted aspect of cancer treatment, not all physicians recommend it or make sure that those who need it get it. And there may be other obstacles. Community hospitals don't always have the necessary resources. Medical care providers may be able to offer several aspects of care, but a specific person may not be responsible for drawing up a rehabilitation plan.

According to a survey by the American Cancer Society, most people do use rehabilitation services when they learn about them. Unfortunately, only about one in every four people with cancer is aware of what resources are available. So it may be partly or even entirely up to you to take the initiative in getting the help and information you need.

If your oncologist or hospital social worker cannot help, the local unit of the American Cancer Society, through its Resource, Information and Guidance program (RIG), may be of assistance.

The Team Approach

Rehabilitation calls for the coordinated efforts of a team of specialists, usually led by a physiatrist, a physician who specializes in rehabilitation techniques. He or she is trained to diagnose and treat neuromuscular and musculoskeletal disorders and can design therapies to restore mobility or compensate for its limitations. A physiatrist also prescribes treatment provided by other members of the team, such as exercise instruction, fitting and training in how to use braces or artificial limbs, breathing assistance, and counseling.

Who Does What

Depending on your situation, your team may include one or several of the following:

- *Physiatrists*, who specialize in rehabilitation medicine.

- *Physical therapists*, who teach exercises and other physical techniques for overcoming disabilities and using artificial limbs or braces, evaluate muscle strength and range of movement in joints, and teach hygienic self-care.

- *Respiratory therapists*, who treat breathing disorders under the direction of a physician and teach techniques to restore lung function.

- *Oncology nurses*, who are specially trained to care for people with cancer and to teach them about their care before, during, and after treatment; who plan at-home care and rehabilitation; and who help families deal with social and emotional issues.

- *Social workers*, who help patients and their families plan treatments and services, guide them to community resources, work with physiatrists or physical or occupational therapists in finding vocational or other counselors, and provide emotional support, psychological guidance, and sometimes stress management. They may evaluate your living environment and suggest how to change it to meet your particular physical needs.

- *Psychologists*, who assess psychological status and problem-solving skills and suggest ways of handling the many challenges of cancer and its treatment, including self-esteem and sexuality issues, family difficulties, and lifestyle changes. They may provide training in stress management techniques and offer behavioral strategies for dealing with certain aspects of treatment. Psychologists also may help evaluate alterations in personality and mental capacity, such as testing memory, perceptual function, and personality.

- *Speech pathologists*, who offer preoperative evaluation and counseling, provide treatment for neurologic communication problems, plan vocal reeducation, and train people with defects in the mouth or without a larynx to acquire and use esophageal speech (see "Learning to Talk").

- *Nutritionists*, who help you maintain good nutrition while dealing with such problems as weight loss, appetite changes, or taste disorders; offer guidance in planning meals; and teach special techniques for supplementary feedings.

- *Vocational rehabilitation counselors*, who evaluate how cancer and its treatment affect life roles and vocational skills and, when necessary, offer counseling regarding career changes. They may serve as a link to placement and training agencies.

- *Maxillofacial prosthodontists*, who are dental specialists who create devices to restore swallowing and speech after surgery.

- *Enterostomal therapists*, who are nurse-specialists who help patients with a stoma (artificial opening for elimination of wastes) to select collection devices and give instructions on how to use them. Therapists may be certified by the International Association for Enterostomal Therapy. (Many therapists have ostomies themselves.)

- *Prosthetist-orthotists*, who evaluate, design, fabricate, and fit braces and *prostheses* (artificial body parts).

- *Recreational therapists*, who help people improve their well-being through music, dance, and art.

- *Volunteers*, who have been trained to provide educational information and support. Many volunteers also are cancer survivors, willing to pass along what they have learned about coping with impairments or other difficulties of living with this disease.

Family Helpers

Some of the most important participants on the rehabilitation team are not medical specialists but your family, a term used collectively in this book to include close personal friends, partners, significant others, and the like. Experience has shown that the people who are most successful in their efforts at recovery and rehabilitation are those whose families make the healthiest adjustment to the cancer, encourage and support efforts toward their recovery, and become involved in rehabilitation whenever appropriate. Nevertheless, people with cancer who are accustomed to being independent may find it especially difficult to share responsibility, let others in on decision making, or sacrifice some of their freedom (see Chapter 32, "Issues for Families and Friends").

Types of Intervention

Rehabilitation may be *preventive*, *restorative*, *supportive*, or *palliative*. Some people may need only one kind; others, two or three. For example, a woman undergoing a mastectomy for breast cancer may get these kinds of rehabilitation care: *preventive*, such as discussion and counseling before treatment, to prepare her for possible complications and to give her emotional support regarding her body image and sexual concerns; *restorative*, which may include exercises to achieve pain-free use of the affected arm as soon as possible after surgery, and possibly reconstructive surgery or breast prosthesis to achieve cosmetic restoration; *supportive*, that is, help in accepting the loss of her breast and coping with fears and anxieties. She may or may not need the fourth type of rehabilitation, *palliative*, which focuses primarily on pain relief and physical and emotional support for the person with advanced cancer.

Preventive Rehabilitation

There are ways to avoid or minimize some of the effects of cancer and its treatment. For example, bed rest may create problems that may be prevented if steps to protect the skin and stimulate circulation are taken early.

Exercises to Do in Bed

The following movements help maintain the full movement of the joints and gently stretch muscles:

Shoulder Rotation

Lie on your back, with knees bent, feet flat on mat. Use as many pillows as you need to feel comfortable. As you progress, you will need to use fewer pillows.

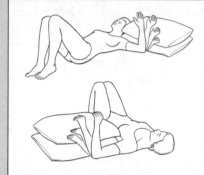

a. Place pillows on left side, next to your head. Slide left arm out to side so that it is as level with shoulder as possible. Bend elbow to 90°. By rotating the shoulder, allow the back of your hand to rest on pillows without pain. *Hold 5 seconds. Relax. Repeat 3 times.*
Repeat exercise with right arm.

b. Position left arm as in figure a, but place pillows next to ribs on that side. By rotating the shoulder, allow the palm of your hand to rest on pillows without pain. *Hold 5 seconds. Relax. Repeat 3 times.*
Repeat exercise with right arm.

Knee to Chest—Side-Lying

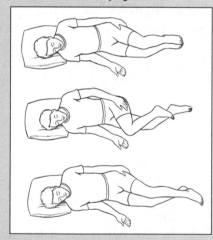

a. Lie on your right side, with knees slightly bent up toward your chest. Place pillow under your head.

b. Slide your left knee up to your chest without straining. At this point, drop the knee onto the floor.

c. Then gently straighten out the leg so that both the hip and knee are straight. Again, drop the leg to the floor so that no effort is used to hold it. Return the leg to the starting position.

Repeat 3 times.
Turn onto your left side and repeat exercise 3 times.

Shoulder Flexion

Sit in a straight-back chair, with feet flat on floor, or lie on your back, with knees bent, feet flat on mat.

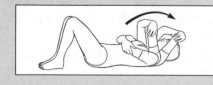

Cradle left arm with right arm, and slowly raise both arms overhead as far as possible. Allow right arm to do most of the work. Do not go past point of pain. *Hold 5 seconds. Relax. Repeat 3 times.*
Reverse arms and repeat exercise 3 times.

Hip Adductor Stretching—Back-Lying

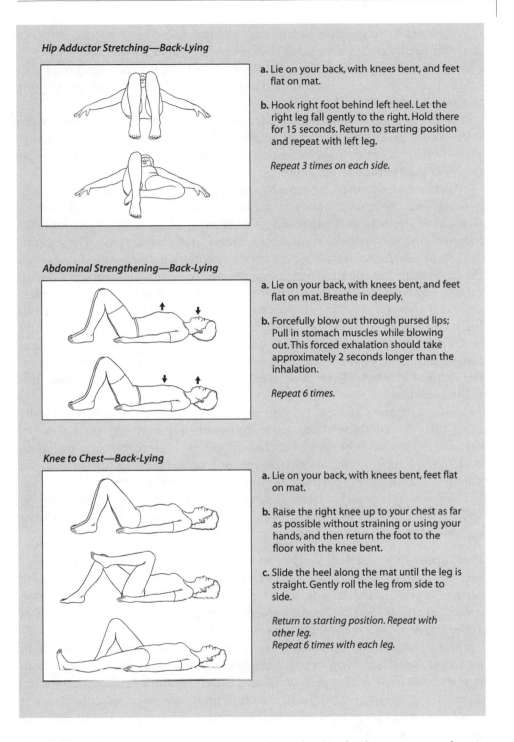

a. Lie on your back, with knees bent, and feet flat on mat.

b. Hook right foot behind left heel. Let the right leg fall gently to the right. Hold there for 15 seconds. Return to starting position and repeat with left leg.

Repeat 3 times on each side.

Abdominal Strengthening—Back-Lying

a. Lie on your back, with knees bent, and feet flat on mat. Breathe in deeply.

b. Forcefully blow out through pursed lips; Pull in stomach muscles while blowing out. This forced exhalation should take approximately 2 seconds longer than the inhalation.

Repeat 6 times.

Knee to Chest—Back-Lying

a. Lie on your back, with knees bent, feet flat on mat.

b. Raise the right knee up to your chest as far as possible without straining or using your hands, and then return the foot to the floor with the knee bent.

c. Slide the heel along the mat until the leg is straight. Gently roll the leg from side to side.

Return to starting position. Repeat with other leg.
Repeat 6 times with each leg.

Immobility. Inactivity causes your muscles and other body systems to deteriorate. You may become weak, and your muscles may tighten and lose their elasticity, further impairing your mobility and slowing your recovery.

Inactivity also produces muscle atrophy (*wasting*) surprisingly soon. A normal muscle that is completely unused loses about 3 to 5 percent of its strength each day. It's estimated that people confined to bed lose half their muscle strength in three to five weeks. Unfortunately, it takes much longer to regain your strength; it may take two months to regain just 10 percent of your lost muscle strength.

When your mobility is restricted, the connective tissues that support the joints don't maintain their ideal length and so become dense from disuse. Because their normal range of motion is compromised, it takes more muscular energy than usual to do anything, which also contributes to fatigue.

Weakness and muscular atrophy may be significantly reduced by simply making sure the muscle undergoes contraction movements several times a day, either opposed or unopposed to resistance. Maintaining joint mobility through exercises helps prevent joint stiffness and contractures. The exercises may be *passive* (a person moves your extremity), *active assisted* (you start the movement but the therapist completes it, taking the joint through its full range), or *active* (you do the entire movement without help). A physical therapist can give you specific exercises to do in and out of bed. You can use pillows appropriately to relieve pressure on the hips and tailbone, use a foot board and back-of-the-leg splints, and do certain exercises in bed several times a day. If necessary, he or she may use electric muscle stimulation, a painless method in which electrodes placed on the skin over the muscles stimulate them to contract.

Soft mattresses and even trying to make yourself more comfortable by using pillows under your knees or behind your neck may aggravate some of the side effects of prolonged bed rest or create other problems, including backaches. Keeping your knees bent for long periods in bed immobilizes leg muscles in a shortened position, further limiting your mobility.

When your normal activity is limited—particularly if you must stay in bed for long periods of time—a physical therapist can teach you and/or the person caring for you several techniques to maintain joint flexibility.

Pretreatment Counseling. Today cancer specialists can anticipate with some precision what lies ahead. For example, if you must have your larynx removed, you should be advised of the several kinds of artificial or aided speech available and talk to a specialist about which one might be most appropriate or easiest for you to use.

If you are having an arm or leg amputated, you need to know about *phantom limb pain.* Most people have heard of this sensation of feeling pain in the space where a missing limb should be, and many who face amputation are afraid it will happen to them. Phantom limb pain is indeed common, but in all but about 15 percent of people it soon goes away, and even those 15 percent can get relief.

Pretreatment counseling also can help those with head and neck cancer. For example, the teeth are particularly susceptible to damage from radiation therapy. The radiation alters the flow of saliva so that bacteria proliferate and contribute to tooth decay. A dental checkup before radiotherapy, with prophylactic treatment if time permits, can prevent cavities. Any essential tooth extractions should be done and allowed to heal before radiation therapy. A

Arm Rehabilitation After Mastectomy

TIPS & ADVICE

Lymphedema (swelling) of the arm on the side of the surgery is a potential complication after mastectomy that not only is inconvenient but can become painful and severely disabling; it can also make the arm more susceptible to infections, which can become quite serious. Preventive steps are based on avoiding excessive use of the arm and protecting the skin and circulation. To do this:

- wear canvas gloves when gardening and rubber gloves when washing dishes.
- use a thimble for sewing.
- keep sleeves loose.
- wash even the smallest break in the skin of the affected arm with soap and water and cover it with a bandage.
- use an electric razor if you shave your underarms.
- keep your arm elevated when sitting down.
- apply a moisturizing body cream several times a day, since dryness encourages skin breaks.
- call your doctor if your arm appears red or feels hot or swollen.
- try to do small tasks requiring manual dexterity, such as typing, sewing, and knitting, as they may hasten physical rehabilitation.

Don't do the following with the affected hand or arm:

- hold a cigarette.
- wear restrictive clothing, a wristwatch, or other jewelry.
- carry your purse or anything heavy.
- cut or pick at cuticles or hangnails.
- work around thorny plants or garden without gloves.
- reach into a hot oven.
- permit injections or vaccinations or blood to be drawn or blood pressure taken.
- get sunburned.
- avoid undue risk performing any task involving balance or depth perception, such as attempting to drive, before you have recovered completely.

program of preventive oral hygiene can maintain the health of the mouth and teeth and lessen the danger of bone damage. Fluoride treatments may help prevent decay and the sensitivity to hot, cold, and sweet foods that sometimes occurs.

Counseling before surgery also is necessary for those who are having part of a lung removed, since their breathing may be seriously compromised. Of course, quitting smoking is a primary goal. An uncomplicated recovery also depends on the ability to cough and expectorate fluid from the lungs. There are methods and exercises to help in learning to cough correctly, expand the remaining lung, and ensure complete filling of the lung with air. It's easier for people to learn breathing exercises before surgery, when they are not hindered by pain from the surgical incision. These techniques help keep the airway clear. Preoperative lessons in effective coughing facilitate drainage, allow sputum to be expelled from the lungs, and keep breathing passages open. Pain at the incision site can be eased with *hand splinting*, a way of holding the chest, and changing position to aid the draining of bronchial secretions.

Restorative Rehabilitation

Restorative rehabilitation is designed to compensate for changes in appearance and function that result from cancer or its treatment. Examples include reconstructive breast surgery, artificial limbs and joints, electronic aids to speech, and exercises to improve muscle strength and joint mobility. Plastic surgery or prostheses may improve or eliminate disfigurement.

Muscle Problems. Cancer or its treatment can directly affect your muscles. For example, in head and neck cancer, surgery sometimes unavoidably affects the nerve that controls the shoulder muscles, which in turn alter alignment and movement. If the nerve is severed, the shoulder will droop, become painful and weak, and be difficult or impossible to raise. Rehabilitation with both passive and active exercise can greatly improve some aspects of shoulder motion even if it cannot restore full function.

Prosthetic Limbs. Amputation of a limb is a major loss that produces a substantial change in mobility, affecting your ability to care for yourself and your independence. It also significantly changes appearance, which may hinder recovery, because of its impact on body image and self-esteem (see Chapter 29, "Body Image and Self-Esteem"). Fortunately, prosthetic design, limb care, and rehabilitation techniques have become quite advanced, and it now is possible to have a well-fitted, smoothly functioning artificial limb.

Appropriate surgical technique is essential, of course, so the rehabilitation team should confer with your medical and surgical team before the operation. The extent of the amputation will determine how much disability you will have and how complex and lengthy your rehabilitation will be. Almost everyone who loses a limb is fitted for an artificial one as soon as possible after surgery, allowing adequate time for stump healing and shrinkage. In some cases, the prosthesis must be molded before surgery. And if you are about to lose a leg, you may get instructions in walking or using crutches before your operation, when your balance is normal and pain doesn't interfere. This preoperative *gait training* will result in your being able to get around quite soon after the operation.

Occupational therapy and training in self-care and dexterity begin soon after an arm amputation. Proper conditioning, including exercises to maintain mobility of the joints near the amputation stump, is essential to using an upper-extremity prosthesis.

Our national enthusiasm for sports has led to some important benefits for amputees. Many have become athletes, and thousands now participate in organized competition. Their determination has helped stimulate research and experimentation to produce some important new devices and aids to activity, for example, energy-storing foot replacements that assist in "pushing off" and devices with specialized grasps for rods, reels, guns, rackets, and gymnastic equipment. The many specialized athletic groups for amputees also are an important source of psychological support and motivation.

Reconstruction. Breasts can be replaced by implants that move and feel like the body's own tissue. The implants may be synthetic—a silicone bag filled with a liquid material such as saline—or your own skin and fat may be used to create a new breast. The breast can be reconstructed at the time of the mastectomy or in a later operation. Because these decisions are complicated and many techniques are available, it's important to consult with at least one specialist—such as a plastic surgeon—before your cancer surgery.

For head and neck cancers, remarkable things can be done with surgery, implantable devices, and prostheses. Healthy tissue from the chest or other parts of the body can be used to repair even large facial defects. Bone "harvested" from the skull or hip can be sculpted to replenish surgically removed bone. Permanently implanted devices can be used to rebuild the nose, cheekbones, and forehead, and artificial material may be combined with grafted bone to make a new jaw.

If you need reconstructive surgery for any reason, a variety of specialists may confer with your surgeon before the operation to make sure the surgery will be done so as to enable the best possible restoration later. A prosthodontist may make impressions and casts so that any devices or repairs made later will fit, look natural, and feel comfortable. It's important to try to be patient during the restoration, though, since some of the procedures must be done in small steps over a period of time.

Supportive Rehabilitation

Regardless of the extent of your disability—even if it is quite severe—you will benefit from rehabilitation by gaining control of the ordinary activities of life, learning to deal with whatever you confront, and regaining at least some degree of independence. For example, people with cancer of the central nervous system that leaves them paralyzed and essentially dependent on others can learn to propel an electric wheelchair with a mouth wand, chin control, or breathing apparatus. There now are devices that let them talk on the telephone and control a television set, light switches, call buttons, and other equipment.

Indeed, techniques that promote self-care and mobility are almost unlimited. People who have lost the use of one hand or arm, for example, can learn one-handed techniques and use such aids as shoes with one-handed closures, Velcro fasteners instead of buttons, silverware for one-handed eating, bathtub or shower benches, and long-handled sponges and grabbers. Patients with paralysis, leg amputations, or other mobility difficulties can learn how to use various kinds of wheelchairs or to walk with a four-legged cane, even on stairs, ramps, and uneven ground. An important part of this learning is knowing safety limits, how to get out of trouble (for example, getting up after a fall), and when to ask for assistance.

Learning to Talk. One of the most dramatic forms of supportive rehabilitation is alternative forms of speech for those unable to talk because of brain tumors, tumors that compress the spinal cord, or removal of the larynx. If you have cancer of the larynx, for instance, you may be offered speech rehabilitation by *esophageal voice*, a voice prosthesis inserted through an opening in the throat, or an *electrolarynx*, a battery-powered tone generator.

To create an esophageal voice, you must learn how to force air into the esophagus, trap it there, and release it in a controlled manner. When done efficiently, this kind of speech sounds remarkably normal. But if you are one of the many who have trouble with it, you may be able to produce esophageal speech by using your fingers or a valve to manipulate air through a tube in your throat. Whether this is the best solution for you depends on your motivation, dexterity, and eyesight; your willingness and ability to maintain the necessary hygiene; and other factors, including cost.

The most commonly used speech aid is the electrolarynx, which conveys sound through the neck tissue into the oral cavity, where it resonates in ways that can be manipulated to produce words.

If you have had surgery that leaves your neck swollen or painful, an electrolarynx isn't feasible. Instead, you can generate the tone inside the oral cavity through a small catheter or tube. The sound is not as good as esophageal speech, but this method has the advantage of allowing speech training to begin almost immediately after surgery.

Even removal of part or all of the tongue does not necessarily result in a permanent loss of speech. People with some tongue left can learn to modify their usual ways of forming words. Those with none can use their lips, cheeks, soft palate, lower jaw, and floor of the mouth as substitutes. You should begin this kind of speech therapy as soon as the wounds have healed, beginning with learning to swallow properly. It may take intensive effort for as long as six to eight weeks, but it can lead to intelligible speech.

Living with an Ostomy. When treatment for intestinal or genitourinary cancer requires an ostomy, you have to confront not only the loss of your previous elimination function but drastically altered feelings about your body and your identity (see Chapter 29, "Body Image and Self-Esteem"). Supportive rehabilitation can address all these issues.

For many people the worst part of dealing with an ostomy is learning that they are going to need one. The best thing you can do for yourself at the very start is to talk to experts. No question should be left unasked or unanswered. A visit from a member of the Ostomy Association (see Appendix I, "Resources") can be informative and reassuring. For example, you will learn that at least half the people who have colostomies develop a regular pattern of evacuation so that they don't even need a collection device. You can also train yourself to evacuate on schedule by irrigating the intestinal tract through the stoma. Your diet needn't necessarily consist of an interminable list of restrictions but can include the foods you tolerate best, and in time you will know what foods to avoid to prevent gassiness. Many people find that not chewing gum, sucking candy, or smoking helps.

Rehabilitation with an ostomy has four important components.

- *Planning before surgery.* By becoming familiar with your emotional state, age, and willingness and ability to learn, your stoma therapist will be better equipped to help you adjust to an ostomy. He or she will tell you what to expect and introduce you to the available appliances.

- *Surgical techniques.* The surgeon and the ostomy therapist confer on the placement and shape of the ostomy, so that it will be well placed and constructed. That way the appliance will be easy to manage and not interfere with your clothing and movement, and your equipment costs will be lower than if these issues were not considered in advance.

- *After surgery.* The stoma therapist will help you choose a skin barrier and a pouch system, making certain that the supplies you need are readily available in your community or, if not, that they can be easily obtained from an alternative source. Wearing your own clothes while still in the hospital will help you get used to the appliance, reassure you that it is not noticeable to others, and make you feel more comfortable and normal.

- *Information and support.* Your stoma therapist and other health care professionals should give you all the information you need about how to take care of yourself at home. Home health care assistance is often available for those who need it. At the very least, you need advice on how to get help in your community. A good rehabilitation effort will motivate you and your family to maintain a positive attitude toward the stoma and its care. As others who have learned to live with a stoma point out, it helps to think of it not as something hateful but as something that allows you to live.

You should be able to go back to your job unless you have serious medical complications or your work requires heavy, prolonged lifting. You can expect few restrictions on travel, recreational activities, or sports—even swimming—as long as the appliance seal is waterproof.

One-on-One Assistance. Some people find it helpful to meet another person who has had the same kind of cancer and has been trained to counsel others on the emotional and practical aspects of their recovery. Several organizations make such services available, such as the American Cancer Society's Reach to Recovery program, whose volunteers have been treated for breast cancer.

The United Ostomy Association, which can provide a volunteer hospital visitor who is about your age and sex and has your kind of ostomy, holds meetings for an exchange of information, moral support, and a discussion of mutual problems. It also provides information and names of people to call for assistance (see Chapter 13, "Your Support Network," and Appendix I, "Resources").

Vocational Rehabilitation

Medical social workers, physical occupational therapists, and vocational counselors can help ease your transition back into the workforce. They can devise ways to adapt your job to the needs of your physical disability or teach you techniques to make you more efficient and productive. Work issues need to be addressed as early as possible in your rehabilitation. Preparing for your return to work also gives you a tangible goal and motivation for your overall rehabilitation effort.

It is very important to try to avoid feeling defeated by job setbacks or rejections. Negative images of yourself as a "has been" at work, fear of colleagues and employers, or thoughts about cancer's limiting the horizons of your working life aren't constructive. At least three-fourths of all cancer patients go back to work. Talking with other cancer survivors about their work experiences and how they surmounted particular difficulties is helpful. (See "Employment Issues" later.)

Palliative Rehabilitation

Many people with advanced cancer or metastatic disease can live and function well for some time even if they cannot be cured. Palliative rehabilitation is designed to provide comfort, emotional support, and assistance in day-to-day functioning.

In fact, palliative rehabilitation can transform lives, in ways ranging from the very simple and ordinary to the dramatic. On the simplest level, you can learn how to move from bed to chair or wheelchair without help, making the difference between being confined to bed and being able to have some independence. Modifying the home or work environment and learning to use tools adapted to specific disabilities can allow you to work and/or participate in leisure activities. All these efforts can cut down on the need for caretakers or the demands on family members.

More far-reaching steps include total joint replacements for people who are susceptible to fractures. The outcome is often additional months of being able to walk or move comfortably. For some people, a destroyed cervical vertebra can be replaced with an artificial one, providing comfort and preventing helplessness.

Pain relief is an important part of palliative rehabilitation, requiring careful choices by the members of your treatment team. They need to take into account the source of your pain, its quality, and its duration; what eases it and what makes it worse; and how it affects your life. It may be mild, moderate, or severe, and it may be relieved by nothing more than heat and aspirin or it may require medication. Like all other aspects of rehabilitation, this requires a customized approach (see Chapters 23, "The Pain Challenge," and 24, "Pain Relief").

Hospice care, which may be considered a part of palliative rehabilitation, has become a good option for those whose cancer is so far advanced that little more can be expected from therapy. Not everyone with advanced cancer needs hospice care, though, and some people don't want it. However, it should be available to all who do. An important advantage and a reason that so many seriously ill people prefer hospice care is that it can allow them to remain at home with their families, rather than in the hospital, to the last (see Chapter 34, "Supportive Care").

Spiritual solace, whether from a religious adviser or other source, is another vital aspect of palliative rehabilitation for many people. Organized religion became directly involved in cancer care almost 20 years ago when the American Cancer Society started offering educational programs for clergy and produced its first training film on pastoral care.

If you are a member of a nonreligious group with a significant spiritual component, such as Alcoholics Anonymous and/or other 12-step programs, it's helpful to stay involved and active, as these groups have proved to be a source of strength during major life crises.

Dealing with Costs

Private insurance policies and managed-care plans usually cover some but rarely all rehabilitation services. Medicare, Medicaid, Social Security disability payments, and Social Security supplementary service income may cover some rehabilitation care. Often people overlook or do not know how to find sources of financial help, so the most important action you can take is to get help in investigating every possibility. Social workers or the staff of your hospital or rehabilitation center can assess your situation and help you apply for various forms of coverage or reimbursement. A social worker may also be able to negotiate the rehabilitation fees for you. Others who have been in your situation may advise you how they got financial help. It is wise to start as early as possible, since the process of investigation, application, and getting assistance may be time-consuming.

Transportation may be a major part of your costs. People over the age of 65 may qualify for senior citizen services, and Medicaid may reimburse some of the costs of driving to and from your rehabilitation facility. The American Cancer Society (ACS) and other volunteer agencies provide some transportation assistance (see Appendix I, "Resources"). Check with any veterans' organizations to which you belong. If transportation to a distant facility is a burden, you might ask your physician if you could be referred to a closer center.

The American Cancer Society in some states contributes to the cost of such essentials as ostomy appliances. Self-care equipment may be provided by the ACS, the Visiting Nurse Association, and various community agencies.

Insurance policies, managed care plans, and government assistance vary widely in their coverage of restorative procedures that may be considered "cosmetic" rather than functional, no matter how obviously necessary they might seem (for example, breast reconstruction or prostheses). Some major medical insurance companies don't cover the cost of a surgical reconstruction but will pay for removable prostheses and bras. You should know beforehand what your coverage is before making decisions about any kind of rehabilitative surgery or procedure.

Employment Issues

In our society, work provides not only financial support but also a sense of identity and self-worth. People with cancer have the same rights as does anybody else to employment befitting their skills, training, and experience; they should not have to accept jobs they never would have considered before their illness; and hiring, promotion, and treatment in the workplace should depend entirely on ability and qualifications. In reality, however, cancer survivors face many employment and workplace discrimination issues for which outside assistance is necessary and available if you search hard for it. Begin by contacting your local chapter of the American Cancer Society (see Appendix I, "Resources").

People with cancer often face a less than ideal situation when they return to work or seek employment. They may feel "locked into" jobs they would like to leave but can't because they're afraid they will never be hired if they have to reveal their cancer on a new job application. Others continue to work at jobs that aren't satisfying or are physically too demanding, or they continue to work beyond a previously planned early retirement date because of financial need.

In addition, despite generally improved attitudes toward and understanding of cancer, some prejudices and wariness in the workplace remain, perhaps produced or exaggerated by competitiveness and economic pressures and fears.

Employers and coworkers may react out of a vague fear or uneasiness about cancer in the abstract, as some kind of lurking, unspecified danger. Many people are bothered by it as an unpleasant reminder of their own mortality. And some people just don't know what to say or how to treat you (see Chapter 31, "Coping Strategies").

Employers' attitudes have been hard to assess, but some may be afraid of lower production or financial losses because of your diminished capability or the occasional need to take time off from work for treatment. Despite these concerns, a Metropolitan Life survey shows that the absentee rate for people with cancer doesn't differ from that of other workers.

Current Legal Protection

Some people with job problems related to cancer are protected by federal legislation such as the Rehabilitation Act and the Americans with Disabilities Act. Nearly all states have laws pertaining to employing people with various illnesses, including some that are specifically aimed at cancer. Some court decisions have been helpful. For example, a ruling in California requires employers to provide reasonable accommodation for medical appointments, including long-term chemotherapy or radiation therapy And by federal law, your health insurance policy cannot be automatically canceled once you lose or leave your job (although of course you'll have to pay for it).

Although the vocational counselor on your rehabilitation team can help with some of your job-related legal questions, you may have to take some initiative in finding out what laws may affect you and how you can deal with any grievances. The American Cancer Society's National Services and Rehabilitation Committee has a work-study group on employment and insurance that provides reference and educational materials through its local divisions (see Appendix I, "Resources").

Vocational Counseling

You may not realize how much your feelings of security and self-worth depend on your being active, productive, and capable of taking care of yourself and others. A loss of self-esteem can be magnified by physical disability or the demands of recovery that make you dependent on family and friends for financial support.

It's vital to find ways of returning to productive work in some capacity. If you cannot return to your job, you may have to learn a new skill, go back to school, or establish a work-at-home career. Vocational counselors and others on the rehabilitation team can help match your skills with available jobs or assist you with job training if necessary.

C H A P T E R

BODY IMAGE AND SELF-ESTEEM

A diagnosis of cancer can feel like a betrayal of your body, inside and out. Especially if you have never been seriously ill before, it's as though the body you had always counted on is now unpredictable, out of control.

The illness and its treatment may result in physical changes that are obvious to everyone or just to you and those closest to you. They may be temporary, such as hair loss, or permanent, such as an amputation. Despite the nature of these changes, cancer draws inordinate attention to the body.

Early in the diagnostic and treatment stages, although most people worry more about survival and recovery, some keep their focus on how they look or how they feel about themselves. But two to six months later, after basic concerns have been addressed, the impact of physical changes and other inroads on self-esteem will have begun to take hold.

How you feel about those changes and how well you are able to incorporate them into your sense of who you are will color the quality of your life from now on.

It is not the specific physical alteration that is most important in coming to terms with your "new" body. Some people with truly devastating and obvious physical changes that result from cancer treatment are able to adjust in time and to maintain a good opinion of themselves. Others, who have had to sustain temporary or relatively minor alterations, may end up hating their bodies and have difficulty regaining their self-esteem.

Recognizing body-image problems and their relation to self-esteem generally, and understanding how to resolve them help men and women of all ages accept themselves during and after cancer treatment. This chapter addresses these concerns by focusing on the following questions:

- What is body image and how does cancer alter it?

- What is the relationship between body image and self-esteem?

- What are the signs of problems with body image and self-esteem?

- How can body image and self-esteem be strengthened?

- What can be done to improve your appearance while being treated for cancer or recovering from it?

- Who can help?

Body Image and Cancer

Body image has two major components: your feelings about how your body *looks* and about how it *functions*. Cancer and its treatment can drastically affect both and in turn can challenge your self-esteem—your entire sense of identity and value as a human being.

Appearance

The loss of a limb or other body part, hair loss, cracking and peeling skin, and facial disfigurement, among others, dramatically change appearance. In a society that emphasizes physical attractiveness, youth, and fitness, people who don't look "normal" can be stigmatized. When the alteration is to the face, which others study first when meeting and communicating with you, their reactions can be especially difficult.

Sometimes the permanent physical change is not so obvious to others— such as a small scar or the indelible marks left after radiation therapy—but serves as a lifelong reminder to you that cancer "invaded" your body.

Body Functioning

The need for an ostomy and alterations in sexual functioning are just two of the many ways that cancer treatment can affect the way the body works. A body that does not function the way it used to (and that you may not be able to take care of by yourself anymore) can be traumatizing and upsetting to your self-concept. Although physical changes may not be seen by strangers, coworkers, or friends, the judgment and reaction of more intimate friends and family is also an issue, since those who do see the altered parts are the very people whose acceptance matters most.

Common Reactions

It is not unusual to feel angry or outraged, depressed, anxious, or hostile toward health care professionals or family members, at least initially. Those to whom appearance is especially important will have a difficult time if their looks are altered, whether by illness or age. Since women are under greater cultural pressure to be attractive, they are more vulnerable to the emotional consequences of looking sick or different. Men may be somewhat more concerned about changes in the way their body functions.

People who fear they are being judged according to their altered appearance may well feel reluctant to leave the house or to interact with others. And although it is possible to conceal a mastectomy scar or ostomy bag, for example, it is common to feel extremely self-conscious, at least for a while, and to wonder whether observers can see the change.

The Process of Adjustment

Most people eventually come to terms with their new body image, but learning to accept the differences takes time and energy. Those who cannot handle the changes right away need to respect their own timetable and work on self-acceptance when the time is right for them. Most people successfully accept and integrate body changes in one to two years following treatment.

There are no predictable stages in coming to terms with such changes, however, because each person copes in a different way. For some people, any perceived defect in their physical appearance is embarrassing and shameful. Others may initially refuse to accept that anything has changed at all. Still others grieve and cry so much that they seem as if they'll never deal with it, yet they eventually are able to look on the bright side. For example, an athletic, fit, and extremely attractive woman in her 50s had disfiguring surgery on her face. For months she grieved over the loss of her looks. Finally, as she told her family, "Well, at least the surgery didn't make me fat. I couldn't deal with that."

As with the diagnosis of the cancer itself, the process of coming to terms with an altered body may include shock and dismay, denial, fear and anxiety, depression, and eventual acceptance. Ultimately, how you handle such body-image issues depends on your general coping skills, family dynamics, social support systems in place before the diagnosis, and the sum total of your self-esteem (see Chapter 31, "Coping Strategies"). These adjustment factors combine with the nature of the change itself—how much of your appearance and/or functioning is lost—and how diminished the alteration makes you feel.

People who are used to feeling good about themselves and who have a solid support network of family and friends generally do manage to incorporate these changes into a positive image of themselves. This doesn't mean that they don't struggle with difficult feelings, of course, or that they don't miss their former appearance or abilities.

People who have problems with self-esteem, a history of depression, and negative feelings about their body beyond the part affected by the illness, or who had no support systems or shaky relationships before treatment, are more likely to find the adjustment difficult. They have fewer resources in dealing with crisis generally. But it can be done, perhaps with professional guidance.

What Does That Part of Your Body *Really* Mean to You?

Chapter 31 ("Coping Strategies") will help you understand your usual style of coping with crisis and stress. In addition, it is helpful to think about the personal significance of the changed body part or function. For example, some women see their breasts as signifying their sexuality and/or motherhood, and so losing one or both may mean to them that they are "no longer women." Others, perhaps those who have already experienced a loss of bodily functions or aesthetics through illness or aging, may adapt to the surgery without damage to their identity as women.

Understanding the highly individual meaning of the change in what your body looks like or what it can no longer do will help you understand the degree of distress you are experiencing. Men with testicular cancer (which usually strikes young men), for example, commonly hear from well-meaning friends and relatives that they don't need that "extra" testicle, since they still have one that works. But having their manhood altered in any way may be devastating, despite their continued ability to function.

Building Up Other Components of Self-Esteem

Body image is only one component of self-esteem. What you do, what you value and believe in, and your relationships with other people are others. As this chapter explains, working to strengthen all these aspects of identity will help you weather not only challenges to your bodily self-image but also the many other ways that cancer can threaten self-esteem.

Although it may be difficult to believe if you are just beginning to face the crisis of cancer, coping with this disease offers an opportunity to gain self-esteem. After enduring the trauma of cancer treatment, many men, women, and children perceive their own strengths for the first time. They now have a new sense of what is and is not important in life and feel empowered by capabilities they never knew they had.

Body Image and Self-Esteem

Self-esteem can be seen as resting on a four-part foundation. The key to recovering from assaults on body image thus is to shore up all aspects of self-worth. The four selves are

- The *body self* (or body image): how your body looks and functions. In addition to specific physical appearance and functioning, the body self can be viewed more broadly. For example, some people emphasize how they look (models, performers), and others are more concerned with what their bodies do (machine operators, police, athletes, artists).

- The *interpersonal self*: how you respond to others (coworkers, friends, lovers, family members) and how they respond to you. Those who are happy with their family relationships, get along easily with others, and have people they can count on usually feel an important sense of connection.

- The *achieving self*: your goals and aspirations. How you perform at anything you do, from work to hobbies to providing for and taking care of your family, contributes to your achieving self.

- The *identification self*: your spiritual or ethical beliefs, values, and behaviors. People who gain strength from spiritual or ethical beliefs usually have a sense of meaning and a sense of fulfillment in their lives.

How Cancer Threatens Self-Esteem

Cancer and its treatment can disrupt self-esteem by undermining any or all of these selves in several ways:

- As discussed in the first part of this chapter, cancer affects your body self by altering your looks and your physical ability to function.

- The illness often disrupts important relationships. For example, the feeling that a mate, lover, child, friends, or a coworker is avoiding you because of your illness can shatter your sense of connection to others.

- A missed promotion at work because of time off for treatment, a role change at home, or the necessity of giving up a favorite sport because of a physical change can make you feel less of a person.

- Cancer can challenge your faith in the fairness of life. If you feel angry at God or at life for allowing such a terrible thing to happen, you may feel spiritually adrift.

Maintaining the Balance

To safeguard your self-esteem during cancer treatment, it is essential to maintain a balance among these four components of yourself, so that if one aspect of self-esteem is diminished, another will be enhanced. For example, when body image is under siege, you can concentrate on how important your friends or family are to you. If treatment has interrupted your work or other important activities, you can pay more attention to your loved ones, spiritual life, or other interests.

The following are two examples of ways in which people who lost a limb balanced their resources and regained their self-esteem:

- A teacher nearing retirement lost a leg to cancer. During his recovery, as two generations of students came forward to show their love and concern for him, he realized what a great teacher he had been. The more he thought about his professional competence and what he had yet to accomplish, the better he felt about himself, despite his difficulty dealing with his amputation. Although he was single, the realization of how important he was to others helped strengthen his faith in people and reassured him that life really had been good to him after all.

- A woman in her forties who had often said she "lived for tennis" lost her right arm, putting an end to her game. While recovering, she spent much more time around the house. At first she was extremely depressed by her amputation and inactivity. She felt she no longer had an outlet for her energy. Then, out of sheer boredom, she started cooking more adventurously than she had before. She found that having one arm did not limit her as much as she had thought it would, and her family was delighted

Charting Self-Esteem

INFORM
YOURSELF

Everybody has a characteristic way of relating in the world—as strong, smart, beautiful, caring, hardworking, and so on. Changes or losses of abilities, looks, roles, or independence resulting from cancer can alter your usual way of obtaining the self-enhancing feedback, or "strokes," that you've always counted on.

This chart can help you identify how you felt about yourself in the four self-esteem areas before cancer and how you feel about yourself now. If you discover that your self-worth before cancer rested heavily on one of the four components now being threatened, try to locate strengths in other aspects of yourself to which you can shift your attention. By recognizing your remaining strengths or where you can turn to renew your sources of self-esteem, you can have a weakened body image and yet still maintain a positive balance of self-esteem.

Circle how much good feeling you had about yourself both before your cancer and now in each of the four components, with 1 indicating very little and 5 quite a lot:

	Before					Now				
Body self	1	2	3	4	5	1	2	3	4	5
Interpersonal self	1	2	3	4	5	1	2	3	4	5
Achieving self	1	2	3	4	5	1	2	3	4	5
Identification self	1	2	3	4	5	1	2	3	4	5

Compare the Before and Now columns for each aspect of self-esteem and notice where there has been a change. Think about why you feel diminished in this area and whether you can do anything to improve the score. Suggestions for building up your feelings about yourself and enhancing your appearance are offered throughout this chapter.

with the food and her newfound culinary creativity. Spending more time with her teenagers helped her realize just how important she was to them, and they to her. Once she was fitted for a prosthesis, she became less self-conscious about her appearance. Jogging eventually replaced the tennis. When she ran her first marathon, she realized she had never in her life felt more vital.

Strengthening Your Body Image and Self-Esteem

The following are suggestions for preventing body-image problems and strengthening self-esteem and relationships with others, which may be challenged during cancer treatment.

Learn as much as you can about your body change and how to manage it. For example, learn to spot the early signs of infection or how to care for an ostomy. Information and knowledge enable most people to feel less frightened or intimidated by physical changes and restore their sense of control over their body and their life.

Begin to touch and look at the altered body site. This is the new you, and you'll need to get used to your new body as it is now. If you can't touch or look at it right away, don't worry about it. You may need to try many times to get comfortable with the change.

Work on becoming more comfortable showing your body to other people like health care professionals, a spouse, or significant other. When you feel comfortable and relaxed about how you look, the people around you generally will feel more comfortable too.

Restore your physical fitness, or start exercising for the first time. People who are committed to fitness as a way of life often have greater mastery over their bodies. As Chapter 27 ("Activity Counts") explains, trainers and physical therapists can devise fitness strategies for all levels of activity, even for the bedridden. Even if you cannot return to your previous activities, you'll appreciate what you still can do to restore your strength and muscle tone. It can also be helpful to focus on what your body can do, rather than on what it can't.

Shift your emphasis to another attractive part of your body. A woman with a mastectomy, for example, might decide to wear skirts or tights to draw attention to her nice legs.

Do something new and different. Another way of taking your mind off a changed body is to find a way to do something that makes you feel capable and valued. Take up golf or pottery, start a journal, do volunteer work—anything that makes you feel competent and worthwhile.

Shift your values. If you cannot continue your career or household responsibilities, turn your attention to something else (another kind of job, gardening, painting). A former carpenter might turn to wood carving, a former secretary might find a new joy in writing poetry, or a woman who can no longer do the physical cleaning for her family might become a fabulous cook. A one-time executive might turn to teaching.

Learn to value your body as a whole. Just because one part of your body has changed in some way does not make you an unattractive person. Wearing an ostomy bag, for example, does not mean you've become worthless. Even if others have a hard time at first looking at your surgically distorted face, this does not mean that you are no longer a sensuous, sexual, athletic, physically vital, interesting person—whatever is true for you.

To distract yourself and others from the problem, create a "healthy illusion." A man who has lost his hair during chemotherapy might have some fun with baseball caps or hats. Many women decide to wear wigs or scarves. (Not everyone feels the need to cover up a cancer-related alteration or to create the illusion of health, however, as we will discuss later in this chapter.)

Try to find some value in what has happened. This may take some real work and growth to accomplish, but a positive attitude can dramatically improve your quality of life. For example, instead of perceiving a stoma as unnatural or embarrassing, think of it as a way of having the freedom to go out in public and interact with others without having to worry about incontinence or frequent trips to the bathroom. If you have a reconstructed breast, instead of thinking of it as asymmetrical, tighter, or harder than your real one, think of it as a way of gaining new freedom in clothes.

In your relationships, how you look and control your own physical functions can affect even your closest ties to other people. In addition, changes to your body may threaten an already poor relationship with an intimate partner. To determine whether body-image problems are causing or contributing to relationship difficulties, see the box on page 359.

Talk about it. Open communication can help alleviate stress and clear up any misconceptions about what the cancer has and has not changed about you.

It is not unusual to discover that your partner is less upset about the changes than you imagined. A husband, for example, may be grateful his wife is alive and not be concerned at all about her mastectomy scar. Furthermore, he may be avoiding his wife not because he is turned off by her body but because he is afraid of causing pain when he hugs or makes love to her. But when partners are afraid of or repulsed by the changes, this is even more reason for them to talk and seek help if they cannot resolve it on their own. Frank discussion is equally important with children, whose fears about a parent need to be explored. (See Chapter 32, "Issues for Families and Friends.")

Look the best you can. Physical appearance can reveal not only how ill you are but also your attitude about yourself. Exercise or dieting can tone and firm your body and make you look healthier and more attractive to others and to yourself. A new hairstyle, clothes, jewelry, perfume or aftershave, although seemingly insignificant, suggest that you are interested in yourself and others again. (For more ideas, see "Appearance Tips" below.)

Start to value new activities with other people. If you can no longer do something you used to do with someone else because of a cancer-related change, put a value on sharing something else. If you can no longer go bowling with friends or ballroom dancing with a spouse, for example, finding other activities that are fun or meaningful is a good way to maintain the relationship. Volunteer with a friend at the senior center or in a literacy program. Take up cards or join a book discussion group—anything that keeps you enjoying your time together. This advice is equally valid for relationships with children and grandchildren.

Appearance Tips

Whether or not it is possible to restore your body to what it was before treatment, you can regain control over your appearance. Feeling attractive and that you look yourself again is important to both men and women as they resume their careers and day-to-day lives. For most people, feeling good about their appearance restores self-confidence and improves interactions with others.

Restoring appearance does not, however, necessarily mean hiding all the physical changes brought on by cancer treatment. Rather, it means expressing positive feelings about yourself through your appearance in whatever feels like "you."

The Option Not to Cover Up

There is a new freedom in today's more accepting social climate that gives women and men the option of being seen in public without covering up a hair loss or a disfigurement. For some people—such as women who choose to go without breast prostheses or reconstructive surgery and not to conform to societal expectations—the cancer experience even enables them to discover and demonstrate their acceptance of who they are. Art photographs of nude women without breasts that have been shown in some magazines and exhibitions prove that sensuality comes from within a person's whole body, not from one particular body part.

In addition, some people are refusing to hide their bald heads or create the illusion that no change has taken place. For some women with breast cancer, the decision is political: They want to call a disinterested public's attention to the desperate need for research to curb the disease.

If you feel more comfortable covering up, however, there are many options available, including the following.

Hair and Complexion

Even though treatment-related baldness is temporary, hair loss can be as devastating for men as it is for women. Although some people are proud of a bald head, others feel more comfortable and self-confident with a wig or some other covering.

If you choose to wear a wig, select one before you lose your hair so that the hairdresser or wig salon can match your color and style. Your local American Cancer Society may have a list of stores experienced in working with cancer patients. Since hair usually falls out in clumps rather abruptly during treatment, it's a good idea to have a wig available when you need it.

There are several other options besides wigs. Women can look appealing and attractive in stylish hats, turbans, or scarves; men can use baseball caps or hats.

Even for those who feel comfortable with no hair, be aware that family and friends may view the baldness as a constant reminder of your illness and feel more comfortable when you're covered up. Discuss it with them and then decide what to do.

Some people like to wear a wig or head covering during lovemaking, whereas others don't. Talk it over as a couple and decide on whatever makes you both comfortable.

An American Cancer Society program called "Look Good . . . Feel Better" teaches women who have undergone cancer treatment how to improve their appearance using cosmetics, wigs, turbans, and scarves. Pampering yourself can improve your attitude, so don't feel embarrassed or vain about attending such a group. For further information, contact your

Metamorphosis, by Judith Hooper

CASE HISTORIES

TRUE STORIES

About two or three weeks into chemotherapy, I began to wake up to a tangled wad of hair on my pillow. Hair fell into my plate as I ate. It fell on my clothes, on the floor, on my son's bed when I read him a bedtime story, prompting him to call, "Mommy, you forgot your hair!" It clogged the vacuum cleaner, filled the plastic, handle-tie garbage bags. When the part in my hair became an inch wide, I knew it was time to visit Audrey's Wigs.

Audrey was in her late 50s, I estimated, and sported a lemon-yellow cascade of hair resembling the hair on a doll I had as a little girl. She confided that the bulk of her clients were chemotherapy patients or country and western singers. I could tell that she disapproved of me, perhaps because I was not wearing makeup or perhaps because my head was too small for most of her wigs. She produced a longish light-brown wig with a shag cut. When I put it on, I looked like a failed cocktail-lounge act. "Do you have anything else?" I asked. Finally we settled on a short, curly wig that didn't look anything like me, but did look vaguely natural. I bought a couple of terry cloth turbans, too. I never wore the wig. I did wear the turbans day in and day out, often coordinating them with my outfits....

My chemotherapy ended in mid-January....By mid-February I had eyebrows and eyelashes, and my skin had returned to normal earthling color. I was even pleased to see tiny hairs appear on my arms and legs. During the late-turban–early-hair phase, which happened to coincide with late winter–early spring, I felt that I was a creature undergoing a profound metamorphosis. I was cocooning, molting, transforming. The new being that would emerge from this process, I visualized, would be beautiful, transcendent. Even while ignorant observers saw an unresplendent woman with sallow skin and an unbecoming hairstyle, I knew I was incubating my reborn self. About the time that blossoms and new pale-green leaves appeared on the trees, I was growing my new foliage.

local American Cancer Society, look for posters in your hospital or clinic, or call 800-395-LOOK (see also Appendix I, "Resources").

Clothing

Clothing says a lot about personality. It still is possible to be fashionable and look your usual self even if you've lost a body part or gained an appliance.

Although you may need to make some adjustments after cancer treatment, you can still dress to look your best. Catheters can be hidden beneath high-neck blouses or shirts or under long sleeves; pleated slacks can hide an ostomy; and breast forms can camouflage a mastectomy. Choose fabrics that are soft and flowing, and select styles that draw the eye away from the changed body part.

If you've lost or gained a lot of weight because of chemotherapy, buy a few new clothes that fit well. Loose or tight clothing draws attention.

Reconstructive Surgery

Reconstructive surgeries—such as breast reconstruction or plastic surgery to correct face or head deformities—are becoming more common and are no longer considered vain or purely cosmetic.

When considering reconstruction, you must decide for yourself whether the benefits of the surgery outweigh the risks. Although reconstructive surgery improves the quality of life for many people, many of these procedures are considered elective and thus may not be covered by insurance. Be sure to discuss this fully with your insurance company or health plan before you agree to any kind of surgery.

Many people feel reconstruction helps them feel whole again and happier about their body image. Some even find that they feel healthier.

Signs of Body-Image Problems

People who are having body-image problems often feel self-conscious, embarrassed, and/or inadequate. They may spend a disproportionate amount of time and energy feeling bitter about their bodies, leaving little time or inclination for more productive activities.

Other indications include no longer wanting to hug or be hugged and avoiding touching or looking at what's different. Switching to unflattering styles of clothing is often a giveaway that someone is struggling with a body-image problem. So is giving up exercising in front of others, for fear of being seen in revealing workout clothes or undressing in a locker room.

Avoiding discussing the body changes, continually displacing anger toward health care professionals or family members, refusing to talk about changes that must be distressing, and denying that anything unfortunate has happened are other signs of problems. (See Chapter 31, "Coping Strategies.")

Body-image difficulties are almost always revealed in sexual avoidance or outright problems with sexual functioning. Fear of rejection or abandonment can make people retreat from intimacy from fear that loved ones have the same negative reactions to their body that they do. Sexual difficulties resulting from cancer treatment, such as anxiety about erections or painful intercourse due to vaginal dryness, can also change people's image of themselves as sexual beings (see Chapter 30, "Sexuality," for a further discussion of sexuality and cancer).

Failing to accept a changed body can lead to problems that extend far beyond the bedroom. People who withdraw from others because of their appearance or because they are depressed about their looks have a substantially reduced quality of life, not because their looks have changed, but because they no longer have vital human companionship. These reactions can become life threatening for those who become so overwhelmed and depressed that they choose not to continue treatment.

Is a Poor Body Image Causing Relationship Problems?

- Do you feel self-conscious when your children, friends, or colleagues look at you or hug you?

- Do your children, friends, or colleagues feel self-conscious when they look at you or hug you?

- Are there subtle signs of negative changes in your relationships with others? Do you argue more or laugh less when you are together?

- Do you feel uncomfortable when your spouse or significant other touches, kisses, or fondles you?

- Does your partner feel uncomfortable when he or she touches, kisses, or fondles you?

- Are you spending less time with your spouse, children, friends, colleagues?

- Are you avoiding sex?

If you answered yes to two or more of these questions, you may wish to talk to someone who can help you to work through these concerns.

Where to Go for Help

When your self-esteem is low, it feels like everyone is staring at, criticizing, or judging you, which can make you feel isolated and alone just when you need other people the most.

People who also have cancer, or the same type of cancer, can often identify best with your problems and can offer the most practical advice, not to mention crucial companionship. Support groups give people with cancer a chance to see that their feelings are normal and shared by others. Exchanging information and ways of coping helps them regain their sense of control and gives them a more positive outlook toward life (see Chapter 13, "Your Support Network").

Several professional mental health resources are available to make the adjustment process smoother or to provide essential help for those who can't cope. An accredited cancer center can put you in touch with a sensitive, trained counselor with expertise in the issues that cancer survivors face.

Body Image and Self-Esteem in the Hospital

Almost everyone would agree that staying in a hospital can be a dehumanizing experience. You can't wear any underwear, and you have to wear dreadful gowns that never tie right in the back. Strangers keep coming in and out of the room to poke and prod your naked body and to discuss private bodily functions. There is a lack of personalization and a lack of sensitivity. You feel more like a piece of meat than a human being.

What to do? Make your part of the hospital room your own personal environment. Bring in things from home that make you feel happy—your own night clothes (if appropriate and allowed), framed photographs, your own pillow case and blanket (that can handle occasional spills), and a tape recorder with your favorite music or meditation tapes.

Establish a relationship with the hospital staff, so that they know your name and not just your room and bed number. Don't be afraid to ask questions of your doctors and nurses. You have a right to know what they're doing to you and why.

Set up visits and/or phone calls from people you love. The support of friends and family can make you feel better.

The aim is to bring you as an individual to the hospital with you, with as many loves, tastes, and quirks as you can fit into the room. In the hospital or at home, at work, anywhere, it's the sum total of who you are, not what you look like, that shines through.

Loving Yourself

You've just finished what is often several months of grueling cancer treatment. You know you should feel happy to be alive, but instead you feel unhappy about the way you look. There is no reason to feel guilty or vain about feeling that way. Your looks have changed, either temporarily or permanently, and you need to grieve for the loss of your old body image—and it may be an enormous loss—before you can accept the new one.

The most important thing you can do for yourself is to grow comfortable with your new body, with both how it looks and how it functions. You need to accept your body as it now is so that you can get on with your life.

One way to do that is to look at yourself in the mirror and become accustomed to your new body. Try it at first with your clothes on, and if you normally wear certain clothing or accessories to disguise the changes occurring from treatment, wear those too. Find at least three positive things about your looks that you like.

Now take off your clothes and face yourself in the mirror. How you look to yourself is more important than how you look (or think you look) to strangers. Examine your scar or appliance. Get used to touching it. Instead of seeing it as ugly, think of it as beautiful—without it, you wouldn't be here. Try considering it as a badge of courage. You had the strength to go through a difficult ordeal and come out the other side. You have every right to feel proud of the breast scar, stoma, lost limb, or new face.

Think about yourself as a whole person, not just a body part. Try to put things into perspective. You have changed, but you still have positive traits and personal attributes that you and others value. Indeed, you may find that the way you are handling the cancer experience has enhanced your personality and made you a better person. The people who truly loved and cared for you before your treatment still love and care for you now, maybe even more.

Whether to conceal a body change is up to you. You need to do whatever makes you feel comfortable. The most important thing is to feel good about yourself as a human being.

SEXUALITY

Sexuality is an important quality-of-life issue in surviving cancer, whether you are young or old, single or paired. Even during advanced illness, the physical expression of caring—a touch, a kiss—can help keep you feeling connected and loved.

Only recently have the effects of cancer on sexuality begun to receive the attention they deserve. It is now widely accepted that, directly or indirectly, cancer and its treatment can affect sexual desire, pleasure, and function in virtually everyone. Nonetheless, according to experts on sexual health, pleasurable feelings and sexual performance can continue in some way for almost everyone. Partners may have to change positions, habits, or notions about how sex "should" be or otherwise adapt to new ways of expressing caring in order to meet each other's need for intimacy.

Men and women with cancer need to deal with their feelings about their bodies and the effects of these changes on their self-esteem, which is the subject of Chapter 29, "Body Image and Self-Esteem." Open discussion about cancer and sexuality among those with cancer, their partners, and their treatment team is crucial. Equally important is getting an accurate diagnosis of any sexual problems that occur.

This chapter explores how cancer affects sexuality generally and then moves on to specific temporary or permanent effects of chemotherapy, radiation, hormone treatments, surgical procedures, and particular male or female cancers. Included too is advice on dealing with ostomies and laryngectomies in intimate situations; restarting and maintaining a sex life when you have cancer; and sex and the single person with cancer.

How Cancer Affects Sexuality

Sexual response depends on a finely tuned balance of physical and emotional factors. Your nerves, blood vessels, muscles, hormones, sex organs, and senses and the brain centers that control sexual response all must function harmoniously. Moreover, you must be able to clear your mind of other concerns (worries, fears, depression, pain, anger) in order to abandon yourself to sexual intimacy. Even in the best of circumstances—in a good relationship with a caring and attractive partner—smooth sexual functioning can be difficult to achieve. For people with cancer, then, for a host of physical and emotional reasons, it can seem impossible, at least temporarily.

The Sexual Response Cycle

Sexual functioning consists of a four-phase cycle consisting of desire, excitement, orgasm, and resolution. *Desire* is having an interest in sex; *excitement* is becoming physically aroused; *orgasm* is the climax; and *resolution* is the body's returning to its unexcited state. Desire and arousal—wanting to have sex and getting mentally and physically "turned on" by it—are the phases most often affected by cancer.

Physical Disruptions

Physically, cancer can disrupt sexual function directly through the disease process itself or, more commonly, through the side effects of treatments. For example, the cancer can damage the blood vessels, organs, glands, or nerves necessary for sexual arousal. Some surgical procedures cut nerves or remove the organs involved in sexual response. Chemotherapy and pelvic radiation can affect a variety of body systems, including hormone levels, vessels that carry blood to the genital areas, and nerves involved in sexual function. Hormone therapy may directly alter the balance of body chemicals necessary to achieve a smooth sexual response. Nausea, fatigue, or pain in the genital areas or in other parts of the body can dampen any interest in sex. Many drugs taken to counteract side effects or symptoms also can interfere with sexual desire or response.

Emotional and Psychological Factors

Psychological and emotional concerns are probably the most common causes of sexual problems in people with cancer. But this is good news, since sexual anxieties can be successfully treated if properly diagnosed.

Cancer produces no end of psychological stresses, or so it often seems. A diagnosis of cancer, for example, can be so emotionally overwhelming that sex is the last thing on your mind. Anxiety about sexual performance after treatment, worry about changing roles at home or at work, or fear of no longer being attractive to your partner all can diminish sexual interest. Depression is also a major contributing factor. One of the classic symptoms of depression is loss of interest in sex.

In addition to leaving physical scars, cancer treatment can alter body or self-image. A man who loses a testicle, a woman who loses a breast, or a person with a facial disfigurement might feel undesirable or embarrassed by the changes in his or her body, causing great reluctance to engage in sexual intimacy. As Chapter 29, "Body Image and Self-Esteem," explains more fully, a negative self-image or the fear of appearing unattractive because of a hair loss or weight changes can change your self-perception and how others see you.

Of course, partners are also powerfully affected by the cancer. They may feel frightened about initiating sex, perhaps for fear of causing pain, or they may find the changes in their loved one's body hard to accept, at least at first. In a troubled relationship, the cancer may worsen an already threatened intimacy. (See Chapter 32, "Issues for Families and Friends.") Or a partner's sadness over a loved one's illness may affect his or her own ability to respond sexually.

The Importance of Diagnosis

Many problems in sexual functioning after cancer can be improved with counseling or medical treatment. Interventions are keyed to an accurate diagnosis of the problem and its causes. Ideally, you should be able to discuss your sexual problems with a doctor, but in reality, not all professionals are comfortable with the subject or are aware of the impact of cancer on sexuality. And not all people have the courage to bring it up.

If you are having some of the problems discussed in this chapter, the suggestions here about dealing with them may be helpful. Just understanding what is causing the sexual difficulties may help you feel better about what is happening. But if difficulties persist and the members of your health care team can offer no solutions, take advantage of the specialists available to diagnose and treat the problem.

Effects of Chemotherapy on Sexuality

The side effects of chemotherapy, including upset stomach and weakness, reduce both the physical energy and the emotional desire for sex. But most people find their sexual desire returns after the side effects go away. It can be frustrating, though, that you may not feel in the mood until it's just about time for the next treatment. After completing the entire course of chemotherapy, however, sexual desire ordinarily returns.

For both men and women, the changes that chemotherapy temporarily causes in appearance can also interfere with feeling sexy or sexual. Not only is hair loss from the head and face upsetting, but it may be hard to get used to losing pubic hair or, for men, chest hair. Weight gain, weight loss, or extremely pale skin also commonly interfere with a person's sexual self-image, even if these side effects do not directly affect the ability to engage in intimate behavior.

For Men

Although there are only a few isolated reports of chemotherapy's permanently affecting erections, some chemotherapy drugs, such as cisplatin (Platinol) or vincristine (Oncovin), may interfere with the nerves that control erection. Most men continue to have normal erections during chemotherapy, although their desire may decrease temporarily, because of the side effects.

Some chemotherapy drugs, including vincristine, can also damage nerves controlling the emission of semen and produce what is known as a dry orgasm, that is, having the feeling of pleasure but no semen (retrograde ejaculation or complete failure of emission, as explained on page 375). This effect, however, is rare. Once in a while, chemotherapy dampens sexual desire and causes erection difficulties by slowing down the production of *testosterone*, a male hormone. The areas in the testicles that produce testosterone are not as easily damaged as those that make sperm cells, however. Some antinausea medications can also disrupt a man's hormonal balance, though it usually return to normal after treatments and medications to manage side effects have ended, restoring the man's desire and erections.

For Women

Although many women lose interest in sex because of the side effects of chemotherapy, understanding that the change is not permanent usually eases the concern.

Premature Menopause. For women of childbearing age, the critical issue affecting sexuality and reproductive capability is premature menopause brought on by chemotherapy drugs that temporarily compromise or permanently destroy the functioning of the ovaries. For example, most women over 35 years old who are treated with combination chemotherapy for breast cancer stop menstruating permanently. Those under 35 are more likely to recover their menstrual periods but may begin menopause sooner than they would have without the chemotherapy. How much the ovaries are damaged depends on the type of drugs used and the size of the doses. Therefore, women who wish to have children should discuss the possible effects of chemotherapy on their reproductive capacity with their doctors before undergoing treatment (see page 377, "Can Your Sexual and Reproductive Functioning Be Spared?").

When the ovaries stop functioning, they no longer produce the hormones *estrogen* and *progesterone*, which control the menstrual cycle. Women thus lose their ability to produce ripe eggs and become pregnant. Symptoms of premature menopause can appear quite suddenly and be more severe than those occurring with natural menopause, which takes place gradually over several years. Hot flashes, vaginal dryness, partial loss of the vagina's capacity to expand, and the absence of menstrual periods are the usual symptoms caused by a lack of estrogen. Vaginal dryness and loss of elasticity can make intercourse painful and are a chief cause of sexual difficulties for women who have undergone chemotherapy. It is not unusual to have a light spotting of blood after intercourse, because of small tears in the vaginal lining, which is not in itself serious but can be frightening if you do not expect it.

Finally, a lack of testosterone (a male hormone that is also present, albeit in lower levels, in women) can result in a loss of desire for sex (see page 373).

Women who have already gone through menopause may not notice so much change after chemotherapy, although those whose cancers are sensitive to estrogen (breast or endometrial cancers) may have to stop taking replace-

Premature Menopause: Some Solutions

Premature menopause can be caused by chemotherapy, radiation treatments to the pelvic area, or surgical removal of the ovaries. After what is often months of treatment, vaginal dryness and hot flashes may seem like the last thing you need, but don't despair. Understanding that these side effects are to be expected is the first step in planning how to cope with them.

Is estrogen replacement for you? Many women who enter menopause naturally decide to take replacement hormones (estrogen alone or in combination with progesterone) to ease the symptoms and to prevent the long-term risks of osteoporosis and heart disease. This may be an option for you, too—unless you have breast or uterine cancer, which are stimulated by these hormones. Most women treated for early-stage uterine cancer can take estrogen safely, but use at any time with breast cancer is much more controversial.

Vaginal Dryness

Vaginal dryness is the most common cause of sexual difficulties. It causes not only physical problems (pain during intercourse) but also emotional ones (you know the intercourse is going to hurt so you lose interest). Vaginal lubricants can sometimes provide enough extra lubrication to make intercourse comfortable. Apply the lubricant inside and around the vaginal area and on your partner's penis. Look for over-the-counter water-based gels rather than Vaseline or other oil-based lubricants that may contribute to yeast infections.

You do not need a prescription to buy vaginal lubricants. You can find them in a drugstore near the contraceptives or sanitary napkins. Some brand names to try are Lubrin, CondomMate suppositories, K-Y Jelly, Ortho Personal Lubricant, Surgilube, Today Personal Lubricant, and Astroglide.

For severe dryness, a vaginal moisturizer called Replens can be used several times a week to keep the vagina moist at all times. Since it is used on a regular basis and not just during intercourse, you don't have to stop in the middle of lovemaking to apply a lubricant. If you still have pain, continue using Replens, but try using a gel lubricant during intercourse.

Self-Help for Symptoms of Menopause

Many self-help books on menopause suggest that exercise, relaxation techniques such as meditation or yoga, and an increase in vitamins C, D, and E may help ease the symptoms. Relaxation techniques are detailed in Chapter 25, "Coping with Stress, Fear, Anxiety, and Depression." The most important thing is to talk to your doctor about any symptoms you may be having and then decide what treatment is right for you. If your doctor offers no solutions, ask for a referral to a specialist.

ment hormones. The lack of estrogen may then become more obvious.

There is much that can be done to make intercourse more comfortable following chemotherapy, as described on pages 368–69. For tips on coping with premature menopause, see "Premature Menopause: Some Solutions," on page 365.

The Risk of Pregnancy. Although many chemotherapy drugs interrupt the menstrual cycle, the ovaries do not necessarily fail totally. A woman therefore may occasionally ovulate and have a period even if she has not menstruated for several months. Thus, it still may be possible to get pregnant while undergoing chemotherapy. Since many chemotherapy drugs can damage the fetus, she should discuss methods of birth control with her doctor.

Infections. Since chemotherapy weakens the immune system, women undergoing chemotherapy are also more vulnerable to yeast infections. Symptoms such as vaginal itching, a whitish discharge, or a burning sensation during intercourse can make a woman less interested in sex. Yeast infections can be easily treated with medication.

For the same reason, genital herpes or warts can flare up if a woman had them before treatment. Any infection can become a problem, so it is important to contact a doctor as soon as symptoms appear. Some chemotherapy drugs can also cause a temporary, painful inflammation of the vaginal lining, just as they may irritate the mouth or other mucous membranes.

Chemotherapy for Bladder Cancer. For cancer of the bladder, chemotherapy drugs are sometimes placed directly into the bladder through a catheter in the urethra. Because the drugs do not circulate to the ovaries, the treatment does not cause menopause, but intercourse can be painful soon after treatment while the bladder and urethra are still irritated.

Effects of Radiation Therapy on Sexuality

Radiation therapy can cause fatigue and weakness toward the end of the course of treatment, leaving little or no energy for sexual activity. In addition, radiation that includes the pelvic area (e.g., that for prostate, bladder, colon, and cervical cancers) causes physical changes that result in sexual problems for both men and women.

For Men

Although radiation to the pelvic area is one of the most common causes of erection difficulties in men with cancer, it is important to know that the majority of men do not have permanent sexual problems after they undergo radiation.

Problems with Erections. The higher the dose of radiation is and the wider the pelvic area that is being treated, the greater the chance of developing this problem will be. Of those men who had good erections before the radiation, about one-quarter will develop permanent difficulties. Those most at risk, however, are men who already had a decline in erections as a result of inade-

Coping with Lost Erections

Erection problems can have either emotional and physical causes or a combination of both. Stress from the diagnosis or treatment, fear of not being able to get an erection or satisfy your partner, or side effects of cancer treatments all can cause problems with erection.

- The first step is get a proper diagnosis to determine whether the cause is medical or psychological. If you find your erection difficulties occur all the time in all situations, the problem is more likely to be medical and perhaps permanent. But if you sometimes awake with an erection, can stimulate your own penis, have an erection during sex with your partner, or get turned on unexpectedly, your problem is probably psychological and temporary.

- Erection problems do not make you less masculine, and you shouldn't feel embarrassed to seek help; sex therapy has been very successful in treating sexual problems caused by anxiety and stress. Even if the problem is medical, a sex therapist can explain things you might not even realize about your own body. For example, many men do not know they can still have an orgasm with a flaccid penis, with manual or oral caressing.

- If your problem is physical, several effective treatments can restore firm erections. Men can learn to inject several types of medications into the penis to make it firm. Although the erections feel and look natural, injection therapy can cause scarring inside the soft tissue of the penis. A less risky option is a plastic vacuum erection pump. A man places a cylinder over his penis and uses a hand- or battery-powered pump to produce a vacuum that draws blood into the penis and makes it firm. A medical doctor (urologist or family practitioner) can prescribe a vacuum erection device if you and your partner would like to try it.

- Although there are also some experimental surgical procedures to correct erection problems due to blockage of the arteries, only a small number of men have realized any long-term improvements. Far more successful are penile prostheses, or implants. The two most common types are a semirigid prosthesis that stays about 80 percent erect all the time or an inflatable penile prosthesis that gives a man the option of having his penis hard or soft, as he chooses. The implant is placed surgically inside the body.

- Be sure to discuss the benefits and risks of any medications, devices, or implants with your own doctor to find which is best. Each of these treatment options can provide firm erections, but none can restore sexual desire or improve skin sensation. Sexual counseling can help you cope with permanent changes in your ability to experience sexual pleasure.

- It's a good idea to include your partner in these talks, so that she or he can understand what's happening to you and how that affects your sex life together.

> • It's important to talk to your partner also about what's happening to your body and find new ways of giving you both pleasure. Sex therapy can help you both in this regard.

quate blood flow before radiation. Heavy smokers or men with high blood pressure are vulnerable, since their arteries may have already been damaged before the treatment.

Ejaculation Difficulties. After radiation to the prostate, some men find that the amount of semen they ejaculate has decreased to only a few drops. Since the urethra has been irritated during radiation, it is not unusual, toward the end of treatment, to feel a sharp pain during ejaculation. Although the semen may not return to previous levels, the pain will fade, and desire will return within several weeks after the treatment has been completed.

Loss of Desire. Once in a while, scattered radiation can affect a man's testicles, decreasing the amount of testosterone produced and resulting in temporary erection problems or a loss of desire. These problems usually improve within a few months, however, as hormone levels recover (see page 373, "Lost Sexual Desire: Is Androgen Replacement Therapy for You?").

For Women

Radiation to a woman's pelvic area affects all organs in the region (but not those outside the target area) and thus can influence her sex and reproductive life in several ways. Radiation can make the lining of the vagina thin and fragile. As a result, some women experience bleeding after intercourse. This is not unusual and can often be prevented by using extra lubricants and more gentle sexual stimulation.

Premature Menopause. Large doses of pelvic radiation stop the ovaries from functioning and cause the same menopause symptoms as do some chemotherapy drugs. Sometimes this effect is temporary, but often it is permanent. For a more complete discussion, see "Premature Menopause," page 364, and "Premature Menopause: Some Solutions," page 365.

Vaginal Irritation and Scarring. Radiation can also inflame or irritate the vagina. As it heals, scar tissue makes its walls less firm and elastic, and sex may become painful. In some cases, the scarring also shortens or narrows the vagina to the point that intercourse becomes impossible.

By using a vaginal dilator several times a week, you can prevent scar tissue from tightening the vagina. A vaginal dilator is a plastic or rubber tube a bit smaller than an erect penis. Available only by doctor's prescription, dilators stretch out the vagina, keeping it a normal size and making intercourse and gynecologic exams more comfortable. Some dilators come in sets of three or four of increasing size. A woman can start with a small dilator and progress to larger ones as she feels more relaxed.

Another way to stretch the vaginal walls is to have sexual intercourse several times a week. This option is not appropriate for all women, however. Women with cervical cancer, for example, may experience considerable bleeding after intercourse until the radiation shrinks the tumor, so frequent intercourse could cause anemia. Because scarring after radiation therapy is a slow process, many gynecologists recommend that to maintain a good vaginal size, women either use a dilator or have intercourse a total of two or three times weekly for the rest of their lives.

Pain from Ulceration. A less common complication is a radiation ulcer in the vagina that causes pain during sexual activity. Although the ulcer can take months to heal, it will eventually disappear.

Effects of Hormone Therapy on Sexuality

Some people with breast, prostate, or uterine cancer receive treatment with sex hormones; although they help treat the cancer, they generally alter sexual functioning in some way.

For Men

If prostate cancer has spread, it is necessary to block testosterone from nourishing the cancer cells, by either removing the testicles or taking hormones. For men, loss of desire is the principal effect of hormone therapy on sexuality. Most men also have trouble getting or keeping an erection or reaching an orgasm. Roughly 20 percent of men taking hormone therapy, usually those aged 65 or younger, stay sexually active after treatment. Experts believe that a motivation to stay sexually active makes a difference in how successfully a man functions during therapy.

For Women

Tamoxifen and progestins prevent cancer cells from using estrogen, which can stimulate certain types of breast and uterine cancer cells. Although these hormones are not as sexually damaging as chemotherapy, they can cause some menopausal symptoms, including hot flashes. Because tamoxifen actually acts like a weak form of estrogen on vaginal tissues, in menopausal women it can have the positive impact of increasing vaginal lubrication.

The hormones themselves can sometimes decrease sexual desire. Women with breast cancer are sometimes treated with *androgens* (so-called male hormones) when other hormone treatments no longer work. Androgen treatments can boost a woman's sexual desire (see page 373) but, in large doses, can also deepen her voice, cause acne, and increase facial hair. Although these virilizing effects can be upsetting, they are not usually severe enough to be very noticeable at the doses used for cancer treatment. It is helpful to keep in mind that the androgen is being given to control the cancer.

Coping with Specific Cancers and Procedures That Affect Female Sexuality and Fertility

INFORM

YOURSELF

| Female Sexual Problems Caused by Cancer Treatment |

Treatment	Low Sexual Desire	Less Vaginal Moisture	Reduced Vaginal Size	Painful Intercourse	Trouble Reaching Orgasm	Infertility
Chemotherapy	Sometimes	Often	Sometimes	Often	Rarely	Often†
Pelvic radiation therapy	Rarely	Often	Often	Often	Rarely	Often†
Radical hysterectomy	Rarely	Often*	Often	Rarely	Rarely	Always
Radical cystectomy	Rarely	Often*	Always	Sometimes	Rarely	Always
Abdominoperineal (A-P) resection	Rarely	Often*	Sometimes	Sometimes	Rarely	Sometimes
Total pelvic exenteration with vaginal reconstruction	Sometimes	Always	Sometimes	Sometimes	Sometimes	Always
Radical vulvectomy	Rarely	Never	Sometimes	Often	Sometimes	Never
Conization of the cervix	Never	Never	Never	Rarely	Never	Rarely
Oophorectomy (removal of one tube and ovary)	Rarely	Never*	Never*	Rarely	Never	Rarely
Oophorectomy (removal of both tubes and ovaries)	Rarely	Often*	Sometimes*	Sometimes*	Rarely	Always
Mastectomy or radiation to the breast	Rarely	Never	Never	Never	Rarely	Never
Anti-estrogen therapy for the breast or uterine cancer	Sometimes	Rarely	Rarely	Rarely	Rarely	Rarely†
Androgen therapy	Never	Never	Never	Never	Never	Uncertain†

* Vaginal dryness and size changes should not occur if one ovary is left in or if hormone replacement therapy is given.

† It is advisable to use birth control to avoid the possibility of pregnancy at this time.

Hysterectomy

A hysterectomy, removal of the uterus, does not change a woman's ability to feel sexual pleasure. Particularly for women of childbearing age, however, the operation can be emotionally difficult, since they no longer can have children. If both ovaries are also removed from a woman under 50, premature menopause will result (see page 365 for coping strategies).

Although several popular self-help books have suggested that a large percentage of women have problems becoming aroused or reaching orgasm after having a hysterectomy, no scientific data substantiate this. Women find that the area around the clitoris and the lining of the vagina remain as sensitive as they were before the surgery, even after a radical hysterectomy, which includes removing part of the upper vagina.

Coping Tips. Although the vagina is shortened during a radical hysterectomy, extra time spent on foreplay makes the most of the natural deepening of the vagina that occurs with sexual excitement. If the vagina still feels short, a woman can close her hands around the base of her partner's penis to give him the feeling of more depth during thrusting. Another method is to put lubricating gel on the tops of the woman's thighs and around the outer genitals and to squeeze the thighs together during intercourse.

Radical Cystectomy

A cystectomy, surgery to remove a cancerous bladder, may also remove up to half the front wall of the vagina. Although the clitoris remains intact, a surgeon must reconstruct the vagina to enable the woman to have intercourse again. One type of vaginal reconstruction makes the vagina narrower, and the other makes it shorter. Although both can result in painful intercourse initially, most women find that it becomes less uncomfortable over time.

It is important to discuss the advantages and disadvantages of both types of reconstruction with the doctor before the surgery. Recently, surgeons have begun to try to spare more of the vaginal tissue when they perform cystectomies.

Coping with Painful Intercourse. Pain during intercourse can be eased by using lubricants (page 365) or dilators (pages 368–69), taking prescribed replacement hormones (page 369), or using estrogen creams, if appropriate. Also try different intercourse positions to find the one that is most comfortable (page 380).

Most women do not realize that they are contributing to the pain by tensing the muscles around the vaginal entrance. The fear that penetration will hurt causes a reflex of muscle tension. These muscles are called the *pubococcygeal*, or *PC*, muscles. They form a ring around the outer third of the vagina, closest to the entrance. Fortunately, there are exercises you can practice that will help you learn to relax these muscles.

To become aware of your PC muscles, the next time that you urinate, notice the squeezing motion you use when you want to shut off the flow of urine. That squeeze tenses the PC muscles around your vaginal entrance. Next, try squeezing them when you are not urinating but just sitting or lying comfortably.

Practice squeezing or relaxing your PC muscles twice daily. Squeeze the PC muscles for a count of 3, and then relax them as much as you can. Do 10 squeezes in a row. It takes only a couple of minutes to do this (and you can do the exercise anywhere, since no one will know you're doing it). Regular practice will help you learn to feel the difference between tension and relaxation in your PC muscles.

Vulvectomy

A radical vulvectomy removes a woman's entire outer genital area, including the inner and outer lips and the clitoris. The sexual consequences can be considerable, as the vulva contributes greatly to a woman's sexual pleasure. Even though the outer third of the vagina, which remains intact, has numerous nerve endings, many women find they have trouble reaching an orgasm without the clitoris. Also, the scarring that results from the surgery can narrow the vaginal opening and make penetration difficult.

Some women may lose sexual interest because they fear that the changes in the appearance of the area around their genitals will disturb their partner, especially for those who enjoy oral sex. If the surgery included removal of lymph nodes in the groin, unsightly leg swelling can also be a continuing problem.

Coping Tips. In some cases, a surgeon can reconstruct the contours of the vulva. Vaginal dilators (pages 368–69) can be used to stretch the vaginal opening, or in severe cases, skin grafts can widen the entrance.

Increasingly, surgeons have been able to spare a woman's sexual functioning by removing only the tumor and adjoining tissue, rather than by performing such radical surgery.

Total Pelvic Exenteration

Removal of the pelvic organs—the uterus, ovaries, bladder, rectum, and vagina—is called total pelvic exenteration. This type of radical pelvic surgery can alter a woman's sexual pleasure and ability to achieve orgasm, even though the sensitive vulva may remain. The vagina must be completely reconstructed to make intercourse possible. The most widely accepted reconstruction procedure uses muscle and skin from the inner thigh to create a closed tube the same size and shape as the vagina. Since the nerves remain attached, the reconstructed vagina is sensitive to touch, but it does not become moist with arousal. Women may have to learn through experience to find intercourse erotic with a reconstructed vagina. Most women also have a colostomy and a urinary ostomy, unless they have internal reconstruction work.

Coping Tips. Even after total pelvic exenteration, it is possible, with determination and motivation, to return to sexual activity. A sex therapist can help. Because the outer genitals, including the clitoris, are usually not removed, some women find they can still feel pleasure and reach an orgasm when caressed in this area.

Mastectomy

Although the removal of one or both breasts, a mastectomy, does not directly influence a woman's ability to have sex, she may feel inhibited or lack interest in it if she is embarrassed by her body or afraid of turning off her partner. Women who enjoy stimulation of their breasts may have trouble enjoying caressing of the remaining breast. When both breasts are removed or reconstructed, women may need to shift their focus to other erotic zones to achieve sexual arousal.

A partial mastectomy may reduce nipple sensation, depending on the location and extent of surgery. A reconstructed breast and nipple do not have the same sensitivity to touch as the natural breast does, but women often find they develop more pleasurable feelings over time.

Coping Tips. If breast caressing becomes less pleasurable, couples can experiment to find other sensitive parts of the body. Spending more time on caressing the body and being creative with various kinds of touch can help. Some women feel more comfortable wearing a breast prosthesis and lingerie during sex. Others find the prosthesis awkward or feel no need to conceal their scar.

Lost Sexual Desire: Is Androgen Replacement for You?

INFORM YOURSELF

Androgens are the hormones believed to control sexual desire in both men and women. Testosterone is a common androgen, and although many people think of it as a male hormone, women's bodies also produce and use it, although in lesser quantities.

For Men

For men experiencing a loss of desire or erection problems, a blood test can determine whether your androgen production has been slowed because of radiation treatment or chemotherapy. If your testosterone level is truly below normal—which is rare—replacement therapy can be helpful in restoring sexual desire. An injection or patch is more effective than hormone pills.

Since a replacement testosterone dosage is designed to return the androgen level to normal and no higher, there are no known risks associated with it. Those men who have prostate cancer or a history of prostrate cancer, however, must avoid testosterone, since it can accelerate the growth of prostate cancer cells.

For Women

According to some experts, many women who go through menopause prematurely have an androgen deficiency and thus lose some desire for sex. A blood test can determine whether decreased androgen production is the problem. If it is, androgen replacement may be a possibility. You don't have to worry about the hormone's making you appear masculine. A small dose, about one-tenth that used to treat men, may boost sexual desire without causing any virilizing effects like lowering your voice or causing facial hair to grow.

Keep in mind that androgen only restores desire. It does not relieve other symptoms of menopause, such as vaginal dryness or loss of elasticity. There are some minor risks for women taking androgen. It can have a mildly negative impact on your cholesterol level and produce oily skin. It also is risky for women with some types of breast cancer to take androgens or any hormones that might make the cancer grow. The benefits and safety of androgen replacement are still somewhat controversial.

Coping with Specific Cancers and Procedures That Affect Male Sexuality and Fertility

INFORM
YOURSELF

Male Sexual Problems Caused by Cancer Treatment

Treatment	Low Sexual Desire	Erection Problems	Lack of Orgasm	Dry Orgasm	Weaker Orgasm	Infertility
Chemotherapy	Sometimes	Rarely	Rarely	Rarely	Rarely	Often
Pelvic radiation therapy	Rarely	Sometimes	Rarely	Rarely	Sometimes	Often
Retroperitoneal lymph node dissection	Rarely	Rarely	Rarely	Often	Sometimes	Often
Abdominoperineal (A-P) resection	Rarely	Often	Rarely	Often	Sometimes	Sometimes*
Radical prostatectomy	Rarely	Often	Rarely	Always	Sometimes	Always**
Radical cystectomy	Rarely	Often	Rarely	Always	Sometimes	Always**
Total pelvic exenteration	Rarely	Often	Rarely	Always	Sometimes	Always
Partial penectomy	Rarely	Rarely	Rarely	Never	Rarely	Never
Total penectomy	Rarely	Always	Sometimes	Never	Sometimes	Usually*
Orchiectomy (removal of one testicle)	Rarely	Rarely	Never	Never	Never	Rarely†
Orchiectomy (removal of both testicles)	Often	Often	Sometimes	Sometimes	Sometimes	Always
Hormone therapy for prostate cancer	Often	Often	Sometimes	Sometimes	Sometimes	Always

* Artificial insemination of a spouse with the man's own semen may be possible.

† Infertile only if remaining testicle is not normal.

** In vitro fertilization using sperm cells retrieved directly from the testicles may be possible, however.

Radical Pelvic Surgery

Radical pelvic surgeries can damage the nerves that control blood flow to the penis. When that happens, it is difficult for men either to achieve or to maintain an erection.

Some operations cause more erection problems than others do. For example, recovery of full erections after *total pelvic exenteration* (removal of the prostate, seminal vesicles, bladder, and rectum) is unheard of, but the surgery is so rare that no statistics are available. After removal of the bladder (*cystectomy*), at least 15 percent of men recover erections firm enough for vaginal intercourse. Erections are more likely to be recovered after *abdominoperineal (A-P) resection* (removal of the lower colon and rectum). In the past decade, nerve-sparing techniques have been developed for radical prostatectomy and are also sometimes used with radical cystectomy or A-P resection. After nerve-sparing prostatectomy, up to 50 percent of men may eventually recover usable erections. Sometimes these erections are not completely firm, however. Recovery often takes up to a year or even two to be as complete as possible.

Coping with Erection Difficulties. The recovery of erections varies from person to person and depends on the man's age, how good his erections were before surgery, and the extent of surgery necessary. In general, young men, especially those under 50 or 60, and men who had good erections before their cancer surgery are more likely to regain full erections than older men are. If a man had difficulties before the operation because of health problems or old age, he will most likely have problems after surgery.

See the boxes "Coping with Lost Erections," pages 367–68, and "Can Your Sexual and Reproductive Functioning Be Spared?," page 377, to determine whether nerve-sparing surgery may be possible for your type or stage of cancer.

Coping with Ejaculation Changes. Radical prostatectomy and radical cystectomy also result in a loss of semen production. Although orgasm occurs, nothing is emitted—a dry orgasm. Some men consider dry orgasms less satisfying, whereas others say they feel completely normal. Although men worry that their partners will miss the semen, most people can't tell the difference during intercourse and no pleasure is lost. The man will not be able to father children, however, although high-technology in vitro fertilization with sperm cells retrieved directly from the testicles may be possible.

An A-P resection for colon cancer also can cause a dry orgasm, but for a different reason. Sometimes *retrograde ejaculation* occurs. Because of surgery-related nerve damage, the valve between the bladder and urethra, which is normally tightly closed during emission, stays open. As a result, the semen goes backward into the bladder instead of out through the penis. Since the semen mixes with the urine, it is not unusual to have cloudy-looking urine after this type of ejaculation. If the man wants to have children, the sperm can sometimes be recovered from the urine and used to make a woman pregnant. Some medications may also restore normal ejaculation temporarily when attempting pregnancy. Retrograde ejaculation is not painful.

Sometimes the nerve damage is more severe, and there is no emission at all; the prostate and seminal vesicles are "paralyzed." Infertility treatments may still be useful, however, and orgasm remains pleasurable.

Testicular Surgery

The sexual and reproductive consequences of surgery for testicular cancer depend on whether one or both testicles are removed.

Coping with the Loss of One Testicle. Testicular cancer almost always affects only one testicle, and so only the abnormal one is removed. Since the remaining testicle compensates for the loss of testosterone and only one testicle is needed for normal hormonal levels, this surgery usually does not physically affect a man's sexual desire. A few men may have some abnormalities in the remaining testicle, however, and need to take a testosterone replacement.

Because one side of the sac looks empty, some men feel embarrassed in front of their partners or in the locker room. A testicular prosthesis, a silicone gel-filled sac that looks and feels like a testicle when implanted by a surgeon, used to be available to help a man feel better about the way he looks and restore his sexual self-confidence. The controversy surrounding the safety of silicone has forced its removal from the market. Ask your urologist whether there are any possibilities for you in the offing.

Coping with the Loss of Two Testicles. Both testicles are sometimes removed from those men whose prostate cancer has spread, to stop the production of testosterone that nourishes the cancer. In this case, the cords at the tops of the testicles are left so that the sacs do not look empty. Since the testicles produce most of a man's testosterone, this surgery can greatly reduce his sexual desire and ability to achieve and maintain erections. As explained in the box "Coping with Lost Erections," pages 367–68, all hope for a sex life is not lost for men who are motivated.

Coping with Lymph Node Dissections for Testicular Cancer (Retroperitoneal Lymphadenectomy). Men with testicular cancer often have surgery to remove the lymph nodes to which the cancer can spread. This surgery frequently damages the nerves that control emission, causing a dry orgasm. As with A-P resection, the problem may be due to retrograde ejaculation or to total paralysis of the emission phase. Again, orgasm is still pleasurable, and infertility treatment is often helpful.

Because men with testicular cancer usually are young and have not completed their families, surgeons may either try to avoid doing a lymph node dissection, or they may remove less tissue, making it more likely that crucial nerves will be spared.

Penectomy

If a man has a *partial penectomy*, which removes only the end of the penis, he can still have an erection, orgasm, and normal ejaculation. If a total penectomy is required, the entire penis is removed. Since the remaining tissues around the genitals still have nerve endings, a man can still experience erotic sensations when the scrotum, the skin behind the scrotum, or the area surrounding the surgical scars is caressed. He can have an orgasm and ejaculate through the opening created for his urinary tube (called a *perineal urethrostomy*).

Coping with the Change. Despite his loss, a motivated man can learn to reach orgasm through sexual fantasies, erotic pictures and stories, or sensitive touching around the scrotum. He can also please his partner in many ways without a penis, using his fingers, oral sex, or a vibrator.

Can Your Sexual and Reproductive Functioning Be Spared?

INFORM

YOURSELF

When faced with a cancer treatment that can damage your sexual or reproductive functioning, be assertive with your health care team in asking whether an alternative procedure is available. In general, radical procedures remove an entire organ. More localized procedures leave some of the organ or tissue and possibly more of its functioning intact.

You must weigh the importance of maintaining your full sexual and reproductive capability and intact appearance against the ability of the treatment to eliminate or control the cancer. You cannot have a good sex life if you are not alive and in reasonably good health, however!

Men can bank their sperm to be frozen and used later to father children. Researchers currently are developing the ability to freeze a woman's unfertilized eggs or ovarian tissue. At present only fertilized embryos, produced by *in vitro* fertilization, can be successfully frozen and thawed. Those men or women who wish to have children may be willing to postpone treatment to allow for sperm banking or *in vitro* (test-tube) fertilization, if that's an option, or to risk a less drastic procedure that may have a somewhat lower cure rate until they are able to have a family.

For Men

If you have been told you need radical surgery, ask your doctor whether you are a candidate for a procedure that spares the nerves responsible for erection or emission.

For Women

Preserving the breast through partial mastectomy or having breast reconstruction can help women with breast cancer feel more whole and attractive, even though most procedures decrease erotic breast sensation.

If you have vulvar cancer, ask your doctor whether you are a good candidate for a local excision that removes only the tumor and some of the surrounding tissue instead of the whole vulva. This type of surgery is less disfiguring, results in less scarring and less painful intercourse, and removes less sensitive tissue, so that sexual pleasure is preserved. Avoiding a groin node dissection also saves considerable discomfort and disfigurement.

For early-stage cervical cancer, a hysterectomy that leaves the ovaries intact is usually as effective as radiation therapy. Neither treatment can preserve a woman's fertility. Some studies indicate that women who undergo a hysterectomy have fewer sexual difficulties than do women who have radiation therapy, although they can no longer have children.

Cancer of the penis is most common in elderly men who may have already stopped having sex because of other health problems. Whether the amputation is partial or total, however, this operation can devastate a man's-self-image, so sexual or psychological counseling may be helpful.

Sex and Other Surgeries

Several surgical procedures may alter your body in ways that do not directly affect your ability to perform or respond sexually but that can cause embarrassment or physical awkwardness in intimate situations. For example, operations on the face can cause changes in appearance that are very hard for you and others to deal with. See Chapter 29, "Body Image and Self-Esteem," for information about coming to terms with body changes and restoring your good feelings about yourself as a person, which are necessary before sexual interest can be rekindled and intimate needs fulfilled.

Other types of surgery do necessitate some kinds of personal care before making love, however, for which specific advice follows.

Urostomy or Colostomy

Both a urostomy (removal of the tubes through which urine leaves the body) and a colostomy (removal of the colon) result in the often permanent need to wear an ostomy bag to collect urine and feces. Some people are comfortable making love with the ostomy bag exposed, but others like to cover it up. Either way, the bag should be emptied and sealed before lovemaking, to reduce the chance of leakage. If the bag does leak, jump in the shower together and try again. Some people use a pouch cover to make the bag look less medical. You can get urinary ostomy pouches made in a smaller size for short-term use during sexual activity. If you have had a colostomy, you may be able to irrigate and regulate your bowel movements so that you can wear a small stoma cap instead of a pouch. Women can wear sexy lingerie to cover the bag, and men can wear a T-shirt.

For some people, touching the ostomy can feel erotic. Too much rubbing or touching, however, can tear or irritate the stoma and should be avoided. Most people are more comfortable during sex if the partner's weight is off the ostomy. Sometimes a small pillow can be used to shift the partner's weight away from the appliance.

Laryngectomy

Since they can no longer breathe through their mouth following a laryngectomy, removal of the voice box, many people worry about how their partners will feel about kissing them. Embarrassment and worry about odors coming from the tube in their neck also can make people lose interest in sex.

Some people find wearing perfume or aftershave and avoiding spicy foods reduce the odors from the stoma. Most people like to wear a stoma cover in their neck during lovemaking. Since talking requires effort and can lessen some of the emotional overtones during lovemaking, communicating any needs and desires before intercourse or through touch while making love can help things go more smoothly.

Maintaining or Restoring Your Sex Life

For everyone, with or without cancer, keeping a sex life going depends on a lot more than the physical ability to perform sexually. But having cancer adds its own issues, which need to be understood and worked through by you and your partner.

How Do You Feel About Your Body?

The first order of business for many people is to restore their self-esteem and body image. Chapter 29 is devoted to this subject, of how to get comfortable with your body now that it has harbored cancer and/or changed in appearance. Many people find that once they get used to seeing themselves naked in a mirror, they can accept themselves as they are and feel more at ease in a sexual situation.

Sexual difficulties resulting from cancer treatment can, of course, jar your self-image. Fear of pain during intercourse or anxiety about erections can interfere with your sexual image of yourself. Learning what can be done to relieve the problems, communicating with your partner, and finding new ways of expressing love and intimacy all can help reassure you that you are still a vital, sexual person.

You may have come to the point that staying sexually active is not so important to you. You may not want to go through the pain or the ordeal involved. This does not mean you are less of a person or less loveable. Talking to your partner and understanding that you still have love and support are important to restoring your sense of wholeness and well-being. As long as you both feel comfortable about it, you can find other ways of staying intimate.

Talk!

Good communication is essential. Cancer puts a lot of strain on each partner in a relationship and on the relationship itself, whether it is of long standing or relatively new. There is much you will need to talk about—each other's fears, needs, anger, yearnings, anguish, and hopes. For example, many partners of people with cancer are afraid to initiate sexual contact for fear of causing pain. Their reluctance often comes across as cold and standoffish and can hurt the very sensitive feelings of the person with cancer. Open discussion can eliminate an unfounded concern or allow both of you to work out more comfortable ways of being close and giving pleasure.

Understand What You Can and Cannot Do

People with cancer and their partners often think that sex will make the cancer worse or make it recur. Some people avoid sex because they think the cancer is contagious. These myths, though common, are untrue. Talking honestly with a doctor or sex therapist can help couples gain a better understanding of what they can and cannot do before, during, and after treatment. The questions on page 381 can help you ask your doctor about the effects of your treatment on your sexuality and what, if any, activities you should avoid at particular phases of treatment.

Take It Easy

Don't expect to "pick up where you left off" sexually. Schedule private time together, and make it relaxed, romantic, and special. Start the lovemaking slowly by gently touching each other's bodies, and concentrate on the feelings of pleasure you are having. Many couples prefer to stay with caressing each other and building up the excitement over days or even weeks before resuming intercourse. And if intercourse is no longer possible or desired, you will have learned much about bringing pleasure to yourself and your partner.

Change Your Routine

Many couples have a favorite position for lovemaking or a routine for their sexual activity. Cancer treatment may cause changes that mean you need to find new ways to be comfortable and to please each other. The drawings below show several positions to try to help you resume intercourse after cancer treatment. There is no right or wrong way. Each couple needs to decide what is right for them.

If your movement is restricted or you are no longer comfortable in your usual ways of making love, experiment to find new positions.

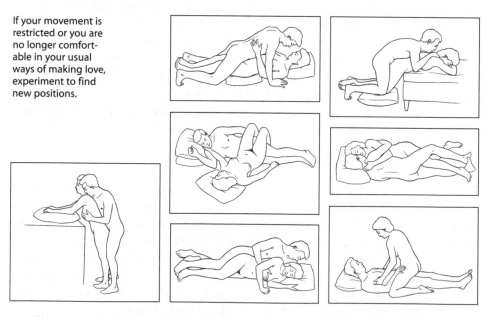

Keep in mind that it is possible to show physical affection and experience sexual pleasure in ways other than conventional intercourse. Intimate touching, for example, remains pleasurable regardless of the type of cancer treatment. Women with vaginal dryness and men with erection problems can still reach orgasm through touching.

Sexual intercourse or physical pleasure is not at the top of everyone's agenda, however. Nonsexual touching—hugging, cuddling, or holding hands—is equally important and keeps couples feeling intimate with each other.

Sex and the Single Person

It is not unusual for single people to worry about being rejected by a future lover or mate because of the cancer. How your partner will react to any changes in body appearance is one concern. Equally important are the anxieties that can keep a single person who has had cancer from committing to a relationship afterward. Fear of not being able to have children because of possible infertility, fear of not living to see their children grow up, or fear of becoming a burden to a future spouse makes single people afraid of drawing someone they love into an uncertain future.

It is important to have honest and open communication with any future lover or mate, but finding a good time to discuss mastectomy scars, an ostomy bag, or a sexual problem can be difficult while dating. Bringing up these concerns too soon may scare the person away. But waiting too long may make the other person feel untrusted or duped. Most people find it is best to wait until a sense of trust has developed and they feel liked and accepted (see also Chapter 31, page 395, "Single with Cancer").

QUESTIONS
TO ASK

Questions to Ask About the Effects of Treatments on Sex

Health care providers seldom bring up the topic of sex. Sometimes they are too busy; sometimes they are too uncomfortable or embarrassed to bring it up. You, however, should try to fight whatever embarrassment you feel and talk to your doctor about sex. The more you know about what sexual changes to expect, the better you can cope with what happens. Everyone has the right to know about his or her own sexual health.

Here are some questions to ask your doctor:

- How will this treatment (surgery, chemotherapy, radiation) affect my desire for sex?
- How will this treatment affect my ability to feel pleasure when my genital areas are touched?
- How will this treatment affect my ability to reach an orgasm?
- Am I likely to have pain during sex as a result of this treatment?
- How will this treatment affect my ability to have an erection and ejaculate semen?
- Will this treatment make me menopausal or interfere with taking replacement estrogen after menopause?
- How will this treatment affect my ability to have children in the future?
- Will the effects be temporary or permanent?
- What will I look like? Can you show me pictures?
- Are any alternatives or options available to me?
- Is there any reason that I should not have sex while undergoing treatment?

Where to Go for Help

A proper diagnosis will determine whether sexual difficulties are caused by physical or emotional problems or both. If sexual problems continue after treatment has ended, it can be helpful to talk to a professional. Some people get referrals from their oncologist, gynecologist, urologist, family doctor, social worker, or nurse. Here are other options to try:

- *A sexual rehabilitation program in a cancer center.* This option may be available only for those treated at that center. Ask the social services department in the hospital in which you were treated whether such a program is available there, or for a referral to another one.

- *Sexual dysfunction clinics.* Some medical schools and private practice groups run comprehensive clinics to diagnose and treat sexual problems. They vary in the range of services and health care specialists they offer.

- *Urologists.* Many of these specialists now have skills in treating erection problems.

- *Gynecologists.* A gynecologist with special expertise in treating pelvic pain or menopause may be available in your community.

- *Sex therapists.* Although most states have no laws regulating this field, a sex therapist should be a trained, certified mental health professional with additional training in sex therapy. A qualified sex therapist *never* suggests having sex with you or observing you having sex.

INFORM

YOURSELF

For Further Assistance

The following are some professional societies that give referrals. Ask for a therapist who is familiar with the sexual difficulties caused by cancer and its treatment.

- American Association of Sex Educators, Counselors, and Therapists (AASECT), 435 North Michigan Avenue, Suite 1717, Chicago, IL 60611-4067; tel. 312-644-0828.

- Society for the Scientific Study of Sex, P.O. Box 208, Mount Vernon, IA 52314; tel. 319-895-8407.

- Society for Sex Therapy and Research (SSTAR), c/o Blanche Freund, Ph.D., Secretary, 316 Poinciana Island Drive, North Miami Beach, FL 33160-4531 (mail inquiries only).

- Marital therapists or other mental health professionals. Frequently the source of a sexual problem after the onset of cancer is in the relationship. It can help to work on these and other personal issues that may be interfering. Remember too that any problems you had before probably will continue or even grow worse under the added pressure of illness. Sex therapists frequently also specialize in marital counseling.

- A support group of others with cancer or of people with your type of cancer. Confide in others who have been through the same experience and seek their practical advice. (See Chapter 13, "Your Support Network.")

COPING STRATEGIES

Not so many years ago, coping with cancer meant preparing for the end. Nowadays, most men, women, and children who have cancer also have a future. For them as well as for their families, coping means learning to maintain the highest quality of life with a chronic illness. And that means preserving self-esteem and being able to find significance and pleasure in life, to be comfortable, and to enjoy important relationships in the face of the emotional and practical challenges of living with cancer, which can be enormous, sometimes overwhelming, from the start.

No two people, no two families, deal with the cancer experience in the same way. All come with their own history of handling crisis, threat, or challenge. Yet as more and more attention is paid to helping individuals and families cope with cancer, researchers report that most people *do* deal with it remarkably well, whether the cancer is severe and unremitting, is successfully cured, or becomes chronic. A number of people with cancer and those close to them even report that the experience helped them improve the quality of their lives. Through this experience, which they never wished upon themselves or their families, they were able to find new meaning in life, solidify relationships, and discover what is important and what is not.

Through the study of how individual people and their networks of family and friends confront the problems that cancer creates, much has been learned about styles of coping and how they help or hinder, which is the subject of this chapter and the next ("Issues for Families and Friends"). Together these two chapters provide help for people with cancer and those who are important to them, related or not, including children, to comprehend and bolster their own ways of dealing with the crisis and challenge of cancer. Both chapters also identify key coping issues and obstacles and provide advice for all concerned.

Factors in Coping

Coping refers to how a person or a family comes to terms with an illness, makes decisions and solves problems as they occur, and adapts to the changes in their lives while still feeling good about themselves. Those who cope well with cancer and those who cope poorly have very different experiences, even if they or their loved one has the identical type of cancer that progresses in the same way.

The following are a number of coping factors from which you can determine your style of dealing with cancer and its effects on your life. There is no "right" approach. However, you can decide whether some of the ways in which you are trying to manage are causing other problems or are simply not working.

Emotions

It is normal and appropriate to experience a range of difficult and mixed feelings throughout your illness and recovery, such as anxiety, anger, depression, guilt, worry, fear, and grief. Managing such distress is essential to successful coping so that you can proceed with treatment and recovery. For example, anyone who experiences continual, overwhelming distress after learning the diagnosis will be unable to focus on gathering the information or making critical decisions. Someone who feels unremitting rage (at the unfairness of it all, at God, at the terrible disruption of present opportunities and future plans) may blame doctors and treatment providers and refuse to follow medical advice or alienate those trying to help. Likewise, a woman or man who is so upset at losing hair because of chemotherapy may avoid the company of others, who could be an important distraction and source of support during the difficult weeks of treatment.

Such people, and indeed anyone with cancer, can benefit from learning emotional regulation or distress-tolerance skills, as well as techniques to manage anxiety, as detailed in Chapter 25, "Coping with Stress, Fear, Anxiety, and Depression." Cancer is a new kind of stress or series of stresses that most people aren't prepared for, and you may need to learn new ways of handling your emotions, thought processes, and behaviors. When the distress is overwhelming, counseling can be helpful (see Chapter 13, "Your Support Network").

Coping with emotions does *not* mean pretending that you're not upset when you are. Never feel that you must bottle up your feelings, be ashamed of them, or feel "positive" all the time (see "Hopefulness and a Positive Outlook," pages 385–86).

Flexibility

In general, those who cope well are flexible and so can adapt to uncertainty and change. For example, although no one wants to have an ostomy, the person who can grieve for the loss of the natural elimination function following surgery but then accept the change as a way of getting on with living will achieve a much higher quality of life than will someone who can't accept his or her altered body. By the same token, someone whose self-image is based on being the family breadwinner and who can't stand having a spouse or child assume this role during his or her illness will suffer far more distress than will someone who perceives that adapting to the changing circumstances is for the good of all.

Control

Having a sense of control over what happens to you and those you love makes a difficult experience easier to bear. Gathering information about the illness, choosing doctors and hospitals, participating in treatment decisions, and knowing what to expect can counteract feelings that you are at the mercy of others and of fate and that nothing can be done to improve the situation. Learning that you can control pain, symptoms, and side effects (see Chapter 25, "Coping with Stress, Fear, Anxiety, and Depression") can be extremely empowering.

It's possible to gather too much information, however, and to feel inundated with details and out of control. Also, coping by seeking information may work well during the diagnostic and treatment phases of illness but may be less effective for dealing with uncertainty after the treatment ends.

Similarly, staying in control of what is happening by being extremely vigilant about symptoms and side effects can become problematic during periods of remission or recovery for those who have become highly sensitive to every bodily sensation.

It is important to learn what you can control and what you cannot. People who are reluctant to let others take control of some matters or do things for them and/or who cannot tolerate the changes taking place in their bodies will suffer stress and anxiety just when they need to devote their energy to taking care of themselves. To compensate for feeling out of control, they may become overly domineering toward family, subordinates at work, and the health care staff, without even realizing it.

It is not necessary to feel that you must relentlessly gather information, ask question after question, and make all the decisions. Rather, you can gain control by making sure you have a treatment team that you can trust to recommend and provide the best care you need.

Hopefulness and a Positive Outlook

Hope has been called "probably the single most important factor needed for living with cancer." Hoping for the best possible outcome often motivates people to take good care of themselves and to follow medical advice. Men and women who are hopeful usually look on the bright side—to see the glass as half full rather than half empty. They therefore can find meaning in situations in which others would find less to live for. Because they believe that things will work out, they attempt to solve the problems that occur. And because they try, they accomplish more than those who don't make an effort.

People who can find something good or meaningful in even the most difficult experiences and who can concentrate on what they still have rather than on what they've lost often feel spiritually enriched, more involved in their daily lives, and more connected to others. They also report that living with cancer has made them better people, showed them who and what really matters, and helped them appreciate life more.

The ability to see something positive in most experiences can be learned. To kindle hope, look around your life and find the smallest things that are worth living for. Set short-term goals that you can achieve, such as attending a child's or grandchild's recital, being around people you care for, or doing something you enjoy during a comfortable hour.

Try to take one day at a time and "live in the now": Focus on what is meaningful and enjoyable in the present rather than on what you risk losing in the future. When you have a bad day, don't read more meaning into it than when you have a good day.

But beware of any coercion you may feel, from yourself or others, that you *must* feel positive and cheerful about what is happening to you or to force a coping style on yourself that just isn't you. Don't fake it. Keeping your true feelings inside and feeling guilty about them will make it much harder to cope with what's going on, to deal with other people honestly and intimately, and to get the help you need. Much of the pressure to be positive comes from the unfounded belief that emotions are what made you sick and what will prevent you from getting better.

Trying to keep a hopeful, positive attitude often lessens the impact of cancer on you and those close to you and may make it easier to solve problems. But it will not make a difference between illness and recovery. Similarly, less than perfect coping will not trigger a recurrence.

Feeling hopeless, powerless, and convinced that you have nothing to live for can be a sign of depression. As Chapter 25, "Coping with Stress, Fear, Anxiety, and Depression," points out, depression can be treated and hope restored even in gravely ill people. Although a fatalistic, resigned attitude cannot foster a fighting spirit or a high quality of life in the early stages of illness, such a coping style is the way some tolerate the approaching end of life.

Note that having a positive attitude is not the same as wishful thinking, which is simply pretending that something good is going to happen rather than doing something about it (see "Denial," page 387).

Fighting Spirit

People with a fighting spirit take on cancer as a battle to be won. At times they may be angry and hostile, just as warriors are, but they direct that energy into finding out everything they can about their illness and demanding their rights to have the best possible care and, of course, to be involved in decisions. They rush headlong toward every hurdle in their path. They believe that they have power over what happens to them and use all "weapons" at hand, including complementary and often nontraditional therapies (see Chapter 22, "Alternative and Complementary Therapies"). With their sense of entitlement, they are not necessarily "good" patients or easy to get along with—they don't passively agree to everything that happens to them, and they forcefully insist on what they want even if it's inconvenient—but they tend to get the best out of their health care system because they insist on it.

Even if you are not by nature a fighter, with your permission a friend or family member who is can accomplish as much on your behalf.

Problem Solving

There are many ways to approach the problems that cancer presents. At one extreme is the style of "taking the bull by the horns" and seeking information and opinions, evaluating the options, setting priorities, considering advantages and disadvantages, and ultimately making choices. If one way doesn't work, the people who employ this problem-solving style try another. Although not everyone can meet this ideal—particularly when feeling ill, anxious, isolated, or sapped of strength—attempting to confront problems as they occur, big ones and everyday ones, keeps them from getting out of hand (see "How to Make an Informed Decision," pages 388–89).

Good problem solvers attempt to reduce problems to a manageable size and solve the larger challenges one step at a time.

The other extreme—doing nothing and passively letting things happen—is rarely satisfying and usually creates more problems, which become harder to resolve.

It often is easier to take a team approach (see Chapter 11, "Getting Help for Cancer: Who, What, Where, and How"). Even if someone else is the information gatherer or decision maker, be sure to make clear your personal opinions and preferences or risk getting stuck with solutions that aren't suitable.

Of course, not all problems can be resolved. "Nevertheless," as one psychiatrist who has studied coping in cancer patients observed, "more problems are solved by awareness and acceptance than by disavowal, avoidance, and denial."

Denial

Denial—the ability to proceed as if you or a family member doesn't have cancer—can be either a helpful or a harmful coping style, depending on the behavior it produces. Denial is destructive when, for instance, a person with a lump or troubling symptoms delays going to a doctor because "there's nothing wrong with me." People who exhibit this kind of *maladaptive* denial don't show up for treatment, don't seek or retain information that they need to know, don't ask questions, don't make necessary plans for themselves or others for whom they are responsible, and sometimes don't experience the emotions that are appropriate to their situation.

Family members or friends who are in denial don't visit or pretend everything is just fine when they do, don't listen, don't provide needed help, and thus strain the relationship. They are in denial because the reality is too terrifying for them to confront.

But the ability to keep the frightening truth at some distance can also be beneficial, as long as you do what needs to be done. Minimizing the seriousness of your diagnosis can provide time for the reality to sink in while you seek second opinions and settle on a treatment plan. Making plans for the future, even if others think they're unrealistic, can be motivating and interesting, as long as you don't set yourself up to fail (see "Coping with

How to Make an Informed Decision

When there's a lot on your mind, it's hard to focus on one problem at a time. It often helps to write things down. Use the following chart to organize your thoughts and to help you take the necessary steps to reach a decision. Write your responses on a separate piece of paper.

1. What are the problems I need to resolve now? (List all that come to mind, in any order.)

2. How important are these problems? (To set priorities, number each item on your list, from most important to least important right now.)

3. Beginning with my highest-priority problem, what are all the alternative solutions I can think of? (List all that come to mind, in any order.)

4. Do I need more information about any of them or about other possible solutions?

If you answered yes to these questions, what can you do or who can you ask to find out more?

5. What are the advantages and disadvantages of each alternative I have thought of? (List all that apply.)

	Advantages	Disadvantages
Solution 1		
Solution 2		

	Advantages	Disadvantages
Solution 3		

6. Considering all the advantages and disadvantages, which option seems to make most sense?

7. Whose help or contribution do I need in order to implement this choice?

8. What do I need to do now to get it going?

9. When will I take the first step? (Set a realistic schedule.)

10. I still can't seem to make up my mind or take action. What's bothering me? (Write down everything that comes to mind. Then relax and try again when you're ready.)

Repeat steps 3 through 10 for every problem on your list, in order of importance.

Disappointment and Frustration," page 392). Going about your life at home or at work as if you or someone close to you doesn't have cancer or as if it's not serious can minimize your fear and anxiety and contribute to a high quality of life. But make sure you do what needs to be done to solve the real-life problems that, denial or no denial, won't go away.

People with cancer as well as their family members need to be aware, however, that the desire to play down the seriousness of the illness may prevent others from providing emotional or practical support. But if overzealous hospital staff, among others, insist to you or your family that you *must* face up to the full reality of your illness and its course, tell them to mind their own business! In the past, staff tended to encourage not telling the truth to the patient. Now the pendulum may have swung too much in the other direction. Each person should be allowed to deal with "the truth" in his or her own way.

Support

Seeking the support, assistance, and companionship of other people is the sine qua non (without which nothing) of coping with cancer. Can you open up to others, ask for help, share your concerns? Many people with cancer have no one close to them. Others would rather keep the diagnosis to themselves or

Forget Your Troubles?

Yes, when you can. Sure, there's plenty to worry about with cancer. But try not to dwell on what can't be changed. And by all means, permit yourself full enjoyment at those times when you're feeling okay. Have fun. Relish a good laugh. Reward yourself after each step you complete in your treatment. Compliment yourself and others for everyone's endurance, determination, strength, and caring. Celebrate birthdays, holidays, and anniversaries just as before.

Besides providing some relief from the concerns of cancer treatment and recovery, these moments of enjoyment and reward can energize you to get through difficult times.

be alone rather than endure uncaring or frightened reactions of others toward their illness (see "Stigma and Unfortunate Reactions from Other People," page 393). Even those who find that others rally around them when they or a family member is ill can benefit from self-help, group support, and professional assistance available for people with cancer. One of the principal advantages of support groups is help with coping (see Chapter 13, "Your Support Network").

Coping Challenges

Although the cancer experience is rarely the same for any two people, there are predictable critical periods that challenge everyone's emotional resources. Chapters throughout this book provide advice on coping with particular problems and issues. Here is an overview of what to expect. If at any time during your illness, your efforts at coping seem to fail, help is always available. You must be able to ask for it. The hospital's social workers, nurses, or chaplain are good people to start with.

Diagnosis

Diagnosis is, of course, a time of enormous shock for most people, except perhaps some who are quite old or have already been in compromised health for a long time. Despite their great emotional distress, all people need to absorb complicated information and make weighty decisions quickly, a task for which most of us, even in the best of health, would not feel equipped. The need for others' support is great, at a time when many people are hesitant to share the news or wish to retreat into themselves; joining a support group or talking with people who have been through this experience can be very helpful.

Treatment

When their treatment commences, many are faced with having to reorganize their family lives and work responsibilities and to deal with insurance and finances, all while preparing to deal with effects of surgery, radiation, chemotherapy, and or other treatments. Those who have a difficult time enduring the treatments, emotionally or physically, may be tempted not to continue and, instead, to "let nature take its course." Body image, self-esteem, sexuality, and intimate relationships may be sorely challenged, and many people feel at this stage that they will never be themselves again.

Coping with the side effects of even the most aggressive treatments is much easier for those who have explored in advance all the new developments in pain and symptom control that have become available in recent years. Some of these methods and technologies may even help prevent unnecessary discomfort and disability. But because they are relatively new, they may not be routinely offered to people who do not know about them and seek them out.

Resuming Normal Routines When Treatment Ends

Although a number of people are greatly relieved to have treatment behind them and to return to their regular lives as best they can, many experience a coping crisis at this time.

Emotional recovery takes longer than physical recovery, a fact that family members, friends and coworkers, and even health care providers may not appreciate. No longer in active treatment, many people feel abandoned by those who have been helping them fight their illness and with whom they were so closely involved for such a long time. "The idea that cancer survivors can resume where they left off is not consistent with the experience of the overwhelming majority of survivors. Instead, the illness often has created a major discontinuity in their lives that brings about lasting changes in which they perceive themselves and their future," one expert in the psychological challenges of cancer acknowledges.*

Cancer survivors feel different even if they appear the same, and they're extremely vulnerable. And everyone who has been treated for cancer fears a recurrence, an anxiety that can become a preoccupation.

People with disabilities resulting from the illness or its treatment are faced with trying to build a new self-image, set new goals, and cope with the difficult practical realities of the impairment. Even without obvious disabilities, however, they may fear the impact of their medical history on their employment, relationships in existing social networks, and certainly with new people who come into their lives. In addition, reestablishing emotional and physical intimacy can be difficult and frightening. As throughout the cancer experience, contact with people who have been through this stage themselves and who understand the anxiety can be very helpful.

Recurrence and Relapse

The return of your cancer produces the same shock and distress of the initial diagnosis, but now the faith that you can win this battle may collapse—even though this is not necessarily the medical reality. Some people blame themselves, as if they could have prevented it with a different sort of behavior or attitude. Even for those who coped well with the initial round of treatment,

---

* Grace Christ, "Psychosocial Tasks Throughout the Cancer Experience." In *Oncology Social Work*, Naomi M. Stearns et al., eds. (Atlanta: The American Cancer Society, 1993), p. 87.

Coping with Disappointment and Frustration

Most disappointment and frustration evolve from unmet expectations. What you hope for is up to you. But if your emotional state depends entirely on test results and physicians' statements, you probably have forgotten your own internal resources.

If you spend all your time worrying about the worst possible outcomes of tests or treatments, you will sap your energy, deplete your strength for dealing with whatever the results may be, and waste precious time that you could use for fun or productivity. And worry won't change the outcome.

You must believe in yourself so that even if things don't go well, you can survive those times with your spirit alive, ready for the next challenge.

Warning Signs

- You are constantly looking into the future, to the total exclusion of the present. (Or conversely, you completely block out anything to do with the future because you might be disappointed.)

- You keep pretending that everything will be all right, when inside you feel just the opposite.

- You avoid positive feelings because you fear being let down.

- You are setting unrealistic goals and then sinking emotionally because you are unable to meet them.

- You feel that only a physical change will make you feel better emotionally.

having to go through it all again, perhaps even more aggressively, can be discouraging. And whatever success you may have had at establishing new directions or taking up where you left off may now come to a halt.

In addition, all the practical problems of being in treatment return, and other people may not be so willing or available to help out this time around. They may be exhausted by their initial efforts or so frightened that they can't face you.

Those who enter clinical trials face still other coping challenges, not least of which is dealing with the uncertainty of a treatment that has not yet proved successful. For people who are involved in blind studies, in which neither they nor their doctor knows whether they are getting the research treatment, the standard therapy, or a placebo, not knowing can create anxiety. Discovering that they did not receive the intervention under study can be very disappointing, no matter how well they may have prepared for it in advance.

Advancing Illness

Maintaining hope while undergoing intensifying treatments and their side effects is a major challenge, especially for those who lack information about the purpose and consequences of continuing treatment. For example, many people are confused between interventions that could cure their cancer and those that relieve symptoms.

Accepting that your life span is limited yet still has meaning is a fundamental coping task. You and your family may be afraid to talk about it and to make appropriate decisions; as a result you may feel distant from one another, frightened, and unprepared.

Pain and other unpleasant symptoms and physical limitations can leave you and your family feeling helpless and overwhelmed. Those people whose coping style is not assertive may not insist on receiving adequate relief, for which many approaches are available.

Information about options and financing for continuing care at this stage of illness is of prime importance. Support groups, social workers, oncology nurses, and the other sources of formal support listed in Chapter 11, "Getting Help for Cancer: Who, What, Where, and How," can be very important. Emotionally and spiritually, groups can help improve your quality of life, alleviate your anxiety and depression, and help maintain your feelings of self-worth and well-being, to which everyone is entitled at all stages of life.

Stigma and Unfortunate Reactions from Other People

Of all the coping challenges to prepare for when living the best you can with cancer, there's one that catches nearly everybody by surprise: the distancing, insensitive, hurtful, and sometimes rude reactions of other people. It seems inexplicable that at a time when you would expect your relatives, friends, neighbors, coworkers, and acquaintances to turn out in force, some never even call or visit. Others won't get too close to you; still others seem to blame you for your illness; and some who do visit are nervous and uncomfortable and won't mention your illness.

The best way to cope with such behavior and to protect your feelings is to understand that many people are afraid of cancer and of their own vulnerability. Hard as it may seem to comprehend, their reaction has little to do with you personally.

Cancer still carries a stigma in some people's minds, and so they may feel embarrassed or uncomfortable around you—or they may pick up on your own worries that you are no longer "socially acceptable." But beyond the stigma is the fear that many people have of their own mortality, which your illness or that of a family member triggers. Or they may be so afraid of their own pain in seeing you suffer or of losing you that they pretend you don't exist, deny that you're ill, or withdraw emotionally from you.

When, What, and Whom to Tell

Telling anyone, from new acquaintances to potential employers, that you have or have had cancer is fraught with risks, from ostracism to outright discrimination. Before telling anyone, however, examine your own feelings about the illness. If you feel down deep that you are "tainted" or unworthy because of your sickness, you will probably communicate these feelings to others and may influence their response.

Dealing with Other People's Reactions

"Get cancer and you'll find out who your friends really are," many people say who have been through it. Indeed, besides continually reminding yourself that others' unfortunate reactions are not a reflection on you, a good coping strategy is to let go of the people who disappoint you and turn toward those who come through for you. You may find that some of the most under-standing and helpful people are those who have had a serious illness them-selves and have no fear of reaching out to you. Support and self-help groups may be good ways of finding people—potential new friends, if you're open to it—who have had such an experience.

Joining such groups may indirectly improve your relationships with those close to you. At times, your family and friends may react insensitively simply because they are so stressed by the disruptions to their own daily lives that they may have limited tolerance for more difficult talk about cancer (see Chapter 32, "Issues for Family and Friends"). Your counterparts in the support group, however, share your intense need to analyze facts and feelings. Other coping strategies include the following:

- Educate others about cancer. Let them know it's not catching, for exam-ple, or a certain death sentence. Accurate information is always a good way to counteract fear and ignorance that fuel inappropriate responses.

- If the person is important to you, try to talk about your feelings of dis-appointment or letdown. Tell the person how he or she can help.

- Encourage others to be there in whatever small ways they can. Ask for something that this person is good at, like choosing interesting books or videos, helping you figure out a bank statement or insurance bill, fix-ing a leaky faucet, or just talking on the telephone.

- Talk about what it's like to have cancer. Some people may be avoiding you because they don't know what to ask or to say or are afraid to bring anything up that may be painful to you. Encourage them to ask ques-tions.

- Understand and forgive. Rather than expending precious energy in anger or hurt feelings, compassion for the person's fear or discomfort may make you feel better.

In Your Personal Life

It probably makes little sense not to tell your friends and family members that you have or have had cancer. Concealing it can be very stressful at a time when you need their emotional and practical support. How they react to you will be a test of your relationship, of course.

Sharing the information with casual or new acquaintances can be quite difficult, considering the stigma attached to the disease. Consider how the other person might interpret or respond to the information. Is his or her response likely to be hurtful or helpful?

Single with Cancer

Particularly among single people who want to go on about their lives as if they have been untouched by the disease, knowing what and when to tell people, including new romantic partners, can be especially difficult. Here's what Susan Nessim, cancer survivor and founder of the Cancervive support group, and coauthor Judith Ellis suggest in their book *Cancervive: The Challenge of Life After Cancer*:

T I P S &

A D V I C E

There is certainly nothing wrong with being forthright; it allows you to set the stage for an honest and sincere relationship. If this approach results in high attrition in your romantic life, however, you might rethink your tactics. It could be that you are using this "first strike" approach as a way of protecting yourself. Or perhaps you are using your history of cancer as a way of testing the other person. "I've had cancer; take me or leave me" is the message implicit in this approach. Try to determine what is motivating your need to tell potential partners of your illness.

On the other side of this issue are the survivors who have found that honesty is not the best policy—at least not on the first or second date. Experience has shown them that most people are threatened when confronted with the topic of cancer early on in a relationship. It could be that you are hitting your friend with too much too soon—before both of you have had a chance to establish bonds of affection and trust.

There is another advantage to waiting. If, somewhere down the road, the two of you part ways, you will have a better idea as to whether it was cancer or simply "bad chemistry" that caused the romance to sputter out. For many survivors, it is important to make this distinction. But that's hard to do if you have made a point of revealing your cancer early in the game.

The issue of disclosure is a personal one; only you can know if and when to share this part of who you are. Most survivors say it all comes down to sizing up the other person and then gauging whether the relationship has potential for longevity.

At Work

Although it may not be wise to volunteer a cancer history at a job interview—because employers may fear that you will not be productive or that you will increase their health insurance costs—always tell the truth if you are asked about your medical history. Provide a brief explanation of the illness and your recovery. Express confidence in your skills, outlook, and energy. Don't overexplain or the interviewer may think that you're trying to conceal something. Be aware that there are laws protecting people with cancer against illegal discrimination, and if you need assistance in understanding the laws in your state, your local chapter of the American Cancer Society can help (see also Chapter 28, "Managing Disabilities and Limitations").

Even if you have no problem getting or keeping a job, be prepared for ignorant and fearful attitudes of coworkers. Educating them about the illness and demonstrating how well you have come through it may help. If you have a new job, you may want to size up your coworkers before confiding in them, in the same way you would before revealing any personal information. If your company has a personnel office and your cancer history is already known, ask for their help to distribute information about cancer should you run into unpleasant reactions.

For your own sake, remember that most people at work know somebody with cancer, probably in their own families. In other words, you're not the only one on the planet with this disease. If you can talk about your history comfortably, you may well encourage their respect, and they may turn to you when they need information.

ISSUES FOR FAMILIES AND FRIENDS

Cancer affects everyone close to the person who becomes ill—the spouses, children, parents, friends, partners, and lovers who constitute the modern-day family. The sickness changes the individual and alters the family. Be prepared: The cumulative stresses will challenge even the best-functioning families or circle of friends. But, depending on how everyone responds, cancer can also bring them closer and provide a deepened appreciation of life and of one another.

This chapter explores the stress factors that are most predictable when there is cancer in the family, and it addresses all of you. It discusses how to cope and communicate. Finally, it explains the needs and reactions of children of parents with cancer and how to help them.

What to Expect

Coping crises for the family tend to mirror those for the individual (see Chapter 31, "Coping Strategies"), beginning with the shock of the diagnosis, the need to make life-altering decisions rapidly, and the extraordinary disruption to life of entering active treatment.

Not everyone reacts in the same way to the distress, of course, or adjusts on the same timetable. For example, the person with cancer may already have made peace with some loss of physical functioning while a spouse or child is still wishing that things were as before. And each person has his or her own concerns. The adult children of a cancer patient may struggle with their sometimes conflicting responsibilities toward their parents and their own children, for instance. Friends may be troubled by concerns about their own health or mortality. Spouses may feel overwhelmed by practical matters, not the least of them financial.

Although there is no one way of coping with cancer in the family that works for everyone, generally the adjustment is easier when all are involved from the start. Everyone, including children (as will be explained later in the chapter) should receive accurate information about the illness and its treatment. Being included in the information and education process and feeling that everyone has a role helps family members comprehend the physical and emotional challenges of the cancer experience, feel more in control, provide support where it counts, and make informed decisions on behalf of all.

Coping Styles

An important element in coping is understanding what to expect from the illness, the treatment, yourself, and everyone else. Everybody has his or her own coping style, and so thinking about how you usually function in a crisis, separately and together, can help forestall surprises.

Some family members, for example, deal with difficulty in their personal lives by throwing themselves into their jobs or hobbies, becoming less available to their families. Although this style may help them escape their distress, it can be misunderstood by others in the family as uncaring, and it may indeed prove inconvenient for those who have to fill in at home or at the hospital. Others, to manage their own anxiety, attempt to take control of all information gathering and decision making, thereby leaving the person with cancer with little voice.

In some families, crisis causes fighting and blaming. Some draw closer to one another, perhaps feeling more of a sense of purpose than when life returns to normal. Some reach out to others for support, whereas others draw in and away from the outside world.

Threats to a family often make everyone behave childishly. Even among grown siblings, old rivalries may surface and threaten the cooperation so necessary at this time. Groups in which everyone is very involved with and dependent on one another may feel more at a loss than do those whose members are more autonomous.

Predictable Dilemmas

Understanding how each family member copes with crisis may help you plan for cancer's predictable assaults on family life. Confusion, anger, frustration, anxiety, or depression can result from any or all of the following:

Role Changes. Almost invariably after a diagnosis of cancer, one or more people in the group has to take over the duties of the person who is ill. Over time, the new responsibilities, on top of what you usually have to do, can be a great burden, for adults and children alike.

The families that seem to adapt best have always been flexible about who does what. When both spouses have worked and shared household chores, by design or necessity they have probably had to learn how to fill in for one another. But in those families in which each member has had a specific, fixed role and the boundaries have rarely overlapped—such as those with the tradition that the man works and the woman keeps house—the adjustment is likely to be more difficult.

Burnout Alert

Caring for someone who is sick, taking over his or her responsibilities, having to change habits and routines, and worrying about what will happen results in fatigue at the very least. At the most, the combined pressures lead to resentment, guilt, exhaustion, depression, even physical illness, and an inability to continue to care for your loved one or friend. This stressed-out condition is sometimes called *burnout*.

Recognize the Signs

- You're exhausted all the time.
- You can't fall asleep, sleep through the night, or get up in the morning.
- You've pulled away from your friends and lost interest in the activities that used to bring pleasure.
- You feel guilty that you're not doing enough or that you don't want to do even more.
- You worry that you don't really care anymore for the person you're caring for.
- You are easily irritated by people who tell you that you should take care of yourself.
- You think the only relief you can get right now is from alcohol, drugs, food, or cigarettes.
- You don't feel well.
- You're sure that nothing good is ever going to happen again; you feel numb; and you don't care.

What to Do

Above all, you must recognize the importance of your own respite and resist feeling guilty for thinking of yourself.

You may need to learn to delegate some of the responsibilities that you think you "should" be doing yourself. Insist, if need be, that out-of-town family members provide their fair share of assistance.

Divide up responsibilities according to each person's strengths, interests, and personalities; some people are better at dealing with paperwork than providing a soothing presence at the bedside, for example. Some may be good at dealing with medical personnel and taking notes, and others can run errands or cook meals. Those who may be unable or unwilling to contribute time might help out financially.

Ask friends, neighbors, people in your church or synagogue, or others in your informal support network for whatever help they can provide (see Chapter 13, "Your Support Network"); people often are glad to be asked.

Recognize your limits and forgive yourself for not being perfect and for not being able to do more for your loved one than is humanly possible.

Practice stress reduction techniques, anything from taking a hot bath to getting some exercise to practicing the relaxation and meditation techniques described in detail in Chapter 25 ("Coping with Stress, Fear, Anxiety, and Depression").

Distract yourself. There's no reason to focus all your thoughts on your friend's or loved one's illness—in fact, there's every reason *not* to. Go out to dinner or the movies. Have a good laugh. Goof off. Play games. Go on a vacation, if only for a day. Remember that if you lighten up, you'll take better care of the person with cancer and make him or her feel less guilty. Sick people are often highly sensitive to the body language and unexpressed feelings of those taking care of them.

Recognize and deal with your depression. Problems with sleeping and eating, irritability, negativity, hopelessness, and loss of energy all are symptomatic of depression. Although these feelings and symptoms tend occur at times of intense distress, if they become your constant companions after the crisis is over, you need to address them for your own health and ability to function.

Shifting the balance of power can be trying too. Frequently, one person in the family is the decision maker or the one on whom everybody relies in a crisis. So when illness strikes this dominant individual, life can be chaotic while everybody tries to sort out who's "in charge." But it can ultimately bring a family closer when those who have been kept in the background are allowed to demonstrate their competence.

For most people, self-esteem is defined at least in part by the roles they fulfill in life. For the sick family member, giving up these roles, even for a short time, can be an enormous loss. It may be possible to exchange some responsibilities—trading the bill paying for the lawn mowing, for example—to enable the person with cancer to feel useful while taking some of the load off those who have been picking up the slack.

It helps to be able to call on others in the extended family or in the community to take over the additional responsibilities. Families that have always prided themselves on their complete self-sufficiency may find coping difficult unless they reach out. When asking for assistance, be specific about what you want and when you want it.

Disruption of Routines. Most people follow fixed routines in their daily lives, patterns that provide structure and predictability. But when cancer is diagnosed, these usual ways of doing things are thrown up in the air. Everyone has to accommodate the demands of the illness and the treatment schedule, yet at the same time, each person has daily responsibilities that may conflict with the needs of the person with cancer. Such disruptions are especially difficult for children, who often react to even minor changes in meal- and bedtimes and types of food and to who helps with homework and who takes them to school.

Never underestimate the amount of stress that results from the conflicts between daily needs of each family member and those of the person with cancer, and don't be surprised if at times someone is feeling angry, resentful, or guilty. A grown son may feel that he's being petty about wanting to get in a golf game rather than going to the hospital. Likewise, a wife may feel guilty for wishing to attend a luncheon rather than be home taking care of her husband. But the desire to relax and enjoy yourself is understandable. Indeed, finding some way to schedule "time off" from a loved one's illness may be essential to avoid burnout.

Future Plans. Every family has dreams and hopes at every stage of life. Perhaps one of the most difficult coping challenges, therefore, is accepting a future that has suddenly become unpredictable, in which all that you've worked for or dreamed about may not come true, at least not in the way you had hoped or within the time frame you had set. Rather than concentrate on what hopes may be lost, try to manage for the time being by setting new short-term goals and making plans for now that you know you can complete. You can continue to add steps to the plan as the course of the illness and the potential for recovery become clearer.

An illness that threatens your ability to pursue important personal goals—such as new career responsibilities, a young adult's planned move away from home, retirement plans—tests the strength of marriage and family bonds. To resolve this potential crisis, try to avoid all-or-nothing solutions, such as forfeiting plans forever. There may be a way to negotiate a temporary compromise among all those whose needs conflict. For example, a child who was about to go away to college and who is now needed at home, or whose family needs the tuition money for expenses, may be able to postpone admission and enroll for one year in a local, less expensive community college.

These conflicts can produce difficult, mixed feelings of guilt and anger. Here you're supposed to be fully supportive of the person who's ill, and all you can do is think of yourself. But you've got important needs of your own, right? At times like these, outside perspectives, from a support group or religious or psychological counselor, can be a great relief.

Relationship Conflicts. Couples, family members, and friends who have forgotten how much they mean to one another may well be brought closer by the experience of cancer. But it can also be the straw that breaks the camel's back: Relationships that were deeply troubled to begin with may not survive. Conflicts and problems that existed before the illness could get worse.

Much depends on your individual and collective style of functioning. Stress can bring out the best or worst in people, usually both. Similarly, it reveals the strengths and vulnerabilities in any relationship.

Loss of Physical Intimacy. For everyone in the network of family and friends, maintaining physical intimacy is important to your sense of closeness. But some people may be afraid of touching or hugging the sick person, perhaps out of a deep-seated fear that the illness is "catching" or simply because the changes to the loved one's body are upsetting. Intimate partners may be con-

Couples and Cancer: How Are We Doing?

It may help to ask yourself questions such as these:

- Does one of you deal with difficult feelings by distancing yourself emotionally or physically from the person who needs you?
- Does one of you tend to minimize a threat, act overly cheerful all the time, or refuse to acknowledge there's a problem?
- Are you resentful that your needs are being pushed under the rug because of the illness?
- Do you tend to blame one another when something terrible happens?
- Does one of you seem unrealistically optimistic or pessimistic in ways that cause conflict and distance?
- Do you feel that your or your partner's level of anxiety or emotionality is hurting your relationship?
- Was your relationship or family life so troubled or chaotic before the diagnosis that you thought it couldn't get any worse—but it did?
- Is the illness so much on your minds that there's just nothing else you can talk about anymore?
- Do you have difficulty talking to and listening to one another?
- Do you feel that cancer has trapped you in a relationship that you wish to escape?

Answering yes to any of these might mean you could use some help, together or separately, to deal with the stresses and strains of cancer.

cerned that sex will injure the person who is ill or recovering. Or sometimes people with cancer are so upset with their own appearance that they reject physical closeness; if such is the case, intimate partners should be aware that their willingness to look at the changes in their loved ones' bodies and to touch them will contribute greatly to their renewed self-acceptance (see Chapter 29, "Body Image and Self-Esteem").

Although cancer and its treatment can profoundly affect sexuality, a return to some form of physical intimacy is virtually always possible. But couples must confront the issues (see Chapter 30, "Sexuality").

The Importance of Communication

The ability to talk and listen to one another is essential to finding solutions to the challenges cancer presents to a couple, family, or group. But even if all have communicated reasonably well before, cancer produces complex and intense feelings that can be difficult to talk about. Family members often use silence as a shield to protect themselves or the person with cancer from their fears. Often they don't want to trouble each other with upsetting thoughts or feelings. Unfortunately, withholding or denying genuine feelings engenders stress and tension and creates an unfortunate distance.

Of course, people have different communication needs at various times.

Cancer in the Morton Family

CASE HISTORIES

TRUE STORIES

Henry Morton had just retired from his oil-supply business, which he had founded nearly 50 years before; then he was diagnosed with melanoma. Henry had always been proud of "never being sick a day in my life." His wife of 48 years, Janelle, and their four adult children had also relied on Henry's strength and hardiness and had never pressured him to get regular medical checkups, since he was always in such good health.

Henry had definitely been the head of the family and its chief decision maker, although Beth, his eldest child who now ran the family business, had come to be the unofficial second in command. Janelle—who had always depended on Henry and, later, her children—was shattered and lost. She felt incompetent to express an opinion about what course of action to take, as did all the children except Beth. Beth insisted on gathering information and getting more opinions, but Henry wouldn't hear of it. He followed the advice of the surgeon to whom their family doctor referred him and had surgery within days.

The family gathered at his bedside. "It was like a wake," Beth remembers. Everyone felt bereft contemplating the potential loss of the family linchpin. Beth was the only one of the siblings who lived in the same city, and she began to feel that she was the only responsible one of the lot—an old resentment. For their part, her sisters and brother felt pushed around by her constant attempts to organize who was going to be at home or at the hospital helping. Yet her siblings, under the pressure of their first family crisis, among themselves blamed Beth for not having forced their father to take better care of his health, so that his cancer would have been discovered at an earlier stage.

None of the Mortons—not even Beth or Henry himself—asked the doctors about the prognosis. The medical team took the lead from the family and did not force information on them that they did not want to know, about the odds against a cure when the cancer was discovered so late. They did encourage Henry to seek regular checkups, which he did.

Henry recovered well from the surgery, and the family followed him, acting as if nothing serious had happened—just a bad scare. At the next Christmas gathering, about six months after the surgery, the siblings were able to talk about how childish they had acted with one another and vowed to forgive and forget.

They were careful not to refer to their father's illness in front of their mother, for fear that she would worry about a recurrence and become depressed. Janelle, however, was extremely anxious about her husband's health but felt that there was no one she could talk to about it. Whenever she tried to raise her concerns with Beth, her daughter would rush to reassure her that everything would be all right. In her isolation and fear, Janelle grew depressed, waiting for "the other shoe to drop."

The first metastasis was discovered nearly a year later, which stripped away the family facade that everything was just fine and that Henry would live forever. This time Henry was willing to let Beth do more research on his behalf and include the whole family in decisions that had to be made. For the first time since he had become ill, they all began to share their concerns, which freed them to express their love for one another more openly. The hospital oncology team encouraged Janelle to join a spouse support group, which she did readily and gratefully.

Beth, who had just had her third child and continued to head the family business, tried again to organize how her siblings would help their parents. This time her brother and sisters were more sensitive to her need to feel in control and recognized that they were used to letting her do all the work. They worked out their responsibilities among themselves and scheduled visits so that one of them would be in town at all times to give support to their parents and to Beth. They even gave Beth a birthday present of a weekend at a spa for her and her husband. Her sisters came to take care of the children.

Everyone in the family wanted to visit so frequently, with their spouses and children, that they began to recognize that the pressure was too great on Henry to entertain them, which was his style. Although the cancer had now spread to Henry's brain, he continued to believe that it was in remission. His sons became convinced that Henry should "face the truth," but the rest of the family, with the help of hospital social workers, were able to convince them that as long as his affairs were in good order, Henry was entitled to his optimism.

It was Beth's idea to have a fiftieth wedding anniversary party for her parents. They hired a caterer and invited relatives and longtime friends. Beth and her brother and sisters told each invited guest that there was only one rule for the evening: Talk about happy times. Despite how ill Henry looked, there was to be no grief.

"I think it was the happiest night of my life," Beth says. "I wouldn't have believed that even though Daddy was so weak, so much joy could exist in one room. I learned things about my dad and mom that I had never known, how inspiring they had been as a young couple to their friends and family, how my dad had started his brother in business, so many things!

"As the evening went on, Dad no longer looked ill or changed to any of us in the room, I'm sure of that. We all were ageless, immortal, happy in our love for one another. What greater meaning could come out of any life?"

Henry remains at home, receiving hospice care. He enjoys the company of his family, and they have found renewal in one another.

The person with cancer may want to talk about the progress of the illness, but a friend or spouse may not be ready to acknowledge what is happening. Or the significant others may be trying to manage their own fears at a time when the sick person is feeling more positive and hopeful. Parents may want to have a long talk about the illness and its consequences with children living at home; children, however, can generally tolerate intense emotions only briefly but may need to revisit them repeatedly over time.

Family members frequently differ in their communication styles. Many men have been raised not to share their feelings; women may be less inclined toward silence. These are broad generalizations, but if family members' ways of sharing feelings and information conflict, each member will experience greater stress in times of crisis if he or she cannot find a way to talk about it.

What to Do

It is better not to try to protect one another but, rather, to have the courage to discuss any concerns and to listen to each other. As research among women who have had mastectomies has shown, the type of support they most valued was their husbands' willingness to listen to them and to talk about the disease.

Everyone in the circle of family or friends needs to try to take in what the other person is saying without minimizing his or her feelings, judging them, or providing false reassurances. When you don't know how to respond, say so, and continue listening. If you lack a solution to a difficult problem, you often don't need to say anything other than to acknowledge that you hear what the other person is saying and are willing to think about it. If the other person seems lost for words, simply ask a question.

Schedule frequent family meetings in which you air all your concerns, large and small, and solve problems before they grow unwieldy. If family members are separated by distance, try to get together frequently. Or send videotapes or audiotapes in which you address one another directly.

Support groups for families of people with cancer provide an important forum. You can unload troubling feelings and concerns in a safe environment and at the same time get feedback about how to approach difficult subjects and solve problems.

Turning to helping professionals—social workers, nurses, psychiatrists, clergy, psychologists—to facilitate communication can also provide needed relief and enable growth through crisis. In families that have had numerous difficulties before the onset of illness, as well as those that have become overwhelmed dealing with the cancer, outside help may be the lifeline they need.

Helping Children Adjust to Cancer in the Family

When cancer strikes families with dependent children, parents often want to protect them as long as possible from the harsh "adult" realities. Or they are so wrapped up in dealing with the illness and treatment that they don't have time to spend with the children. In any case, even very small children will know that something is terribly wrong. They perceive their parents' moods and anxieties, unusual absences, secrecy, and even the slightest alterations in the daily routines that regulate their lives. Children are good lie detectors, often better than adults. But if they aren't given an honest explanation, they will arrive at their own conclusions, which spring from their imaginations and immature intellects. Very often children feel rejected and conclude that Mommy or Daddy is away, secretive, or staying in bed because he or she

Don't Avoid It—Talk About It

The great strain of dealing with cancer can disrupt the communication skills even of families that are used to being open with one another. Conversation can become stiff and awkward, particularly when family members become overprotective of one another. All too commonly, they are reluctant to talk about the disease and its effects with the person who has it and with others closely involved. Those who feel uncomfortable with the subject may avoid it at all costs, even switching off the television if the word cancer is mentioned. Many people fear that if they talk about death, they will sound like they have given up, which would upset or depress the person with cancer.

- Drop the charade! It won't work, and it's a handicap.

- Be kind to yourself; understand that the stress of your situation has led to your overprotective attitudes and actions.

- Realize that you are not really protecting the person with cancer. People have an innate sense of physical self and usually are aware of their own states of health—sometimes even before the diagnoses are made. Keeping secrets or avoiding the subject is just silencing any form of communication you may be able to have.

- Understand that being honest does not mean being blunt or tactless or unkind. It means discussing real events and projected events and sharing emotional reactions to those events.

- Start slowly. Discussions about truly important issues—no matter what they may be—are always difficult. So don't rush. And don't let silences scare you away from the issues. It's often hard to find the right words to describe feelings.

- Listen. Don't interpret another's response and then change it into something it wasn't meant to be. If you're uncertain about the meaning of what's said to you, ask for clarification.

- Be honest. Don't pretend that you're not concerned or afraid or angry if you are. Try to explain what you are really feeling to the person with cancer or another family member. Allow that person to help you.

- Talking about death can be hard for everyone. The point is to talk about your feelings. "I am afraid of losing you" is a way to express your concern that your loved one may die. The important thing is to let each other know how much you care.

- If it seems useful, seek help from a nonfamily member to guide conversations that are difficult for you.

doesn't love them anymore or as punishment for their "bad" behavior.

The way their parents cope with these emotional and practical disruptions sets the stage for how their children deal with them. Cancer may be the first family crisis the children have faced. How youngsters adapt is important to their social and emotional development and can influence how they will deal with difficulty in the future. If they've already experienced loss or serious illness in the family constellation, their previous fears and anxieties will probably affect their coping now.

On the parents' side, the fact that they have to help their children adjust can be a powerful incentive to manage themselves as constructively as possible. If they are not overwhelmed by the current crisis, they may welcome being able to shift their focus to their youngsters, with whom they may feel a greater sense of effectiveness and control.

Tell Them

As with adults, information demystifies cancer and helps children feel less helpless. Thus, the first and most important step is to give the children accurate information about the illness *immediately*. Tell them the name of the disease, where it is located, and how it will be treated. Keep them posted throughout the illness about what is going on in the present and what is likely to happen in the near future.

A parent or relative who is very close to the children should convey the news, in familiar surroundings.

Explain the effects of the illness and the side effects of the treatment—such as fatigue, hair loss, weight loss, surgical alterations, moods—so that the children are not left to fantasize why these things are happening.

How you tell them will depend on their age, of course. Use simple, age-appropriate language based on what is really happening. Begin by asking what they understand or think about the illness. Using dolls or drawing pictures can help, but don't use fairy tales to help little ones understand, because these can get their imaginations going in unforeseen directions.

Remember that children are familiar with being sick, going to doctors, and taking medicines, but be careful about saying things such as, "It's like when you had a sore throat and had to go to the doctor," because they might conclude that their sore throat caused the parent's illness or that the next time their throat hurts, it means that they also have cancer.

Although they may not respond right away, be prepared to answer whatever questions the children have and allow them to react emotionally. Keep in mind that they may react more to how you are behaving than to what you are saying.

Parents often avoid useful discussions with their children because they're afraid of such pointed and difficult questions as "Will you die?" The answers to all questions should be honest but as optimistic as the situation allows—for example: "This is a serious illness, but we are getting the best possible treatment and the doctor thinks I am responding very well." When optimism seems quite unrealistic, parents need to acknowledge how difficult it is to live with uncertainty and to emphasize their determination to confront whatever happens together as a family. Be sure to let children know when death is near, and if possible, allow a final leave-taking.

Children need continuous reassurance that they'll be safe, secure, and loved. Because cancer and its treatment necessitate frequent absences from home, and/or leaving youngsters in the care of others for periods of time, reassure them that they are not being abandoned and that their parents are always going to make sure that they are all right, no matter what happens. Allow them to be angry. Address their daily needs and activities: They'll still get their favorite sandwiches for lunch, go to Little League, play with their friends, and so on.

It is important to let children know that the parent's illness is not their fault. Children dwell at the center of their small universes and often think that bad things happen because they were naughty.

Keep in mind that communicating with young people about cancer is not a one-time event; it is a process that will continue over time. Should the illness go into an extended remission or continue as a chronic problem, children will require updates tailored to their own changing understanding and emotional needs as they develop.

You may want to ask a social worker, school counselor, or other parents in your position how they have explained cancer to children that are your youngsters' ages. In any case, tell the child's teachers about the parent's illness so that they can be alert to problems that crop up in school as a result.

What They Can Do

Children often must take on additional chores and responsibilities when a parent is ill. Providing tasks for them can help them feel involved and necessary in the parent's recovery, at a time when children often feel left out. Small children can bring the mail to the parent or paint pictures to send to the hospital, for example.

Older children will probably have to help out more than usual around the house or even take jobs to contribute to the family finances. Especially if there is no other adult living at home, they may even have to assume parental roles that they are not prepared for, such as cooking or caring for younger siblings. This can be a great burden at a time when they are learning to be independent. Even more than adult helpers, teenagers need time off and frequent expressions of appreciation.

Life as Normal

Life is anything but normal when a parent has cancer. Seeing to children's emotional and physical needs can be extraordinarily difficult in the face of illness-related absences or disability, especially in a single-parent household or if the other parent has to work extra hours to compensate for lost earnings or increased costs. It may be necessary to call on friends and relatives to provide child care. Child care can be a parent's greatest problem even in the best of times, and if adequate supervision for children cannot be found now, investigate community resources, such as those listed in Chapter 13, "Your Support Network."

Because of the many disruptions, maintaining children's normal routines and allowing them their usual activities in and out of school are important, to give the children the security they need to stay on their developmental track. Adolescents, in particular, need to spend time with their peers and have their privacy.

Maintain normal discipline as well. Children need to know their limits, especially at times of upheaval.

Becky's Mom Has Cancer

When Maureen Tyler was diagnosed with breast cancer, her daughter, Becky, had just turned five and was about to enter kindergarten. Becky was too young to understand any threat to her mother's life, although she heard the fear in her parents' voices as they discussed the diagnosis.

Maureen sat down with Becky and told her about the lump in her breast. Becky knew that she had been breast-fed as a baby, and it was hard for her to understand that this nurturing part of her mother had something wrong with it. Her mother let her feel the lump and explained that Grandma would come to take care of Becky while she was in the hospital to have the breast with the lump taken away. She also explained that she would be tired for a while after she came back from the hospital but that she would still be the same loving mommy except for the change in one part of her body.

That night, when Becky's father put her to bed, she asked him to tell her the whole story again, and they acted it out with teddy bears. When her mother left for the hospital, Becky clung to her for a minute and then patted her mother's breast and said goodbye to it.

Because she was so young, Becky was not allowed to visit her mother in the hospital, but she and her grandmother drove by it and looked up, trying to imagine which window was Mommy's. Her mother called her every evening on the telephone, and Becky drew lots of pictures expressing her childlike understanding of what had happened.

When her mother came home, she tired easily, and Becky had to learn to bring her mother a glass of water or the morning mail. She also had to learn to play alone more. She wanted to see where the surgery had been, and she touched the scar gently. She continued to reenact the surgery from time to time with her teddy bears, but gradually she lost interest as Mommy seemed more like her old self.

Signs of Problems

Any distressing family situation or threat to their security is likely to be revealed in children's behavior at home, in school, and with friends. Kids who were having problems before will probably have a worse time now, so counseling may be needed to help them manage their increased distress without prolonged consequences for their schoolwork and peer relationships.

Children of all ages may have trouble sleeping or have nightmares, lose their appetites, develop physical complaints, become unusually quiet or fearful, and/or begin to fail at tasks at which they are usually successful.

Preschool and School-Age Children. Small children often become babyish, resume wetting, become clingy, talk baby talk, refuse to go to day care, and so on. School-age children may resist going to school, have problems with schoolwork, or develop difficulties in relationships with siblings and peers. Because they now rely so much on the well parent, they may also react strongly, perhaps angrily when the well parent cries or otherwise seems fragile. They may not seem as sympathetic or supportive as parents might hope them to be. Indeed, they may be furious at the sick parent and critical of his or her changed appearance and failure to attend to their needs.

Teenagers. Adolescents, as befits their complex developmental period, can have a range of complicated reactions. In the process of testing their parents' limits and breaking away, they may feel very ambivalent about their sick parent, wanting to help and yet feeling angry and guilty about wanting to flee. Their reaction can be especially difficult for them, and everybody around them, if they were not getting along with the parent before the illness.

More aware than younger children of cancer news in the media and developmentally able to think of the future, teens may be extremely frightened of death and loss. They may feel utterly alone and abandoned. More capable of empathy, older adolescents may feel overwhelmed by the parents' pain and their own helplessness in dealing with it; as a result, some may become aloof, others anxiously overinvolved in the parent's care.

Some more mature teens cope as adults do, seeking and evaluating information and turning to friends and counselors for help. Some, however, may act out aggressively and destructively, whereas others may begin to fail in school, even if they've been trying to keep up. They may start developing headaches, rashes, and other psychosomatic problems. Some may abandon their social outlets and retreat into their rooms.

What to Do

Always inform teachers that there's cancer in the family so that they can keep track of how the children are performing and report any problems. Any significant changes in their behavior that persist for more than a couple of weeks are warning signs that children are having difficulty. And if children start talking about wanting to die or suddenly begin giving away favorite possessions, seek help from a mental health professional immediately.

Additional attention from their parents may be all that young children need to get them back on track. Talk to them, try to get them to verbalize their feelings, and always express your love. Remember that kids need to know that the surviving parent will be there to take care of them.

When problems persist or are destructive to the children or to others, parents or other responsible adults must intervene. Always try to ascertain the children's understanding of the illness. Despite your best attempts, they may have imagined something that is deeply disturbing to them. This may be true even for older children.

Even with less severe problems, talking to the school guidance counselor or seeking help through the social work department at your hospital or through other resources can relieve the pressure on you when your own capacity to cope with your children's reactions is limited. Ask about support groups just for children of parents with cancer.

There's Something to Celebrate

Celebrating holidays and family occasions and milestones—religious rituals, birthdays, graduations, athletic or academic accomplishments, steps in the parent's recovery—and pursuing shared activities as a group take on increased significance when there's cancer in the family. Allowing yourselves to mark important events and to channel your energies away from fear and sadness offers a welcome distraction from the serious concerns that have probably been dominating your family life.

Most of all, celebrations are a way to recall how much you mean to one another, to bolster hope and restore energy, and to confirm that each person in the family is special. You'll see that even if one of you is ill, you have a future as a family. And memories last forever.

ADVANCING
ILLNESS

METASTASIS AND RECURRENCE

The initial course of therapy is successful for about half the people diagnosed with a malignancy, and they never have to fight another battle with the disease. For others, however, at the time of diagnosis, the cancer has already spread to other parts of their bodies, or *metastasized*. And for some there is no evidence of disease for a long time after the initial treatment; then it recurs.

Whether metastasis is present when a cancer is initially diagnosed or becomes obvious months after the treatment has been completed, the term conveys a similar message: Cancer cells have escaped into the system, and the disease has advanced beyond an early stage. That does not mean, however, that control is impossible. Much can be done to continue the battle and prolong a high quality of life with surgery, chemotherapy, radiation therapy, and/or biological therapy. Optimism, hope, and effective coping strategies are great allies as well. And in those cases in which the cancer cells are very sensitive to chemotherapy—such as testicular cancer, Hodgkin's disease, and some childhood cancers—additional therapy may cure the disease.

Certainly, the spread or return of cancer is a significant challenge. This chapter explains what metastasis and recurrence are, why they happen, what is known about preventing them, and how to deal with them emotionally.

Understanding the Language

The terms used to describe the various transitions in cancer development have different connotations that can sometimes be confusing. The meanings can be clouded too by the person—a doctor or a layperson—who uses them. It's important that you and your oncologist speak the same language, so don't hesitate to ask exactly what he or she means by terms like *advanced, spread,* and *recurrence*.

Words You May Hear

The names of tumors typically refer to their site of origin, that is, the place or organ where they began. For example, a malignancy in the lung is called *lung cancer,* and even when those cells spread to the liver, the cancer is still called lung cancer or sometimes *lung cancer metastatic to the liver.*

Cancer terms convey information about a tumor's location in other ways as well:

- A *localized cancer* is a solitary tumor in one organ, and a *localized recurrence* is one or more tumors that recur in the original site but with no involvement of nearby lymph nodes or tissue.

- A *regional cancer* refers to the spread of the original cancer to the nearest lymph nodes. A *regional recurrence* is the appearance of a tumor in the lymph nodes or in tissue near the original location. In this case the recurrence is always a *metastatic* lesion, meaning that it consists of a cluster of cancer cells that have spread from the primary site.

- *Metastatic cancer* indicates that cancer cells from the original tumor are elsewhere in the body, having spread from the original or primary site.

- A *direct extension* is a cancer that has grown, or extended, directly from the original tumor.

- *Primary* tumors are original tumors, and the *primary site* is the location of the original tumor.

- *Secondary* tumors are the result of the metastatic process, that is, the spread of a cancer. A *secondary site* is the location of metastatic cells or a tumor at a site other than the primary one.

- A *recurrence* is any reemergence of a tumor after any treatment that initially removed or destroyed all the recognized tumor cells. A recurrence may occur in the original site (local recurrence), in the nearby lymph nodes or adjacent soft tissues (regional recurrence), or in organs or tissues far removed from the initial tumor site (distant metastases).

- During the disease-free interval, the cancer is said to be in *remission.* Remission may last for months or years. (Of course, if the cancer never grows back, a person is said to be cured.) If cancer recurs at all, the most likely period is within the first two years following treatment.

- *Advanced cancer* is sometimes medically defined as cancer that has affected at least one organ to the point that it is not functioning. However, it is more commonly used to describe a cancer that for all practical purposes is incurable and usually indicates that life expectancy is limited to a period of months, but people with advanced cancer may sometimes live much longer.

How Cancer Spreads

Although malignant tumors grow at different rates and spread in different ways, cancer typically progresses in a series of somewhat predictable steps. This sequence of events is called the *metastatic cascade.* It's important to understand the phenomenon because physicians may refer to one or more of these steps—and the factors that influence them—when discussing treatment options.

Dormant State

Cancer cells vary in their aggressiveness and tendency to spread, depending on their type and location. Your oncologist will be able to make an educated guess regarding the likelihood that your particular cancer will spread or recur based on knowledge about your type of cancer, its stage when it was diagnosed, and specific characteristics of the cells identified by the pathologist examining tissue from your tumor under the microscope (see Chapter 8, "Diagnostic Tests").

When discussing your cancer with your oncologist or looking at your pathologist's report, you may encounter the terms *differentiated* or *undifferentiated* to describe the cancer cells. Undifferentiated usually means that the cells are not well developed, that they have a tendency to multiply very quickly. In contrast, differentiated cells appear similar to the tissue from the original site and usually grow slowly (see Chapter 2, "The Language of Cancer").

A malignancy may develop slowly and remain inactive for years. Prostate cancer, for example, is usually a slow-growing cancer, so some men who have it die of old age or from other causes before their cancer causes any symptoms or is detected.

In general—but not always—as the cancer cells multiply and the tumor grows larger, the likelihood of metastasis increases. It is known, for example, that in fewer than 10 percent of women, breast tumors detected and removed when they are less than 1 cm in diameter have already spread to the lymph nodes. But if the tumor is larger than 5 cm at the time of diagnosis, there is an 80 percent chance that some lymph nodes will already be involved.

Growth Phase

As a tumor grows, a blood supply develops to nourish the increasing mass. (These new blood vessels also give the cells access to the body's general circulation.) This process of forming new capillaries to connect the tumor to nearby blood vessels is called *neovascularization*. Currently, researchers are investigating various ways of assessing a tumor's blood supply. That is, they are evaluating angiogenesis, the creation of new blood vessels, as a measure of a tumor's potential to metastasize. Researchers are also trying to determine whether angiogenesis can be used as a guide to predict outcomes and create novel treatments.

Invasion

Cancer cells spread to areas of the body beyond the original tumor in two ways. Most commonly—about 80 percent of the time—single cells break away from the initial tumor and enter the surrounding blood vessels. Clumps of cancer cells lodge in the tiny capillaries close to the primary site; some cells manage to enter the general circulation; and others enter the nearby lymphatic system as lymph flows in and out of the bloodstream.

Cells that enter the circulatory and lymphatic systems follow the paths of those vessels and often travel to predictable sites in the body. For example, cancer cells eventually make their way to the lungs and the liver because these are the main organs through which blood flows, carrying with it the cancer cells.

Less often, cancer spreads directly to tissue adjacent to the primary site. The process is similar to the way ivy grows on a wall. A tumor on the outside of an ovary, for example, may grow large enough to shed cells that come to rest on the surface of the nearby uterus. Some of these cells will then put down roots into the wall of the uterus and start a new growth.

A New Tumor

Once the invading cells reach receptive tissue, some of them develop into secondary tumors (metastases). To ensure the cells' survival, these secondary tumors, like the primary tumors, begin to develop a new blood supply.

Map of the Lymph System

The lymph system consists of capillaries and larger vessels, glands known as lymph nodes, and several organs: the spleen, tonsils, and thymus. A clear fluid, called lymph, flows through the capillaries and vessels, which branch throughout the entire body. When cancer cells enter this fluid, they usually become trapped in the nodes and are prevented from spreading further, but sometimes they make their way to distant organs. The illustration shows the network of lymph capillaries and the location of the major lymph nodes and organs.

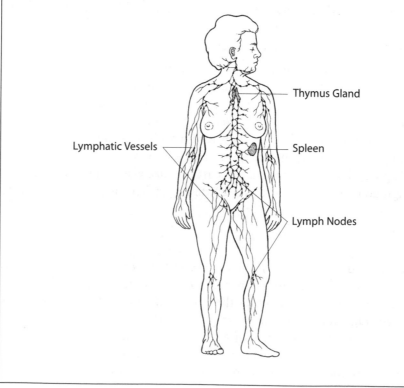

Thymus Gland

Lymphatic Vessels

Spleen

Lymph Nodes

Where Cancer Goes

Cancer tends to spread to specific organs or tissues, usually depending on the path the blood and lymph vessels take from the original site. Also, some tissues provide a more favorable environment for certain tumor cells to flourish.

If you know where your cancer is likely to travel, you can be more alert for symptoms. Of course, it's difficult not to worry about every unusual discomfort or to imagine that it spells disaster. Still, it is better to have your symptoms evaluated and be reassured or, if necessary, receive treatment, than to let a possible metastasis or recurrence go unchecked.

Primary Tumor	Common Sites of Metastasis*
Breast	Axillary lymph nodes, opposite breast, lungs, liver, bones, brain, adrenal glands, spleen, and ovaries
Colon	Regional lymph nodes, liver, and lungs
Kidney	Lungs, liver, and bones
Lung	Regional lymph nodes, pleura, diaphragm, liver, bones, brain, and adrenal glands
Ovary	Peritoneum, regional lymph nodes, uterus, omentum, intestines, lungs, and liver
Prostate	Bones of spine and pelvis, regional lymph nodes
Stomach	Regional lymph nodes, liver, and lungs
Testis	Regional lymph nodes, lungs, and liver
Urinary bladder	Regional lymph nodes, bones, lungs, peritoneum, pleura, liver, and brain
Uterus	Regional lymph nodes, lungs, and liver

* This does not include organs that may be affected by direct extension of the cancer from its original site.

Although fewer than one-tenth of 1 percent of the circulating cancer cells live long enough to establish themselves in another part of the body, about 50 percent of cancers have already spread at the time of diagnosis, depending on the organ in which the cancer originated. In many cases, the secondary tumor, metastases, or involvement in the lymph nodes is too small to be detected. This is why after surgery to remove your primary tumor, your oncologist may recommend adjuvant therapy with radiation or chemotherapy even when there is no evidence of metastasis (see Chapters 14, "Principles of Treatment," and 20, "Combination Treatments"). Furthermore, studies have shown that chemotherapy and/or radiation therapy may be much more effective against occult cancer, or *micrometastases*—that is, undetectably small cancers—than either treatment is when the secondary tumors are large enough to be detected.

Spotting—and Stopping—Wandering Cells

A *metastatic work-up* is a series of tests and evaluations to determine the extent of the disease beyond the region of the primary cancer and to detect any distant metastases. Some of these tests are done at the time of diagnosis, and some are done—or performed for the first time—at subsequent checkups. They may be repeated if symptoms of spread appear (see Chapter 8, "Diagnostic Tests").

At the time of diagnosis, your oncologist may order a series of tests, such as various x-rays and imaging. Which tests are necessary and the extent of the evaluation to detect possible metastases depend on the site and stage of the cancer. An advanced cancer and/or a cancer known to grow rapidly or to spread early in the course of its development may require a more comprehensive group of tests. Doctors do not always agree on the choice, timeliness, or usefulness of the tests. Nevertheless, practice guidelines or managed care providers may require a certain sequence of tests.

The surgeon who removes the primary tumor usually requests that the tumor tissue be examined by a pathologist for certain *prognostic factors,* characteristics of the cells that indicate whether the tumor is fast growing (aggressive and with a potential for metastasizing) or slow growing (see "How Cancer Spreads," page 416). This information will help your doctor decide on the immediate treatment, and it may be useful later if metastases are found or the cancer recurs.

For example, when the primary tumor is removed, breast cancer tissue is examined for the presence of hormone receptors. If the receptors are present, therapy with hormone-blocking drugs may be prescribed to prevent a recurrence.

Preventing New Cancers

At the time of diagnosis, your oncologist may recommend certain other steps to take in the hopes of preventing any further development of the disease. Although clinical studies are currently under way to determine which drugs or nutrients might prevent cancer—an intervention called *chemoprevention*—there now is no certainty that any treatment will be preventive. Nevertheless, there are several steps you can take to increase the odds of preventing metastasis and recurrence.

Combating Cancer Again

If tests reveal that the cancer has recurred and/or has spread to the lymph nodes or other organs, oncologists usually want to begin treatment, although in some cases, they may not (see "Watch and Wait," in "Prostate" in the Encyclopedia). When it's possible to remove a recurrent cancer or secondary tumor, sometimes surgery alone can cure the disease. But if a secondary tumor cannot be removed or in cases of advanced disease, the oncologist may recommend chemotherapy or radiation therapy or both in an attempt to arrest or slow the cancer's growth (see Chapter 20, "Combination Treatments"). In some cases, particularly when there is disagreement over the effectiveness or choice of treatment and also when it may cause side effects that will affect your quality of life, experts advise a second opinion regarding the therapy (see Chapter 12, "How Many Opinions Do You Need?").

Preventing Metastasis and Recurrence

Adjuvant therapy is designed to prevent cancer from spreading or recurring (see Chapter 20, "Combination Treatments"). In addition, the best advice is to follow the recommendations usually given to avoid cancer in the first place. Generally, that means making lifestyle changes (see Chapter 10, "Cancer Causes and Risks").

Some of these changes are well known. Smokers who break the habit reduce their risk of not only lung cancer but also cancers of the mouth, throat, esophagus, larynx, pancreas, kidney, and bladder. Eating a diet rich in fiber, as found in fruits and grains, reduces the risk of colon cancer. Exercise and a low-fat diet help control weight and may reduce the risk of endometrial, breast, and colon cancers. Protecting yourself from exposure to the sun lowers the chances of developing skin cancer.

Although it is impossible to avoid stress entirely, it's helpful to learn ways of coping with upsetting situations. Investigations are being conducted to determine whether stress reduction techniques have a beneficial effect on outcome of cancer treatment (see Chapter 25, "Coping with Stress, Fear, Anxiety, and Depression").

When the cancer has advanced beyond an early stage or has spread to distant sites, the organs affected can produce symptoms that require immediate attention, particularly if they are vital organs such as the brain, heart, lungs, liver, or kidney. Bone metastasis, which occurs in about 70 percent of people with cancer, does not threaten life, but it can eventually cause pain and lead to fractures, called *pathologic* or *insufficiency* fractures. Consequently, immediate treatment is almost always suggested.

Cancer Emergencies

In addition to treating the cancer itself—that is, arresting or slowing the growth of metastatic lesions—the treatment team must manage the consequences when the vital organs cannot function normally. For example, about 30 percent of people with cancer develop lung metastases. Often, though, depending on where the cancer originates, these lesions can be removed, and cure is possible. However, in advanced disease when surgery is impossible or has failed, fluid may accumulate in the space between the lungs and the tissue covering them. In many cases, this condition—called *pleural effusion*—causes no discomfort, but when the fluid buildup is extreme, the patient may develop a nagging cough, become short of breath, or have pain. A procedure to drain the fluid is then necessary.

Other conditions—such as bowel obstruction, pathologic fractures, jaundice caused by blockage of the bile duct, or too much calcium in the bloodstream—require immediate treatment to relieve discomfort and perhaps save life.

Obviously, a person with advanced cancer is aware of the situation and needs to discuss with his or her doctor the signs and symptoms of potential emergencies. As in any medical crisis, an awareness of the signs of distress allows you to take the appropriate steps to resolve the problem before it becomes life threatening. In most cases, the complications can be treated, and the person may return home once the emergency has passed (see Chapter 34, "Supportive Care").

When Cancer Comes Back

A remission may last for decades, but some people experience a recurrence of disease within a few years of the treatment of the original cancer. Of course, no matter how well prepared you may be, hearing your physician tell you that your cancer has returned is extremely distressing, and you are immediately forced to confront and cope again with powerful emotions.

You should expect to shed tears of grief over losing your health. If you had a difficult time with the treatment when your cancer was first diagnosed, you may be distraught at having to repeat the process. Some people express feelings of betrayal, by a body that appeared to be healthy, by a medical system that seemed to have failed, by treatments that now seem to have been ineffective. Doubts arise about what treatment can accomplish, and feelings of guilt or self-blame are common. You may question whether you did something to cause the recurrence or didn't do something to improve your resistance to the disease. It's important to dispel these feelings of guilt or irresponsibility by understanding that you have done nothing to cause the cancer metastases or recurrence.

Those who have been through this time of profound disappointment and emotional turmoil and the professionals who have cared for them say that realizing that these myriad feelings are normal is the first step in coping with them.

Keeping Up the Fight

Survivors of cancer suggest that for many people, thinking of the disease as a long-term, chronic condition can help in coping with the fear of recurrence. That is, instead of thinking that you had a cancer that might return at any moment, you should regard yourself as having a cancer that can be managed by taking care of yourself and following your doctor's advice.

You can learn to live with and adjust to having cancer, just as a person learns to live with other serious conditions such as diabetes or high blood pressure. If your disease is in remission, it's essential to follow your doctor's recommended schedule of follow-up visits to detect any signs of metastasis or recurrence. You may be given certain physical exams and blood tests, x-rays, and CT or MRI scans. In addition, your oncologist may request that you have other procedures, not because he or she is worried about anything new, but because these are the steps to follow in managing a chronic condition.

It often is easier to make lifestyle changes, such as altering your diet or stopping smoking, if you think of them as a way to keep yourself in the best possible condition given the challenges of your health history. And if your cancer should return, you will know about it early and take the next appropriate steps for your care. Cancer survivors often say that keeping fully abreast of their conditions throughout their illness is crucial to gaining control of their fear and anxiety and allowing them to make important decisions about their future treatment.

Dealing with the Bad News

Hearing that cancer has reached an advanced stage obviously is a shock. You no longer can deny the existence of the disease, as so often happens after the initial diagnosis. Gradually, though, your expectations will shift. You may find yourself becoming more cautious about your prognosis. Rather than believing the disease will not affect your life span, you may begin to see the future as finite because of your cancer.

Most people who face cancer learn that the battle is as much a mental one as a physical one. For many, greater knowledge about their disease, treatment choices, and prognosis can boost their capacities to handle any setbacks. Those who seem to cope best are the best informed, and recent studies suggest a link between improved survival and effective coping skills (see Chapter 31, "Coping Strategies").

Sharing the Stress

Enlisting support from family and friends may never be quite so important. Old issues may resurface, accompanied by new concerns and fears. Being reassured and supported by close friends and loved ones is the best foundation for handling a recurrence and the even more difficult challenges of advanced disease. Many people find joining a support group extremely helpful at these times. Family members too may find it beneficial to talk, in a support group, to other people coping with the same situation (see Chapter 13, "Your Support Network").

People who have been in remission for a long time sometimes have problems asking for help again. No matter how caring the support was the first time around, relying on others once more can generate feelings of failure and fear of being a burden. It's a difficult time for family members and friends as well. They may be hesitant to approach you and worry that they will do or say something wrong. They may also have a hard time coming to terms with their own feelings about your illness (see Chapter 32, "Issues for Families and Friends").

This is why the best way to get support is to ask directly, and in an open and trusting way, for whatever you need. You must be very clear about what you want, and those offering support should be equally clear about what they can give. Everyone should realize that needs—and someone's ability to fulfill them—may change as the situation changes.

SUPPORTIVE CARE

At some point, it may no longer be possible to alter the course of your cancer significantly. But at no time should anyone ever be told that "there is nothing more we can do." Indeed, something can always be done to relieve symptoms, ease distress, provide comfort, and in other ways improve the quality of life of someone with advanced cancer. This is called *palliative care.*

Treatment measures initiated at this time are designed to help you maintain the best possible level of physical, emotional, mental, spiritual, and social life—regardless of how far your disease has progressed. Palliative care also addresses the family's needs throughout the course of the advanced illness and afterward.

You may hear other terms, such as *supportive care, comfort care,* and *hospice care.* The distinctions among them are not always clear. To avoid confusion, this chapter uses *palliative care* to describe all treatments for advanced cancer that are meant to improve your quality of life. *Hospice care* is used to mean a specific approach to care during the final stages of life, when it is clear that the time remaining is limited. This chapter explains the many decisions you may need to make and the available options.

One of the most important things that you or those close to you can do is to discover what kind of palliative care is available and to make sure you get it. You can discuss your feelings and needs with your primary caregivers and come to an understanding about how you want to be treated. Your primary physician may help provide palliative care or refer you to and work with a palliative care team.

Many experts think that these discussions should start at the time of diagnosis and continue throughout the course of the disease. Keep in mind, too, that palliative care—that is, care aimed at controlling symptoms and improving the quality of life—is important at any stage of the disease.

The Crucial Turning Point

Deciding to shift the focus of treatment from cure to comfort can be extremely difficult. People with cancer, their families, and even their physicians often have trouble accepting that the therapy directed against the disease is not going to halt it.

The reasons for coming to this conclusion include the following:

- The treatment's side effects are debilitating.

- The disease is not responding to treatment.

- The treatment has a detrimental effect on life quality.

When the conclusion is reached that treatment cannot stop the disease, the usual response is to discontinue ineffective treatments and to give greater attention to managing such symptoms as pain, anxiety, or depression. Sometimes these measures may entail surgery, chemotherapy, or radiation therapy, but with the purpose of palliation, not cure. It is important to learn both what a treatment can accomplish at this time—and what not to expect.

You may have to make a number of decisions concerning this shift from treatment focused on curing the disease to palliative therapy directed toward controlling symptoms and maintaining a good quality of life. Some choices are difficult, partly because others may see the issue from different points of view and react according to their own needs, concerns, or fears. For example, some physicians are trained to take an aggressive stance against disease and so are uncomfortable about doing anything that seems like "giving up." Family members may have similar beliefs (see Chapter 32, "Issues for Families and Friends").

The final decisions must rest with you, but your family and your primary care physician, oncologist, and/or palliative care staff should also discuss the issues honestly and help reach a consensus.

Quality of Life

The terms *quality of life* and *meaningful life* have a variety of meanings. No specific standard or set of guidelines regarding quality of life is widely accepted by the lay public or medical or psychiatric communities. The common notion of a "good" quality of life often includes such things as independence,

---

Questions to Ask About Treatment

When deciding whether it is appropriate to continue treatment targeted against the disease or to focus the treatment on symptom control and maintaining the quality of life, you can discuss the following questions with your doctor, caregivers, and family:

- Is it possible for this treatment to cure the disease?
- Will the treatment slow the progress of the disease?
- Will the treatment improve the quality of my life?

QUESTIONS
TO ASK

full functioning of body and senses, sexual activity, and freedom from anxiety. But quality of life is really a very personal issue. For example, many people who are confined to a wheelchair have very fulfilling lives. For a person with advanced cancer, though, a reasonable quality of life requires at the very least: relief from pain and other uncomfortable symptoms; relief from anxiety and depression, including the fear of pain; and a sense of security that assistance will be readily available whenever needed. All are possible.

For you, acceptable life quality may also require being treated with the respect and consideration that would be expected if you were not sick. It may mean maintaining your personal integrity and self-worth and a sense of meaning and purpose, such as continuing to be consulted on family and perhaps business issues. It may hinge on having some sense of control over events. You may want only a little authority, preferring to feel that others are taking charge and thus freeing you from having to make difficult decisions. Or you may prefer to stay in charge. A good supportive care program should provide just the degree of control that each person needs, which may mean helping overcontrollers to relax their grip a little and accept needed help.

Care and Communication

Most palliative and hospice care is provided in your home, sometimes with intermittent visits to the hospital or a specialty unit if fine-tuning of treatment to control symptoms is required. It may be supervised by your private physician and/or the physicians of your community hospital. In addition, some hospitals and cancer centers now have palliative care services, hospice, or supportive care teams. In most cases, your day-to-day palliative care needs are managed by a nurse working closely with your physician and other members of the team. Since your relationship with your nurse is critical, he or she must be skilled in pain management, symptom control, and end-of-life issues. This person is often your link to the others involved in your care and—most important—can help you communicate what is happening so that you can get what you need.

People who have used palliative or hospice services say that it gave them hope that they would be looked after, without fear of uncontrollable pain or other symptoms. Other advantages that people have mentioned are as follows:

- It's an approach to care that includes the family. Families are encouraged to ask questions and to participate actively in caregiving and decision making.

- Personnel are attuned to details and recognize that you and your family are part of the team. Everyone works together, even though members of the team may have different priorities. For instance, your doctor may be concerned with correctly measuring your response to therapy, but you are more involved in decisions about a distressing family situation. Your family may be worried about the costs of the treatment or managing your care at home. A social worker on the team can be helpful in this case.

- Rules and regulations are relaxed. Instead of making you and your family fit the system, it is adjusted to your needs. If you are in a freestanding hospice or a hospice unit in a hospital, the visiting hours will be flexible.

Pets are sometimes allowed, as is any activity that doesn't embarrass or disturb other patients.

- Palliative care is highly skilled and compassionate care, and it is linked to medical resources. It adds security and keeps people from feeling pushed away or abandoned when cure-related treatments are no longer appropriate or helpful.

- Testing is kept to a minimum. The hospital may be especially fatiguing to people with cancer because typically it is where they are constantly being examined and tested. Palliative caregivers monitor you carefully by talking with you, keeping in touch, and making sure you are comfortable.

- Treatment is focused on relieving distressing symptoms.

- Twenty-four-hour telephone availability is present.

- Care is provided by an interdisciplinary team. All the people involved with your care meet frequently to make sure they are working toward the same goals.

- Nurses participate fully, collaborating with your physician and social worker in addressing your needs. Specially trained volunteers working with their social work colleagues are available also to help you and your family.

- Finally, spiritual resources are available.

One of the most important aspects of palliative care is its emphasis on communication. It isn't always easy to talk to professionals about your day-to-day or even moment-to-moment difficulties and needs. For one thing, you may be anxious and frightened. Many people with advanced cancer constantly monitor their bodies for any sign of something wrong. They worry about what's going to happen later. Although these fears are not unusual, many feel uncomfortable mentioning such things to others. Your caregiver can deal with each worry specifically and concretely, keeping you informed of the treatments and choices available to you. Getting a more realistic idea of your future can provide some relief from worry and make a big difference in both your physical and emotional conditions.

For another thing, you may not know how to talk about your symptoms. You've never had this experience before, so you have no practice in communicating in these circumstances. Your caregivers can teach you how.

Sometimes other people have to learn new ways of communicating too. In some families, especially among married couples, it is common for one person to be the "communicator." If your husband (or wife, son, daughter, or friend) has usually spoken for you, it may be especially hard for you to speak for yourself now. Palliative care specialists suggest that the other person can continue to be your spokesperson—as long as you are able to discuss things clearly with that person and he or she learns how to describe your experience to your caregivers.

Relieving Symptoms

Palliative care specialists have focused considerable attention on what kind of support can best improve the well-being of people with advanced cancer.

Their concerns are controlling symptoms and maintaining a reasonable quality of life for you and your family.

Pain

One of the first things people with advanced cancer worry about is pain. But cancer does not always cause pain. Although 60 percent of people with advanced cancer have some pain, it can be controlled. (More detailed discussions can be found in Chapters 23, "The Pain Challenge"; 24, "Pain Relief"; and 25, "Coping with Stress, Fear, Anxiety, and Depression.")

Gastrointestinal Problems

Nausea and vomiting may be associated with the disease or with the medicines used to control symptoms. Your palliative care team will evaluate the symptom and arrive at an appropriate treatment.

Constipation is usual with pain medicines, so a program of treatment to prevent or relieve it is started at the same time as the pain medicine. Constipation is a common cause of distress in people receiving narcotics for pain, and it should be treated as aggressively as the pain itself.

Dry Mouth

A dry mouth is a common side effect of certain drugs. It can be alleviated in several ways. Cleaning your mouth and rinsing it with water every two hours; using a room humidifier; sucking on ice cubes, lemon candy, pineapple pieces,

TIPS & ADVICE

Talking About Your Needs

People can't help you if they don't know what you need or want. Specialists in palliative care say the best guideline is "Be specific." For example:

It's not enough just to say, "I'm nauseated." Instead, you are encouraged to supply specific details. You might say, "I don't feel nauseated when I lie still, but as soon as I move my head I get sick and vomit." Or, "I vomit once, twice, five times a day. The color is green. I'm always nauseated when I feel upset." This tells your caregiver what may be contributing to your nausea and helps him or her determine what medicine or other measures, such as relaxation techniques, are most likely to alleviate the discomfort.

"The pain is worse" could mean anything from a little more discomfort all the way to severe. Caregivers can respond more effectively if you say instead, "The pain is mild when I keep still but becomes severe when I try to walk. The pain is in my hip and back." Or, "The pain is worse when I wake up in the morning and improves during the day after I take my pain medication and walk around." Some caregivers encourage you to rate the intensity of your pain on a scale of 0 to 10, or they may give you a list of words to help you describe your problem more precisely (see Chapter 23, "The Pain Challenge").

or frozen tonic water; and chewing sugarless gum are some solutions. It is important that the nurse examine your mouth periodically for signs of infection, which may also cause your mouth to feel dry.

Respiratory Problems

If you cough or have some shortness of breath, your palliative care physician and nurse will evaluate the symptom and start appropriate treatment to make you more comfortable. Sometimes you will be given medicine to help your cough; at other times you will be given medicine to dry up the secretions. Sometimes oxygen is helpful; sometimes morphine in combination with other medication is used. The important thing is to let your physician or nurse know you have some breathing problems so that the symptom can be relieved.

Loss of Appetite

One of the most distressing accompaniments of advanced cancer may be loss of appetite. Some people develop an aversion to certain foods and/or eat less. Others begin to hate meat, fish, chicken, and eggs. Still others stop liking foods that have always been their favorites. The palliative care or hospice nurse or nutritionist can tell you how to make meals more attractive and suggest appropriate substitutes. For example, those who no longer enjoy eating meat may get their protein from yogurt or cheese. Frequent, small meals may be more appetizing than large, three-course ones. Cold foods are often more acceptable than hot. Foods with strong aromas can be avoided. People who don't feel like eating in the morning may be more interested by the afternoon. Poor oral hygiene, often a factor in eating problems, can be overcome with proper instruction in mouth care. Sometimes dentures that no longer fit properly impede a person's ability to eat.

Remember, eating less is normal at the end of life and should not become a focus of stress for the family (see Chapter 26, "Food and Nutrition").

Sleeplessness

Sleep-wake patterns may change when people are sick or nearing the end of their life. You may sleep more during the day, when others are around, and feel more secure than you do in the silence of the night. Again, it is important to find out the cause of the sleeplessness. Is it because of pain, anxiety, other symptoms, depression? Once the cause is known, appropriate steps can be taken, such as providing better pain control, taking a sedative, airing fears, listening to relaxation tapes at night and/or keeping a night light on.

Weakness and Fatigue

As the illness progresses, a generalized weakness can make you and your caregivers feel discouraged. Weakness and fatigue can be caused by many things, including the progress of the disease, certain treatments, or depression. Once again, understanding the cause of these symptoms is essential to obtaining appropriate treatment, which is the function of the palliative care team. Some things are reversible; others are not. Pacing yourself and setting goals that can be achieved can be helpful to some.

Forms of Treatment

It is important to understand that the same treatments given when cure was the goal—surgery, chemotherapy, and radiation therapy—may be used in advanced cancer solely to relieve symptoms or to prevent complications (see Chapter 14, "Principles of Treatment"). This is the time for you and your family to discuss with your physician and nurse the goals, risks, and benefits of palliative treatment. What are the side effects, and how long will they last; and what are the benefits, and how long will they last? When you have the answers, you can decide. Remember that although the decision is yours, many people can help you make it. Many of these treatments are not burdensome and can make a big difference in your quality of life. For example, radiation therapy to reduce the size of a tumor pressing on a nerve and causing pain can be helpful. Chemotherapy can also be used in some instances to reduce the size of a tumor and relieve pain.

Always ask your physician whether this treatment will improve your quality of life or whether its side effects will diminish it and, therefore, outweigh the benefit.

Palliative Care at Home

In a major national survey, 86 percent of the people questioned said that if they had advanced disease with no likelihood of cure, they would rather be cared for at home or in the home of a family member than at a hospital. The same percentage said they would be interested in a comprehensive program of care at home by physicians, nurses, counselors, or other health care professionals. When choosing between supportive care in a hospital (or other inpatient facility) or at home, you need to understand the advantages and disadvantages of each. It is a very personal decision that depends on a great many variables. Furthermore, there is no right or wrong choice, only what feels best for you.

A hospital unit or freestanding hospice has 24-hour nurse support. At home, a nurse may visit you once or twice a day. In a unit, you are more separated from your family and familiar surroundings. At home, you are more likely to be at the center of the household. In a unit, family members can visit and help in modest ways, whereas they must carry the major burden of home care. In each setting, however, you have a team available to you and your family. Your physician continues to play as important a role in your care as he or she did when the objective of treatment was cure.

Sometimes arrangements can be made to take advantage of both settings at different stages. You and your family should discuss the issues thoroughly with your doctor, nurse, and social worker before you make any decisions. It's important to understand what home care entails. Some families underestimate its difficulties, but others discover that it is well within their capabilities. Including your nurse or social worker in these discussions is important,

Choosing a Treatment

When a doctor recommends medication, surgery, chemotherapy, radiation therapy, or another treatment to relieve symptoms, you may want to ask such questions as the following:

- Will this treatment prolong my life?
- Will this treatment improve the quality of my life?
- Will it do both?
- Will it do neither?

QUESTIONS

TO ASK

because your doctor may be unaware of the options available for home care or of the insurance and financial issues.

Hospice Programs

In the Middle Ages, a hospice was a way station for travelers. The term is used today to reflect the philosophy that the final stage of disease is still a part of life's journey. Accepting death is central to the hospice philosophy, yet the emphasis on care reflects the positive aspects of living. Hospice programs continue to provide palliative care but focus on the last days, weeks, or months of life.

The growth of hospice care is part of a grassroots movement toward social reform that began in the late 1960s. People began to wonder whether life-prolonging technology was valuable or even useful in every instance. They questioned the notion, "If it can be done, it should be done." There was a general movement toward more humane approaches to health care, and values and ethics in medical practice gained new importance. The growing concern with human and social values included a new examination of how to care for people in the final phase of illness.

Professionals and the public alike have come to recognize that too often in the past, people with very advanced disease were allowed to suffer and were isolated when they could have lived relatively well until the end. Some began to express anger and frustration over the widely accepted belief that pain was inevitable. Inspired by St. Christopher's Hospice in England and the pioneering efforts of its founder Cicely Saunders and her colleagues, a variety of special programs have been developed in the United States and Canada for both the inpatient and outpatient care of people with terminal diseases, most often very advanced cancer, and their families.

Hospice care focuses on working with your family to provide home care and on your physical, emotional, and spiritual needs. Although the emphasis is on helping your family take care of you, hospice care is also provided in some nursing homes and hospitals that have hospice units. There are a few freestanding hospice programs as explained below. If most of your hospice care will be at home, you may be admitted to a local hospital or hospice unit for a few days to bring a symptom under control or to provide respite for your family. Whatever the setting, hospice care is widely available and is covered by Medicare, Medicaid in many states, and some private insurance companies. Ask if your managed-care plan includes it.

One of the greatest differences between hospice and the usual hospital care is that so few things are done "routinely" in a hospice setting. For example, diagnostic tests and procedures are ordered only if the information they provide will lead to measures that will increase your comfort.

Many people may be nervous about discontinuing the therapy for their disease because they're afraid their doctor may no longer keep them as a patient. This is the time to make sure that your social worker and nurse are aware of your feelings. They can assure that you will continue to receive excellent medical care.

Admission

You may seek to enter a hospice program on your own initiative or be referred by a family member, physician, social worker, visiting nurse, friend, or clergy member. Typically, there is an initial assessment visit, when a member of the hospice team takes your medical history, evaluates your emotional state and needs, and discusses nursing concerns with you and your family. The admission criteria may vary, but hospices usually accept only those people with a limited life expectancy (usually six months or less). Home hospice programs may require that you live within a defined area; have access to a caregiver among your immediate family, relatives, friends, and neighbors; and want to remain at home during the last stages of your illness. Hospices that are reimbursed by Medicare or Medicaid have similar but slightly more restrictive admission standards.

Hospice at Home

The choice between home and institutional care is where America has largely departed from the British hospice model, where more people are cared for at inpatient facilities. British hospices are noted for being cheerful and homelike and for having a high ratio of nurses to patients. The staff are carefully chosen and are generally calm, well trained to control symptoms, unhurried, enthusiastic, and remarkably cheerful. There is surprisingly little of the usual paraphernalia of hospitals. People wear their own clothes, decorate their areas with personal items, give themselves their own medications, and are allowed prescribed alcoholic drinks. Family members are encouraged to bring meals and give personal care and may remain overnight. Guests, including pets and children, may come at any time. Such hospices can be found in America, but they are uncommon. Instead, for the most part, special areas of hospitals are redesigned to incorporate some of the British features, in much the same way that many hospitals have done with birthing rooms. Home care is by far the more favored hospice model in the United States, largely because so many people want it, but also because of economic pressures.

Some people prefer to die at home; others feel safer in a hospital setting. What is most important for you and your family to recognize is that there are no "right" or "wrong" choices, only personal ones that are best for you. Just because home hospice care is popular in this country doesn't mean it will be right for you. *You* don't have to choose it. It's just one of your options. And sometimes you may make a decision and then change your mind.

The Hospice Team

A hospice team is similar to a palliative care team and usually includes physicians, nurses, psychologists or social workers, clergy, bereavement specialists, and volunteers. The hospice is the only Medicare-supported program that uses volunteers; in fact, Medicare requires that 5 percent of the patient care be given by volunteers.

What makes the hospice team unique is its heightened spiritual component and focus on controlling pain. Another essential part of the hospice approach is recognition of the central role of the family in taking care of their family member.

Body, Mind, and Spirit

People with advanced illness inevitably undergo a psychological crisis, and no person or intervention can eliminate all the distress. But people can be greatly relieved of their loneliness, feelings of vulnerability, practical worries, and spiritual fears and can be helped to cope with their concerns.

In advanced disease, people often turn to their physicians for cure or palliation but seek understanding and consolation elsewhere. Sometimes it helps just to have someone around who makes you physically comfortable and creates a supportive, personally satisfying environment. Of course, your existing support networks—family, friends, clergy, and the like—are vital. But different and special benefits come from talking to those who are not emotionally entangled: your physician, nurse, social worker, or volunteer trained to serve as a "friendly listener."

People with advanced cancer need to talk. The hospice or palliative care team can give you opportunities to openly discuss your feelings, especially those that you may not want to reveal to family members for fear of increasing their burden. The team can also help you understand and deal with your family members' discomfort in engaging in these conversations. Respecting your need to talk can be good for them as well as you, because it prevents later feelings of guilt or unfinished business and starts the necessary process of grieving.

Your Family and You

Anticipatory grieving by loved ones can be extremely difficult and painful, but it is a healthy response to advanced illness. Unexpressed or unresolved grief is a frequent source of psychological trouble for family members. Supportive care experts have specific criteria for recognizing the difference between normal and dysfunctional grief.

Under the stress of grief, strains among family members may appear, or old ones may reappear, thus depriving people of mutual support when it is most needed and causing further pain to everyone. Most conflicts can be alle-

To Die in Loving Arms, by Lois B. Morris

My Mother, Faye Nathan Borkan, died August 22, 1979, at the age of 67 from cancer that began in her lung and traveled to her liver. This is the story of two weeks of her life, her last two, and how the intervention of some of the kindest people I have ever met made her death worth living.

My mother's illness entered its final stages in early August. She and my father were living in Tucson, Arizona, where they had recently retired. My brother, sister, and I lived in separate locations from coast to coast, and throughout the year we had taken turns being with Mother. I was there when she was hospitalized yet again and it became clear that there was no hope left for recovery. Yet there she lay in the hospital bed while the doctors continued to perform painful tests and useless procedures.

What to do? My family and I, as my mother's condition deteriorated, felt increasingly out of control. At last, a young doctor at the hospital told us, "Call Hillhaven Hospice. They'll help you."

I had heard a little about hospices. A concept imported from England. Places for the terminally ill. A humane way to die.

"They'll help you take care of her at home," the doctor said, "and if you find you can't cope there, you can move her into their facility." He said he would have the hospital social service department contact the hospice on our behalf.

I thanked him gratefully—for the first time in months and months I felt we could do something for Mother.

I went back into her room. "Mother," I said, "how would you like to go home?"

Her eyes opened wide. "Yes!" she said with surprising vigor.

Armed with oxygen and pain medication, my father and I took my mother home, where we were met by her sister Belle. Immediately, Mother's spirits improved. And I felt somewhat more comfortable about returning to my job back East.

My sister, Susan, arrived the day after I left. Shortly, my family's first contact with the hospice was established. A nurse named Joan drove out to assess the situation and to begin so marvelously—almost miraculously—to serve our needs.

Joan's initial advice—after explaining the hospice's home-care, in-patient, and bereavement follow-up services—was that we needed skilled help at home—someone who could handle mother's symptoms and to help prepare meals, to relieve some of the burden so that we could be free to attend to emotional and spiritual needs.

Very matter-of-factly she explained exactly what to expect. She talked about everything from dry lips, to pain, to Mother's rage at becoming increasingly helpless, to incontinence, to coma, to death. Somehow, after a year in which our family faced the inevitable with increasing horror, Joan made it sound acceptable, natural, right.

Joan, as did all hospice personnel, spoke to my mother with honesty, compassion, and love, and she spent a lot of time talking—just talking—to my father and sister.

On her second visit, Joan told Susan and Dad that it was time to say our final goodbyes. "Say the things you never got around to saying, all the things you know she wants to hear. Express your love."

"Mother loved it!" Susan remembers. "She was much more lucid than she'd been for some time. There were a lot of tears—and a lot of smiles."

My brother Gene and I said our goodbyes by phone. Mother responded with sounds of comprehension and by frequently repeating our names.

Now Mother was dying fast. My sister and Joan agreed it was time to move Mother to the hospice. Dad resisted at first, equating the hospice with a nursing home, in his mind the cold place in which his mother had died long before.

Joan suggested that Susan and Dad visit the hospice. "See how it feels," she said.

Immediately upon entering, Susan explains, "there was such a pleasant feeling! Even though each of the fifteen or so patients was dying of cancer, there were signs of life there! A bunch of kids came running out of one of the rooms playing tag. People were smiling. All the doors were open. You had the feeling there was nothing to hide from."

Yes, my father said after Joan had given them a full tour, this was the right place. They went home to talk to Mother, who, after initially refusing to go—she kept saying "hospital!" with repugnance—was convinced by Dad, Susan, and Aunt Belle that she would be much more comfortable there.

Once at the hospice, the family was showered with attention and care. Mother was placed in a room with a view of a peaceful courtyard. The staff—doctors and nurses—tended immediately to her, paying overwhelming attention, as they did throughout those last five days, to her comfort. That meant, first of all, treating her pain so that she could be totally free of it yet not so doped up that she had no wits at all about her. The staff observed her constantly, ready at the first sign of any discomfort to drop everything and run to her side.

Very soon after she got there, Mother became frightened. She asked, "What is this place?" Joan answered simply, "This is a hospice, where everybody is very ill like you. We take care of people."

Later, during a moment of consciousness, Mother wet the bed. "Why am I doing this?" she cried out. There was a nurse in the room, "Because you're ill," she answered with a naturalness and simple directness that, Susan reports, relaxed Mother visibly.

Again she became more clearheaded, delighting in recognizing the close friends and family who were gathering to be with her, and each other, during her final hours. The staff attended to the family's needs thoroughly. They encouraged everyone to speak openly, to air their concerns, fears, and worries, to attend to burial and funeral plans, to seek the comfort of our religion, to think of the future. They were exquisitely sensitive.

Susan, who needed to cope with the situation by being "in charge," says, "They didn't deprive me of my role. They understood me." And when Susan mentioned that Mother preferred health foods, they cheerfully made up one of her favorite concoctions according to Susan's precise instructions—though by that time, Mother was beyond eating anything.

The first day, the doctor told the family that death would likely occur within 24 to 48 hours. Gene arrived with his family the next day, at the hospice's suggestion allowing his children the run of the place. By the time I arrived two nights later, the kids, eight and three and a half, were very matter of fact about "Grammy." "She doesn't have any teeth any more, "the younger one told me in the car coming from the airport. "She's sleeping." "No she's not," said the eight-year-old. "She's in a coma."

I asked how she knew that, and she replied, "The nurse told me. That's why her eyes are open. I get to help take care of her."

When I arrived at my mother's bedside, a nurse came up and put her arms around me. That's all—just put her arms around me, and I knew, feeling those arms, that though my mother was dying, it was okay.

A while later I turned to leave the room. The nurse urged me to stay. "She's alive," she said. "Talk to her. Touch her. Comfort her."

"Can she hear me?" I asked. Though she was moving in the bed, she didn't seem responsive.

"Possibly," the nurse said. "Many people who have come out of comas much deeper than this report having heard everything that was said. Put your lips up close to her ears. Say whatever you want." Then she leaned down, took my mother's hand, and said kindly, "Faye, Lois is here. Now they're all here." My mother made a sound that I still believe was one of recognition and welcome.

I slept at the hospice that night, as my brother had been doing. The next morning, a nurse asked me if there was anything else that I wanted to say to my mother.

"Yes," I said. "I want to tell her to stop fighting, to let go, to be peaceful. But I feel guilty—should I say a thing like that?"

"By all means," said the nurse. "Maybe you'll help her."

So I sat there, urging my mother to be peaceful. I kissed her, stroked her, loved her. I had never felt so close to her since I was a small child. It is a feeling—so close, so warm—that I know will be with me always.

That afternoon, with only my father and his sister present in the room, my mother very quietly died. The family gathered around her. We sighed and cried. But there was no wailing, no breast beating, no sense of tragedy. Her life had been completed. She had died in loving arms, the same arms that enfolded us all.

After the death, the hospice presence became very discreet: they had seen in all their watchfulness that now we needed each other. Quietly they took care of the final details. When we left a few hours later, I thought our experience with Hillhaven Hospice was ended. But at the funeral two days later, I spotted a hospice nurse and social worker among those who came to pay their respects. With us all the way, I remember thinking.

And that wasn't the end of it. About six weeks later, when all the attention paid my father was beginning to fade away, a hospice worker phoned my father and asked whether he might like to join a discussion group of widows and widowers weekly at the hospice. Dad gratefully accepted. It's free and he can attend as long as he wants to.

Recently when I told my father that I was going to write this story, I asked if he could characterize the hospice experience for me.

"Oh," he answered immediately, "it's out of this world!"

How right he is.

Hillhaven Hospice, which was operating in Tucson as a freestanding facility at the time this story was written, in 1980, has since closed. Hospice care remains widely available throughout Tucson, however, as elsewhere in the United States.

viated by talking openly about such practical matters as obtaining equipment and services in the home, providing for minor children, settling financial affairs, and paying medical bills. Some people want to talk about their funeral, prayers to be said, where they want their ashes scattered, or what they would like to be buried in. This is normal. Various hospice or palliative care team members can help you with each of these concerns.

Occasionally, family members may exhibit unhealthy coping patterns or reactions, such as extreme denial, pathological anxiety, depression, excessive or abnormal grieving, sexual disorders, or other signs of poor adjustment. They can get specialized psychological help from a mental health professional trained to work with the very ill and bereaved (see Chapter 32, "Issues for Families and Friends").

Those who are carrying the largest responsibility for home care may need extra emotional support. Even when everyone in the family may agree that you should be at home, many people are understandably frightened and daunted by the prospect, thinking that they can't possibly learn how to take care of you or have the strength to do it. The supportive caregiver or hospice or palliative care team can give your family the necessary information and help them deal with these concerns. They also can provide an emotional safety net by listening to your family's fears and frustrations.

Certainly home care can be a hardship, especially if the caregiver has a job, children, or other major responsibilities. But many family members discover what's best about themselves in the process, and most find it an enormous comfort to know that they are doing everything they can, that they are deeply involved in making their loved one as comfortable as possible, and that they are really "there" for you.

One of the most difficult situations is that of a person with advanced cancer who has young children. Few parents have experience in knowing how to tell young children what is happening in ways that are appropriate to each child's age. The hospice social worker can help you talk to your children and guide you and your family in the best way to help the youngsters through this period. It's also important to involve school counselors and other key personnel. Parents may benefit from professional advice regarding when and under what circumstances children should visit a parent in the hospital. (See also "Helping Children Adjust to Cancer in the Family," pages 405–11, in Chapter 32.)

Dealing with these issues when it is the child who has cancer, which many consider one of the most painful circumstances anyone could ever encounter, is discussed in Chapter 35, "Cancer in Children."

Nearing the End

Experience has shown that many people are better able to deal with the end of life if they are able to acknowledge what is happening. This awareness allows them to resolve old issues and say the things they've always wanted to say to those they love. Finally, it lets people plan and take charge of practical matters, such as providing for their children's education or making certain that their possessions will go to those they wish to have them.

Each person reacts to advanced disease in his or her own way, but often there is a pattern of emotions that follow one another: shock and disbelief that this could be happening, anger that it is happening at this time, a period of mental "bargaining" with God or fate, and finally an acceptance of the reality.

A range of worries often emerges as you begin to imagine the ending of life and what will happen to those you love. You may be concerned about how your family will manage. As your body changes and you become more dependent on others for help, you may worry about becoming a burden or not contributing to the family in the usual way. Sometimes you may feel very alone, that no one could possibly understand what you are going through. This can also be a time for inner growth, leading to a sense of profound peace. As you look back over your life, you may gain insights into yourself and an understanding of some of the events and relationships you experienced.

This is a critical time for clear communication among you, your caregiving staff, and your family. For example, you should let others know whether openly expressing their grief gives you comfort and reassurance of their love or whether it makes you more anxious and distressed. It also is important for family and friends to understand that you may behave differently during these periods of changing emotions. Some people enter a stage of detachment, during which they may seem cool to their family and friends. It will help both you and your family to understand that this is not a real rejection but an attempt to ease away from emotional attachments that are difficult to handle.

Not everyone experiences all these feelings, but when they do arise, it is important to know that ignoring them does not make them go away. Disturbing thoughts often become easier to deal with if you can find a way to express them to someone who is experienced and caring. Various professionals—nurses, social workers, chaplains, and psychologists—can listen, help you put your feelings in perspective, and organize any additional help you might wish.

Family and friends also experience a range of emotions. They share the shock and disbelief, the feelings of unfairness and anger, and the overwhelming sense of helplessness to change the outcome. Some may feel guilty for having trouble with these feelings and for wanting the inevitable to be over with. They may be afraid about having to manage alone and begin to realize that the world will never be the same again. If families can reveal their feelings and share what their lives together have meant, it can strengthen relationships and give everyone courage.

The fundamental principle for family and friends during a loved one's late stage of cancer is to be guided by that person's needs and wishes. Some people want to talk about certain topics; others don't. Some want to know that their loved ones are already grieving for them; others are frightened and upset by this. Some of the greatest comfort can come from nonverbal expressions of love, such as a back rub or offering to bring special foods or other treats.

Some of the most significant decisions to be made at this stage are closely related: first, whether to refuse heroic measures for prolonging life, and second, if you are in a hospital, whether to go home for your last days. When considering these options, it is important to remember that there will be various points at which you can change your mind about almost any decision.

Life-Prolonging Measures

In the past, people with advanced disease had few choices. Today, because technology allows extraordinary things to be done to prolong life, people are forced to make extraordinary decisions. Certainly one of the most difficult is deciding whether or not to use life-prolonging measures, including cardiac resuscitation and mechanical breathing assistance in the final stages of life.

Certain measures are carried out routinely unless you have made clear in advance that you don't want them. For example, cardiopulmonary resuscitation (CPR) will be administered in the event of cardiac arrest, unless the physician in charge—under the patient's or health proxy's (or surrogate's) direction—has issued a "Do Not Resuscitate" order.

To make their own decisions and increase the chances of having their wishes carried out, many people are turning to an *advance directive,* which includes a living will, a health care proxy or surrogate or medical power of attorney, or a document that combines both.

A *living will* specifies what kind of treatment you do or don't want in case of terminal illness, coma, or a near-death situation in which you may be unable to state your wishes. This is not legally binding but allows your health care providers, the person you designate as your health care proxy or surrogate to whom you grant medical power of attorney, and others to know your wishes. A *health care proxy* or *surrogate* is a legally binding document and indicates who should make medical decisions or carry out your advance directives when you are unable to do so; it is also referred to as a *medical power of attorney.* You can get samples of these from your state board of health; from Choice in Dying (200 Varick Street, New York, NY 10014-4810, tel. 800-898-WILL or 212-366-5540); from the *Harvard Health Letter* (by writing HMS Health Publications Group, Department MD-MED, P.O. Box 380, Boston, MA 02117 and including a check for $5 made out to Harvard Medical School and a self-addressed stamped business letter-size envelope); and from Society for the Right to Die (250 West 57th Street, New York, NY 10107; tel. 212-246-6973).

Although the directives may be general, for example, "Do not resuscitate" or "No heroic measures," most experts advise that the documents be quite specific. For example, a directive described by the *Harvard Health Letter* outlines six different medical situations in which decisions have to be made for people who can no longer speak for themselves. A personal preference regarding each of these can be made specific and clear in a detailed advance directive. Since 1991, hospitals have been required by law to inform people that they are entitled to an advance directive.

Unfortunately, there are some cloudy areas in which it is difficult to make a decision because of inadequate information about what would happen if a particular treatment were stopped. There is no confusion about the effects of avoiding or stopping such treatments as cardiopulmonary resuscitation, endotracheal tubes, and mechanical breathing devices. Medical, legal, and religious groups all agree that people have a right to reject these procedures for themselves or for relatives for whom they are empowered to speak.

SPECIAL

!

CONCERNS

A Living Will

Living wills differ in every state. The following is an example of a living will for the state of Florida.*

Declaration made this _____ day of _____, 19_____

I,_____, willfully and voluntarily make known my desire that my dying not be artificially prolonged under the circumstances set forth below, and I do hereby declare:

If at any time I have a terminal condition and if my attending or treating physician and another consulting physician have determined that there is no medical probability of my recovery from such condition, I direct that life-prolonging procedures be withheld or withdrawn when the application of such procedures would serve only to prolong artificially the process of dying, and that I be permitted to die naturally with only the administration of medication or the performance of any medical procedure deemed necessary to provide me with comfort care or to alleviate pain.

It is my intention that this declaration be honored by my family and physician as the final expression of my legal right to refuse medical or surgical treatment and to accept the consequences for such refusal.

In the event that I have been determined to be unable to provide express and informed consent regarding the withholding, withdrawal, or continuation of life-prolonging procedures, I wish to designate, as my surrogate to carry out the provisions of this declaration:

Name: _____
Address: _____
_____ Zip Code: _____
Phone: _____

I wish to designate the following person as my alternate surrogate, to carry out the provisions of this declaration should my surrogate be unwilling or unable to act on my behalf:

Name: _____
Address: _____
_____ Zip Code: _____
Phone: _____

* Reprinted by permission of Choice in Dying.

Additional Instructions (optional):

I understand the full importance of this declaration, and I am emotionally and mentally competent to make this declaration.

Signed:_____

Witness 1:
Signed:_____
Address:_____

Witness 2:
Signed:_____
Address:_____

Designation of Health Care Surrogate

The following is a sample of a form used to designate a health care proxy in the state of Florida.*

Name:_____
　　　　　Last　　　　　　　First　　　　　　Middle Initial

In the event that I have been determined to be incapacitated to provide informed consent for medical treatment and surgical and diagnostic procedures, I wish to designate as my surrogate for health care decisions:

Name: _____
Address: _____
_____ Zip Code: _____
Phone: _____

If my surrogate is unwilling or unable to perform his duties, I wish to designate as my alternate surrogate:

Name: _____
Address: _____
_____ Zip Code: _____
Phone: _____

SPECIAL

CONCERNS

* Reprinted by permission of Choice in Dying.

I fully understand that this designation will permit my designee to make health care decisions and to provide, withhold, or withdraw consent on my behalf; to apply for public benefits to defray the cost of my health care; and to authorize my admission to or transfer from a health care facility.

Additional instructions (optional):

I further affirm that this designation is not being made as a condition of treatment or admission to a health care facility. I will notify and send copy of this document to the following persons other than my surrogate, so they may know who my surrogate is:

Name: _____
Address: _____

Name: _____
Address: _____

Signed: _____
Date: _____

Witness 1:
Signed: _____
Address: _____

Witness 2:
Signed: _____
Address: _____

A person also has the right to decline food and fluids given by tube. Eating and drinking less and less as one nears the end of one's life is natural.

Going Home

What used to be the normal course of events—for people to end their days at home in their own beds—has become more rare in this technological era. But like the movement toward palliative, supportive, and hospice care, it is becoming an increasingly preferred option.

There are definite advantages. Most people are psychologically more comfortable in familiar surroundings, with caring friends and family nearby. Staying home lets you continue to enjoy hobbies or personal projects as long as you are physically able. It gives you greater control over the details of your life, such as sleeping and eating when you are tired or hungry, not when the hospital schedule requires. It makes it easier to refuse or avoid invasive pro-

Artificial Nutrition and Hydration

The most important issue, of course, is *what you want.* But you may not be sure; you may not even know on what basis to make your decision. Some points that may be helpful to discuss when deciding whether to use artificial nutrition and hydration are as follows:

- What is the goal or purpose of artificial feeding? Will it cure or arrest the cancer? Will it prolong life? Will it maintain an acceptable quality of life? Will it make you more comfortable?
- Will it have *any* benefits?
- What burdens will it create?
- Do your cultural, religious, or personal values affect your choice?

cedures. These things—along with the greater peace and quiet of home—can go a long way toward providing emotional well-being. Some people, however, feel safer in the hospital, and that should be respected.

There also are disadvantages. The family may not be available. The needs of the ill person may be too great for family resources. The family may be unable to handle the emotional or physical stress of home care. For some people, being without immediate medical supervision or backup can be frightening. If they have been in the hospital, the physician who had been caring for them there may not be able to continue as their primary caregiver, and so they may be referred to a new doctor at a crucial time.

However, hospice care at home is an option that may eliminate or reduce these disadvantages. Another important aid to families is to have a "care plan" provided by the hospital, which outlines a specific schedule of medication and indicates under what circumstances and whom to call for professional assistance. It should also include information on whom to call in an emergency, with backup numbers, and what constitutes an emergency in that person's situation.

Focusing on Comfort

Advanced cancer is emotionally painful for everyone, and some problems associated with it may test the ingenuity, patience, and strength of everyone involved. In general, however, simple remedies, common sense, good nursing care, the liberal use of carefully selected pain relief—anything designed to comfort, not cure—can help reduce your suffering and that of your loved ones. Specialists in palliative care realize that they can't "make everything perfect," but they do have a great many options and alternatives that allow them to make most things much better. The central and most important message of palliative/hospice care providers should be "We will always do our absolute best for you. If one thing doesn't work well for you, we will try another. You will never be abandoned."

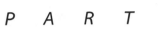

SPECIAL NEEDS

CANCER IN CHILDREN

Cancer in children is significantly different from cancer in later life in many ways, but one of the most important is that the outlook is far better for them than for adults. The median age at diagnosis of cancer in children is 6; for adults it is 67. So most adults who are cured of cancer are given added years of life, but children who are cured of cancer are given their whole lives.

Today, two-thirds of children diagnosed with cancer are cured, many by the very first attempt at treatment. For instance, about 70 percent of those with acute lymphoblastic anemia (ALL), the most common form of childhood cancer, are alive and free of disease five years after diagnosis. This is a major advance, considering that in the 1950s, almost all children with the disease died. In 1970, fewer than one-third of those with non-Hodgkin's lymphoma achieved long-term, disease-free survival. Now more than two-thirds are considered cured.

Another important difference is that many adults with cancer also have additional health problems that complicate their treatment. Children who have cancer usually are otherwise healthy. Of course, this also means that the diagnosis of cancer comes as a particularly severe shock.

The initial signs of cancer and even those that prompt a visit to the doctor may be very much like those of any ordinary childhood illness. Sometimes the cancer may be discovered on a routine doctor's visit. Without warning, parents who thought everything was normal are told that their child's life may be in danger. It may be hard to pinpoint a diagnosis, so there is uncertainty and delay, which aggravate the parents' already great stress and anxiety.

Parents must have information if they are to handle the impact of diagnosis, tell the child what is happening, make decisions, and take care of the child and themselves through treatment and recovery. And whether the diagnosis is good or guarded, they need the support of family, friends, and other parents who know that life-threatening illness in a child is one of the most emotionally difficult experiences they will ever go through. This chapter deals specifically with childhood cancer: the various kinds, their treatment, possible medical and emotional problems, possible long-term outcome, and resources available.

Special Treatment

One of the most important differences between adults and children with cancer is where and how they are treated. Approximately 80 percent of all adults with cancer are cared for in their own communities by their family doctor or primary physician, with referrals to whatever specialists are available locally. Most adults do not go to major medical institutions or specialized centers.

Most pediatricians and general and family physicians do not treat childhood cancer. It is so rare that they may not have had experience diagnosing it and may be uninformed of the recent advances in its treatment. Furthermore, they may not have access to needed resources, such as cancer specialists and diagnostic and treatment technology.

Doctors in general practice usually refer children suspected of having cancer to a specialized center, which may be a children's hospital, the pediatrics department of a nearby university hospital, or a major cancer institution. For example, 90 percent of children under 15 with acute lymphoblastic leukemia are treated in a major pediatric medical institution with special programs for children with cancer. Fortunately, there are such centers for childhood cancer all over the United States (see Appendix I, "Resources").

These centers are unique; they are staffed by physicians and other health care specialists who have been trained not just in a particular specialty—such as cancer chemotherapy, body imaging, radiation therapy, tissue pathology—but in those areas *in children*. The radiation therapist, for example, knows not only that treatment requirements for children are different from those for adults but also that those for infants differ from those for older children and teens. Pediatric surgeons in special centers are trained to operate on children, and many devote themselves exclusively to those with cancer. These specialists are part of a multidisciplinary team that covers every aspect of childhood cancer, from diagnosis to play therapy to preparation to return to school.

Childhood cancer treatment centers are most likely to be involved in clinical trials, which employ the latest and most sophisticated treatments. Only 2 percent of all cancers are diagnosed among children, but at least 70 percent of children with cancer are treated in clinical trial programs. By contrast, 98 percent of cancer patients are adults, and only 3 percent of them are enrolled in clinical trials. Managed health care plans may be unwilling to cover clinical trials or even to permit referrals to specialists in pediatric cancer or to childhood cancer centers, which my be outside their own network. (See "Getting the Best Cancer Care from Managed Care" on pages 94–95 in Chapter 11, "Getting Help for Cancer: Who, What, Where, and How.")

The Different Kinds of Cancer in Children

There are fewer different kinds of cancer among children than among adults.

- Nearly half the 8,000 to 10,000 children less than 15 years of age diagnosed with cancer each year have leukemia; of this number, three-fourths have the acute lymphoblastic type (ALL).

- Solid tumors (for example, neuroblastoma and osteogenic sarcoma) constitute about 40 percent of childhood malignancies. Tumors of the nervous system, including brain cancer, are the most common of these solid tumors among children.

- Although a few childhood cancers are similar to the adult disease of the same name, children usually do not have the same kinds of cancer that affect adults. Most childhood cancers affect only a specific site or a limited number of organs. Carcinomas (see Chapter 2, "The Language of Cancer") are more common in adults and can affect any organ or site in the body.

- Some childhood cancers are observed soon after birth; others are detected during major periods of growth and development, such as adolescence. Solid tumors have their peak incidence in children under 5. But two common solid tumors, those of the brain and bone, are most often diagnosed in adolescence.

- Age also affects outcome; children younger than a year who have neuroblastoma, for example, do better than those over 2. The incidence of childhood cancer in the United States is slightly higher in males, for no known reason, and is lower in black children, largely because of a lower incidence of acute leukemia, lymphoma, Ewing's sarcoma, and malignant melanoma.

- The incidence of some childhood cancers worldwide varies enormously, depending on geography: Retinoblastoma is relatively rare in America but common in India; Burkitt's lymphoma accounts for nearly half of all childhood cancer in Uganda but is quite rare in the rest of the world.

Detecting Childhood Cancer

The signs of childhood cancer are often subtle or vague, but any of the following symptoms, in the absence of an obvious cause, calls for a prompt and thorough examination:

- A new or growing mass or lump;
- Unexplained bruising or bleeding;
- Unexplained pain;
- Lengthy or recurrent infection;
- Prolonged fever;
- Prolonged paleness, fatigue, and/or weakness;
- Weight loss accompanying any of these symptoms;

• Night sweats that soak the body;

• Persistently swollen glands.

The symptoms may be so suggestive of cancer that the child is immediately referred to an oncologist, but if there's only a vague suspicion, the pediatrician may examine for swelling or lumps in the neck, underarms, and groin and may order x-rays, a CT scan, or a biopsy (see Chapter 8, "Diagnostic Tests"). Sometimes a biopsy can't be done at this time, but the location of the tumor, along with urine or serum tests, can lead to a diagnosis.

Specific Cancers That Affect Children

Childhood cancers fall into one of two general categories: (a) solid tumors, including tumors of the brain and central nervous system and other solid organs in the body such as the bones, liver, and kidneys; and (b) leukemias and lymphomas. Each childhood cancer is treated by a specific plan, but the treatment follows general principles no matter what kind of cancer is involved. Most significant is the fact that childhood cancers are often fast growing and may have spread to distant parts of the body even before diagnosis. However, they are usually susceptible to treatments (described later in this chapter).

The types of childhood cancers are described briefly in the following pages. More information is available in the Encyclopedia; here the focus is on the symptoms in and effects on children. See Appendix I, "Resources," for more sources of infomation.

Leukemias and Lymphomas

Leukemia is the most common malignancy in children, affecting some 4,000 children each year in the United States. Three-fourths of them have *acute lymphoblastic anemia (ALL)*; the rest have *acute nonlymphocytic leukemia (ANLL)*, except for a very few who have *chronic myelogenous leukemia.*

Acute Lymphoblastic Anemia (ALL). ALL is most common between the ages of 2 and 6; the other leukemias occur at any age. The most common signs of ALL are fever, pallor and fatigue, loss of appetite, bleeding (which shows up as bruising or tiny purplish spots like little hemorrhages under the skin), swollen glands, enlarged spleen, and bone pain, which often makes the child limp or even refuse to walk. These symptoms may be confused with a number of other childhood illnesses, including mononucleosis and certain viral infections. ALL commonly spreads to the central nervous system and the testes.

Children between 2 and 10 have the best outlook for recovery. Treatment aims first at remission, then at blocking the cancer's spread to the central nervous system, and finally at preventing a recurrence. Bone marrow relapse, a frequent problem, may be treated with chemotherapy or bone marrow transplantation.

Acute Nonlymphocytic Leukemia (ANLL). ANLL has symptoms similar to those of ALL and its treatment is similar if not identical. Unfortunately, largely because of the greater danger of nervous system involvement, the prognosis for ANLL is not as good as that for ALL.

Lymphomas. Hodgkin's disease is rare in children. It affects mostly those between the ages of 4 and 11. There is no apparent cause, although it is known that children and young adults taking phenytoin to control seizures are at risk for the disease—a risk that stops when the drug is discontinued. The treatment usually is chemotherapy. Removal of the spleen is now rarely necessary. Hodgkin's disease has one of the best outcomes of all tumors.

Several other kinds of lymphomas are classified as *non-Hodgkin's lymphoma,* including *T-cell lymphoma,* usually found in preadolescent or adolescent males; *large cell,* in children over 5; and *small cell (Burkitt's* or *non-Burkitt's).* All children receive chemotherapy, sometimes with radiation treatment and surgical removal of the tumor tissue. Chemotherapy has dramatically improved disease control and survival.

Solid Tumors

Three of the main types of solid tumors in children—neuroblastoma, Wilms' tumor, and retinoblastoma—are almost exclusively diseases of childhood.

Central Nervous System Tumors. Tumors of the nervous system and the brain are the most common solid tumors in children, accounting for 20 percent of such cancers. They may occur at any time in childhood, and age doesn't seem to have anything to do with outcome. Symptoms, caused by increased intracranial pressure, include headaches (especially repeated, frequent, or worsening), nausea and vomiting (especially in the morning), and visual problems. In infants, the symptoms may be vomiting, unsteadiness, lethargy, and irritability. Older children, but rarely newborns, may have seizures. A CT or MRI scan may be used to locate the tumor mass. An MRI takes about 45 minutes and requires that the child remain still, which sometimes necessitates sedation. A lumbar puncture (commonly called a spinal tap) may be done after a scan. (See Chapter 8, "Diagnostic Tests.")

Brain tumors in children are far less threatening than those in adults, partly because children rarely have the most dangerous types, nor do their brain cancers usually spread. But there are other special problems. First, childhood brain tumors are so rare that the average pediatrician will see no more than one or two in his or her entire career. So when a child comes in with any of the symptoms of a brain tumor, doctors are likely to think instead of all the other things those symptoms might represent; therefore, a correct diagnosis may be delayed. Second, current treatments can succeed in eliminating the tumor but at the same time may damage the developing brain.

Almost all brain tumors in children require surgery for diagnosis and for removal of some or all of the tumor. Although radiation is often the best therapy for adult brain tumors, surgery is favored in children under 2, because radiation is so likely to harm the developing brain. Chemotherapy drugs are sometimes injected directly into the tumor or the cerebrospinal fluid.

A child with a brain tumor must be observed regularly for years to make sure the treatment has been effective and to identify any complications. This may mean radiographic imaging of the brain every three to six months for two years, annually for a couple of years, and then every other year or every third year. Children who are successfully treated may still suffer long-term effects, including intellectual deficits, endocrine imbalance, and neurologic handicaps. A few children treated by irradiation may have a recurring tumor 10 or 20 years later.

Neuroblastoma. Neuroblastoma is the third most common childhood cancer. Symptoms include a mass in the neck or abdomen, bone pain (if the cancer has spread), a "bruising" pattern around the eyes, irritability, and loss of appetite. Surgery may be the only treatment necessary. Sometimes the tumor can't be surgically removed and so is treated by combined chemotherapy and radiation therapy. The prognosis is excellent for many infants but very poor for older children with widespread disease.

Wilms' Tumor. Wilms' tumor, a cancer of the kidney, is mostly seen in children about 3 to 4 years old and is usually diagnosed when a parent discovers an abdominal mass. It may affect one or both kidneys and almost always calls for *exploratory surgery*—an operation to examine the area directly and possibly remove the tumor—followed by chemotherapy and sometimes radiation. Relapses may occur, mostly during the first two years after treatment, so frequent follow-up is important. The overall cure rate is now more than 80 percent.

Retinoblastoma. Retinoblastoma is a rare cancer and may affect one or both eyes. When it is in both eyes, it is known to be inherited, and other children in the family should be carefully monitored. Retinoblastoma in one eye usually has no genetic basis. A child who suddenly becomes cross-eyed or starts to squint should be examined by a specialist. Radiation treatment cures 90 percent of children. Vision change is common, but vision loss is unusual.

Rhabdomyosarcoma. In almost half the cases, rhabdomyosarcoma occurs in the head and neck. It can also appear in the genitourinary region, the trunk, and/or the limbs. Radiation therapy and surgery, followed by chemotherapy, are combined in ways that try to preserve both function and appearance. (Radiation is not used for the testicular disease.) Rhabdomyosarcoma of the tissues around the eye requires only biopsy and chemotherapy, and vision is often saved. Younger children tend to fare better than older ones, but the prognosis varies widely depending on the site.

Osteogenic Sarcoma. Cancer affecting the bone always requires surgery, but not necessarily amputation, and chemotherapy. A principal concern is this cancer's tendency to spread to the lungs, which calls for careful diagnosis and prompt treatment. The long-term survival rate has been vastly improved over the years and is now better than 50 percent.

Ewing's Sarcoma. Ewing's sarcoma is a rare tumor of the bone that usually occurs in adolescence and is more common in girls than boys. It is most often found when the child has pain (generally in the femur or thigh bone), often with a soft-tissue lump. This cancer requires careful diagnostic evaluation by several methods, followed by intensive treatment. The prognosis is best if the disease has not spread.

Treatment Approaches

Childhood and adult cancers are treated with similar methods, such as surgery, chemotherapy, and radiation therapy (see Chapter 14, "Principles of Treatment"), but there are some special concerns and modifications for children, who are still growing and developing.

Local Treatment

Surgery or radiation is used for solid tumors (bone or soft-tissue tumors or abdominal masses) to control or remove the main tumor mass. Although amputation used to be almost routinely required for certain cancers of the limbs, today limb-sparing techniques allow surgeons to remove cancerous bone and tissue and replace it with a prosthesis (see Chapter 15, "Surgery"). Years ago, some children would not have surgery if their disease was considered too far advanced to benefit, but today, as a result of much improved survival rates, doctors attempt to treat every child, regardless of the stage of his or her disease. Surgery can cure a small percentage of children's cancer. Others require additional local or systemic treatment.

Radiation therapy, also used for local control and in combination with surgery and/or chemotherapy, requires precise evaluation by experts in pediatric radiation therapy because of its potential long-term effects on the child's ability to learn, growth, development, and organ function (see Chapter 16, "Radiation"). It also may be used for systemic control when the entire body is irradiated in preparation for a bone marrow transplant.

Systemic Control

Chemotherapy most often includes a combination of agents that work in different ways to destroy cancer cells. The schedule usually entails initial therapy to halt the cancer, followed by maintenance therapy for months or even years to keep it under control or prevent its recurrence (see Chapter 17, "Chemotherapy").

Bone marrow transplantation allows doctors to deliver extremely high doses of chemotherapy or radiation, both of which have the greatest effect on cancer but profoundly diminish the marrow's ability to fend off infections and perform other vital functions. The transplanted marrow may be the child's own, taken during remission and then frozen and stored until needed, or it may be from a donor, usually a sibling or close relative. Increasingly, donor marrow can now be found through registries (see Appendix I, "Resources") of unrelated donors that have been carefully typed so that a close match can be made (see Chapter 19, "Bone Marrow Transplant").

Biological therapies are the newest treatment methods, consisting of agents that affect the body's immunity and its blood-building system. They are most often used to encourage renewal of bone marrow destroyed by chemotherapy and to reduce such side effects as susceptibility to severe infections. Some are now being evaluated for their ability to attack cancer cells directly (see Chapter 18, "Biological Therapies").

Supportive Care

Various treatments are used primarily to counteract the adverse effects of cancer treatment (such as excess potassium in the system, depressed bone marrow activity, bacterial and fungal infections, pain, nausea, and vomiting) and to give support and encouragement to the child and family.

The Demands of Treatment

Treating cancer in children is often strenuous, invasive, and difficult. Treatment may be more painful than the cancer itself. Constant research regularly produces new methods or levels of treatment and new agents to counteract some of these problems. Nevertheless, the current approaches to therapy, though often highly successful, place tremendous demands on the child, the family, and the medical staff.

Because children are still developing, the side effects of treatment are more complex than those that adults experience. Although many of them are acute but temporary, some may be chronic—or create chronic problems—and hinder growth and development. A few are incapacitating.

If the cancer treatment team does not tell you what to expect in the course of treatment, ask them what your child may encounter and for specific advice on how you can help him or her get through the experience and what they can offer to relieve your child's discomfort.

The most common side effects are similar to those for adults: nausea, vomiting, and hair loss from chemotherapy and radiation therapy; skin irritation; and fatigue. Some children become highly susceptible to fungal infections from the antibiotics given to combat symptoms or drug effects. Children with Hodgkin's disease are susceptible to herpes zoster (shingles) and *Pneumocystis carinii* pneumonia and to severe infection if their spleen has been removed.

Pain and Anxiety

Children don't "get used to" unpleasant or painful diagnostic and treatment procedures; in fact, the more they have to endure, the more fearful they may become and the more emotional distress they may suffer.

Aside from the pain caused directly by the illness or by diagnostic and treatment procedures, children may suffer terror reactions to things that suggest treatment (needles, bottles) and anxiety and other symptoms in anticipation of treatment (such as nausea and vomiting *before* a chemotherapy session).

Individual differences, including age, are important. Some children are unusually stoic and undergo painful procedures with little outward reaction, while others begin to cry and protest the minute they enter the examining or treatment room. Younger children don't typically control their responses and may be especially anxious and frightened because they don't know why things are happening to them. Many think they are being punished; some fear that even a minor procedure could cause them to die.

Medications to reduce pain and anxiety in children with cancer are available, and for the majority the dose ranges for effective pain relief are known. However, individual reactions may vary. The risks of analgesics and anesthetics for children may be far greater than their benefits. The possible dangers include slowed breathing and toxicity to the central nervous system, liver, and kidneys. Also, many children seem to have an aversion to these medications and are unwilling to be regularly sedated.

There are a few myths about children and pain that have been proved untrue. For example, one erroneous belief is that children don't feel pain as acutely as adults do and promptly forget it. It also is unlikely that children will become addicted to narcotic pain relievers. Unfortunately, some health care givers still subscribe to these ideas, so it may take some effort on your part to persuade them to give your child enough medication to be effective. (See Chapters 23, "The Pain Challenge," and 24, "Pain Relief.")

A Child's Mind-Body Interactions

Cognitive/behavioral techniques—which help children think different thoughts and learn new coping skills—can be useful in reducing pain or the anxiety that triggers or magnifies it. Depending on the child's age, these may include simple praise or rewards (stars on a chart, points that can be traded for toys); distraction with storytelling, fantasy play, and games; positive imagery (telling the child a story that identifies him or her with a favorite fictional hero); hypnosis; breathing exercises; "rehearsing" a feared procedure; and role playing (with the child or a doll acting the parts of doctor, nurse, and patient). Experience has shown that when properly used, these techniques can reduce anxiety and pain and even the nausea associated with chemotherapy. You can consult a social worker at your treatment center for a referral to an expert in pediatric behavioral medicine, who can instruct you on the use of these techniques. (See Chapter 25, "Coping with Stress, Fear, Anxiety, and Depression.")

How Parents Can Help Children Deal with Discomfort and Distress

Treatments may continue even after the child has stopped feeling sick or no longer has other symptoms. When children have to undergo therapy without understanding the need for it, they may become rebellious and uncooperative.

Children's feelings and behavior may be made worse by their "sixth sense" for parental anxiety. Children instinctively look to their parents for cues on how they should feel. If a parent is calm and relaxed, often the child will be reassured. A steady voice, strong posture, firm touch, and straight gaze send powerful messages to a child. Likewise, nervousness, erratic behavior, and avoidance activity (pacing the room, turning away from the child, or closing your eyes when a procedure is beginning) make children feel insecure.

Of course, parents need to react to what is happening. It is a mistake to downplay the child's distress and not to offer comfort in the hopes that the child will calm down. Children are most assured when their parents recognize and respond accurately to their level of distress.

When the pain grows worse and the parents increase their efforts to explain, distract, or soothe, the child handles it better. But if a parent is too active in comforting when the distress is minor, the child may become more upset. (See also "Coping with the Family Crisis" later in this chapter.)

Recovery After Therapy

When the planned course of treatment has ended (anywhere from a few months to a few years) and the remission has been continuous or renewed, the therapy ends. Some parents and children celebrate, but others also suffer a letdown. Ending the therapy suggests cure, but it doesn't insure against relapse and recurrence, and parents and children often feel abandoned and vulnerable. Without impending treatments to occupy their attention, many children turn their full attention to changes in appearance that now become horrifying to them.

In older children (preadolescents and adolescents), the posttreatment period of elation may be followed by a period of something resembling grief: They lose confidence, feel sad and lost, and can't concentrate.

Adolescents in particular struggle with body-image issues, although most manage otherwise to take their illness in stride and to cope, adapt, and get back into the mainstream of life with surprising ease.

Many young people who have cancer seem to become mature beyond their years, which may be good or bad. Some will have gained a better sense of self through their survival and will be eager to make new friends and reach for higher goals. Others will feel isolated, inferior, and dependent and may try to fight off their feelings by taking inappropriate risks or indulging in unacceptable behavior.

Survivors of childhood cancer may have a lasting sense of vulnerability that makes it hard for them to deal with simple illnesses or physical complaints. Some become overly concerned about physical symptoms. Some find it difficult to talk about their cancer. Younger children may become fearful about every trip to the doctor or hospital. Older children may worry that having had cancer will jeopardize future employment or relationship possibilities. Many, however, speak of gaining confidence, compassion for others, and a greater appreciation of life.

Overall, it is important for parents to recognize that the wide range of reactions to ending treatment is normal. If the child does not seem able to adapt to life as a cancer survivor, by all means seek help from a mental health professional with expertise in reactions of children and adolescents to serious illness.

Long-Term Effects

Most children with cancer may be cured and survive even aggressive treatment amazingly well, but a small percentage—perhaps 3 percent—have long-term effects from the disease or its treatment. Whether physical, psychological, or social, these repercussions can vary widely from one child to the next. Periodic assessment by cancer specialists is always wise. Doctors are prepared for possible late effects, complications, and recurrences and know what to do about them.

For example, some studies suggest that children who have had leukemia have more than the usual problems with school absenteeism, academic achievement, health complaints, and social skills.

Some children develop a second cancer in the same place as the first or elsewhere. In some cases, the second cancer is due to radiation therapy or chemotherapy or a combination of the two. Whatever their cause, these cancers can be treated just as successfully as the primary ones.

Chemotherapy or radiation treatment to the brain for leukemia can impair mental functioning and memory. Some of the intellectual difficulties—short attention span, inability to pursue a task to its conclusion or to move easily from one task to another—can be treated by specialists in rehabilitation after cancer.

Causes: What's Known and What Isn't

Physicians usually cannot assign a precise reason for cancer in any particular child, which can be quite frustrating to parents who desperately seek some explanation. Researchers have found that the ability of both parents and children to cope with cancer has much to do with why they believe the disease occurred. Specifically, the people they studied who blamed themselves—for example, by assuming the cancer was inherited or is a punishment for their past wrongs—did not cope well with the crisis. Although doctors have a general understanding of the causes of at least some childhood cancers, they can often say more about what is not the cause than what is. For example, if a mother has cancer, it will not be transmitted across the placenta to the fetus. Nor are there any universally accepted statistics linking childhood cancers to the use of diagnostic x-rays before birth. Proof of this comes from studies of offspring of women who were pregnant at the time they were exposed to huge doses of radiation from the atomic bombs dropped on Japan. The incidence of cancer was no greater in those children. But there was a greater incidence of leukemia in those who were young children at the time of the nuclear explosions.

Doctors have identified some statistical "associations" and risk factors, but these have not yet proved to be direct causes. For instance, children with certain chromosomal disorders are at greater risk for certain cancers such as retinoblastoma and Wilms' tumor, but only rarely have underlying inherited disorders been clearly identified as a specific cause of childhood cancer.

It is known that when a child has cancer, the risk for his or her siblings is about double that of the general population. If two siblings get cancer, the risk for other siblings may be even more than double. In rare cases, cancer occurs repeatedly in families, sometimes with more than 25 percent of their members developing a malignancy at some time in their lives. It cannot usually be determined whether this results from direct heredity, a genetic susceptibility, exposure to carcinogens, or a combination of factors. One thing is definitely known, however: cancer is not "catching." (See Chapter 1, "What Is Cancer?")

Cancer in children has been linked to several drugs and chemicals that their mothers took while pregnant, including the drug diethylstilbestrol (DES), which produced cancer of the vagina or cervix in daughters of women treated early in their pregnancy in the 1950s. *Seminomas* (tumors of the testis) were found in some males exposed to DES before birth. There also are links between *fetal alcohol syndrome*—which results from the mother's alcohol use during the critical development stages of pregnancy—and neuroblastoma, adrenocortical carcinoma, and cancer of the liver.

Several chemicals, including drugs, are associated with the development of cancer. For example, vitamin A and related compounds may cause birth defects. Certain chemicals may affect young children through medical therapy. For instance, chemotherapeutic agents, especially VP-16 (epipodophyllotoxins), used to treat other cancers may cause secondary leukemia. However, there are fewer associations between cancer and the environment in children than in adults, partly because children are not so often exposed to such things as industrial carcinogens. Even skin cancer from sun exposure is rare in the young.

Children with a compromised immune system, either because of a congenital immune deficiency disorder or infection with HIV (the AIDS virus), also are at risk for certain cancers, particularly the leukemias and lymphomas.

Various causes have been suggested for leukemia, such as the environment, genetics, viruses, or immune disorders. An abnormal risk of leukemia (ALL) has been associated with chronic exposure to chemicals (for example, benzene) and radiation therapy to treat enlarged thymus in the newborn, tinea capitis infection, and ankylosing spondylitis. Children with Down's syndrome are at higher risk for other congenital abnormalities and for leukemia (15 times higher than normal). The many reports of "leukemia clusters" appear to be a clue, but they have not been confirmed. The striking differences in the incidence of such cancers as Burkitt's lymphoma may be due to some special combination of genetics and environment.

Viruses and parasites have been linked to a few cancers, notably Epstein-Barr virus (EBV) and lymphoproliferative disease. An infectious cause has been suggested for Hodgkin's disease but has never been documented.

See Chapter 10, "Cancer Causes and Risks."

Coping with the Family Crisis

Childhood cancer is a family crisis. Normal daily life is turned inside out, and the future is unknown, uncertain, and frightening. Parents are faced with major tasks at a time when they have suffered a terrible shock. They have to get information from doctors, health care staff, and others about the medical, emotional, and financial dimensions of the diagnosis. They have to decide how much of this information the child should be told, by whom, and how. They have to develop a working relationship with those who will be responsible for their child's health and life, and they have to confront and deal with all their own feelings while trying to give their child emotional support and attend to the needs of their other children.

Just as their parents do, children with cancer feel threatened, and their emotional discomfort is made worse by pain and other symptoms, strange and frightening surroundings, examinations and manipulation by unfamiliar people. They may react with unusual behavior and moods as a result of the diagnosis or the pain, discomfort, tedium of long-term treatment, and disruption in their normal lives. Their behavior often has much to do with how their parents react. Children are reassured when their parents act with confidence, give them clear and straightforward explanations, and calmly help them prepare for medical procedures. Likewise, they feel anxious and fearful when the signals from their parents are hesitant, uncertain, or contradictory.

It is important for parents to maintain a normal life for the entire family, especially in regard to discipline. Although it is difficult to resist the tempta-

Emotional Realities

SPECIAL

CONCERNS

Nearly all parents and family members feel similar emotions on learning that a child has cancer. As Margot Joan Fromer discusses in *Surviving Childhood Cancer: A Guide for Families* (American Psychiatric Press), don't be surprised by any of the following:

- *Anger at the unfairness of getting the disease and at the cancer for causing pain, frightening everyone, and stealing part of childhood.* Spouses blame each other. Sick children get angry at their parents for not protecting them and at their siblings for being healthy. Siblings in turn get angry at the sick child for getting all the attention, for "ruining" their previously happy family life. Illogical as it may seem—and although parents may not realize what's behind their reaction—they get angry at the child for being in danger as well as for causing so much anguish and expense. The whole family is angry at other people who don't understand, who don't help, who are insensitive, and who can't deal with the cancer and abandon them. Much of their anger stems from fear.

- *Depression, which has been called "fear and anger turned inward."* Parents fear the loss of the child. They also may be frightened because they are used to protecting their children and "fixing" things for them but now feel helpless and, therefore, depressed. The depression may be expressed in obvious ways, such as sadness and crying, but it may also be shown in other ways that might not be immediately recognized as depression, such as irritability, insomnia, increased or decreased appetite, restlessness, boredom, and diminished sexual interest or physical energy (see Chapter 25, "Coping with Stress, Fear, Anxiety, and Depression").

- *Denial, which is a powerful tool that may or may not be healthy* (see Chapter 31, "Coping Strategies"). It can protect both parents and children from their feelings or cushion the shock of devastating news until they can gather the strength to deal with it, but denial may also prevent those who need help from getting it. Denial can be very dangerous in adolescents, who are at an age at which they feel immortal, if it leads them to refuse or discontinue treatment.

- *Grief not only because of the possibility of death but also for a lost carefree youth, physical well-being, innocence, simplicity in relationships.* A universal feeling among families is that "things will never be the same."

tion to overindulge a child who is seriously ill, doing so threatens the healthy development not only of the ill child but of other children in the family. Giving in to the sick child's every whim and tolerating misbehavior create resentment and may be a serious problem when the child recovers.

Age-Related Issues for Parents and Children

How parents handle their emotions is greatly influenced by the age of the child with cancer.

Infancy. Cancers that occur in the first year or two of life often have high cure rates, but they can cause parents special anxieties. They can't protect small infants from pain, can't help them cope with it through words of comfort or explanation, and can't emotionally or intellectually ease the way for them when they are about to have an uncomfortable diagnostic or treatment session.

Infants and very young children communicate pain or fear only by crying, and so parents have no way of determining whether the child has severe pain or is only frightened. Naturally, they often assume the worst.

Toddlers. Children aged 2 to 4 are beginning to be rebellious and are often stubborn. They often loudly and actively object to unpleasant events or situations such as examinations and treatment. This makes parents feel ineffective and uneasy, which tends to make the child's behavior worse. Paradoxically, separation from their mothers causes these independent children to suffer more than do younger, more dependent infants. Being in the hospital can produce strong reactions, ranging from lethargy to hysteria. Some toddlers may regress to infantile behavior.

By the age of 3 or 4, children are beginning to "wean away" from their mothers; their constant cry is, "I can do it myself!" Accordingly, they may become frustrated and bad tempered when illness interrupts this movement toward independence.

Young Children. By the time a child is about 7, his or her independence and life outside the home are well established, and so the life disruption of the illness may cause distress. By this time too the child is old enough to understand the gravity of the illness and its possible implications.

Older Children. By age 10 and throughout adolescence, physical appearance plays a significant role in the child's sense of self. For prepubescent and pubescent children, just the threat of hair loss, weight gain, or anything abnormal or attention getting—even something as innocuous, say, as a slight limp—can arouse a lot of anxiety and make them feel isolated.

Coping Skills and Support

Nothing in the normal experience of parents can prepare them for learning that their child has cancer, and not many have the skills needed for dealing with something so unexpected and so devastating. Even friends and relatives cannot really understand what parents are going through. This is why the most helpful people are often those who are undergoing or have gone through

How Parents Cope: Test Yourself

Studies of how parents deal with childhood cancer have revealed a number of strategies, some healthy and some ineffective. To see how you handle such a situation, try taking the following test:

Circle the number of each statement that describes you:

1. For me, laughing is a good way to keep from feeling bad.

2. I notice people around who are worse off than we are.

3. I get easily provoked and fight with those around me.

4. It is important for me to learn what I can do about my child's illness.

5. I refuse to believe this has happened.

6. I turn to someone else for emotional support.

7. I stay busy to keep myself from worrying about things.

8. I go over the problem again and again in my mind to try to understand it.

9. I won't go somewhere if my child's illness will be the topic of conversation.

10. Although I never asked for this, as a result of this experience, I found new faith or some important truth about life.

Scoring. Give yourself one point each if you circled items 1, 2, 4, 6, 7, and 10. Deduct one point each for a circle on items 3, 5, 8, and 9. Hardly anybody gets a perfect score (6). But the higher your score is, the better your coping tactics are. A low or negative score indicates that you could benefit from support or counseling.

the same experience. Parents of children with cancer, who often feel separated and disconnected from others, can therefore benefit greatly from parent support groups. They'll find reassurance that it is normal and acceptable to be angry, to grieve in anticipation, and to feel unable to deal with the pain. This "validation" is considered by many experts to be essential to emotional balance in such situations. A support group provides a safe place for parents to "let go" from time to time, to stop putting on the brave front that needs to be presented to the sick child and other children, and to cry or express anger. Sharing practical experiences—negotiating the health care system, finding ancillary support (home tutoring, for example, or correspondence courses), or finding a good source for children's wigs—also is helpful (see Chapter 13, "Your Support Network").

In addition, supportive relatives; strong spiritual, religious, or philosophical beliefs; and a willingness to ask for and accept emotional and practical help from others can enhance parents' coping skills. Those families that seem to cope best are flexible in adapting to disrupted schedules, financial pressures, and family conflicts. They try to plan for potential problems rather than let events overtake them by surprise, and they understand that there is much to learn about the meaning of life from this painful experience. (See Chapter 32, "Issues for Families and Friends.")

Families who have difficulty mobilizing their resources may benefit from the support of social workers who are part of the treatment team in most pediatric centers. These specialists can help establish an open and trusting relationship among family members that allows important issues to be addressed. Counseling may be provided at the treatment center or by referral to mental health professionals elsewhere.

Communicating with Children

Explaining cancer to children helps make them less anxious, because without information, their imaginations run wild. Informed children seem to comply better with the demands of treatment, and honest communication creates a better relationship between parents and child.

Before telling your child that he or she has cancer, you may want to consult first with counselors and advisers. These experts can suggest, for example, different ways of communicating—depending on the child's age, level of development, and ability to understand information about illness, which may be very different from what you think.

Talk Openly with Health Care Providers

Speaking easily and clearly with children begins with a good understanding between parents and medical staff. If you are confused or misinformed, if your understanding of the diagnosis, treatment, and the most likely outcome is mistaken, then what you communicate to the child also will be wrong. And if you fear the worst and have preconceived, pessimistic notions about cancer, your discussions with your sick child will be far too negative and anxiety provoking.

Early and open exchanges of information with the treatment team will give you greater control over the situation and allow you to make rational decisions, anticipate some of the side effects of treatment and other problems, and discuss these matters more clearly and confidently with your child.

Parents who can learn how and when to ask for help and are able to form a trusting relationship with members of the treatment team are better able to deal with the medical and emotional crises of childhood cancer and nurture the family's strength and hope.

What to Say to a Child

Because not enough is known about children's understanding of cancer, there are no guidelines for deciding who should tell the child and what that person should say. Parents should be aware that there is no established right or wrong way to handle this matter.

What is said to the child depends on his or her age. A 3-year-old can't be expected to grasp the concept of unrestricted cell division or the principles of cancer chemotherapy. An 8-year-old may be satisfied by a simple description of a procedure to be done, but an older child will want to know why the test or treatment is necessary. It may be better to discuss the details of treatments, procedures, schedules, and other concrete matters than to communicate the seriousness of the disease and how long it may be a problem. Young children in particular may cope with illness better and have more motivation for recovery if they don't realize how serious their disease is.

Using metaphors or stories as explanations doesn't necessarily help children handle medical information and may even create more problems than it solves. For example, a child may be told that her body is like a garden and that the bad cells are like weeds crowding out the good cells, the flowers. Certain children at certain ages may find this a familiar and comfortable notion, but another child at another age may believe that this literally means that weeds are growing inside her.

It helps to take your cue from your child. For example, some children enjoy the doctor, nurse, and patient dolls and toys sometimes used to help "act out" an explanation of illness. But others may not like this kind of play, and they shouldn't be pressured into it; other ways can be found for them, perhaps with the help of social workers, nurses, or other parents who have been through this difficult experience.

School and Social Issues

More than 80 percent of children with cancer have to leave school at least temporarily. Some miss short periods that can be made up with homework or tutoring, whereas others may be held back as much as a year. Most children know that everybody goes to school and that it is essential to normal life. It is important, therefore, to talk as early as possible about the interruption in schooling and especially what plans are being made for getting back on track. Even if parents are preoccupied with more immediate demands and worries, their children's first reactions to their illness will include concerns about missing school, falling behind their friends, and how they will look when they go back. If parents and others don't talk and act as if school attendance is important, a child may think that everyone has given up.

Get Outside Help

To deal with school issues, parents would be wise to consult the treatment team or other professionals promptly. They or the parents may need to talk to the school authorities about how to fit the schedule of treatment appointments into the child's school requirements.

Many pediatric cancer centers include hospital teachers as part of the pediatric cancer team. Along with social workers and nurses, such teachers can gauge the children's learning level and help prepare for the return to school following discharge from the hospital. Children should be asked whether they want someone to explain the situation to their classmates. Some would rather do it themselves. Some treatment centers have school visiting programs in which members of the treatment team go to the school and meet with the sick child's teachers, nurse, class, or student assembly.

In any case, parents should try to arrange some regular contact with their child's school and classmates, through homework assignments, exchanges of letters or cards, and visits from friends, teachers, and school counselors.

Many fully accredited colleges have correspondence courses that allow students to earn credits toward both high school and college degrees. (Information can be obtained from individual colleges or *The Independent Study Catalogue,* available in most public libraries, or *Peterson's Guides,* P.O. Box 2123, Princeton, NJ 08540.)

Going Back to School

Returning to school can be painful and difficult, because of fears about seeing teachers and friends again and worry over what people will think. Children are apprehensive about their appearance and about being behind everyone else in schoolwork. Having to miss days repeatedly because of medical appointments makes them feel different from their classmates. Young people can be surprisingly cruel, intentionally or not, and children should be prepared for awkward questions, stares, snubs, and a variety of potentially hurtful encounters.

Know Your Rights

Continuing symptoms or the demands of treatment may require a prolonged absence from school. Some local boards of education provide tutoring; some treatment centers have school programs for children; or private tutors can be arranged.

It is important to know that the federal "Education for All the Handicapped" law requires the states to provide education for handicapped people between 3 and 21, including those with cancer. Even so, it may be up to the parents to persuade school authorities that cancer constitutes a handicap for their child. It requires that an individual education plan be developed for the child and that those who physically cannot get to school be educated. If the physician signs a certificate of need, the school system should (in some states it *must*) provide home teachers, sometimes with the additional help of telephone conferences, closed-circuit television, or computer programs. The law also mandates training for both regular and special-education teachers in handling handicaps.

Loss and Grief

Perhaps at no time during a child's illness with cancer is it more important for families to maintain a close and constant relationship with the health care team than when it becomes clear the child is not going to recover. You will need help in accepting the terrible fact so that you can begin to deal with its reality and confront some extremely difficult decisions. Perhaps the most difficult choice is whether to try even more aggressive therapy or to turn to palliative care—that is, to end therapy directed toward cure as gently as possible while continuing to provide every bit of pain relief and other comforts the child may need or want. (See Chapter 34, "Supportive Care.") It is a time when it is most valuable to be able to talk about what is going to happen, deal with practical problems, and begin the process of mourning.

Evaluating Care Options

An important issue is whether the child should leave the hospital, go to a hospice, or have hospice care at home. Many families have found that having the child at home is rewarding and comforting for all, if they can manage the required care. Taking care of the child and maintaining as normal a home life as possible helps ease the family's emotional stress and discomfort. Even if the treatment has ended, the child may feel relatively well and need no elaborate medical care. Being at home allows the child to enjoy the good moments when they come along, surrounded by caring family in a familiar place. Schooling and social life may even continue for some time. However, it is wise to discuss with a counselor any disadvantages of home care, such as later associating the home always with the child's death.

Bereavement

It is almost universally agreed that the loss of a child is the most painful thing a parent can experience. The traditional pattern of grief and healing that follows the death of another loved person does not apply. Parents may continue to grieve and have difficulty coping with their loss far longer, and they may have trouble talking about their loss, controlling sudden unexpected feelings of sadness, planning for the future, and dealing with other family members.

Bereavement support services provide help not only for parents but also for siblings and other family members who are touched by the loss. Often, counseling and support groups are sponsored by hospitals, cancer organizations, social service agencies, hospices, counseling centers, or religious institutions (see Appendix I, "Resources").

Healing

Each parent has his or her own way of reacting and trying to cope with something that seems unbearable, but certain approaches seem to offer solace and direction. Strong religious, spiritual, or philosophical beliefs allow many parents to come to terms with a child's death. Here are some suggestions some parents have found to be helpful.

TIPS &
ADVICE

- Create something new for your child, especially something beautiful or lasting, such as music, a painting, or a garden.

- Live as fully as possible, in recognition of how precious life is and as a memorial to your child.

- Work toward realizing your greatest potential, being the best person you can be, or finding satisfaction in achievement other than parenthood.

- Dedicate yourself to a cause, especially one related to the child's death, such as doing volunteer work at a children's hospital or some other activity designed to leave the world a better place.

AIDS-Related Cancers

Acquired immune deficiency syndrome (AIDS) is a devastating illness in which the white blood cells, or *lymphocytes,* are destroyed by the *human immunodeficiency virus (HIV),* also known as the human T-cell lymphotropic virus III, or HTLV-III. This situation is sometimes referred to as *immunosuppression.* People with AIDS are susceptible to deadly infections of virtually every tissue in the body, especially the skin, lungs, gastrointestinal tract, and central nervous system, including the brain. And they are not able to defend themselves against certain cancers.

Ironically, now that people infected with the HIV virus are living longer, the incidence of cancer among them is increasing. About 40 percent of people with AIDS also develop certain forms of cancer, such as Kaposi's sarcoma, various lymphomas, or cervical cancer. Because a full discussion of AIDS and its treatment is beyond the scope of this brief chapter, we will concentrate mostly on the occurrence and treatment of AIDS-related cancers.

What Is AIDS?

Although some cases probably occurred earlier, the first AIDS cases were officially diagnosed in 1981. As knowledge of the disease has increased over the years, its definition has evolved.

In most cases, HIV is transmitted through the exchange of body fluids (blood, semen, and vaginal secretions), as happens with sexual intercourse or through the use of shared needles during intravenous drug use. Certain sexual practices, such as receptive anal sex, increase the risk that the virus will penetrate delicate or torn tissues. Pregnant women can pass the virus to the growing fetus. And people may be infected if they receive a transfusion of HIV-contaminated blood. However, since 1985 all blood donors have been screened for HIV, and the risk of getting HIV from blood has been almost completely eliminated.

The terms *HIV* and *AIDS* are not synonymous. People whose blood tests reveal the presence of the virus are told they are *HIV positive* (i.e., that they are carrying the virus), but they may not develop any symptoms or AIDS-related diseases for as long as 10 years. Gradually, however, as the virus continues to obliterate immune cells (specifically the T4 or CD4 lymphocytes of the white blood cells), these people become vulnerable to infection.

Because people may be HIV positive and not know it, and they don't feel sick, they may unknowingly pass the virus on to other people. Once symptoms of infection appear, such people are said to have AIDS.

A diagnosis of AIDS is made when a person (1) is HIV positive and has a low T4-lymphocyte count (fewer than 200 per cubic millimeter) and (2) has an infection or disease usually associated with AIDS, which is sometimes called an indicative disease.

The U.S. Public Health Service estimated that by 1994, there were 1 million HIV-positive people in this country and approximately 442,000 diagnosed cases of AIDS. Since it was first identified, AIDS has killed between 270,000 and 400,000 Americans. It is estimated that 20 to 25 percent of all HIV-infected people will develop some form of cancer.

The trends are as frightening as the numbers. AIDS has become the fourth leading cause of death among women aged 25 to 44, and the incidence of the disease is rising faster among women than among men. It also is increasing

Indicative Diseases Associated with AIDS

- Cancer
    - Kaposi's sarcoma
    - Lymphoma
    - Non-Hodgkin's lymphoma
    - Hodgkin's disease
    - Primary central nervous system lymphoma
    - Cervical cancer
- Pneumonia (especially recurrent bacterial pneumonia)
- *Pneumocystis carinii* pneumonia
- Tuberculosis
- Salmonella blood poisoning
- Blindness caused by cytomegalovirus
- Fungal infections caused by *Candida,* a nonpulmonary *Cryptococcus mycobacterium* avium
- Gastrointestinal disorders (e.g., cryptosporidiosis with persistent diarrhea)
- Severe viral infection of the brain (*progressive multifocal leukoencephalopathy*)

CANCER
BASICS

among adolescent girls: The disease affects 4.2 girls in 1,000, compared with 2.0 boys in 1,000. AIDS is the sixth leading cause of death among 15- to 24-year-olds in the United States. Although AIDS is usually perceived to be a disease of homosexuals, the proportion of cases of heterosexual transmission rose from 2 to 9 percent between 1985 and 1993.

There also has been a rapid increase among intravenous drug users. One estimate found that three-quarters of the 40,000 new HIV infections reported in 1994 occurred in this group.

The rate among minorities also is rising. Between 1989 and 1994, the incidence among gay African-American men rose from 21 cases to more than 37 cases per 100,000, an increase of 79 percent. (In the South, there was a 109 percent increase.) Among Latinos during the same period, the rate rose by 61 percent, from 14 to 23 cases per 100,000. Meanwhile, the incidence among Caucasians appears to be decreasing.

Although the *proportion* of AIDS cases arising from homosexual contact declined from 66 to 47 percent between 1985 and 1993 in the United States, the highest rate of transmission continues to be among this population. Between 1989 and 1994, the actual *number* of cases of AIDS in this group rose by 31 percent.

AIDS and Cancer

Certain cancers occur so often in AIDS that they are considered part of the definition of the disease. In fact, one of the first signs that this new illness had emerged was the sudden increase in the incidence of Kaposi's sarcoma. Previously, this uncommon skin cancer had afflicted primarily elderly Jewish men from central Europe. Then, in the early 1980s, there was a sudden increase in reported cases, mostly among young gay men. Today there is an upsurge in Kaposi's sarcoma and lymphoma coinciding with the start of the AIDS epidemic.

The other two cancers whose presence indicates the progression to AIDS in an HIV-positive person are aggressive lymphoma of the central nervous system and cervical cancer. People with AIDS do not seem to develop other cancers—such as breast, colon, or lung cancer—in greater numbers than does the general population. However, because of the breakdown of normal immune protection, there are reports that those with ARC (AIDS-related cancer) have more aggressive forms of cancer than the general population. Their treatment is directed at relieving or curing the cancer while AIDS therapy continues.

Scientists are not sure how immunosuppression resulting from HIV infection leads to cancer, but there are several theories. The most likely explanation is that HIV is easily able to attach itself to a protein on the surface of the T4 lymphocytes, penetrating and destroying them. As their number is depleted, their ability to take part in the complex immune response is diminished. Because its defense system has failed, the body becomes more prone to the development of cancer and more vulnerable to infections.

Factors other than immunosuppression may be involved. For example, some people may be born with genes that make them more susceptible to illnesses like Kaposi's sarcoma. There may be an organism (for example, a herpeslike virus) that causes Kaposi's sarcoma that is transmitted sexually along with HIV. Similarly, Epstein-Barr virus (EBV) may contribute to lymphoma, and human papillomavirus (HPV), the virus that causes genital warts, is implicated in cervical cancer (see Chapter 9, "Who Gets Cancer?").

Other immune deficiency conditions besides AIDS also pose an increased risk of cancer. These include organ transplantation (because of the need for immunosuppressive drugs to prevent rejection of the organ) and congenital immune abnormalities. But because of the association between AIDS—an infectious disease—and certain cancers, many people are afraid that they might catch cancer through casual contact (see Chapter 1, "What Is Cancer?"). This mistaken notion increases the stigma of the disease, further isolating those with AIDS and contributing needlessly to their suffering. Cancer is not a contagious illness. Rather, people with AIDS develop cancers because their immune system cannot launch a defense against abnormal cells.

Treatment of AIDS

At this time, there is no cure for AIDS, nor is there an effective vaccine. Still, treatment can provide some benefits, including symptom relief and improved quality of life, and, with the newest drug regimens, possibly life can be extended considerably. A drug called AZT (zidovudine) was the first agent developed to reduce the levels of HIV in the blood, increase the levels of T4 cells, and relieve some symptoms. Clinical trials show that early treatment of HIV infection slows the onset of AIDS-related diseases. AZT also appears to reduce the risk of dementia and of mother-to-fetus transmission.

Recently, the focus in AIDS treatment has been on combining different drugs to achieve better results. For example, the addition of a new class of drugs called *protease inhibitors* may reverse the course of the disease, either by destroying HIV or boosting the immune response against infection. The early results of these drugs and combinations of them are encouraging. On occasion, the virus can be reduced to an undetectable level. One concern is that the AIDS virus appears to evolve rapidly. That is, a drug that is effective today may not work against a new strain that emerges tomorrow.

The best measure is prevention, such as practicing safer sex (including using condoms) and not sharing needles when injecting drugs.

Since AIDS cannot yet be eliminated, the targets of treatment are the ailments that accompany it. Antibiotics, for example, address recurring pneumonia or gastrointestinal problems, and antifungal medications relieve fungal infections. As described later, surgery, chemotherapy, and radiation therapy are sometimes used separately or in combination to treat AIDS-related cancers.

If you have AIDS and develop cancer, you may want to consult with an AIDS oncologist. You may also want to consider looking into one of the many clinical trials evaluating new chemotherapy agents and biological therapies (see Chapter 21, "Investigational Treatments").

Kaposi's Sarcoma (KS)

In the early 1980s, Kaposi's sarcoma occurred in about 40 percent of AIDS cases. For unknown reasons, the rate has fallen, and today the incidence is around 14 percent. About 95 percent of AIDS-KS cases occur in homosexual or bisexual men.

Signs and Symptoms

Before AIDS, Kaposi's sarcoma was considered a disease of elderly men, one that produced purple, red, or brown *lesions,* sometimes called *plaques,* on the skin, usually on the lower legs. This classic form of Kaposi's is not usually life threatening (see "Bone and Connective Tissue" in the Encyclopedia).

AIDS-KS is different. The average age of onset is about 34. The tumors are widespread and often affect the skin on the trunk, arms, head, and neck; the mucous membranes of the mouth or genitals; and internal structures (the gastrointestinal tract and lungs). In fact, KS can affect all tissues, though rarely the brain.

The symptoms depend on where the lesions are. Swollen lymph nodes are common. Some people experience pain in the chest, stomach, or rectum. There may be loss of blood, diarrhea, cramps, weight loss, shortness of breath, fever, and cough. Although most cases of AIDS-KS occur in men, the women with this cancer tend to have more aggressive disease of internal organs.

AIDS-KS can progress rapidly, involving extensive areas. How long a person with AIDS can survive with KS depends on such factors as the severity of other symptoms (including opportunistic infection) and on the T4–lymphocyte cell counts. One study found that people with AIDS who had KS alone and high T4 counts (<lt>300) survived for 32 months. Those with no other symptoms and lower counts survived for 24 months, and those with symptoms and counts below 200 survived for one year.

Treatment

Occasionally, people with AIDS-KS survive many years with little or no treatment. Usually, if the disease appears to progress slowly or is localized, no therapy is required for cosmetic reasons.

Lesions can be removed by cryotherapy (freezing) or direct injections of chemotherapeutic agents (see Chapters 15, "Surgery," and 17, "Chemotherapy"). Lesions located on such areas as the palms, face, or mouth usually respond to radiation therapy (see Chapter 16, "Radiation"). Low doses of radiation can prevent the oral side effects—dry mouth, infections, and changes in taste. There is a risk also that radiation will cause the skin to darken (*hyperpigmentation*). In such cases, surgery or injections with a minute quantity of vincristine (Oncovin), vinblastine (Velban), or alpha-interferon (see Chapter 18, "Biological Therapies") may be the alternative.

People with AIDS-KS who have a high T4 count and no current opportunistic infections may get better and live longer with high doses of biological response modifiers, specifically recombinant alpha-interferon. Interferon plus AZT (zidovudine) seems to produce even better results.

If the sarcoma is widespread in the viscera or is progressing rapidly, systemic chemotherapy with vinblastine, alone or alternating with vincristine, may produce some improvement in about one-third of cases. Other systemic agents include etoposide (VePesid), bleomycin (Blenoxane), and doxorubicin (Adriamycin). Combination therapy with doxorubicin, bleomycin (Blenoxane), and vincristine is helpful about 80 percent of the time, but the benefit is usually limited to six to 12 months.

Non-Hodgkin's Lymphoma

Because AIDS assaults the cells of the lymphatic system, it is not surprising that people with AIDS are apt to develop one of the various lymphomas, or cancers of the lymph system. Non-Hodgkin's lymphoma (NHL) is the most common form of these cancers in people with HIV (see "Non-Hodgkin's Lymphoma" in the Encyclopedia). Estimates are that about 3 percent of people with AIDS develop NHL, a rate that is between 60 and 100 times that of the general population. Women with AIDS develop lymphomas at a slightly lower rate than men do. The longer a person with AIDS survives, the more likely it is that he or she will develop lymphoma.

Scientists believe that the Epstein-Barr virus is involved in many B-cell lymphomas, but its exact role in AIDS-related lymphoma is not clear. Perhaps the presence of both EBV and HIV causes abnormal B cells to proliferate.

Signs and Symptoms

The lymphoma usually emerges some time after other AIDS complications, such as Kaposi's sarcoma, and is already well advanced (stage III or IV) when it is diagnosed. Or the lymphoma may be present but is not detected until after death. Symptoms include painless swelling in the lymph nodes, persistent fever, night sweats, fatigue, weight loss, and itchy skin.

Most AIDS-related lymphomas are classified like other lymphomas, but the intermediate or high grade predominates. This means that it grows faster and is more likely to spread to other places outside the lymph nodes, especially the central nervous system, bone marrow, gastrointestinal tract, and liver.

Treatment

People with the disease respond to treatment differently from people with NHL who do not have AIDS. They receive lower doses of drugs, because these agents often are immunosuppressive and can compromise the body's defense mechanism still further and increase the chance of infection.

The standard approach is systemic chemotherapy with the regimen known as M-BACOD (methotrexate, bleomycin, cytosine arabinoside, cyclophosphamide [Cytoxan], vincristine, and doxorubicin). Lower than usual doses of this combination chemotherapy have recently shown in clinical trials to have similar efficacy but fewer complications, such as low white cell count and infection. Some evidence suggests that adding granulocyte macrophage colony–stimulating factor (GM–CSF) to the CHOP regimen (doxorubicin, vincristine, and prednisone) is also beneficial, but the chemotherapy has not extended survival time. In addition to drugs, external-beam radiation is also used to treat either the bulky tumor or lymphoma in central nervous system cells.

Unfortunately, people with AIDS-related NHL do not usually respond well to treatment, and relapse is common. In about half the cases, death is due directly to the lymphoma.

Primary Central Nervous System Lymphoma (PCL)

AIDS-related PCL, a non-Hodgkin's lymphatic cancer that has started in the brain (see "Brain" in the Encyclopedia), occurs in about 6 percent of AIDS cases.

Signs and Symptoms

PCL typically emerges late in the course of the HIV infection. The symptoms include headache, palsy (shaking), and seizures, along with changes in mental ability or personality. Brain scans show lesions pressing on a delicate part of the brain.

Treatment

The standard treatment is radiation therapy to the whole brain, along with corticosteroid medication. About half the patients do not respond to therapy, and their survival time is about one to six months. Survival is longer in those who do respond, but remission typically does not last long. Chemotherapy is complicated by the fact that many cancer drugs cannot penetrate the brain's protective membrane.

Hodgkin's Disease

Hodgkin's disease (HD) is a form of lymphoma that probably affects the lymphocytes, allowing certain ones to proliferate. It occurs at about the same rate in people with AIDS as in people without HIV, but it tends to be more aggressive in the AIDS group and to produce a somewhat different clinical picture (see "Hodgkin's Disease" in the Encyclopedia).

Signs and Symptoms

About 85 percent of AIDS-related HD cases are diagnosed at a more advanced stage III or IV, compared with 40 percent in the general population. AIDS-related HD is more likely to involve the bone marrow or to spread to unusual sites, such as the lung, gastrointestinal tract, and skin.

Treatment

The treatment is the same as that for people who do not have AIDS.

Cervical Cancer

It has long been known that sexually transmitted diseases, such as herpes and genital warts, can make women susceptible to precancerous cervical abnormalities (*dysplasia*) and cervical cancer. Women who are HIV positive have ten times the risk of developing cervical lesions as do women in the general population. In 1993, the Centers for Disease Control, recognizing the high incidence of cervical cancer among HIV-positive women, added this cancer to its list of AIDS-defining diseases. Many experts now believe that whenever cervical lesions are detected, the patient should also be tested for HIV infection.

The exact cause of AIDS-related cervical cancer isn't known. However, some studies have found that women with HIV (who by definition are immuno-suppressed) are also very likely to be severely infected with human papillo-mavirus (HPV), which is a suspected risk factor for cervical cancer (see Chapter 10, "Cancer Causes and Risks"). If these findings are confirmed, it may be that HIV allows HPV to flourish, which in turn leads to cervical lesions.

Fortunately, when detected early, cervical dysplasia and cervical cancer can often be cured (see "Cervix" in the Encyclopedia).

Psychological Implications

About one-fifth of the people with AIDS die of cancer, especially lymphoma or Kaposi's sarcoma. An essential aspect of treatment is supportive care. People with AIDS must cope not just with the pain and suffering but also with their emotional response to a shortened life. Making matters worse, they are often shunned and isolated because of other people's ignorance or fear of the disease. Because AIDS frequently spreads by means of sexual practices or IV drug use, it raises questions of morality and responsibility. Many families and even health care providers thus confront personal issues when dealing with people with AIDS, such as coming to terms with homosexuality or drug addiction. Financial problems are an added complication, because many with AIDS lose their jobs and consequently their health care. Some are even evict-ed from their homes. And in a terrible irony, although new AIDS treatments are available, their cost is beyond the reach of many people who would ben-efit from them.

The point is that, given the broader picture, the plan of cancer treatment for people with AIDS must include consideration of these realities.

A person with AIDS with a poor prognosis needs to be made as comfort-able as possible, physically and emotionally. Whenever feasible, care should be provided at home with hospice support or in a hospice (see Chapter 34, "Supportive Care"). Psychological and spiritual counseling services may be of enormous benefit in helping such people come to grips with their situation. Friends and families can take advantage of these services. Community sup-port networks may be activated to ease the enormous emotional, physical, and financial burdens of caring for people with AIDS. However, many experts believe that for better treatment, a person with AIDS who has a good prog-nosis might consider an experimental program.

The greatest lesson of the AIDS epidemic may well be that in the end love, support, compassion, and faith are the most important medicines of all.

AN ENCYCLOPEDIA OF COMMON AND UNCOMMON CANCERS

HOW TO USE THIS ENCYCLOPEDIA

Cancer is a disease with at least 100 different forms, depending on where it begins and the tissues and cells involved. The previous chapters provide information applicable to all types of cancer. This Encyclopedia discusses individual cancers specifically. You will find all the relevant information here about the cancer that concerns you. To use the Encyclopedia sections to best advantage, it is important to read the following instructions first:

- Most of the cancers are arranged by site (that is, where they initially occur in the body, such as the skin, breast, kidney, and so on). The sites are organized by physiologic system. To look for a particular cancer, consult the index at the back of the book. In general, the cancers that occur within a particular organ system are grouped together. Thus, for example, all the cancers that affect the digestive system—esophagus, stomach, colon and rectum, liver, gallbladder and bile ducts—are discussed one after the other. Of course, some cancers affect an entire system or a type of tissue found throughout the body. In these cases, the diseases are listed by their proper names: leukemia, Hodgkin's disease, multiple myeloma, and so on. These systemwide cancers are presented first.

- Each Encyclopedia section is organized similarly, beginning with a general introduction about cancers of that kind or in that particular site. In most cases an illustration will help you understand the basic anatomy involved. Additional categories of information include:

  Who Is at Risk?, which describes characteristics common to people who get the cancer.

  Screening Tests, which include any procedures that tend to be routinely provided to large numbers of people, whether or not your doctor suspects cancer (such as mammography for breast tumors or PSA test for prostate cancer); details about screening tests are provided at length in Chapters 5 and 6. You will be told where to turn if you want more information.

  Types of Cancer, including all varieties that originate at that site.

Signs and Symptoms, through which the cancer may give warning.

Diagnostic and Staging Tests, meaning those that will determine definitively whether cancer is present, where precisely, and its level of development. Because many of these tests are used to diagnose and stage different cancers, details are provided in Chapter 8.

Tests Unique to the Cancer, providing complete descriptions of the procedures, which are discussed in no other place in the book.

Staging, or level of development of the cancer, which is important to you because treatment recommendations are typically based on the stage of disease. In most cases, the staging is based on the American Joint Committee on Cancer TNM system. *T* indicates the size or invasiveness of the tumor. *N* means the number, size, and location of lymph nodes involved. *M* indicates the presence of metastasis (see Chapter 2, "The Language of Cancer").

Treatment, including recommended individual and combination therapies, for all stages of disease. Investigational or experimental therapies are found in "Ask About" (see later).

Survival, giving prognostic projections of the likelihood of surviving five years with a cancer diagnosed at a particular stage and treated with the standard therapy recommended at the time these statistical analyses were made. At best, these are very generalized estimates, which may give you an idea of the aggressiveness of the disease, but *they do not accurately predict how long any individual will live.*

Special Needs, alerting you to services you will require or want or issues to consider, such as diet.

Ask About, alerting you to any emerging treatments, controversies, and clinical trials, which will enable you to communicate most effectively with your doctors.

• The Encyclopedia entries provide information in lists and short paragraphs, with numerous cross references to earlier chapters in the book. Do not be alarmed if you do not understand what a particular test or procedure or term means; if you see a chapter reference or page number, turn to it for all relevant details and instructions or for additional information that you may find useful.

ACUTE LEUKEMIA

Leukemias are cancers of the blood-forming system, which includes the bone marrow and the lymphatic system. They account for about 2 percent of all cancers. Because leukemia is the most common form of childhood cancer, it is often thought of as a disease of childhood. However, leukemia of all types affects nine times as many adults as children. Half the cases occur in people over the age of 60, and the incidence among the elderly is increasing. The incidence of acute and chronic leukemia is about the same.

Acute leukemia affects the bone marrow, disrupting the blood cells' maturation and causing immature ones to proliferate rapidly. These immature cells crowd out mature white blood cells. In time, abnormal cells accumulate in various organs and tissues, disrupting their normal functions. In the bone marrow, the proliferation of abnormal white blood cells interferes with the production of red blood cells and platelets. Without an adequate supply of mature cells in the blood, the body loses much of its ability to combat infection and the person is at risk of developing anemia or internal bleeding.

The cause of leukemia is unknown, although there appear to be some links to genetic abnormalities. Viral infection may predispose a person to leukemia, and exposure to excessive radiation and certain chemicals may induce leukemia many years later.

Advances in treatment have improved the survival rate enormously. Today about half of people with leukemia survive five years or more after diagnosis.

Red and white blood cells and platelets originate in the bone marrow. Some of these cells mature in the marrow; others migrate through blood vessels and lymph channels to various organs, where they mature.

About half of blood is *plasma*, a pale yellow fluid that is mostly water. The rest consists of cells with specific purposes: erythrocytes, or *red cells*, which carry oxygen from the lungs to tissues throughout the body; *platelets*, which help form clots; and *leukocytes*, or *white cells*, which protect the body against infection. All these cells are derived from stem cells in the bone marrow. Among stem cells are those that develop into *proerythroblasts*, which eventually become red blood cells; *lymphoblasts*, which become lymphocytes; and *myeloblasts* and *monoblasts*, which form different types of white blood cells.

Most types of leukemia cause production of abnormal white blood cells, called *blast cells*. Because blood circulates throughout the body, leukemia affects virtually all tissues.

Who Is at Risk?

- Acute lymphoid leukemia (ALL) is more common among Caucasians than among African-Americans; while acute myeloid leukemia (AML) affects Caucasians and African-Americans equally. Men develop acute leukemia slightly more often than women;

- People of Jewish ancestry are slightly more likely to have leukemia than others;

- People who have prolonged exposure to high doses of radiation, including x-rays;

- People with prolonged exposure to toxic organic chemicals, such as benzene;

- People with a history of other diseases that damage bone marrow, such as aplastic anemia or myelofibrosis;

- People who have a history of other cancers of the lymphatic system;

- Those who have used such drugs as the antibiotic chloramphenicol; anticancer medications, including those used in treatment of Hodgkin's disease; and immunosuppressants.

Screening Tests

There are no screening tests. Early detection is difficult and usually occurs by chance during a routine physical examination.

Types of Acute Leukemia

Many people with leukemia do not know they have it until the late stages of the disease when symptoms occur. Acute leukemia rarely produces visible or painful tumors. Instead the proliferation of immature blood cells keeps the blood and other organs from carrying out their functions.

Acute leukemias are divided into types and subtypes, depending on which cells fail to mature.

Acute Myeloid Leukemia

About 80 percent of adult acute leukemias are of the myeloid type. On average, the incidence of AML ranges from one per 100,000 among people under 30 to 14 per 100,000 in those over 75. AML (also called *acute myelogenous*, *acute myeloblastic*, and *acute granulocytic leukemia*) affects white blood cells that contain distinctive *particles* or *granules*, which appear as beadlike sacs under the microscope and contain enzymes, histamine, and other substances. Researchers have identified at least seven subtypes of AML, including *acute myelogenous* or *myeloblastic*, *acute monocytic* or *monoblastic* (AMOL), *acute myelomonocytic* (AMML), and *acute promyelocytic* (APL).

About 25 percent of people with AML have serious infections, and about 33 percent have bruising or hemorrhage when the diagnosis is made.

The spleen or liver enlarges in less than one out of four cases. Lymph node swelling is even less frequent. Many people with leukemia complain about shortness of breath, which usually results from a secondary lung infection, such as pneumonia.

In rare cases people with AML develop solid masses of leukemia cells called *granulocytic sarcomas*. These masses usually occur in the skin or bones (especially the *sternum* or breast bone, ribs, or eye sockets), but they may involve any organ, especially the breasts, ovaries, or testicles. In severe cases of AML, distinctive spots may appear on the retina.

At the time of diagnosis, perhaps two cases out of 100 involve the central nervous system (brain and spinal cord), causing neurologic problems, including vomiting and headaches. People with AML may develop heart problems, such as murmurs, congestive heart failure, and abnormal rhythms. These conditions are usually a consequence of problems with red blood cells, such as anemia.

Acute Lymphoid Leukemia

An estimated 20 percent of adult acute leukemias are of the lymphoid type. ALL (also called *acute lymphocytic* and *lymphoblastic leukemia*) affects white blood cells that are characterized by an absence of particles or granules. It is the most common childhood cancer (see Chapter 35, "Cancer in Children").

At the time of diagnosis, people with ALL, especially children, may complain of pain in the bones or joints. About one out of three have infection or hemorrhage, and half have swelling of the lymph nodes, spleen, or liver. Chest x-rays reveal a mass in the thymus in about 15 percent of cases. Central nervous system problems arise in 5 to 10 percent of adults with ALL, causing palsy, headache, or pressure on the optic nerve.

Other Types

Erythroleukemia affects red blood cells, precursor cells, or procrythroblasts. The paradoxical name (also called *red leukemia*) indicates that this form of leukemia disrupts the maturation process of red cells.

Myelodysplastic syndrome (MDS) is a preleukemic blood disorder that develops into AML in about half of cases. Some experts regard MDS as an early stage of leukemia.

Signs and Symptoms

If a person with leukemia experiences any symptoms, they are usually vague and nonspecific. The more common are:

- Generalized weakness and fatigue;
- Fever;
- Weight loss;
- Frequent infections;
- Easy bruising;
- Bleeding of gums or nose;
- Blood in urine or stools;
- Paleness;
- Enlarged lymph glands, liver, and/or spleen;
- Abdominal fullness;
- Bone pain;
- Headaches;
- Skin rash;
- Breast masses.

Diagnostic and Staging Tests

(For more details on the following tests, see Chapter 8, "Diagnostic Tests.")

- Physical examination to detect enlarged lymph nodes, swollen gums, enlarged liver or spleen, bruises, small pinpoint red rashes (petechiae);
- Blood tests, including a complete blood count, blood typing, blood chemistry, and coagulation studies;

- Urine test;
- Bone marrow test and/or biopsy;
- Lumbar puncture;
- Antibody tests to determine immune status;
- Immunologic tissue typing (see Chapter 19, "Bone Marrow Transplant");
- Blood typing of the person with leukemia and of family members willing to serve as blood or bone marrow donors.

Tests Unique to Acute Leukemia

- Bone marrow test or fine-needle aspiration;
- Bone marrow biopsy;
- Chromosomal or DNA analysis of the bone marrow to identify the type of leukemia and to look for the presence of the Philadelphia chromosome and other chromosomal abnormalities (see "Survival");
- Blood work-up with special stains to determine unique features of the blood cells involved.

Staging

There is no staging system for the acute leukemias.

Treatment

Treatment depends on whether the leukemia is untreated, in remission (controlled by treatment), or relapsed (the leukemia has returned after a period of remission).

Chemotherapy to relieve symptoms and achieve a complete and long-term remission is the standard treatment. Typically, the oncologist combines two to five drugs in three or four phases (see Chapter 17, "Chemotherapy").

Acute Myeloid Leukemia

Therapy for AML may also occur in phases, but the effectiveness of consolidation chemotherapy and maintenance chemotherapy is not as predictable as it is for ALL.

Induction Chemotherapy. Intravenous treatment with daunorubicin (Cerubidine) for several days followed with cytarabine (Cytosar-U) for a few more days produces complete remission in about 65 percent of adults. Because these drugs tend to be more toxic than those used for ALL and because the bone marrow of people with AML recovers more slowly than that of those with ALL, frequent blood tests are needed. Hospitalization is usually necessary. Other regimes include thioguanine or etoposide (Ve Pesid) or replacing daunorubicin (Cerubidine) with idarubicin (Idamycin).

People treated for AML are very susceptible to infections, bleeding, and severe nausea and vomiting. Signs of improvement usually appear two to three weeks after induction chemotherapy is complete, and 80 percent of those who will have complete remission do so within a month. Bone marrow studies determine whether a second phase of induction chemotherapy is needed.

The roles of consolidation chemotherapy and maintenance chemotherapy are still under investigation for AML. Most treatment centers will offer one or the other on an outpatient basis. Chemotherapy regimens include different drugs from those used in previous phases of treatment. Thioguanine may be administered every 12 hours. The treatment is repeated every few months for up to one year.

Cytarabine (Cytosar-U) may be given subcutaneously or intravenously over the course of an hour, every 12 hours for a total of 12 doses. A second course begins as soon as blood counts return to normal. Treatment is given typically every four weeks, depending on the blood counts. The second course rarely continues for more than a year.

Prophylaxis Chemotherapy. Children with AML may receive this treatment, but it is not usually a part of treatment for adults. Standard intravenous chemotherapy with high doses of cytarabine (Cytosar-U) appears to be effective in preventing brain involvement.

Acute Lymphoid Leukemia

Induction Chemotherapy. The first phase of treatment is designed to produce remission.

The combination of drugs commonly used during induction is intravenous vincristine (Oncovin) and oral prednisone. Combinations may also include intravenous doxorubicin (Adriamycin), intravenous asparaginase (Elspar), cyclophosphamide (Cytoxan), methotrexate, and cytarabine (Cytosar-U).

Because chemotherapy reduces the number of normal white blood cells and platelets, the risk of infection or bleeding increases. To minimize these complications, induction chemotherapy usually begins in the hospital. Although complete remission requires about three weeks, improvement is often good enough within several days to allow the person to complete the treatment on an outpatient basis.

Consolidation Chemotherapy. The oncologist often uses the same drugs as those used in induction chemotherapy to eliminate residual disease or may add other drugs such as methotrexate. Consolidation treatment on an outpatient basis may continue for several weeks even during remission.

Prophylaxis Chemotherapy. Prophylaxis chemotherapy is a preventive course of treatment. For example, methotrexate may be injected into the spinal fluid or infused into it from a tiny reservoir implanted under the scalp. Radiation therapy may accompany chemotherapy to reduce the risk that the leukemia will involve the central nervous system. Prophylaxis chemotherapy, performed on an outpatient basis, begins immediately before or after consolidation therapy.

Maintenance Chemotherapy. Different drugs in doses that vary from those used in other phases of treatment continue for 36 to 60 months with prednisone and various chemotherapy drugs to prolong the remission. Patients can receive maintenance treatment on an outpatient basis.

Bone Marrow Transplantation. Replacing defective bone marrow with healthy marrow may prevent the formation of leukemic cells (see Chapter 19, "Bone Marrow Transplant").

Allogenic bone marrow transplant (BMT), which uses bone marrow from a sibling, is now an accepted approach if previous induction treatment succeeded in producing remission and the patient is under age 50. Cure rates under these circumstances are substantially higher than those with standard doses of chemotherapy alone.

Erythroleukemia

Management of erythroleukemia is more varied, with some physicians using drugs similar to those used to treat AML. Others occasionally use radiation therapy to shrink enlarged lymph nodes or the spleen.

Myelodysplastic Syndrome

A transfusion of blood cells or platelets every few weeks may be beneficial as supportive therapy, but it does not keep the disease from progressing. Eventually, chemotherapy is initiated if symptoms of progression to leukemia appear.

Survival

Because of improved treatments, survival rates for those with leukemia have increased dramatically. In the early 1960s the five-year survival rate was 4 percent; by the 1970s it was 28 percent; and by the mid-1980s, more than 50 percent of people with leukemia survived five or more years. The younger the individual, the better the response to treatment and the greater the chance of remission. Remission in adults lasts for a shorter time than that in children.

Survival rates vary according to the type of leukemia. Adults with ALL generally have an 80 percent chance of achieving remission and a 35 to 45 percent chance of surviving five years or more. (The survival rate ranges from 1 to 85 percent, depending on the subtype of leukemia involved.) Those who stay in remission for more than four years rarely relapse, and therapy can be discontinued. Seventy to 80 percent of children with ALL survive five years.

Those with AML have an overall 60 to 70 percent chance of remission. About 20 percent of those who attain remission can expect to survive three years or more with a possibility of being cured. If left untreated, AML can be fatal within a few months.

A form of ALL involving a specific chromosomal abnormality, the *Philadelphia chromosome*, has a prognosis similar to that of AML.

Special Needs

Induction chemotherapy usually requires care at a major cancer care facility, because community hospitals often lack experience with the complex, highly toxic regimens and their potential complications.

When BMT is an option, care at a facility with the expertise to perform the procedure is essential. Insurance and health plans do not always cover the costs, which can be extraordinary.

Supportive therapy, which includes blood and platelet transfusions and antibiotic treatment to lower the risk of bleeding problems and infections, also often requires hospitalization.

Many experts suggest a low-bacteria diet (cooked food only) to reduce the risk of infection. Adequate nutrition is a concern, because symptoms of the disease and the side effects of chemotherapy (for example, nausea, vomiting, diarrhea) can affect appetite. Some physicians no longer believe that people hospitalized for leukemia need to be kept in complete, sterile isolation to reduce risk of infection.

As the cancer progresses, circulating leukemia cells tend to concentrate in sanctuary organs. In men, the testicles can be a sanctuary organ. Men with leukemia who may wish to father children in the future are often encouraged to deposit sperm in sperm banks.

Long-term follow-up and close observation are essential. After remission patients have blood counts every one to two months to detect signs of lingering or recurring disease.

Ask About

Research is ongoing to test new drugs and different combinations of standard and new chemotherapy drugs. An exciting development in leukemia treatment involves a growing awareness of the different cell abnormalities and increased ability to identify them. Precise identification of these blood cells is making it possible to identify which type of leukemia is present and what therapy is most likely to cure it.

If you have acute leukemia, ask your oncologist about clinical trials investigating new combinations of drugs. You may also discuss maintenance therapy with your doctor if you have AML, because the need for long-term therapy is in dispute.

Drugs are being designed to target specific cells affected by the subtypes of acute leukemia. For example, monoclonal antibodies can seek out and bind to certain leukemic cells. These antibodies can carry cytotoxic drugs that penetrate the membranes of the leukemic cells and destroy them.

If your doctor suggests bone marrow transplant, ask about growth factors, such as granulocyte/macrophage colony-stimulating factor (GM-CSF) or granulocyte colony-stimulating factor (G-CSF), which are injected intravenously or subcutaneously to stimulate the bone marrow and thus help leukocytes reach maturity (see Chapter 18, "Biological Therapies"). New drugs that produce similar effects are also under investigation.

The use of a person's own bone marrow, or autologous BMT, is under study. In this approach, bone marrow is removed when the person with leukemia is in remission, is treated with anticancer drugs in the lab, and is returned to the individual after he or she has received high-dose chemotherapy.

The technique could enhance the chance of a cure and eliminate the difficulty of finding a suitable donor, which limits the use of allogenic BMT.

If you have ALL or AML and have had a relapse, discuss with your doctor the possibility of entering a bone marrow transplant clinical trial.

If your child has acute leukemia, it's important that treatment is coordinated by a specialist in childhood cancer at a center equipped to deliver supportive care. You may want to ask your pediatric oncologist about the availability of nationwide studies: The Pediatric Oncology Group and the Children's Cancer Group are both studying the use of autologous bone marrow transplantation and chemotherapy. Studies are also under way evaluating allogenic bone marrow transplant and using biological response modifiers (see Chapter 18, "Biological Therapies") as well as new chemotherapy agents.

CHRONIC LEUKEMIA

Leukemias are cancers of the blood-forming system, which includes the bone marrow and the lymphatic system. They account for about 2 percent of all cancers. Because leukemia is the most common form of childhood cancer, it is often thought of as a disease of childhood. However, it affects nine times as many adults as children. Half of all cases occur in people over the age of 60, and the disease is increasing among the elderly. The incidence of acute and chronic leukemias is approximately equal.

Chronic leukemia involves cells in an advanced stage of development. Although they may appear to be mature, they cannot perform their vital functions.

Chronic leukemia accounts for roughly 1.2 percent of all cancers. It is the most common leukemia, affecting about three out of every 100,000 people.

Although the cause is unknown, chronic leukemia is linked to genetic abnormalities and environmental factors. For example, there is an association between chronic lymphoid leukemia (CLL) (see "Types") and exposure to benzene or high doses of radiation. CLL also occurs in some people with retrovirus infections such as that caused by the human T-lymphocyte virus (HTLV-I and HTLV-II).

Genetic abnormalities, especially the Philadelphia chromosome, are detected in the vast majority of those with chronic myeloid leukemia (CML) (see "Types"), but whether chromosome changes cause CML or result from the disease is unclear.

Advances in treatment have improved the survival rate enormously. Today about half of those with leukemia survive five years or more after diagnosis.

Who Is at Risk?

- People who have prolonged exposure to high doses of radiation, including X-rays;

- People who have long-term exposure to toxic organic chemicals, such as benzene;

- People with a hereditary disposition to cancer of any kind.

Chronic Lymphoid Leukemia

- Those over 50 (90 percent of cases, with the average age of onset about 65; incidence increases with age; rare in people under age 30 and almost never seen in children);

- Men, who develop CLL twice as often as women;

- People with a family history of CLL (16 times more likely to develop the disease than those without such a history).

Hairy Cell Leukemia

- Men (affected four times as often as women), especially those over 50;

- People over 30.

Chronic Myeloid Leukemia

- Those in their mid-40s;

- Men, who develop CML at a slightly higher rate than women.

Screening Tests

There are no screening tests.

Types of Chronic Leukemia

Chronic leukemia is divided into types, depending on the characteristics of the cells involved. Because, unlike acute leukemia, the blood cells affected by chronic leukemia are mature or nearly so, they often appear normal. Close scrutiny under a microscope, however, reveals important distinctions.

Chronic Lymphoid Leukemia

Chronic lymphoid leukemia (CLL; also known as *chronic lymphocytic leukemia*) affects *lymphoid cells*, white cells that lack cellular granules or particles (see "Acute Leukemia"). It accounts for 30 percent of all leukemias. There are several subtypes of CLL, the most common of which is B-cell CLL, which involves the immune cells, or *lymphocytes*, that produce antibodies. About 5 to 10 percent of people with CLL have the T-cell type, which affects the lymphocytes that regulate the actions of B cells. Hairy cell leukemia (HCL), which is a subtype of CLL and accounts for 2 percent of leukemias, gives lymphocytes of both types a characteristic "hairy" appearance under the microscope.

In CLL, lymphocytes proliferate that cannot fight infection. So not only is the body more vulnerable to bacteria, but the unhealthy cells crowd out the healthy ones. Eventually, the bone marrow may contain only lymphocytes. CLL is incurable, but chemotherapy can produce lengthy remission.

The lymphocytes of people with CLL accumulate in the lymph nodes and cause swelling. The spleen enlarges, and lymphatic tissue may appear in unusual areas, such as the scalp, orbit of the eye, pharynx, lung, gastrointestinal tract, and in men, in the prostate and gonads. The liver may also enlarge and cause the person to become jaundiced.

Chronic Myeloid Leukemia

Chronic myeloid leukemia (also known as *chronic myelogenous leukemia* and *chronic granulocytic leukemia*) affects *myeloid cells,* white cells that have granules (see "Acute Leukemia"). It accounts for 20 to 30 percent of adult leukemia. In most cases, DNA analysis reveals the presence of an abnormal chromosome called the Philadelphia chromosome.

The affected cells in the bone marrow of the person with CML may overproduce to the point that few, if any, normal cells remain. Excess cells in the blood collect in the spleen and liver, enlarging these organs and interfering with their functions.

Signs and Symptoms

As with acute leukemia, symptoms are often vague and nonspecific.

Chronic Lymphoid Leukemia

Early Stage
- Minimal nontender swollen lymph nodes;
- Enlarged spleen (noted as a feeling of fullness or presence of a mass on the left side of the abdomen; some people notice that they feel full early on during a meal and may have weight loss, swelling in the legs, and pain in the left shoulder);
- Fatigue;
- Malaise;
- Occasional fever;
- Night sweats.

Later Stages
- Weight loss;
- Uncomfortable, large lymph nodes.

Hairy Cell Leukemia
- Frequent infections;
- Pancytopenia (a decrease in most types of blood cells; any symptoms may be due to these blood changes).

Chronic Myeloid Leukemia

Early Stage
- Enlarged spleen (see symptom description under "Chronic Lymphoid Leukemia").

Later Stages
- Bone pain;
- Bleeding problems;
- Mucous membrane irritation;
- Infection;
- Pallor;
- Swollen lymph glands;
- Fever;
- Night sweats.

Diagnostic and Staging Tests

See "Acute Leukemia."

Tests Unique to Chronic Leukemia

See "Acute Leukemia."

Staging

Chronic Lymphoid Leukemia

Two systems exist for staging CLL, the Rai system and the International Staging System. Both define stages according to signs and symptoms plus abnormalities detected in lab tests. Excessive numbers of lymphocytes (*lymphocytosis*) occur at all stages in both systems.

The Rai system (named after the physician who created it) identifies five stages:
- Stage 0: lymphocytosis only;
- Stage I: enlarged lymph nodes;
- Stage II: enlarged spleen and/or liver;
- Stage III: anemia;
- Stage IV: low platelet count (thrombocytopenia).

The International Staging System identifies three stages:
- Stage A: enlargement of fewer than three lymph node groups (Rai stages 0, I, or II);
- Stage B: enlargement of more than three lymph node groups (Rai stages I or II);
- Stage C: anemia or thrombocytopenia

regardless of lymph enlargement (Rai stages III or IV).

Chronic Myeloid Leukemia

Chronic (or Stable) Phase
- Mild and nonspecific symptoms such as fatigue and weight loss;
- Mildly enlarged spleen;
- Elevated white blood count;
- High platelet counts (some patients have normal counts);
- Less than 10 percent immature bone marrow cells.

Accelerated Phase
- Same symptoms as in chronic phase, but moderately severe;
- Possible increase in spleen size;
- Erratic white blood cell count;
- Erratic platelet counts;
- Between 10 percent and 30 percent immature bone marrow.

Acute Phase (Blast Crisis).
This phase consists of the transformation of CML into an acute terminal stage. A *blast crisis* occurs when large numbers of blast cells are produced and other bone marrow cells and substances decline; features of the acute phase include:
- Same symptoms as preceding, but severe;
- Marked increase in spleen size;
- High or low white blood cell count;
- Low platelet count;
- Blast cells constituting more than 30 percent of bone marrow cells;
- Presence of granulocytic sarcomas (accumulations of leukemic cells)—most often found in the bones or lymph nodes but also found in the skin, brain membranes (meninges), or the gastrointestinal tract.

Treatment

The treatment depends on the specific type of chronic leukemia and its stage. Chemotherapy is the standard approach to both CLL and CML (see Chapter 17, "Chemotherapy"). In CLL, radiation therapy is sometimes added (see Chapter 16, "Radiation"). Supportive therapy includes blood transfusions, antibiotics, and immunoglobulins to boost the immune system.

Bone marrow transplantation (BMT) is becoming the treatment of choice during the chronic stage of CML because it has the possibility of curing the illness (see Chapter 19, "Bone Marrow Transplant"). When CML progresses to the acute phase, the treatment is similar to that for acute leukemia (see "Acute Leukemia").

BMT is not usually an option in treating CLL, primarily because CLL affects people over the age of 60, who are not considered candidates for the procedure. The following are specific approaches to treatment:

Chronic Lymphoid Leukemia
- Stage A (Rai stage 0): no treatment.
- Stage B (Rai stages I–II): single-agent drugs such as chlorambucil (Leukeran) to interfere with cell proliferation, with or without corticosteroids. Remission occurs in 70 percent of cases.
- Stage C (Rai stages III–IV): more intensive chemotherapy with CVP (cyclophosphamide [Cytoxan], vincristine [Oncovin], and prednisone). Adding doxorubicin (Adriamycin) may improve survival rates.

Other Treatments
- Palliative radiation therapy to the spleen or enlarged lymph nodes;
- Removal of the spleen to prevent symptoms and improve blood counts;
- Vaccinations against influenza and pneumonia;
- Low-dose, total body radiation therapy.

Hairy Cell Leukemia
- 2-Chlorodeoxyadenosine (2-CDA) (the treatment of choice; evidence suggests 2-CDA may cure HCL);
- Alpha interferon or pentostatin.

T-Cell ALL

- Topical drugs may make lesions disappear.

- Systemic chemotherapy with the same drugs that are used for CLL is needed for advanced disease.

Chronic Myeloid Leukemia

Chronic Phase
- Bone marrow transplantation (BMT) with matched donor marrow (allogenic BMT) offers the only potential cure and is the treatment of choice;

- hydroxyurea (Hydrea), to control white blood cell count and platelet count;

- busulfan (Myleran) (a greater risk of serious toxicity than hydroxyurea);

- Palliative radiation therapy of the spleen.

Accelerated Phase
- Bone marrow transplant;

- Spleen removal (splenectomy) for control of pain and to improve blood problems.

Acute (Blast Crisis) Phase
- Aggressive treatment with doxorubicin (Adriamycin), daunorubicin (Cerubidine), and cytarabine (Cytosar-U);

- Vincristine (Oncovin) and steroids, alone or with other agents such as asparaginase (Elspar) (induces transient remissions in approximately 60 percent of cases).

Survival

Chronic Lymphoid Leukemia

Median survival overall is around nine years. International stage A survival is 10 years or more; stage B is five years; stage C is two years. Most fatalities in people with CLL result from infections or other illnesses that occur as a consequence of the leukemia.

Hairy Cell Leukemia

Up to 20 percent of people with HCL may have prolonged survival without any treatment. The rate of partial or complete response to interfer-

on is as high as 80 percent; the response may last for 12 to 18 months. Cure is unlikely, but repeat treatment can produce additional remission. Survival with 2-CDA or pentostatin is excellent, and most people remain free of disease for many years, apparently cured.

T-cell CLL. Median survival is less than a year, even with aggressive treatment.

Chronic Myeloid Leukemia

Chronic Phase. In patients under 40, BMT during the chronic phase produces long-term (three-year) survival rates of 50 to 60 percent when the procedure is performed within one to three years of diagnosis. The longer BMT is delayed, the poorer the prognosis; the three-year survival rate is 38 percent when the transplant takes place three years or more after diagnosis.

Accelerated Phase. Average survival time from diagnosis of accelerated phase is only three months.

Acute Phase. If the blast crisis involves lymphoid cells, complete remission can occur in 67 percent of people and can last seven or eight months. Those who respond to treatment survive an average of 15.7 months; nonresponders survive an average of four months. Less aggressive treatment results in median survival of 30 weeks.

If the blast crisis involves myeloid cells, the outlook is poorer: Remission rates are less than 20 percent. The survival rate among those who do not respond to treatment is about two months; those who enter a second, chronic phase have a survival rate of about six months.

Special Needs

People undergoing BMT need to be monitored carefully to minimize risk of complications, including graft vs. host disease, relapse, and pneumonitis (see Chapter 19, "Bone Marrow Transplant").

People in remission need to visit physicians every one to three months to detect any changes in blood or immune values. The earlier changes are detected, the sooner treatment can be adjusted.

Ask About

Some experts advocate aggressive treatment with the standard combinations of chemotherapy drugs to lower white blood counts, whether or not the person with leukemia experiences symptoms. However, this approach is not considered standard therapy at this time.

As in acute leukemia, the exciting development in chronic leukemia treatment is a growing awareness of the different cell abnormalities produced by different forms of the disease. The more precisely molecular biologists can describe leukemic cells, the better able they are to design treatments targeted for a particular subtype. For instance, by distinguishing the more aggressive forms of chronic leukemia from the types that are slower to develop, physicians may tailor therapy to produce the best results with the lowest risk of adverse effects.

If you have CML, you will want to discuss the risks and benefits of BMT, because it may cure the disease, whereas chemotherapy can do no more than induce remission, except in some cases of hairy cell leukemia. Trials are under way to determine whether BMT will work in CLL. Unfortunately, this form of leukemia strikes elderly people who may be unable to withstand the demands of the procedure.

Evidence is growing that new approaches to drug therapy will prove useful in chronic leukemia. For example, you may want to ask your oncologist about interferon (see Chapters 18, "Biological Therapies," and 21, "Investigational Treatments"). Investigators have shown that interferon has a clear role in CML, inducing remission in up to 80 percent of cases. It is becoming the treatment of choice over the previous standard treatment, a drug called busulfan (Myleran). Unfortunately, the side effects of interferon can be quite unpleasant and may seriously compromise your quality of life, so it's helpful to discuss it with your doctor before beginning therapy. Cost is another issue.

Fludarabine phosphate (Fludara) is a promising agent for advanced CLL, especially when prior therapy has failed.

New drugs, such as 2-chlorodeoxyadenosine (2-CDA), have produced complete long-lasting remission in cases of HCL, giving rise to the hope that such treatments may produce cures. Research shows that treatment with alpha interferon and pentostatin in some cases may eliminate hairy cells and produce a higher rate of longer-lasting remissions.

If you have stage II, III, or IV CLL, you may want to talk with your oncologist about participating in a clinical trial evaluating biological response modifiers.

HODGKIN'S DISEASE

Hodgkin's disease (HD), named for Thomas Hodgkin, the British physician who identified it in 1832, is a rare cancer and accounts for only about 14 percent of all lymphatic cancers or *lymphomas* (see "Non-Hodgkin's Lymphoma"). Although HD is detected in only three of every 100,000 people each year, it most often affects men and women in their late 20s. (HD rarely affects children and almost never strikes those under 5.)

Fortunately, because of advances in treatment, survival rates have improved remarkably. About 45 years ago the average length of survival from onset to death was 30 months. Today 80 to 90 percent of people with HD survive five years, and 60 to 70 percent survive 10 years or more. Knowledge of what causes the disease is advancing rapidly, and even higher cure rates are expected when that mystery is solved.

Many researchers suspect there is a relationship between HD and a virus—most commonly the Epstein-Barr virus, which is responsible for several infections that typically strike in late adolescence, such as infectious mononucleosis.

When cancer affects the lymphocytes, certain types of lymph cells proliferate. In HD, this abundance of abnormal lymphocytes creates a situation that closely resembles an infection: the glands swell, though they are not painful, and there may be a fever and fatigue. At the same time, the body's ability to defend against infection is seriously compromised.

When cells from the swollen lymph nodes are examined under the microscope, their abnormalities are identified and the pathologist can distinguish between infection, HD, and the other lymphomas. For example, one characteristic common to most types of HD (see "Types," later) but not non-Hodgkin's lymphoma is the presence of unusually large cells called *Reed-Sternberg* cells.

The *lymphatic system* (illustrated on page 418) is a network of vessels that carry *lymph* away from body tissues. *Lymph* is a watery fluid containing immune cells called *lymphocytes*. These cells help fight infection and participate in immune processes such as allergies. Lymph collects in small lymph vessels the size of capillaries in the tissues.

Located along the lymph vessels like pearls on a string are *lymph nodes*, small, bean-shaped structures that filter the lymph fluid, identify *antigens* (proteins, viruses, foreign material), and serve as storage sites for lymph cells. Lymph passing through the lymph nodes eventually arrives at the thoracic duct, from which it enters the bloodstream.

Lymph nodes exist at many sites in the body, including the underarms, groin, neck, and abdomen. The other major organs of the lymphatic system are the *thymus*, which stores lymphocytes until they mature, and the *spleen*, which stores lymphocytes and other blood cells. The spleen also filters impurities from the blood.

Who Is at Risk?

- People between 15 and 34 and 55 and 70;

- Men;

- Siblings of those with HD (three to seven times more likely to develop the disease than those with unaffected siblings);

- People with acquired immune deficiency syndrome (AIDS);

- People taking drugs that suppress the immune system following organ transplant;

- People who have been treated with chemotherapy.

Screening Tests

There are no screening tests.

Types of Hodgkin's Disease

There are four main types of HD that vary according to the cells present. Accurate identification of the type is important because some forms are more aggressive than others and are treated differently.

- *Nodular sclerosis*: Bands of scarlike tissue in the lymph nodes separate pockets of abnormal cells containing Reed-Sternberg cells. These cells, named for the doctors who discovered them, are abnormally large immune cells that are characteristic of HD. (They may rarely be present in some benign conditions, such as infectious mononucleosis.) This is the most common type of HD.

- *Lymphocyte predominant*: Cells called reactive lymphocytes are present; Reed-Sternberg cells are rarely detected. This rare type is the least aggressive form of HD.

- *Mixed cellularity*: Reed-Sternberg cells and inflammatory white blood cells and lymphocytes are present. About one case in four of HD is this type.

- *Lymphocyte depleted*: Scarlike tissue may be diffuse, and there may be few lymphocytes. Reed-Sternberg cells are abundant. In a variation of this type, malignant cells vary in size. This is the most aggressive form of HD.

HD causes lymphocytes to proliferate in the lymph nodes, most often in the neck, underarm, or groin, resulting in painless swelling. The swelling may progress from one lymph node to a neighboring node on the same side of the body (ipsilateral spread) or to nodes on the opposite side (contralateral spread). The swelling typically extends from the neck to the collarbone, to the underarms, and finally to the chest. The disease rarely "skips" from one node group to another at a distant location, as non-Hodgkin's lymphoma does.

Abnormal cells may leave the lymph nodes and pass into the bloodstream, where they migrate to other organs, particularly the spleen, liver, lungs, bone, and bone marrow. Where these cells cluster together, they disrupt the ability of those organs to function. The cells rarely spread to the central nervous system (the spinal cord and brain).

Clusters of cells can become large enough to produce a noticeable lump, or *tumor mass*. The term *bulky disease* refers to cases in which several large node masses are grouped together.

Signs and Symptoms

Often there are no symptoms, but about 40 percent of people will have some vague signs of disease. If symptoms do occur, they may include

- Persistent, painless swelling of lymph nodes, especially in the neck, underarm, or groin;
- Unexplained fevers, tiredness, night sweats, weight loss, and itching;
- Cough, shortness of breath, chest discomfort;
- Enlarged spleen.

Diagnostic and Staging Tests

(For more details on the following tests, see Chapter 8, "Diagnostic Tests.")
- Lymph node biopsy, which is essential;
- Physical examination;
- Blood tests to detect signs of disease, high

enzyme levels (which may indicate liver or bone involvement), or other clues, such as high levels of antibodies;

- X-rays of chest, bones, liver, spleen;
- Liver biopsy;
- Bone marrow biopsy;
- Lymphangiography (see later);
- Computed tomography (CT) scan of the abdomen;
- Laparotomy (also called staging laparotomy; surgical exploration of the abdomen, sometimes involving lymph node or liver biopsies or removal of the spleen; usually done only if the disease may be present below the diaphragm and if the doctors believe the procedure will aid in planning treatment).

Tests Unique to Hodgkin's Disease

Lymphangiography is a procedure for obtaining x-ray images of the lymph nodes. After the person receives an anesthetic to numb the feet, the physician makes an incision over one of the vessels on each foot and uses a needle to inject a contrast dye, or medium, into the lymph vessel. The medium travels up the legs to the groin, abdomen, and chest. A radiologist then takes x-rays, which reveal any abnormalities in the lymph nodes and vessels. The contrast medium remains in the lymph system for several months, allowing doctors to monitor the disease and its response to treatment. In recent years, CT and MRI scans, which can produce images of soft tissues, has largely supplanted the need for lymphangiography.

Staging

- Stage I: involvement of a single lymph node region (stage I), or a single organ or site other than the lymph nodes (stage IE; E stands for extralymphatic or extension);
- Stage II: involvement of two or more lymph node regions on the same side of the diaphragm (above or below) (stage II), or localized involvement of a extralymphatic organ or site (IIE);

- Stage III: involvement of lymph node regions on both sides of the diaphragm (III), and possible localized involvement of an extralymphatic site (IIIE), the spleen (IIIS), or both (IIISE);

- Stage IV: Widespread involvement of one or more sites other than lymph nodes, with or without associated lymph node involvement, or isolated extralymphatic involvement with distant lymph node involvement.

Each of these stages is subclassified as either A (symptoms absent) or B (symptoms present, including fever, sweats, and weight loss greater than 10 percent of body weight).

In addition, stages I and II may be further classified as favorable (no bulky tumor mass present) or unfavorable (a bulky tumor mass greater than 10 centimeters in diameter is present).

Treatment

HD was one of the first cancers cured with chemotherapy (see Chapter 17, "Chemotherapy"). Today the standard approach is to use radiation therapy alone in the early stages (see Chapter 16, "Radiation") and radiation therapy and/or combination chemotherapy in the later stages.

The radiologist directs the radiation to sites known to harbor the disease (where abnormal cells have formed clusters and/or masses), and often to adjacent regions of nodes (called fields), where the disease may be or might develop later. Radiation therapy for early-stage disease usually lasts three to six months with intervals of rest between courses. Chemotherapy is given in courses, usually at monthly intervals. Treatment usually lasts nine months to a year, depending on the person's response in the first six months.

Stage IA and IIA, Favorable. Standard treatment is radiation to the chest and lymph nodes and/or spleen in the abdomen. If radiation therapy is to be the only treatment, frequently a surgeon will perform a staging laparotomy to determine if any disease is present in the abdomen (see Chapter 15, "Surgery"). Radiation therapy can either be *total* (aimed at all the lymph nodes) or *subtotal* (aimed at most nodes). Some physicians

may recommend either radiation therapy plus chemotherapy (see Chapter 20, "Combination Treatments") or combination chemotherapy alone. Combination chemotherapy commonly involves one of the following regimens:

- MOPP [mechlorethamine (nitrogen mustard) + vincristine (Oncovin) + procarbazine (Matulane) + prednisone];

- ABVD [doxorubicin (Adriamycin) + bleomycin (Blenoxane) + vincristine + dacarbazine (DTIC-Dome)];

- MOPP + ABV (no dacarbazine);

- Alternating MOPP and ABVD cycles;

- Cyclophosphamide (Cytoxan) + MOPP (C-MOPP).

Stage IB and IIB, Favorable. Physicians usually recommend combination chemotherapy using MOPP, ABVD, or some variation instead. In some cases the patient may receive radiation therapy and chemotherapy. These choices take into account the patient's age, general health, extent of disease, and other factors.

Stages I and II, Unfavorable. Staging laparotomy is not necessary. Combination chemotherapy (see earlier) plus radiation therapy to the involved sites is the standard approach.

Stage IIIA. When staging laparotomy reveals little involvement of the spleen, and no liver disease, radiation therapy to all lymph nodes in the body may be recommended. People with extensive involvement of the spleen, or those who have been staged clinically (that is, without laparotomy) will probably receive combination chemotherapy (MOPP, ABVD, or MOPP-ABV). People with bulky disease usually receive both radiation therapy and chemotherapy.

Stages IIIB and Stage IV. Standard therapy is combination chemotherapy (MOPP, ABVD, MOPP-ABV, or MOPP alternating with ABVD). In addition, patients with large tumor masses may receive radiation therapy to those areas.

Physicians usually treat children with HD

somewhat differently. In stages I and II, chemotherapy plus low-dose radiation therapy is the standard of care. If relapse occurs following radiation therapy, combination chemotherapy usually produces a second remission. Those with stage III or IV disease receive chemotherapy and, if bulky disease is present, radiation therapy.

Survival

Some experts hesitate to cite 10-year survival rates because HD is so often a disease of young adults who may live for many years after treatment. Furthermore, not enough time has passed since significant advances in treatment to know for certain what the long-term survival rate will be for those treated with the new therapies. However, current data on five-year survival do show very positive outcomes for all stages. About 90 percent of people with stage IA or IIA favorable HD will survive five years or longer. Those with stage IB or IIB favorable, or stage I or II unfavorable, have a 75 to 90 percent chance of surviving five years. Stage IIIA disease has a 65 to 85 percent five-year survival, and even the most advanced form of HD, stages IIIB and stage IV, has a survival rate of 60 to 80 percent.

Special Needs

People who have received chemotherapy for HD are at increased risk of developing other forms of cancer, especially non-Hodgkin's lymphoma and leukemia. Radiation treatment also increases the risk of other cancers, especially cancer of the skin, breast, stomach, bone, and lung. Therefore, follow-up visits continue for several years after treatment.

Physicians typically order x-rays, blood tests, and other laboratory tests to detect a recurrence of HD or occurrence of a new cancer. Those treated with limited radiation therapy usually have annual abdominal CT scans. If the thyroid received radiation therapy, the doctor will order annual thyroid function tests and may prescribe thyroid hormone replacement therapy.

Permanent sterility in men and infertility or premature menopause in women occurs in nearly everyone with HD who receives six or more cycles of MOPP.

Because HD weakens immune resistance, people with this form of cancer are susceptible to infections. Therefore, it is important to avoid exposure to contagious illnesses. Most deaths from this disease result from severe infection.

People who have had their spleen removed are particularly vulnerable to pneumonia and pneumococcal sepsis, because without a spleen there are fewer ways to destroy the bacteria. Use of a vaccine called Pneumovax prior to the surgery to remove the spleen helps prevent this complication. Doctors often prescribe antibiotics if symptoms of infection develop in those who did not receive the vaccine.

Because children are still growing, physicians take precautions to preserve the integrity of their bones and connective tissue. To minimize the risk of adverse effects, children with HD usually receive doses of radiation therapy that are lower than the doses used in adults. In many cases, children with stage I or II disease receive combination chemotherapy to supplement radiation therapy. This is different from treatment of adults, most of whom do not receive chemotherapy unless the disease progresses to stage III or IV.

Ask About

Although treatment of Hodgkin's disease is well established, opinions differ on the best approach to the intermediate stages, especially stage IIIA. Seriously consider a second opinion (see Chapter 12, "How Many Opinions Do You Need?") and discuss with the consultant the total dose of radiation therapy he or she recommends, how much tissue will be irradiated, whether both radiation therapy and chemotherapy will be helpful, and what drugs and/or combinations of drugs will work best in treating your particular type of HD.

If you have stage IV disease or you have had a relapse, you may want to inquire about the risks and benefits of high-dose chemotherapy and bone marrow transplant (see Chapter 19, "Bone Marrow Transplant"). Several clinical trials are comparing the effects of this option with the current standard care (see Chapter 21, "Investigational Treatments").

Disease that has spread to the liver or bone marrow presents the greatest challenge. The current trend is to use higher doses of chemotherapy in these cases, but some physicians still prefer to reserve this approach for those who relapse.

NON-HODGKIN'S LYMPHOMA

News reports about the *lymphomas* (non-Hodgkin's lymphoma and Hodgkin's disease)—cancers of the lymphatic system—are sometimes confusing. On the one hand, this group of cancers is relatively rare, accounting for about 3 percent of all malignancies. On the other, the incidence of non-Hodgkin's lymphoma (NHL) is escalating in the United States.

Since the 1970s the number of cases of NHL has risen by more than 65 percent, making its rate of increase the third highest of all cancers, just behind that of lung cancer in women and skin cancer in both sexes. About eight men in 100,000 and nearly six women in 100,000 have NHL, and about 25 percent of cases occur between the ages of 50 and 59. It is even more common among people 60 to 69.

The leap in NHL incidence is due in part to improved diagnostic techniques, but it also reflects the dramatic rise in the number of people with compromised immunity as a result of infection with HIV, the virus that causes AIDS, and the use of immune-suppressing drugs by organ transplant patients. Certain conditions may also weaken the immune system.

Although scientists do not know for certain what causes the lymph system to become cancerous, evidence strongly suggests that viruses—particularly the Epstein-Barr virus—are partly to blame. Experts believe that inherited genetic deficiencies also play a role.

The good news is that improvements in chemotherapy and radiation therapy over the past few decades and, more recently, bone marrow transplant, have led to an improved cure rate of about 40 to 45 percent.

Doctors distinguish NHL from Hodgkin's Disease (HD) by the absence of abnormally large lymph cells called Reed-Sternberg cells (see "Hodgkin's Disease"). All forms of lymphoma that are not Hodgkin's disease (HD) are considered to be NHL. There are several types of NHL, depending on the size and shape of the lymph cells (see "Types," later).

Who Is at Risk?

- Men, who develop NHL 30 percent more often than women;

- Those between 50 and 69;

- Caucasian children (slightly greater risk

than African-American children);

- People with inherited immune deficiencies, such as Klinefelter's syndrome, Chediak-Higashi syndrome, ataxia telangiectasia syndrome; acquired hypogammaglobulinemia; Swiss-type agammaglobulinemia; Xlinked lymphoproliferative syndrome;

- People with autoimmune disease, such as rheumatoid arthritis or systemic lupus erythematosus;

- People infected with the virus that causes AIDS;

- People taking immunosuppressant drugs following organ transplant;

- People who have received radiation therapy and/or chemotherapy;

- People who work extensively with or are otherwise exposed to chemicals, such as pesticides or some fertilizers.

Screening Tests

There are no screening tests.

Types of Non-Hodgkin's Lymphoma

The most recent classification system, the Working Formulation, groups the different types of NHL according to the rate at which they grow. Low-grade NHLs grow the slowest, high-grade the fastest. Doctors sometimes refer to low-grade NHL as *indolent* and to the intermediate and high-grade forms as *aggressive*.

It is important not to confuse low-grade with less serious, despite the difference in aggressiveness. Low-grade lymphoma can be fatal, whereas high-grade lymphoma may respond well to chemotherapy and those with this disease may have a good chance of being cured.

Within each grade of NHL are several subtypes (see the following table) that vary according to characteristics of the lymphocytes involved. In about one out of five cases, a person has a mixed lymphoma with two or more subtypes at the same time.

Low Grade	Intermediate Grade	High Grade
Small lymphocytic	Follicular large cell	Immunoblastic large cell
Follicular small cleaved	Diffuse small cleaved	Lymphoblastic
Follicular mixed cell	Diffuse mixed cell	Small non-cleaved (Burkitt's or non-Burkitt's)

Another type of NHL is *cutaneous T-cell lymphoma* (CTCL), which is sometimes called *mycosis fungoides*. This low-grade lymphoma, which affects T-lymphocytes, is rare, causing about 600 cases per year in this country.

Miscellaneous forms of NHL—composite, histiocytic, and unclassifiable—that do not fit into these categories are also rare.

In contrast to HD, in which the cancer typically progresses from one lymph node to its neighboring node on the same side of the body or to the opposing node on the other side of the body, NHL is more likely to "skip" from one node to other nodes at more distant locations as it progresses.

NHL usually spreads throughout the lymphatic system, frequently to other tissues such as the liver, bone marrow, gastrointestinal tract, and, in men, the testicles. Spread to the central nervous system (spinal cord and brain) is rare, although one form of the disease, called *primary central nervous system lymphoma*, originates in the brain and is responsible for about 2 percent of all lymphomas (see "Brain"). About 10 percent of people with diffuse large-cell lymphoma develop leukemia.

Studies show that 30 to 60 percent of cases of low-grade NHL develop into a more aggressive form. This process is called conversion. Some subtypes of NHL are more likely to convert than others. The most common example is the conversion from low-grade follicular small cell lymphoma to intermediate-grade diffuse large cell lymphoma or high-grade immunoblastic large cell lymphoma.

Signs and Symptoms

Often the first sign of NHL is a swelling of the lymph nodes, usually in the neck, underarm, or groin. However, because the enlargement is painless, the symptom is easily ignored.

Only about 20 percent of those with NHL have systemic symptoms. When they do occur, symptoms include

- Fever that doesn't go away;

- Night sweats;

- Constant tiredness;

- Unexplained weight loss;
- Itching.

Because there are so many forms of NHL involving different organs, signs and symptoms vary, often depending on the areas of the body or systems affected.

Advanced Lymphoma

- Enlarged liver;
- Enlarged spleen, resulting in abdominal distension.

Lymphoma Involving the Gastrointestinal Tract

- Palpable abdominal mass;
- Abdominal pain;
- Nausea;
- Vomiting;
- Intestinal obstruction;
- Gastrointestinal bleeding.

Lymphoma Involving the Bone Marrow

- Symptoms of anemia, such as pallor, difficulty breathing, fatigue, and rapid heart beat;
- Recurrent infections;
- Increased bruising;
- Petechiae (tiny red spots on the skin).

Lymphoma Involving the Urinary Tract

Lymphoma of the urinary tract can cause renal failure, the symptoms of which are
- Fatigue;
- Loss of appetite;
- Anemia.

Cutaneous T-Cell Lymphoma (CTCL)

- Redness;
- Itching;
- Flat, raised patches on the skin (plaques);
- Skin tumors of various types (for example, isolated dark patches, raised thick nodules, or oozing ulcerated lesions), depending on

the exact type of CTCL and the stage of growth.

Diagnostic and Staging Tests

See "Hodgkin's Disease."

Tests Unique to Non-Hodgkin's Lymphoma

Immune markers in blood or tissue samples that identify particular types of tumor cells are becoming widely available.

Staging

Staging of the lymphomas is more complicated than in other forms of cancer. There are many different types, and the prognosis and treatment of the disease depends on the patient's age and general health, the presence and size of masses in the abdomen, or the rate of growth of the cells as measured by the amount of an enzyme called lactose dehydrogenase (LDH). A high level of LDH indicates advanced disease.

The traditional staging system, known as the Ann Arbor system, follows.

- Stage I: involvement of a single lymph node region (stage I) or of a single organ or site other than the lymph nodes.

- Stage II: involvement of two or more lymph node regions on the same side of the diaphragm (above or below), or localized involvement of an extralymphatic organ or site.

- Stage III: involvement of lymph node regions on both sides of the diaphragm and possible localized involvement of an extra-lymphatic site, the spleen, or both.

- Stage IV: Widespread involvement of one or more sites other than lymph nodes, with or without lymph node involvement, or isolated extralymphatic involvement with distant lymph node involvement.

- Relapsed: The cancer has returned after treatment, either in the original site or in another part of the body.

Often the staging designation includes a letter to indicate the degree of symptoms present. A means no general symptoms. B means the patient has unexplained loss of more than 10 percent of body weight in the six months prior to diagnosis, unexplained fever, or night sweats. E indicates disease has spread to nearby tissues.

Cutaneous T-Cell Lymphoma

Doctors stage cutaneous T-cell lymphoma (CTCL) differently from other types of NHL. There are three clinical stages:

- Stage I, the *premyotic* or *erythematous* stage, produces general itching and superficial skin eruptions. These lesions may come and go spontaneously, sometimes for several years before a physician diagnoses the condition.

- Stage II, the *plaque* stage, involves irregular thickening of the skin; itchiness; raised, irregularly shaped plaques; palpable lymph nodes; and lesions that do not go away. Fissures may develop on palms and soles; lesions on the scalp may lead to hair loss.

- Stage III involves skin tumors and other mass lesions, usually in the lymph nodes in areas such as the underarms, groin, neck, and/or in other organs, including the liver and breasts.

Treatment

The staging system used in assessing NHL, although good for identifying types of the disease, is not very useful in determining treatment. For that reason researchers at the National Cancer Institute have created a simpler system called *treatment staging*. The choice of treatment depends on the type of cells involved, the stage of the disease, whether it is low-grade or aggressive, and the age and overall health of the person.

Low-Grade Lymphoma

There are two treatment groups. Group I (combining Ann Arbor stages I and II) indicates that local radiation therapy may cure the disease (see Chapter 16, "Radiation"). Group II (combining Ann Arbor stages III and IV) requires

systemic chemotherapy (see Chapter 17, "Chemotherapy").

Radiation Therapy. A person with Ann Arbor stage I or II disease receives radiation therapy to places where there is demonstrated disease. Although controversy remains, growing evidence suggests that this treatment may cure localized disease. In some studies, 54 percent of people given local radiation therapy were free of disease after 10 years; the cure rate may be higher among those treated with total lymphoid radiation, but doctors have limited experience with this treatment, and it should be given only through a clinical trial.

There are many therapeutic options in advanced (Ann Arbor stage III or IV) low-grade lymphomas, ranging from no treatment at all but close observation of patients with no symptoms to combination chemotherapy plus biological therapy using interferon (see Chapter 18, "Biological Therapies"). These treatments rarely cure the disease, but they can induce remission, which typically lasts about two years.

Chemotherapy. Single-agent chemotherapy usually involves cyclophosphamide (Cytoxan) or chlorambucil (Leukeran), with or without prednisone. People who receive this treatment usually take longer to achieve complete remission than those who receive more aggressive combination therapy.

Among the combination chemotherapy regimens are:

- CVP (cyclophosphamide [Cytoxan], vincristine [Oncovin], prednisone;

- COPP (CVP + procarbazine [Matulane]);

- CHOP (CVP + doxorubicin [Adriamycin]);

- CHOP-Bleo (CHOP + bleomycin [Blenoxane]);

- BACOP (CVP + bleomycin [Blenoxane] and doxorubicin [Adriamycin]);

- MOPP (mechlorethamine [Mustargen], vincristine [Oncovin], procarbazine, prednisone).

Different treatment centers may use different dosages of these agents and may give them in different intervals.

Combination Therapy. An approach that is currently being investigated combines chemotherapy and radiation therapy, and involves giving three or four cycles of chemotherapy, then radiation therapy directed at all involved lymph nodes, then three or four additional cycles of chemotherapy (see Chapter 20, "Combination Treatments"). If the disease converts from one stage or type to another, doctors perform biopsies of lymph nodes to determine whether and how to change the approach to therapy.

Intermediate-Grade Lymphomas

Some experts consider a three-group system to be more useful in guiding treatment options. Under this rubric, group I is the same as Ann Arbor stage I. Group II describes cases involving two or more lymph node regions or a nonlymph site, and in which there are no factors such as a high level of lactose dehydrogenase (LDH) in the bloodstream, B symptoms have occurred, or bulky tumors are present, suggesting a poor prognosis. Group III includes all other Ann Arbor groups and anyone with group II disease who has one or more poor-prognosis factors (such as the B symptoms).

Radiation Therapy. Although radiation therapy alone can halt localized aggressive lymphoma, results are almost always better with combination chemotherapy.

Chemotherapy. Among the many combination chemotherapy regimens used in treating aggressive lymphomas are BACOP or CHOP (described earlier) and the following:

- C-MOPP [cyclophosphamide (Cytoxan), vincristine (Oncovin), procarbazine (Matulane), prednisone];

- HOP [doxorubicin (Adriamycin), vincristine (Oncovin), prednisone];

- COP-BLAM [cyclophosphamide (Cytoxan), vincristine (Oncovin), prednisone, bleomycin (Blenoxane), doxorubicin (Adriamycin), procarbazine (Matulane)];

- M-BACOD [methotrexate, leucovorin, bleomycin (Blenoxane), doxorubicin (Adriamycin), cyclophosphamide (Cytoxan), vincristine (Oncovin), dexamethasone (Decadron)];

- ProMACE-MOPP [prednisone, methotrexate, leucovorin, doxorubicin (Adriamycin), cyclophosphamide (Cytoxan), epipodophyllotoxin alternating with cycles of mechlorethamine (Mustargen), vincristine (Oncovin), procarbazine (Matulane), and prednisone].

When MOPP and C-MOPP regimens were introduced in the 1970s, the complete remission rate rose from 0 to 45 percent; many people who achieved remission have remained disease-free for up to 24 years. Further refinements in chemotherapy have shown that in some studies about 75 percent of people with aggressive lymphoma can achieve complete remission.

Different centers will administer these agents at different doses and according to different schedules. For example, some experts give four to six cycles of CHOP or ProMACE-MOPP to people with fewer than three sites of disease and no bulky masses; if response is lower than expected, they add radiation therapy directed only at the specific site of the disease.

High-Grade Lymphoma

The preferred choice for treatment of high-grade lymphoma is high-dose combination chemotherapy. The prognosis is better if there are no tumor masses present greater than 10 cm in diameter; if the gastrointestinal tract is not involved; if a tumor is found in no more than one extra nodal site; and if the amount of lactose dehydrogenase (LDH) in the blood is low.

The exact selection of drugs depends on the preference and experience of the oncologist and the form of disease. Generally, treatment includes several courses of high doses of one of the regimens described earlier, followed by evaluation of the response to therapy. Those individuals with residual disease may be given more chemotherapy to eliminate any recurring disease, plus prophylaxis of the central nervous system to prevent spread.

Cutaneous T-Cell Lymphoma (Mycosis Fungoides)

Treatment for CTCL involves topical and systemic chemotherapy, radiation therapy, and biological agents such as interferon or monoclonal antibodies (see Chapter 18, "Biological Therapies").

Survival

Overall, the five-year survival rate of NHL is about 50 percent. Studies of patients with low-grade lymphomas have found that the five-year survival rates are approximately 60 to 80 percent.

Combination chemotherapy for aggressive NHL produces complete responses in 41 to 74 percent of cases, with long-term survival of 40 to 60 percent.

Special Needs

People treated for NHL need checkups every three or four months for the first two years after treatment, and every four to six months for five years after diagnosis. Most oncologists suggest x-rays and blood tests at every visit, and ultrasound or CT scans of the abdomen and pelvis once a year.

In cases where the lymphoma involves the stomach area, the physician may recommend a partial or total gastrectomy, removal of part or all of the stomach, to reduce the bulk of the disease (see "Stomach").

Individuals with CTCL may have disfiguring lesions on the skin and can benefit from instruction about skin care, control of infection, and nutrition. They may also need additional therapy to cope with the impact of a disease that alters personal appearance (see Chapter 29, "Body Image and Self-Esteem").

Ask About

Since so many regimens are available for treating NHL, some oncologists strongly encourage two or more opinions before you make a treatment decision (see Chapter 12, "How Many Opinions Do You Need?"). If you have high-grade lymphoma or low-grade stage III or IV disease, you might consider volunteering for a clinical trial. Although some researchers are evaluating new drugs and/or new combinations, others are exploring ways to refine widely used combinations to produce optimal results (see Chapter 21, "Investigational Treatments").

For example, because one concern is that the lymphoma can become resistant to one or more drugs in a regimen (see Chapter 17, "Chemotherapy"), oncologists are evaluating whether giving doses of certain drugs on different days may minimize resistance and thus improve the response. Another approach is to boost the doses, by increasing the amount of drug given at one time, by reducing the time of the cycle over which the drug is administered (for example, decreasing the number of weeks from 12 to six), or both. These adjustments appear to be improving responses in selected groups that, according to some studies, show remission in 80 percent of cases, with about two-thirds of people exhibiting long-term survival.

Increasing the dose intensity of chemotherapy appears to offer hope for improving the cure rate. (Intensity is determined by the amount of drug given and the interval between doses.) Research is under way to determine how best to increase the intensity of combination regimens while keeping side effects to a minimum.

Bone marrow transplantation allows for very high doses of chemotherapy, and clinical trials are under way for patients with high-grade lymphoma who have a poor prognosis, and those who have had a relapse (see Chapter 19, "Bone Marrow Transplant").

You may want to consider volunteering for a clinical trial in which one of several biological therapies is currently being evaluated, if you are eligible (see Chapter 18, "Biological Therapies," and Chapter 21, "Investigational Treatments"). For instance, interferon may be useful in low-grade lymphoma; a few people with NHL have shown improvement after treatment with interleukin-2; and experiments suggest that vaccines may improve outcome by triggering a person's immune response to lymphoma cells.

MULTIPLE MYELOMA

Multiple myeloma is the most common of a group of cancers known as *plasma cell neoplasms*, also called *plasma cell dyscrasias*, or PCD. (The word dyscrasia, from the Greek for "bad mix," means an imbalance.)

Plasma cells are the most mature form of B-lymphocytes and normally cannot multiply. But PCD causes one specific family of plasma cells to proliferate and produce too many antibodies, called *immunoglobulins* (Ig). The abundant and abnormal cells are called *myeloma cells*. They collect in multiple sites in bone marrow and the outer part of bones, sometimes forming tumors called *plasmacytoma*. At this stage the disorder is called *multiple myeloma*.

PCD can be either benign or malignant. Although it is uncommon, causing roughly 1 percent of all cancers and 10 to 15 percent of the blood cancers, its incidence is increasing, perhaps because of improvements in diagnosis. Today it is more common than Hodgkin's disease. (The plasma cell cancers are different from lymphomas [see "Hodgkin's Disease" and "Non-Hodgkin's Lymphoma"] because PCD affects lymphocytes at a later stage of maturity.) About 75 percent of PCD cases are multiple myelomas. Another 20 percent are *Waldenström's macroglobulinemia*. The remaining types are quite rare (see "Types," later).

Scientists do not know what causes multiple myeloma, and the course of the disease varies widely among those who have it. Some experts suspect that exposure to radiation or such chemicals as those used to manufacture paper pulp or plastics may be a factor, but there is little evidence to prove the link.

Fortunately, in the past two decades, there have been significant advances in treatment, and the pain and disability that once characterized the disease are often avoidable.

Multiple myeloma affects plasma cells, a type of lymphocyte that produces antibodies to help the body fight infections. When an antibody latches onto a bacteria or virus, it triggers a complex immune response that destroys the organism. Each type of plasma cell recognizes only a single foreign substance, and when activated, it produces a large amount of an antibody specifically against that invader. Thus, to defend against the many potentially infectious agents, the body produces an infinite variety of plasma cells.

Who Is at Risk?

- The elderly (average age of onset is 60; rarely occurs before 40; the incidence rises steadily to age 80);

- African-Americans, who develop the disease twice as often as Caucasians;

- People who have been exposed to radiation;

- People who have been exposed to such materials as asbestos, benzene, pesticides, and others used in rubber manufacturing;

- People with a history of a single plasmacytoma (presence of this form of PCD is a precursor to multiple myeloma in about 60 percent of cases).

Screening Tests

There are no screening tests. Routine tests may detect abnormal M-protein levels in blood or urine. If unusual concentrations of protein are found, further diagnostic tests are done (see later).

Types

Multiple Myeloma

- Smoldering multiple myeloma;
- Nonsecretory myeloma;
- Osteosclerotic myeloma;
- Plasma cell leukemia;
- Solitary plasmacytoma (sometimes called solitary myeloma of bone);
- Extramedullary plasmacytoma (myeloma that occurs in soft tissues, such as the tonsils, nose, or throat, rather than in the bones).

Other Forms of Plasma Cell Dyscrasia (PCD)

- Waldenström's macroglobulinemia;
- Monoclonal gammopathy of undetermined significance (MGUS);
- Benign monoclonal gammopathy (BMG).

Signs and Symptoms

Multiple myeloma produces no noticeable symptoms initially. As the number of myeloma cells increases, they destroy the hard part of the bone, causing pain. In about two-thirds of cases, bone pain, especially in the back or chest, is the first symptom that prompts a person to seek treatment. Eventually, as the bones dissolve at a faster rate than the body can rebuild them, lesions and holes develop. Fractures can occur, producing additional pain. If the disease affects the spine, the vertebrae can compress and damage the nerves. The overproduction of plasma cells may crowd out red blood cells, causing anemia, which produces symptoms of fatigue and general weakness.

The breakdown of bone leads to high levels of calcium in the blood, which causes such symptoms as weakness or nausea.

The myeloma cells continue to produce large amounts of certain antibodies and disrupt the ability of normal plasma cells to produce normal antibodies. As a result, people with multiple myeloma are susceptible to bacterial infections.

Left unchecked, abnormal M-protein levels in the blood circulate to all parts of the body, causing fatigue, mental changes, and/or damage to the retina of the eye. The proteins cause some people to become extremely sensitive to cold and may result in damage to the delicate filtering tubes in the kidneys, a condition called myeloma kidney. The damage may be irreversible and ultimately leads to kidney failure. If the disease affects the spine, the vertebrae can compress and cause nerve damage.

- Bone pain usually in the back or chest, sometimes in arms or legs;
- Pain that worsens with movement;
- Pain that diminishes at night;
- Pain that is mild and transient initially but that becomes severe, especially if abrupt movement causes fracture;
- Occasional bleeding from nose or gums;
- Easy bruising.

Advanced or Untreated Disease

- Bone deformities, especially in ribs and breastbone;
- Collapsed vertebrae, resulting in loss of height, sometimes as much as 5 inches;
- Vulnerability to severe infections, especially pneumonia and meningitis;
- Symptoms of anemia or high calcium levels, including:
- Weakness or numbness, especially in the legs;
- Fatigue;
- Loss of appetite;
- Nausea and vomiting;
- Excessive thirst;
- Mental confusion;
- Constipation;
- Increased urination.

Osteosclerotic myeloma produces a set of unique symptoms:

- Bone pain;
- Numbness, burning, and tingling in associated areas due to nerve injury;
- Weakness;

- Enlarged spleen and liver;

- Darkening of skin;

- Increased body hair growth;

- Enlarged breasts or reduced testicle size.

Diagnostic and Staging Tests

(For more details on the following tests, see Chapter 8, "Diagnostic Tests.")

- Blood tests;

- Urine tests;

- X-rays;

- Bone marrow biopsy (presence of more than 30 percent plasma cells in marrow usually indicates myeloma);

- MRI and CT scans.

Tests Unique to Multiple Myeloma

- Blood tests to identify specific immunoglobulins. Almost all people with multiple myeloma have M-protein in the blood or urine.

Staging

- Stage I: low tumor burden (few myeloma cells have spread throughout the bone marrow), and no destructive bone lesions are found. Number of red blood cells and calcium levels are normal; amount of M-protein in blood or urine is low. There may be no symptoms.

- Stage II: a relatively higher number of myeloma cells in the bone marrow.

- Stage III: relatively large number of myeloma cells. One or more other criteria may be present: decrease in number of red blood cells (*anemia*); high calcium levels; and more than three bone tumors. Abnormally high levels of M-protein in blood or urine.

All three stages have substages, depending on kidney function, which is determined by the level of a blood substance called creatinine. They may be low (normal or substage A) or high (abnormal or substage B).

The other forms of PCD do not have staging systems.

Treatment

Multiple Myeloma

In most cases, the goal of treatment for myeloma is to kill myeloma cells, control the growth of bone tumors, and relieve pain. The specific approach depends on the stage, whether symptoms have appeared, the person's age, and other factors.

If symptoms are not present, doctors monitor the person carefully but usually do not prescribe therapy. Evidence does not show that early treatment prolongs survival.

The standard approach to treating symptomatic multiple myeloma is four- to six-week courses of chemotherapy treatment with one oral alkylating agent plus prednisone (see Chapter 17, "Chemotherapy"). Typically, the agent of choice is melphalan (Alkeran). About 70 percent of people on this regimen experience a partial response—that is, they have at least some relief of symptoms. Two measures of improvement are a lower tumor burden and blood tests showing a decrease of at least 75 percent in the level of M-protein. The complete or nearly complete remission rate is usually no more than 10 percent.

Other drug options include chlorambucil (Leukeran) or cyclophosphamide (Cytoxan); success rates with these agents are similar to that of melphalan (Alkeran). Treatment usually lasts no more than six months to a year, because any response to the drug will occur during this time. Prolonged chemotherapy does not improve survival and could increase the risk of leukemia. People who do not respond to melphalan (Alkeran) sometimes receive other drugs and high doses of dexamethasone (Decadron).

Physicians treat local areas of disease in the bone with radiation therapy (see Chapter 16, "Radiation").

People whose myeloma relapses after an initial course of treatment may respond to therapy using the VAD regimen. This involves continuous infusion of vincristine (Oncovin) and doxorubicin (Adriamycin) plus oral high-dose dexamethasone. Response rates are about 60 to 70 percent, but the regimen is highly toxic.

Other forms of PCD

The treatment of choice for isolated plasmacytoma of bone is radiation therapy directed at the single bone tumor. However, most people will relapse with systemic disease, for which chemotherapy is an option.

People with myeloma in soft tissues (extramedullary plasmacytoma) usually receive external beam radiation therapy; sometimes radiation therapy follows surgery to remove a tumor. Chemotherapy may be suggested if symptoms appear (see Chapter 20, "Combination Treatments").

If people with Waldenström's macroglobulinemia do not experience symptoms, they usually receive no treatment. Should symptoms develop, treatment options include chemotherapy or removing a quantity of blood, filtering it to remove the abnormal protein, and reinfusing the blood cells (*plasmapheresis*).

People with monoclonal gammopathy of undetermined significance (MGUS) do not receive treatment, but physicians monitor them closely to watch for signs that another form of PCD or lymphoma is developing.

Survival

Before the advent of chemotherapy, survival following diagnosis of multiple myeloma was only six or seven months. With the use of melphalan plus prednisone, average survival is now three years.

- Five-year survival for stage I cancer is 25 to 40 percent.

- Five-year survival for stage II cancer is 15 to 30 percent.

- Five-year survival for stage III cancer is 10 to 25 percent.

- More than 50 percent of people with isolated plasmacytoma of the bone treated with radiation therapy survive for 10 years or more.

- Median survival among people with extramedullary plasmacytoma treated with radiation therapy is more than eight years.

- Macroglobulinemia has a median survival of approximately five years.

- MGUS is not usually fatal, but people with this form of PCD have about a 30 percent risk of developing myeloma or lymphoma within 15 years.

Special Needs

People with multiple myeloma are very susceptible to infections and should receive vaccinations against such diseases as pneumonia. The vaccines must be the killed or attenuated type, because vaccines that contain live viruses increase the risk of causing the illness they are designed to prevent.

People with PCD are at risk for bone fractures. Myeloma usually afflicts the elderly, and older women may already have brittle bones as the result of osteoporosis. Special precautions to avoid falls and fractures are important. At the same time, it is important to stay active, because moderate exercise helps keep bones strong.

Ask About

Some evidence suggests that those who respond well to initial chemotherapy may have a prolonged response when they receive long-term maintenance treatment with interferon, which boosts the immune system. Also under study is combination chemotherapy in alternating cycles with alpha interferon. Preliminary studies have found a partial response rate of 80 percent for this regimen and a 46 percent rate of complete or nearly complete response, significantly better than combination therapy alone (see Chapter 18, "Biological Therapies").

If you are under 60, you may want to discuss current clinical trials evaluating bone marrow transplant with your oncologist (see Chapters 19, "Bone Marrow Transplant," and 21, "Investigational Treatments").

There is some indication that allogenic BMT (bone marrow transplantation from a matched donor) combined with high-dose chemotherapy and total body radiation therapy may cure myeloma. However, multiple myeloma is primarily a disease of the elderly, who may be unable to withstand the demands of the procedure.

High-dose chemotherapy combined with autologous BMT (reinfusing the patient's own bone marrow) has promise and may be available to older people, because the procedure is tolerated by those in their 60s. Some studies found that this approach reduced the size and number of tumors by up to 75 percent in about half of the cases. Adding radiation therapy to the entire body increased the response rate to 85 percent.

Other steps, such as administering colony-stimulating factor (CSF) may speed the time it takes to respond to treatment and prevent complications. Controversy exists, however, about whether this technique cures the disease or prolongs remission.

Molecular biology holds great promise in the field of myeloma. It is becoming possible to identify specific types of abnormal plasma cells, which will enable scientists to design specific agents, such as monoclonal antibodies, to attach to and deliver cytotoxic agents, healthy genes, or other substances to the cell surfaces. These could curb, or even reverse, proliferation of cancer cells.

A study is under way to test the effectiveness of gene therapy. In this technique, doctors alter viruses in the lab and inject them into the person with myeloma. The viruses carry healthy genes into the bone marrow that correct defects in the immature B cells and thus prevent them from developing into myeloma cells.

Some evidence suggests that the presence of interleukin-6 (IL-6) may play a role in triggering the proliferation of myeloma cells. If so, then designing antibodies that disrupt the activity of IL-6 may help reduce the number of abnormal plasma cells. Studies testing this hypothesis are in progress.

BONE AND CONNECTIVE TISSUE

Sarcoma is a general term for cancer that originates from bone, cartilage, fibrous tissue, fat, or muscle in the broad category of "connective tissues." Although there are many different kinds of sarcoma, they account for only about 1 percent of all cancers.

Many of the more common types of cancer often spread to bones rather than originate there. This section deals with primary cancer that starts in the bones and connective tissues.

In bone, most tumors are benign; only the malignant ones are labeled sarcomas. About one-quarter of all sarcomas in adults are bone sarcomas. They can develop from any bone, but the arms and legs are the most common sites.

The most common bone cancer is *osteosarcoma*, a malignant tumor arising in the extremities, most often in adolescents and young adults. The second most common bone sarcoma, *chondrosarcoma*, begins in cartilage and is usually found in the pelvis, upper leg, or shoulder. The third most common primary bone sarcoma, though relatively rare, is *Ewing's sarcoma*, most often found in the pelvis or lower extremities.

Soft-tissue sarcomas can arise in many sites of the body, with 60 to 65 percent arising from the soft tissues of the extremities. Other anatomic sites include the trunk (15 percent), the head and neck region (9 percent), and the retroperitoneum (13 percent), the back wall of the abdominal cavity. Because connective tissue is distributed throughout the body, it's possible, though uncommon, for soft-tissue sarcomas to arise from almost any other site. They are given different names or "subtitles," depending on their presumed cell of origin, which is determined by a pathologist who examines the cells through a microscope. Their treatment, however, is similar, whatever their category. Most soft-tissue sarcoma in adults appear as a growing solitary tumor mass in the soft tissues.

One exception to the preceding description of soft-tissue sarcomas is Kaposi's sarcoma, a type that arises from blood vessels and often appears as tumors occurring in multiple sites. The classic form begins on the skin of the lower extremities and is usually accompanied by chronic swelling. The other form is associated with acquired immune deficiency syndrome (AIDS) or occurs in people whose immune system is suppressed by drugs required for organ transplantation or other reasons (immunosuppression) (see Chapter 36, "AIDS-Related Cancers"). Lesions associated with this latter form are more widely dispersed throughout the body, and the disease usually grows more rapidly than the classic form.

The cause of most sarcomas is unknown. There is no clear evidence that sarcomas are linked to viruses (with a possible exception of Kaposi's sarcoma) or to injury. Nor is there evidence that people inherit a predisposition to develop the disease except for the very small number of patients with sarcoma who have rare inherited syndromes. A few sarcomas are related to prior radiation and to some chemical exposures.

Sarcoma is distinct from multiple myeloma, which starts in plasma cells that are normally found inside the marrow (see "Multiple Myeloma"). It is distinct also from leukemia, a cancer of blood cells that is found inside the marrow as well as in the circulating blood (see "Acute Leukemia" and "Chronic Leukemia").

The connective tissues include bone, cartilage, muscle, tendon, ligament, and fat tissues as well as the many blood vessels in the body. The bones of the human skeleton support weight, allow movement, and protect the internal organs, such as the brain, the heart, and the lungs. The outermost layer of bone is hard and compact, almost like a nonliving structure, but bony tissue is continually being replaced by metabolic processes in the body. The inside structure of bones is a more porous, spongy tissue called *cancellous* bone. In many of the bones there is tissue in this inner region called *marrow* that produces blood cells. Newly formed and still-growing bone is called *osteoid* tissue. When bones make contact with other bones, at a joint, they are covered with a layer of cushionlike tissue called cartilage. The other connective tissues of the body serve many functions, ranging from moving the limbs (muscles), to holding bones and other structures together (ligaments), to circulating blood (blood vessels). Even fat is considered a connective tissue. Any cancer originating from these tissues is termed a soft-tissue sarcoma.

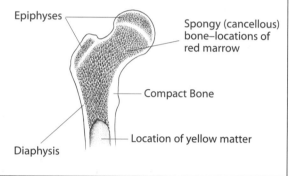

Who Is at Risk?

Both children and adults of all ages can develop sarcomas, but the frequency of the various subcategories varies with age. For example:

- The most common type of soft-tissue sarcoma in children is thought to arise from cells related to the skeletal muscle (childhood rhabdomyosarcoma; see Chapter 35, "Cancer in Children").

- Osteosarcoma and Ewing's sarcoma tend to occur in adolescents and young adults, with the latter occurring in a slightly younger group than the osteosarcomas (see Chapter 35, "Cancer in Children").

- Most types of soft-tissue sarcoma occur over a wide range of age groups.

In proportion to other cancers developing in each age group, sarcoma is a more frequent type of malignant tumor in children than in adults.

A small proportion of sarcomas occur in the area of the body that received radiation treatments for a different cancer.

Sarcomas have been disproportionately associated with some inherited diseases such as neurofibromatosis or Gardiner's syndrome (multiple colon polyps).

Jewish or Mediterranean heritage has been associated with the classic form of Kaposi's sarcoma, and both AIDS and immunosuppression for organ transplantation have been associated with the more widespread form of Kaposi's sarcoma.

Because all the preceding risk factors are uncommon causes of sarcoma, no risk factors are present in most patients.

Screening Tests

There are no screening tests.

Types of Bone and Soft-Tissue Sarcomas

There are many subcategories of the various types of sarcoma. The chart that follows summarizes these types.

Bone Sarcomas	Tissue of Origin
Osteosarcoma	Osteoid tissue
Chondrosarcoma	Cartilage
Ewing's sarcoma	Connective tissue in marrow cavity
Malignant giant cell tumor	Connective tissue in marrow cavity
Fibrosarcoma of bone	Connective tissue in marrow cavity
Chordoma	Cellular remnants of fetal spinal cord
Periosteal sarcoma	Bone surface layer that produces bone tissue (periosteum)

Soft-Tissue Sarcomas (Examples of Various Subtypes)	Tissue of Origin
Angiosarcoma; hemangiosarcoma	Blood vessels
Fibrosarcoma	Fibrous connective tissue
Kaposi's sarcoma	Blood vessels
Leiomyosarcoma	Smooth muscle
Liposarcoma	Fat cells
Lymphangiosarcoma	Lymph vessels
Neurilemmoma	Nerve fiber sheaths
Rhabdomyosarcoma	Skeletal muscle
Synovial sarcoma	Membranes lining joints or around tendons

Bone sarcomas grow like a balloon being inflated. There is usually a distortion of the bone, and the tumor has a shell of tissue (or capsule) around it as it extends into the adjacent soft tissues. These tumor extensions may invade normal tissues, including nerves, which cause pain. Destruction of adjacent normal bone may make the bone susceptible to fracture. The abnormal growth allows spread of the sarcoma to other areas, either through the spongy areas of the bone in the bone marrow cavity or through the bloodstream to distant locations, particularly the lungs.

Soft-tissue sarcomas usually appear first as masses that cause no discomfort until they become fairly large; consequently, they often go unnoticed. Like bone sarcomas, they grow along the path of least resistance. If the tumor compresses major nerves or blood vessels, the person may experience pain, weakness, or even circula-

tory problems, but this is uncommon. In a few cases, the tumor blocks the bowel or the urinary tract, causing problems in these areas. As with bone sarcomas, the soft-tissue sarcoma may spread through the circulatory system to other organs, particularly the lungs, and in a small proportion of patients to nearby lymph glands.

Signs and Symptoms

Bone Sarcomas

- Swelling or firm lump intimately associated with a bone or joint;
- Pain in the area of swelling, often worse at night;
- Stiffness or tenderness in the affected area;
- Fractures of a bone after minimal injury or movement.

Soft-Tissue Sarcomas

- Enlarging, nontender swelling or mass in superficial or deep soft tissues, with minimal discomfort;
- Discomfort from local pressure of a mass pressing against adjacent nerves or muscles.

Kaposi's Sarcoma

- Multiple dark lesions appearing simultaneously in or under the skin of swollen, lower extremities (classic form), or over much of the body and oral cavity (as with AIDS);
- Enlarged lymph glands in the area where the skin lesions have been noted;
- Generalized symptoms of AIDS (diarrhea, malnutrition, fever, etc.).

Diagnostic and Staging Tests

(For more details on the following tests, see Chapter 8, "Diagnostic Tests.")

Bone Sarcoma

- X-ray of the bone and the chest;
- CT or MRI scan;

- Bone scan;

- Biopsy of the suspected sarcoma.

Soft-Tissue Sarcomas

- CT or MRI scan;

- Chest x-ray;

- Biopsy of the suspected sarcoma.

Tests Unique to Bone Cancer and Connective Tissue Cancer

No tests are available.

Staging

Bone Sarcomas

Bone sarcomas are staged according to several factors:

- Grade (G), the microscopic grade is an indication of the rate and pattern of growth;

- Low-grade tumors (G1 & G2) may grow large but are not as likely to metastasize as the higher-grade tumors;

- High-grade tumors (G3 & G4) tend to grow more rapidly, often spread into neighboring tissues, and are more likely to spread to other sites of the body than the low-grade tumors. Ewing's sarcomas are always classified as G4.

Bone sarcomas are also staged according to the TNM system established by the American Joint Committee on Cancer. T is the local extent of the tumor in relation to the cortex, the outer compact shell of the bone. M indicates metastasis. And N indicates lymph node involvement.

- Stage IA is a grade 1 or 2 tumor that is confined within the cortex. There is no lymph node involvement and no metastasis. Stage IB is a grade 1 or 2 tumor that has invaded beyond the cortex.

- Stage IIA is a grade 3 or 4 tumor that is confined within the cortex. There is no lymph node involvement and no metastasis. Stage IIB is a grade 3 or 4 tumor that has invaded beyond the cortex.

- Stage III has not been defined.

- Stage IVA is a tumor of a grade or extent that has spread to the local lymph nodes. There is no metastasis. Stage IVB indicates metastasis has occurred.

Soft-Tissue Sarcomas

The staging system for soft-tissue sarcomas is similar to that used for bone sarcomas and uses a TNM system with microscopic grade added also. The stages of soft-tissue sarcoma depend primarily on tumor size and microscopic grade, because enlargement of local lymph nodes is uncommon. This staging system does not apply to Kaposi's sarcoma.

Grade (G) indicates the assessment of the microscopic appearance (G1, G2, or G3).

- Stage IA is a grade 1 tumor that is less than 5 cm at its greatest dimension. Stage IB is a grade 1 tumor that is larger than 5 cm at its greatest dimension. In either stage there is no lymph node involvement and no metastasis.

- Stage IIA is a grade 2 tumor that is less than 5 cm at its greatest dimension. Stage IIB is a grade 2 tumor that is larger than 5 cm at its greatest dimension. In either stage there is no lymph node involvement and no metastasis.

- Stage IIIA is a grade 3 or 4 tumor that is less than 5 cm at its greatest dimension. Stage IIIB is a grade 3 or 4 tumor that is larger than 5 cm at its greatest dimension. There is no lymph node involvement and no metastasis.

- Stage IVA is any grade tumor of any size with lymph node involvement but no metastasis. Stage IVB is any grade tumor of any size with any lymph node involvement and distant metastasis.

Treatment

All sarcomas require operative treatment of some kind. High-grade tumors typically require surgery and radiation and/or chemotherapy, depending on the type. (See Chapters 15, "Surgery"; 16, "Radiation"; 17, "Chemotherapy"; 20, "Combination Treatments"; and 35, "Cancer in Children".)

Bone Sarcomas

The extent of surgery depends on the stage of the tumor. Benign or unusually low-grade tumors, involving only a short segment of a long bone, can be removed by simple excision or curettage (careful scraping of the bone). Surgeons attempt to remove all the affected tissue plus a margin of healthy tissue to reduce the risk of regrowth. Sometimes, to kill any remaining tumor cells, cryosurgery, a tissue-freezing technique, follows curettage. These conservative approaches are not appropriate for most bone sarcomas because very few of them are low grade.

For most bone sarcomas of limited extent (except Ewing's sarcoma), surgeons can remove a complete segment of bone along with the soft tissue surrounding the tumor. If the sarcoma is in an arm or a leg, the involved bone can be replaced by a metal prosthetic device, or a bone graft from a cadaver. Muscles and other connective tissues may be reattached to allow limb function. This approach, called limb-sparing surgery, can cure up to 80 percent of sarcomas that are anatomically suited for this approach. This is an option if the tumor does not involve adjacent major nerves or blood vessels, and if it is possible to remove adjacent soft tissue and healthy bone on either side of the tumor. This limb-sparing technique routinely employs a program of chemotherapy (with or without radiation therapy) before surgery. This approach is more of a problem in children whose bones are still growing. However, sometimes surgeons can implant a special type of prosthesis that can be expanded in subsequent operations.

Amputation of the affected limb is the only feasible treatment in some circumstances, such as when the tumor has spread too far locally, if the surgery would leave behind a nonworking limb, or if the patient is younger than seven. In this case, an artificial limb is necessary.

For limb-sparing treatment of bone sarcoma, various chemotherapy regimes are administered prior to surgery. Drugs include doxorubicin (Adriamycin), cyclophosphamide (Cytoxan), and methotrexate. Clinical trials have established improved survival when chemotherapy follows surgery, whether limb-sparing treatment is employed or not. The role of radiation therapy is unclear because osteosarcoma is not particularly responsive to it. However, radiation therapy is used before surgery in some cases (for example, osteosarcoma of the jaw).

Ewing's Sarcoma

Chemotherapy plus radiation therapy to the area of the tumor, followed by postradiation chemotherapy, is the standard treatment for Ewing's sarcoma. However, surgical removal of the affected bone is sometimes feasible after the initial combined treatment with chemotherapy and radiation. One effective chemotherapy regime includes vincristine (Oncovin), doxorubicin (Adriamycin), cyclophosphamide (Cytoxan), and actinomycin D in multiple cycles over a one-year period. Recent approaches also include chemotherapy with etoposide (VePesid) and ifosfamide (IFEX). Clinical trials are attempting to determine the optimal regime.

Soft-Tissue Sarcomas

The treatment of choice for soft-tissue sarcomas is complete surgical removal of the tumor along with an envelope of normal tissue around it. Surgery appears to be sufficient for low-grade sarcomas. But if excision cannot be completely accomplished, radiation therapy may control growth of any remaining tumor cells.

For intermediate or high-grade sarcomas, radiation therapy is employed before or after surgery. Even if removal appears complete, radiation therapy may be suggested to destroy any sarcoma cells that remain at the edge of the excision site. In some circumstances, such as after amputation of a limb that removes a generous margin of normal tissue above the tumor, radiation therapy is not considered necessary, even if the sarcoma is a high-grade one.

The optimal timing and method of radiation therapy for high grade soft-tissue sarcomas are not established. Radiation therapy prior to surgery is sometimes preferred by radiation oncologists because of the greater tolerance of normal tissues to the radiation and the possibility of treating a smaller area. Radiation therapy after surgery is often preferred by surgeons because it makes the surgery a bit easier. Implanting small tubes (catheters) at the time of the operation for later intermittent administration of radioactive materials in these catheters may improve the distribution of the radiation somewhat as well as shorten the treatment time.

Radiation therapy combined with surgical removal of the tumor has led to much better results than surgery alone. This combination treatment has also been a key feature in the feasibility of limb-sparing surgery for soft-tissue sarcomas. Radiation therapy has compensated for the often necessary narrow surgical margins around the tumor when the limb is being spared.

The role of chemotherapy in the management of soft-tissue sarcomas is unclear at this time. All clinical trials attempting to improve survival of patients by adding various chemotherapy regimes after surgery (with or without radiation therapy) have failed to do so. Current trials continue to explore possible benefits of different agents and combinations, as a supplement to standard surgery and radiation therapy. However, there is no established role for chemotherapy if the local soft-tissue sarcoma appears controlled by other treatments to the area.

Chemotherapeutic drugs have been administered by injection into the arteries supplying the sarcoma for about 35 years. This procedure has been shown to shrink tumors in some cases, but complete elimination of the cancer cells has not been achieved, and no definite benefit has been demonstrated from using this method prior to radiation and/or surgery.

Kaposi's Sarcoma

Radiation therapy to the involved areas is used for the classic form of Kaposi's sarcoma and for disease of limited extent. More widespread disease usually calls for combining radiation therapy and chemotherapy.

When the Kaposi's sarcoma is associated with AIDS, treatment options are more limited because the outlook is so grave. Combination chemotherapy with doxorubicin (Adriamyacin), bleomycin (Blenoxane), vinblastine (Velban), and/or etoposide (VePesid) has been used, as has interferon (see Chapter 36, "AIDS-Related Cancers").

Survival

Osteosarcoma (Without Distant Metastasis)

- Two-year survival after tumor removal (including amputation) as the only treatment ranges from 18 to 40 percent.
- Two-year survival for osteosarcoma treated with surgery and some form of chemotherapy ranges from 56 to 90 percent. Five-year survival is similar.

Ewing's Sarcoma (Without Distant Metastasis)

- Five-year survival ranges from 35 to 70 percent with treatment programs combining radiation and chemotherapy, with or without surgical removal.

Soft-Tissue Sarcomas (Without Distant Metastasis)

- Five-year survival for extremity, trunk, and head and neck sarcomas ranges from 60 to 70 percent.
- Retroperitoneal soft-tissue sarcomas have a five-year survival rate of 50 percent, but if complete surgical removal is accomplished, results are similar to those obtained with sarcomas in other sites.
- Low-grade soft-tissue sarcomas have much better survival statistics than high-grade sarcomas in all anatomic sites.

Limited Lung Metastasis (Both Bone and Soft-Tissue Sarcomas)

- Five-year survival is approximately 30 percent if gross lung metastasis can be removed.

Metastatic Sarcoma (Not Removable)

- Survival is generally short and is affected by grade. There is a limited response to nonsurgical treatments.

Special Needs

Follow-up examinations recommended include chest x-rays at six- to 12-month intervals, and CT scans of the lungs at longer intervals, because later spread of the sarcoma to the lungs can be completely curtailed by removing a portion of the lung in many instances. This applies to patients with either bone or soft-tissue sarcomas.

Many cases of bone and soft-tissue sarcoma occur in young people. The disease and its treatment may involve amputation, or other changes in physical appearance or function. Traumatic at any age, these events may be particularly so to young people trying to establish their identities and their place in the world. In addition to the need for vigorous physical rehabilitation or appropriate prosthetic help, counseling can help them adjust to the necessary changes in their bodies and help them cope with the problems of self-esteem (see Chapters 28, "Managing Disabilities and Limitations"; 29, "Body Image and Self-Esteem"; and 35, "Cancer in Children").

Ask About

Improvements in surgery of bone sarcomas using preoperative chemotherapy and reconstruction with prosthetic implants are making it possible to reduce the number of amputations for bone sarcomas when they occur on the extremities. Greater appreciation of the important role of added radiation therapy has improved the surgical results for soft-tissue sarcoma and has increased the likelihood of limb-sparing surgery. If amputation is suggested to you, ask about the possibility of limb-sparing surgery. It is also useful to get a second opinion (see Chapter 12, "How Many Opinions Do You Need?").

Because sarcomas are rare, you may want to discuss with your doctor being treated at a large cancer treatment and research center. At these centers, researchers explore the use of different drug combinations for treatment after surgery of soft-tissue sarcomas (see Chapter 21, "Investigational Treatments"). A survival benefit like that achieved in the treatment of osteosarcoma may be possible. Studies are also under way to learn whether some people with Ewing's sarcoma might benefit from very high doses of chemotherapy, which is made possible by bone marrow transplant (see Chapter 19, "Bone Marrow Transplant").

BRAIN

There are approximately 50 types of central nervous system (CNS) tumors, each affecting different types of cells and/or tissues. About 15 percent of these lesions arise in the spinal cord; the rest develop within the brain.

Primary brain cancer—cancer that arises originally in the brain—is the second most common cancer in children (see Chapter 35, "Cancer in Children") and ranks eighth among adult cancers. Secondary brain cancer, which results from metastasis of a primary cancer elsewhere in the body, accounts for 10 percent of all cases. This section is concerned with primary brain tumors.

The incidence of brain tumor peaks twice in childhood—between birth and age 4 and again between 15 and 24. Then the incidence drops to about two people in 100,000; but it begins climbing again after age 50. By 65, the rate rises to 18 people in 100,000. For unknown reasons, the incidence of CNS tumors is increasing, especially among the elderly. In most cases, the cause is unknown.

The brain is the control center for every physiological system within the body and is the organ of thought, language, and emotion. The brain and the *spinal cord*, a nerve "cable" that runs from the base of the brain through the spine, make up the *central nervous system* (CNS). The spinal cord collects nerve signals from throughout the body and directs them to the brain, which processes the information and sends back signals in response.

Joining the brain to the spinal cord are the *brain stem*, the *medulla oblongata*, and the *cerebellum*. The nerve tissues in these structures process such essential functions as breathing and maintaining blood pressure. A number of small glands are nearby. The *pituitary gland* secretes hormones that travel to other organs and that regulate their function. The *pineal gland* regulates the body's "biological clock" by secreting a hormone called *melatonin*.

Wrapped around the central structures is the *cerebrum*, which makes up about 70 percent of the brain's 3-pound weight and handles conscious thought, speech, and memory. The outer surface of the cerebrum, the *cerebral cortex* (also known as the "gray matter"), contains brain cells called *neurons*. These cells transmit nerve impulses within the brain. Cells that support and nourish the neurons are called *glial cells*. The wrinkles and folds in the gray matter create separate lobes within the brain; generally, different mental processes (for example, thought, speech, and memory) take place in different parts of these lobes.

Inside the gray matter is *white matter*, a band of nerve fibers and cells that transmit brain functions. Wrapped around the brain and the spinal cord are membranes called the *meninges*. *Cerebrospinal fluid* (CSF) circulates between the layers of the meninges and within the cavities of the brain; those cavities (also called *ventricles*) are surrounded by a membrane called the *ependyma*.

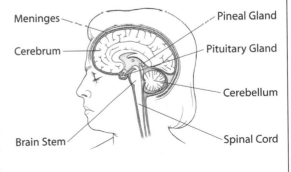

Meninges · Pineal Gland · Cerebrum · Pituitary Gland · Cerebellum · Brain Stem · Spinal Cord

Who Is at Risk?

- Children and the elderly;

- Men (except for meningioma, which occurs most often among women 30 to 50);

- People exposed to x-rays;

- People exposed to chemicals in their work, such as solvents, pesticides, oil products, and rubber;

- People exposed to vinyl chloride (at risk of developing gliomas);

- People with rare genetic conditions (for example, von Hippel-Lindau disease, tuberous sclerosis, Turcot's syndrome, Osler-Weber-Rendu syndrome, and neurofibromatosis);

- People infected with Epstein-Barr (at risk of developing primary brain lymphoma);

- People with compromised immune systems (for example, those taking immunosuppressant drugs following organ transplantation or those with acquired immune deficiency syndrome [AIDS]).

Screening Tests

There are no screening tests.

Types

Brain tumors are different from most other cancers in several ways. Because they develop within the confined space of the skull and there is little room for them to grow, even a small tumor can cause serious problems.

When they are used to describe a brain tumor the terms benign and malignant have different meanings from those used to describe other abnormal growths. In this case, *benign* means the tumor is relatively slow-growing; *malignant* means the tumor is aggressive or fast-growing. Most types of CNS tumors can be either benign or malignant. The important point, however, is that a benign CNS tumor can be just as dangerous over time as a malignant one if it begins to press on a vital area of brain tissue.

Generally, there are two types of primary brain tumors: gliomas and nonglial tumors.

Gliomas

Gliomas arise in glial cells and account for about 50 to 60 percent of CNS tumors. There are several types and subtypes of glial cells, and various kinds of tumors can develop in each subtype:

- *Astrocytoma*, the most common form of glioma, usually develops within the cerebrum. A fast-growing malignant type of astrocytoma is called *glioblastoma multiforme* and accounts for about a third of all brain tumors.

- *Brain stem glioma* develops in glial cells found in the brain stem.

- *Ependymoma* arises within the ependyma.

- *Oligodendroglioma* is a rare tumor that develops in the cells that form a protective sheath (myelin) around nerves in the white matter.

- *Mixed tumors* involve more than one of the glial cell types.

Nonglial Tumors

Nonglial tumors arise in brain cells and structures other than glial cells.

- Acoustic neurinoma, which affects the acoustic nerve, accounts for about 7 percent of primary brain tumors.

- Craniopharyngioma is a tumor arising within a structure near the pituitary gland.

- Medulloblastoma is a tumor that occurs in developing nerve cells in the cerebellum.

- Meningioma is a tumor developing from the meninges.

- Pineal parenchymal tumor is a malignant tumor of the tissues of the pineal gland. Slow-growing ones are called pineocytomas, and fast-growing ones are pineoblastomas.

- Primary brain lymphoma is a form of lymphoma classified as a CNS cancer because it first develops in CNS tissues and can occur even when lymphoma is not present elsewhere in the body.

Some brain tumors—especially glioblastomas, astrocytomas, and medulloblastomas—can quickly infiltrate nearby areas of the brain; these aggressive tumors are often called *high-*

grade tumors. Also, cells from certain cancers, such as medulloblastomas, meningiomas, and glioblastomas, are likely to spread from the brain through the spinal fluid to the spinal cord. Slow-growing (sometimes called *low-grade)* tumors, such as meningiomas, acoustic neurinomas, pituitary adenomas, and cranio-pharyngiomas, are less likely to infiltrate other areas and, if caught in time, can be treated with surgery. They may grow so slowly that symptoms don't occur for years.

Tumor cells rarely spread to other parts of the body through the bloodstream.

Signs and Symptoms

General Symptoms

- Headache, often not limited to a specific site in the head (typically, but not always, these headaches are persistent and severe, and they tend to get worse with activity, at night, or in the early morning);

- Vomiting with or without nausea (most common in children);

- Seizures (in a person over 40 with no prior history of seizures, this is often a strong indication of a brain tumor);

- Changes, often subtle, in mental ability, memory, and personality;

- Lethargy.

Symptoms Specific to Location of Tumor

- Pressure in specific ventricles of the brain, causing headache, nausea, vomiting, and loss of coordination or balance;

- Swelling of the optic nerve (papilledema) due to buildup of spinal fluid, causing blurred or double vision;

- Weakness in various body parts, especially legs or arms, often on only one side;

- Memory impairment;

- Slurred or difficult speech;

- Difficulty swallowing;

- Sensory changes, such as loss of smell or ringing in the ear;

- Inability to gaze upward (pineal tumor).

Diagnostic and Staging Tests

(For more details on the following tests, see Chapter 8, "Diagnostic Tests.")

- MRI or CT scans, which can detect more than 95 percent of all lesions, allowing the neuroradiologist to locate the tumor site and see anatomic detail;

- Positron emission tomography (PET) scans;

- Neurologic tests to evaluate muscle and brain function (memory, vision, etc.);

- Blood tests to look for specific markers of certain tumors (for example, hormone imbalances caused by pituitary tumors; abnormal alpha-fetoprotein or human chorionic gonadotropin levels caused by pineal tumors);

- Eye exam to detect signs of tumor (for example, tumor pressure causing swelling of the optic nerve);

- Hearing test to detect hearing loss, which can result from tumor of the auditory nerve, or to rule out other possible causes of ringing in the ears;

- Lumbar puncture ("spinal tap") to withdraw spinal fluid for examination for malignant cells, increased protein levels, or evidence of blood. (Today an MRI and/or CT scan is often done before—or instead of—a lumbar puncture to diagnose the cancer. A lumbar puncture is not recommended if the person has headaches or other signs of pressure, because a sudden drop in spinal fluid level can cause the tumor to shift in a potentially dangerous way.)

Tests Unique to Brain Tumors

- Diagnostic neurosurgery, a surgical procedure to remove a tumor, enables the pathologist to examine a tissue sample and establish a definitive diagnosis of the type and aggressiveness of the tumor.

- *Stereotactic neurosurgery* or *biopsy* uses computer-directed targeting of a tumor in

516 Informed Decisions: Encyclopedia

the brain. Guided by a CT or MRI scan, a needle is inserted to a precise location, and a tissue sample is retrieved through it.

- Myelography is an x-ray of the spine after injection of a contrast medium directly into the space surrounding the spinal cord. A spinal tap always precedes the test. (Note: An MRI is often performed instead of myelography because it is easier and more accurate, but this test may still be needed if MRI is unavailable or if other specific information is needed.)

- *Electroencephalography (EEG)* evaluates the electrical activity of the brain. It is a painless procedure in which electrodes are attached to various places on the person's skull while he or she lies very still. The signals are recorded on a strip of paper that a neurologist interprets to detect abnormalities.

- *Cerebral arteriogram* is a series of x-rays of the head following injection of a contrast medium into a major artery of the neck, groin, or arm. A local anesthetic is given to numb the area around the injection site. The contrast medium outlines the blood vessels in the brain so they are visible on x-ray. There is a burning sensation when the dye is injected, and some people experience nausea and/or headache.

- *Brain scan* (such as radionuclide scanning, SPECT scan, or gamma encephalography) involves injection of a radioactive substance into the bloodstream. The isotope circulates to the tumor site and is absorbed by the cancer cells, if there are any; an image is then made that reveals how much of the substance was absorbed.

Staging

The American Joint Committee on Cancer has developed a staging system for brain tumors that is based on signs and symptoms and the results of various diagnostic tests. It includes the grade of the tumor, which ranges from low (1) to high (4), depending on the degree of cell abnormality and rate of growth.

- Stage I is a grade 1 tumor that may be as large as 5 centimeters and is limited to one side of the brain. Or it is a grade 1 tumor that invades or encroaches on the ventricular system. There is no metastasis.

- Stage II is a grade 2 tumor that may be as large as 5 centimeters and is limited to one side of the brain, or a grade 2 tumor that invades or encroaches on the ventricular system. There is no metastasis.

- Stage III is a grade 3 tumor that may be as large as 5 centimeters and is limited to one side of the brain or invades, or a grade 3 tumor that encroaches on the ventricular system. There is no metastasis.

- Stage IV is a tumor of any grade that invades the opposite side of the brain and/or has metastasized.

Treatment

Any CNS tumor needs to be treated promptly, because as a tumor grows, it can cause swelling and a buildup of fluid (hydrocephalus). The pressure can block the circulation of blood and spinal fluid, which in turn robs the cells of the brain and spinal cord of necessary nutrients and the cushioning the organ requires to function optimally.

Surgery

Nearly half of primary brain tumors can be cured, usually with surgery (see Chapter 15, "Surgery"). It is often the only step in treating primary brain tumors. Besides removing or reducing the size of the tumor, surgery can relieve pressure within the skull and alleviates symptoms. Surgery also provides tumor tissue for lab analysis, the results of which may help determine whether radiation therapy or chemotherapy will be useful. Advances in technology, including imaging devices, microsurgery, and lasers, allow surgeons to remove tumors that were considered inoperable a decade ago.

For some types of tumors, such as meningiomas and acoustic neurinomas, the goal is total removal and possible cure. For other types, such as the gliomas, partial surgery is performed to reduce the tumor size and relieve pressure.

Surgery usually means a *craniotomy*, which is performed under general or, occasionally, local anesthesia. This procedure involves cutting a bone flap, a kind of window, in the skull through which the surgeon can reach the brain. After the tumor is removed, the surgeon replaces the bone flap and sutures the skin closed over it. Although a craniotomy sounds frightening, it has become relatively routine and is one of the great successes of modern medicine. In most cases, the operation does not change the person's appearance.

In recent years a technology called *stereotaxis* has become available. It uses CT and MRI scans to provide extremely precise three-dimensional images of the tumor. Physicians use stereotactic surgery to biopsy and remove tumors (see "Diagnostic and Staging Tests," earlier).

Radiation Therapy. Aggressive malignant tumors spread rapidly and cannot be cured through surgery alone, but their progress may be slowed with a combination of surgery and radiation therapy (see Chapter 16, "Radiation," and Chapter 20, "Combination Treatments"). However, this combined approach is not an option if the dosage of radiation needed to kill tumor cells risks damaging the sensitive brain tissues. Generally, radiation therapy is not given to children under 8, because their nerve cells are still developing. In older children, treatment of medulloblastomas with combined chemotherapy and radiation therapy is sometimes effective.

Stereotactic radiosurgery involves highly focused doses of radiation precisely delivered to an area deep inside the brain. The location of the tumor is determined by a CT or MRI scan, and the radiation is directed by a computer to the tumor, avoiding contact with healthy brain tissue. Although the technique has proved useful in treating small benign tumors, it is still being investigated for malignant ones.

Brachytherapy (or internal radiation therapy) involves delivering radioactive agents through a tiny catheter inserted directly into the tumor over several days. This technique, which is most often used to treat recurrence of cancer, is used along with external beam radiation therapy.

Chemotherapy. The brain is protected by the blood-brain barrier, a system of thin membranes and other structures that filter chemical molecules from the bloodstream, including many drugs. One reason brain tumors are difficult to treat with anticancer drugs is that there are so many different kinds of CNS tumor cells, several of which become resistant to drugs as the tumor grows (see Chapter 17, "Chemotherapy").

Controversy exists about which anticancer drugs can penetrate the barrier and overcome cell resistance. Some drugs that may be of benefit are nitrosureas, hydroxyureas, and diazoquinone (AZQ). The alkylating agents carmustine (BCNU) and lomustine (CCNU) are commonly given. Certain agents—such as bleomycin (Blenoxane), doxorubicin (Adriamycin), cisplatin (Platinol), vincristine (Oncovin), and plicamycin (Mithramycin)—may be more effective against certain childhood tumors.

People with brain tumors may receive corticosteroids to reduce swelling and relieve inflammation, which in turn helps restore normal brain function.

Sometimes, to overcome the blood-brain barrier, doctors inject anticancer drugs directly into the cerebrospinal fluid or directly into a tumor through a tiny tube. These methods are known as *intrathecal* and *regional delivery*.

Survival

Fortunately, advances in diagnosing and treating CNS cancers in the past two decades have improved survival rates.

Glial Tumors

Astrocytoma	Five-year survival by grade: I, 90 percent; II, 50 percent; III, 10–20 percent
Brain stem glioma	Five-year survival 30 percent–60 percent
Ependymoma	Five-year survival 40–60 percent
Glioblastoma multiforme	One-year survival less than 20 percent after symptom onset
Oligodendroglioma	Five-year survival 90 percent
Metastatic brain tumor	Less than six months—occasional survivors up to two years

Nonglial Tumors

Acoustic neurinoma	Surgery usually results in cure
Craniopharyngioma	Five-year survival 80–90 percent
Medulloblastoma	Five-year survival 60 percent
Meningioma	Following complete surgical removal, five-year survival 90–100 percent; following partial removal, 60–80 percent
Pineal tumor	Long-term survival following treatment is 33–90 percent, depending on extent of disease
Pituitary tumor	Surgery cures 90 percent of cases
Primary CNS lymphoma	One-year survival 66 percent; five-year survival 3–7 percent

Special Needs

Brain tumors can cause many severe and debilitating problems, including pain, headaches, seizures, mood changes, loss of consciousness, and incontinence. The treatment plan must include supportive care to anticipate and deal with these problems.

Some people with brain tumors who experience seizures may require anticonvulsant medication, such as phenytoin sodium (Dilantin).

Ask About

If you have a brain tumor that is considered inoperable or of a type that is not often curable, you may want to discuss with your oncologist the possibility of entering a clinical trial. A variety of treatments are being used experimentally; depending on the type of tumor you have, one of the following new approaches may be helpful (see Chapter 21, "Investigational Treatments").

Some radiologists are using hyperfractionation, the technique of administering smaller doses of radiation more often, to improve results. New aggressive regimens are being designed to treat children that include surgery and postoperative chemotherapy later followed by radiation therapy.

Studies are under way to explore ways to modify the blood-brain barrier so that it allows more drugs to pass through and reach CNS tumors.

Stereotactic radiosurgery is being tested for use on tumors near the brain stem or optic nerves, where radiation poses significant hazards. Brachytherapy, which is often used as treatment for recurrence, is being studied as an initial therapy (see "Treatment," earlier).

Also being studied is the use of photodynamic therapy, in which the person receives a light-sensitive drug that accumulates in the tumor. During surgery, a laser is aimed at the tumor, activating the drug and killing the tumor cells.

Gene therapy is also being explored. In this approach, physicians replace the damaged genes in tumor cells with healthy genes, which take over the cell's function to stop their uncontrolled growth (see Chapter 18, "Biological Therapies").

Children with tumors involving the lower part of the brain stem (medulloblastomas) or with malignant glioma who do not get better following surgery, radiation therapy, and chemotherapy may respond to treatment with aggressive chemotherapy and autologous bone marrow transplantation. Studies are also assessing the value of stereotactic radiotherapy in children with low-grade tumors, such as inoperable nonmalignant gliomas (see Chapter 35, "Cancer in Children").

Immunotherapy may have some value in treating malignant glioma. Active immunotherapy involves removing the patient's own tumor cells, treating them in the lab to create antitumor antibodies, and then injecting the antibodies into the patient. *Restorative immunotherapy* uses such agents as interferon to boost the patient's immune system. *Adoptive immunotherapy* employs the patient's own white cells that have been treated in the lab and that are then injected directly into the tumor, either alone or in combination with interleukin-2 (see Chapter 18, "Biological Therapies").

BREAST

Excluding cancers of the skin, breast cancer is the most common type of cancer in women in the United States, accounting for one of every three cancer diagnoses. (Fewer than 1 percent of breast cancer cases develop in men. The treatment is similar to that in women.) Even though the incidence of the disease in women increased from 88.6 per 100,000 in the early 1970s to 109.8 in the early 1990s, it appears to be reaching a plateau.

Experts believe that the increased incidence of breast cancer may be due partly to increased detection because of the growing use of mammography, an x-ray of the breast that can detect suspicious lesions often before they can be felt. Earlier detection combined with advances in treatment may also be responsible for the increase in five-year survival rate for breast cancer from 78 percent in the 1940s to the current 83.2 percent. The mortality rate has declined; however, it has varied according to race: The five-year survival rate for Caucasian women under 50 is 81.7; it is 66.3 percent for African-American women under 50.

The causes of breast cancer are unknown, although studies suggest that estrogen, the female hormone produced by the ovaries, is involved. One reason for suspecting estrogen is the association of breast cancer to certain reproductive system changes in a woman's life. The longer a woman is exposed to the hormone (for instance, if she starts to menstruate early, has a late menopause, and/or has children later than age 30, or not at all), the greater her risk. In fact, a current controversy is whether continuing estrogen exposure after menopause by taking estrogen replacement therapy increases a woman's risk. The studies completed thus far have yielded conflicting results. Therefore, women in consultation with their doctors must weigh their individual risk of heart disease and osteoporosis, which estrogen helps prevent, against their risk of developing breast cancer. Studies are being conducted that researchers hope will resolve the debate.

Several studies have looked at breast cancer risk and the use of oral contraceptives. Although most women are unaffected by oral contraceptives, several subgroups of women may be increasing their risk. These include women under age 45 who took the Pill before age 25 or before their first child was born, those who had their first child after age 30, and women with a history of benign breast disorders or with a family history of breast cancer.

About 5 percent of all breast cancers are inherited. A test that determines whether or not a woman carries a mutated gene for the disease may become widely available in the near future. Recently, two breast cancer susceptibility genes have been identified: BRCA1 (a flaw in this gene is common to those who have breast and ovarian cancer) and BRCA2 (a defect in this gene is associated with breast cancer alone). Carriers of a mutated BRCA1 gene have an 86 percent risk of developing breast cancer by age 70.

It has already been established that women with first-degree relatives who have had breast cancer are at greater risk of getting it themselves. These women are encouraged to have screening tests earlier and sometimes more often than women without such a family history.

There are many associations for risk, but the most notable is age. The probability of a 60-year-old woman developing breast cancer is 14 times that of a 30-year-old. One reason may be the cumulative effect of estrogen exposure that was discussed earlier.

The link to dietary fat has not been established. Large population studies comparing breast cancer rates among countries show that women in Japan who have a relatively low-fat diet have less breast cancer. When these women immigrate to a country where dietary fat is more prevalent, their rates of breast cancer eventually tend to match those of the host country. However, a review of several large studies on diet and breast cancer found no link between cancer and level of fat intake.

Obesity has also been associated with breast cancer. The link may be due to the fact that fat cells store estrogen.

Exposure to other environmental factors, such as pesticides and electromagnetic radiation, hair dyes, and cigarette smoking have been suspected, but no studies have proved an association (see "Who Is at Risk?," which follows).

It is important to note that *most breast cancers occur in women who are not known to be at high risk*. Therefore, it is important for every woman to learn the proper screening schedules.

The breasts in an adult woman are milk-producing, tear-shaped glands. They are supported by and attached to the front of the chest wall on either side of the breast bone or *sternum* by ligaments. The breasts rest on the major chest muscle, the *pectoralis major*. Each breast contains 15 to 20 lobes arranged like wheel spokes around a hub, coming together just under the nipple. The fat that covers the lobes gives the breast its size and shape. Each lobe is comprised of many lobules, at the end of which are tiny bulblike glands, or sacs, where milk is produced in response to hormonal signals. *Ducts* connect the lobes, lobules, and glands; in nursing mothers, these ducts deliver milk to openings in the nipple. The *areola* is the darker-pigmented area around the nipple. Blood and lymph vessels form a network throughout each breast. Lymph nodes are found under the arm, above the collarbone, and in the chest.

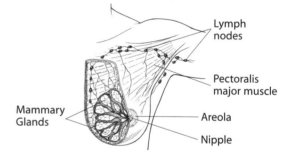

Who Is at Risk?

- Women (100 times more likely to get breast cancer than men);

- Women over 40;

- Those who experienced menarche (beginning of menstruation) at or before age 12;

- Women with their first pregnancy after 30;

- Women who have never had a full-term pregnancy;

- Women who have a late menopause (55 or older);

- Women who are obese;

- Those with a family history of breast cancer in a first-degree relative (mother, sister, daughter—two to three times the risk of the general population; those with both a mother and a sister affected with the disease are at very high risk);

- Women with a genetic predisposition for developing the disease, notably those with a specific genetic mutation;

- Women with a history of cancer in one breast (a three- to fourfold risk of developing cancer in the opposite breast);

- Women with a history of endometrial or ovarian cancer;

- Those with a history of *atypical hyperplasia*, one type of benign breast disease in which cells begin to divide abnormally;

- Women who take hormone replacement therapy for a prolonged period of time (more than five years) may have a moderately increased risk.

Screening Tests

- Monthly breast self-examination (BSE) beginning at puberty to feel for any lumps or signs of breast changes (see Chapter 7, "Examining Yourself");

- Clinical breast examination, an exam done by a doctor or nurse practitioner trained to palpate the breasts and specific lymph nodes to detect abnormalities at least every three years between ages 20 and 40 and every year over 40 (see Chapter 4, "The Cancer Checkup");

- Regular screening mammograms every one or two years beginning at age 40 until age 49, then annually after age 50 (in women with prior breast cancer, mammography screening is individualized based on the doctor's recommendations; see Chapters 5, "Screening for Cancer," and 6, "Routine Tests").

Types of Breast Cancer

Ninety percent of breast cancers are *adenocarcinomas*, which arise from glandular tissue. Within this broad category there is a great degree of variation. For instance, there are about 30 different subtypes of adenocarcinomas.

Cancer that begins in the lobes or lobules is called *lobular (small cell) carcinoma* and is more likely to be found in both breasts. Both ductal and lobular carcinomas can be either *in situ*, or self-contained; or *infiltrating*, meaning penetrating the wall of the duct or lobe and spreading to adjacent tissue. *In situ* carcinomas comprise about 15 to 20 percent of all breast cancers. The course of the disease and its treatment differ, depending on whether it is lobular or ductal carcinoma *in situ*, sometimes called *intraductal carcinoma* (see "Treatment," later).

Five percent of breast cancers are *medullary*, and a small percentage are *mucinous, tubular*, or *papillary*.

Paget's disease is a type of cancer that begins in the nipple. It can occur in conjunction with intraductal carcinoma. Another very rare type of breast cancer is *inflammatory* breast cancer, an aggressive, fast-growing cancer that is characterized by swollen, red breasts and a red rash called *peau d'orange*.

Tumors in breasts grow at different rates. Some may double in size every few days; others may take years to double. Some may grow at different rates at different stages in their development, speeding up their doubling rate as time goes on. But, in general, the typical breast cancer doubles in size about every 100 days, and may not be detectable for several years.

A lump may be detectable on a mammogram before it grows to 1 centimeter, but it is not *palpable*, or able to be felt, until it reaches that size. As the cancer cells multiply, they may invade adjacent tissue. Breast cancer cells commonly spread to the *axillary*, or underarm lymph nodes, the *cervical* lymph nodes in the neck, and the *supra-clavicular* or infraclavicular lymph nodes, found above and just below the collarbone.

The most common sites of distant breast cancer metastases are the skin, distant lymph nodes, bone, lung, and liver. When cancer recurs in the same breast, it may appear around a lumpectomy or mastectomy scar.

Signs and Symptoms

- A persistent lump or thickening that does not change in or near the breast or under the arm;

- Change in the size or shape of the breast;

- Nipple tenderness;

- Nipple discharge;

- Persistent ulceration of or lesion on the nipple;

- Nipples that become inverted;

- Skin irritation;

- Warm, red, swollen breasts with a rash called *peau d'orange*;

- Puckering, dimpling, scaliness;

- Pain in the breast (not usually a symptom, but any pain, particularly that which does not accompany monthly hormonal changes, should be reported to the doctor).

Diagnostic and Staging Tests

(For more details on the following tests, see Chapter 8, "Diagnostic Tests.")

- Palpation of breasts and lymph nodes, including those under the arms;

- Ultrasound (may help distinguish fluid-filled, and probably benign, cysts from solid tumors—used in conjunction with, *not instead of*, mammography). A new type of ultrasound, *high-definition imaging* (HDI) ultrasound shows a clear image of lumps larger than 1 centimeter and may prevent some unnecessary biopsies.

- Fine-needle aspiration (FNA) in which fluid and cells are withdrawn through a thin needle for analysis;

- A needle-core biopsy (uses a wider needle guided by mammography or ultrasound [see later] to remove breast tissue for analysis);

- Needle localization (a technique in which a wire, guided by x-ray, is threaded through a hollow needle inserted into the suspicious area of the breast). (A tiny hook on the end of the wire holds it in place to allow the surgeon to remove a tissue sample. This can be done on an outpatient basis with local anesthesia.)

- Biopsy (may be incisional [removing part of the lump] or excisional [removing the entire lump]);

- Skin biopsy;

- Chest x-ray;

- Bone scan;

- Blood tests;

- Assessments for *thymidine-labeling indices*, *flow cytometry* to determine *S-phase fraction* (or how many cells are in the S-phase of division), or *ploidy* (also called DNA index), which helps determine how well defined the tumor is. It is believed that the less defined a tumor is, the more aggressive and fast-growing it is (see Chapter 14, "Principles of Treatment"). The usefulness of these and other prognostic indicators is controversial.

Tests Unique to Breast Cancer

- Mammography employs two low-dose x-rays of each breast. If a woman has breast implants, multiple views are recommended, using a specific technique for positioning the breasts between the two plastic plates of the x-ray machine.

- *Stereotactic fine-needle biopsy* uses a technique that combines x-ray and computer technology to precisely locate and retrieve a tissue sample with a needle for biopsy.

- Tumor markers such as carcinoembryonic antigen (CEA) and CA 15-3 may indicate if cancer has metastasized and/or recurred.

- Estrogen receptor (ER) and progesterone receptor (PR) tests are performed on excised tissue to determine whether the tumor cells respond to the hormones. This information is important in planning treatment. (In general, estrogen or progesterone receptor-positive tumors will respond to hormone therapy. Also, the greater the percentage of receptor-positive cells, the slower the tumor's growth.)

Staging

Breast cancer is classified according to the tumor-nodes-metastasis (TNM) system of the American Joint Committee on Cancer Staging. The size of the primary tumor (T) at the time of diagnosis is an important indicator of the cancer's invasiveness and the person's prognosis. The surgeon will determine the tumor's size before any tissue is removed for other tests, such as those done to measure estrogen and progesterone receptors.

- Stage 0 breast cancer includes ductal or lobular carcinoma in situ, or Paget's disease with no evidence of tumor. An in situ cancer does not involve the lymph nodes or metastases.

- Stage I includes tumors up to 2 centimeters but no larger, which are also further classified (a, b, or c) according to whether the tumor is 0.5 centimeter or less, between 0.5 and 1 centimeter, or 1 to 2 centimeters.

Lymph nodes are not involved, and there is no spread of the cancer at this early stage.

- Stage IIA breast cancer includes a tumor no larger than 2 centimeters, which has spread to the movable lymph nodes in the armpit on the same side as the involved breast; a 2- to 5-centimeter tumor without lymph node involvement or metastasis; the presence of cancer cells in the lymph nodes under the arm, without evidence of a primary breast tumor.

- Stage IIB carcinoma includes a tumor from 2 to 5 centimeters at its largest dimension, spread to the movable lymph nodes under the arm on the same side as the involved breast, and no distant metastasis; or a tumor more than 5 centimeters, without lymph node involvement or spread to other sites.

- Stage IIIA includes five groupings of tumors measuring 2 to 5 centimeters, and with various stages of spread to the lymph nodes on the same side as the affected breasts. There may be no evidence of a primary tumor but cancer is detected in lymph nodes under an arm that are fixed to a structure or to each other; a tumor no greater than 2 centimeters combined with spread to fixed lymph nodes; a tumor 2 to 5 centimeters with spread to fixed lymph nodes; a tumor larger than 5 centimeters with spread to the movable lymph nodes; and tumors larger than 5 centimeters with spread to fixed lymph nodes. (Spread to movable lymph nodes is not as serious as spread to fixed lymph nodes, because in movable nodes, the cancer is often encapsulated and so is unlikely to have spread further.)

- Stage IIIB breast cancer includes tumors of any size that have extended directly to the chest wall or the skin, and any level of lymph node involvement; or any size tumor with spread to the internal mammary (under the sternum or breast bone) lymph nodes of the same side as the affected breast.

- Stage IV breast cancer includes any size tumor, any lymph node involvement, and spread to distant sites, including the lymph nodes along the collar bone.

Treatment

The treatment of this cancer is among the most widely studied of all cancer therapies. New approaches to therapy and refinements in accepted regimens are constantly being evaluated. What is recommended today may change by next year. The treatment plan widely used in one part of the country may not be suggested by doctors in another. Controversy abounds. And many individual factors further complicate the issues. In fact, the decision-making process can be so complex that at least 18 states now require disclosure of breast cancer treatment and alternatives as part of the informed consent process. Only one thing is certain: Local control of cancer is most likely when the tumor is small and can be completely removed by surgery. Except in the most advanced stages, therapy begins with excision of the tumor or destruction of the tumor by radiation therapy. Surgery is almost always accompanied by some type of adjuvant treatment—radiation therapy; hormonal therapy; chemotherapy; and, in experimental situations, biological therapy and bone marrow transplant (see Chapter 14, "Principles of Treatment").

Surgery. In the past, surgery often immediately followed a positive biopsy, in what is called a one-step procedure (see Chapter 8, "Diagnostic Tests"). Now it is known that there is no danger in waiting a week or two between the time a biopsy confirms that a tumor is malignant and its removal. Separating the diagnostic test from the surgery is called a two-step procedure. Although it requires another visit to a hospital and a second procedure, which some women consider a major disadvantage, there are several advantages. A two-step procedure allows a woman and her doctor to discuss and contemplate her treatment options. Moreover, there is time to seek a second opinion (see Chapter 12, "How Many Opinions Do You Need?"). Furthermore, more definitive laboratory analysis of the biopsied tissue can be done during this time. However, it is important to understand that in some cases, when the tumor is very small, it may be completely removed by a biopsy alone.

When planning therapy, an oncologist and/or surgeon considers the following factors: the stage of the cancer (that is, the size of the tumor, whether or not the lymph nodes are involved, and the presence of metastases); the tumor's hormone status; the woman's age and menopausal status; and her general health, including whether she has any serious and/or chronic illnesses or conditions, such as heart disease, that might be complicated by treatment. In some cases, doctors will want to consider other prognostic factors that indicate the tumor's aggressiveness and likelihood of recurrence (see Chapter 14, "Principles of Treatment").

Surgical possibilities have expanded greatly since the turn of the century, when the *Halsted radical mastectomy* was first done. In this operation, which was commonly used until the 1950s, the breast, chest muscles, all the underarm lymph nodes, and additional fat and skin are removed. Today this extensive operation is performed with far less frequency.

When the breast must be removed by mastectomy, there are several possibilities (see the following chart). Whenever possible, the surgeon tries to remove as little normal, healthy tissue as possible. Of course the extent of surgery will influence the likelihood of complications, long-term side effects, and recovery time (see Chapters 15, "Surgery," and 28, "Managing Disabilities and Limitations").

For early-stage cancers (usually less than 4 to 5 centimeters with no distant metastases or fixed nodes under the arm), including ductal carcinoma in situ, *breast-conserving* therapy—such as a *lumpectomy*, removal of the tumor and a margin of tissue around it, followed by radiation therapy—has proved as successful as a radical mastectomy for local control of cancer. Many women are unaware that a lumpectomy may involve removing a substantial part of the breast, and there may be a considerable cosmetic change. In fact, a lumpectomy may not be a good option if a woman has very small breasts (see Chapter 15, "Surgery").

Other conditions—some of which are not directly related to the cancer—may rule out lumpectomy. These include early pregnancy, because the required postoperative radiation

Types of Breast Cancer Surgery

- **Lumpectomy**

  The cancerous lump and a margin of normal tissue around it are removed.

- **Partial or segmental mastectomy, or quadrantectomy**

  The tumor, a wedge of normal tissue around the tumor, as well as the lining over the chest muscles under the tumor are removed.

- **Total or simple mastectomy**

  The entire breast is removed.

- **Modified radical mastectomy**

  The breast, some of the underarm lymph nodes, and the lining over the chest muscles are removed. One of the chest muscles (usually the smaller one) may also be removed.

- **Radical or Halsted radical mastectomy**

  The breast, chest muscles, all lymph nodes under the arm, and additional fat and skin are removed.

therapy could be harmful to the developing fetus; previous radiation therapy to the breast; unwillingness or inability to undergo several weeks of almost daily radiation therapy; and two or more malignancies in different breast quadrants or several microcalcifications, as is typical in lobular carcinoma in situ.

When a mastectomy is necessary, some women choose to have the breast reconstructed in one of several ways. They may decide to have a saline or silicone implant inserted under the chest muscle that matches the size of the opposite breast. (There is currently a moratorium in the United States on the use of silicone gel-filled implants for cosmetic augmentation purposes because of suspected health problems that have been reported if the silicone leaks into the body. The implant is permitted for breast reconstruction if a woman is enrolled in a clinical trial. Although saline-filled implants are still not approved by the FDA, they are permitted for cosmetic and reconstructive purposes.) In situations where there is not enough tissue to cover an implant, a special balloon-like expander placed under the muscle is filled every one to two weeks for a month or two. It gradually stretches the tissue and eventually is replaced with an implant.

It is now possible for a woman to avoid a synthetic implant entirely and have her removed breast rebuilt using her own fatty tissue, muscle, and skin from her back (*latissimus dorsi procedure*) or abdomen (*TRAM—transverse rectus abdominis musculocutaneous—flap procedure*) in an operation called *autologous reconstruction.*

Nipple and areola reconstruction are usually done later. The timing of the reconstruction surgery varies: It may take place at the same time as the mastectomy, months after the mastectomy wound has healed, or even years later. Reconstruction is an option for most women except those with very advanced disease, although the procedure may not be covered by insurance.

Radiation Therapy. After lumpectomy, radiation therapy to the breast and sometimes the underarm five days a week for four to six weeks is typical (see Chapters 16, "Radiation," and 20, "Combination Treatments"). A concentrated "boost" dose of radiation may be delivered by special implants containing radioactive beads or external beam to end the therapy. (Radiation therapy is also used to treat advanced breast cancer that has spread to the chest wall.)

Such intense exposure to radiation does have unavoidable side effects, particularly fatigue, swelling, and skin changes, which gradually disappear over the following year in most women. More serious side effects include heart and lung damage and a risk of second malignancies.

Chemotherapy. When a tumor is large, identi-fied as aggressive, and/or involves the lymph nodes, some form of systemic adjuvant treatment is often recommended after surgery to destroy cancer cells that have escaped into the lymph and blood vessels and to diminish the likelihood of recurrence (see Chapter 17, "Chemotherapy"). The specific drugs suggested—hormone therapy (see later), chemotherapy drugs, or both—depend on several variables and are individualized. It's very important to ask your doctor to explain the recommendations and to consider a second or even a third opinion (see Chapter 12, "How Many Opinions Do You Need?").

Despite the many options, some general principles have evolved. For example, studies have shown that a combination of chemotherapy drugs is more effective than a single agent. The combination that has been favored for many years is CMF (cyclophosphamide [Cytoxan], methotrexate, and fluorouracil [5-FU]). Alternating CMF with a therapy that is Adriamycin-based, called CAF (cyclophosphamide [Cytoxan], Doxorubicin (Adriamycin), and fluorouracil [5-FU]), is becoming more common, as research reveals good response rates. There are several other variations that include vincristine (Oncovin) and prednisone. Women who enter clinical trials (see "Ask About" later) may be offered new drugs and/or different combinations of widely used ones (see Chapter 21, "Investigational Treatments").

The next decision is when to begin chemotherapy and how long treatment should last. This recommendation, too, is very individualized and may vary from one doctor to another. Some combinations may be given in cycles lasting only two to six months; others are given for a year or even two.

Investigators are looking at whether giving chemotherapy before surgery can shrink a larger tumor enough not only to permit a lumpectomy instead of a mastectomy but also to destroy cancer cells that have spread to other areas.

Hormone Therapy. A critical pathology test on a sample of tumor tissue will reveal if the cancer has receptors for estrogen and progesterone. If it has estrogen receptors, it is said to be estrogen-receptor positive; if not, it is said to be estrogen-receptor negative. The same is true of progesterone receptors.

Research has shown that if a tumor is estrogen-receptor positive, anti-estrogen therapy, such as the drug tamoxifen (Nolvadex), will block the receptor and prevent growth of cancer. Tamoxifen is used with and without chemotherapy primarily to treat women over 50. Some experts say it is reasonable to give tamoxifen alone to low-risk, postmenopausal women and along with chemotherapy to high-risk, postmenopausal women.

Since the drug causes side effects similar to those of menopause—weight gain, hot flashes, and mood swings—younger women may choose not to take it. Most women continue on hormone therapy for two to five years, but research has not yet determined the optimal and safe duration of therapy. The National Cancer Institute (NCI) has warned against prolonged use of the drug.

There are obvious benefits to tamoxifen, but it is not without risk. Some studies have shown there may be an increased risk of endometrial cancer. Large studies are now being conducted to determine if tamoxifen will prevent cancer entirely in high-risk women.

In some rare cases, removal of the ovaries is recommended, resulting in a surgically created menopause.

Controversies. There is still no definitive cure for breast cancer that has spread beyond the breast and regional lymph nodes, so controversies regarding certain treatments are still common. For instance, the debates about chemotherapy revolve around timing and duration of the therapy; length of hormone therapy with or without chemotherapy; the sequencing of chemotherapy after primary treatment; the intensity of dosages; and who should or should not receive adjuvant systemic therapy. So although the treatments described here are typical, your physician may discuss different treatments with you. Some surgeons and medical oncologists will be more aggressive in treating cancers, in hopes of preventing recurrence.

You may or may not be comfortable with the treatment(s) offered, and may feel you need additional information about treatment options before you make a decision (see Chapter 12, "How Many Opinions Do You Need?").

Treatment of ductal carcinoma in situ (DCIS) is currently quite controversial and a consensus has not yet been reached. DCIS may be treated in several ways: excision of the tumor with a wide margin of tissue alone or followed by radiation therapy or total mastectomy (see Chapter 12, "How Many Opinions Do You Need?").

Since lobular carcinoma in situ (LCIS) carries a 25 percent risk of later development of invasive carcinoma, frequent periodic follow-up with a clinical breast examination and mammography is advised. A mastectomy may be done, but neither radiation therapy nor chemotherapy is recommended. LCIS is more likely to occur in both breasts, either simultaneously or concurrently, but it is a rare cancer.

Survival

- Five-year survival for stage 0 (in situ) breast cancer is more than 95 percent.

- Five-year survival for stage I breast cancer is 85 percent.

- Five-year survival for stage II breast cancer is 66 percent.

- Five-year survival for stage III breast cancer is 41 percent.

- Five-year survival for stage IV breast cancer is 10 percent.

Special Needs

Many support groups exist to address the potentially complex psychological challenges of dealing with breast cancer (see Appendix I, "Resources"). Because a woman's breasts often define her sexuality, having breast surgery can have an impact on her sexual desire and ability to be intimate with her partner (see Chapters 29, "Body Image and Self-Esteem," and 30, "Sexuality").

Chemotherapy-induced menopausal symptoms may be very troublesome. If hot flashes, sweating, and vaginal dryness become very uncomfortable, some physicians may prescribe hormone replacement therapy. However, this can interfere with the beneficial effects of chemotherapy, so the side effects of each must be carefully weighed. Women may want to inquire about such nonhormonal drugs as clonidine, which may help with the hot flashes brought on by tamoxifen (Nolvadex).

Special attention should be given to rehabilitation if the lymph nodes have been removed. Swelling of the arm on the affected side, a condition called lymphedema, is often a problem (see Chapter 28, "Managing Disabilities and Limitations").

Women with large breasts may experience neck and shoulder soreness caused by a weight shift after removal of one breast. A suitable prosthesis or reconstructive surgery can help with this problem, as can exercises to help a woman regain strength in her arm and shoulder. Some women choose to have reduction surgery on the unaffected breast.

Pregnancy following breast cancer does not affect recurrence or survival rates. Doctors recommend that women wait at least one year after ending treatment to become pregnant. Breast-feeding a baby from the unaffected breast may be possible if that breast has not been radiated.

Ask About

Numerous clinical trials are ongoing, for every stage of breast cancer (see Chapter 21, "Investigational Treatments"). These involve new biological agents (see Chapter 18, "Biological Therapies"); high-dose chemotherapy with either autologous bone marrow transplantation, stem cell support, or growth factor for advanced disease; or neoadjuvant (preoperative) chemotherapy to shrink the tumor and allow breast conservation surgery in cases where it wouldn't otherwise be feasible.

Bone marrow transplantation (BMT) is currently being investigated for treatment of metastatic disease as well as for aggressive early-stage disease. Some investigators believe that BMT offers a chance for long-term disease control and cure because it permits very-high-dose chemotherapy. Autologous (from the person's own body) marrow is more commonly used than that from a donor (see Chapter 19, "Bone Marrow Transplant"). At this time, however, there is no definitive evidence that high-dose chemotherapy and BMT are more effective than standard therapy.

ADRENAL

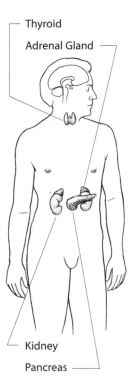

Thyroid

Adrenal Gland

Kidney

Pancreas

The adrenal glands produce *hormones*, chemicals that regulate a wide variety of body processes, from fluid balance to sexual characteristics. Therefore, any growth—benign or malignant—that affects one or both of these glands may disturb vital functions. Tumors that produce excess amounts of hormones are called *functioning tumors*; those that do not are called *nonfunctioning tumors*.

Although it has been estimated that as many as 8 percent of people develop benign tumors of the adrenal glands, malignant tumors are quite rare. When they are discovered early (5 centimeters or less at their greatest dimension), they are likely to be cured with surgery. The adrenal glands are a common site for *secondary* or metastatic cancer—that is, cancer that has spread to one or both glands from other sites (see Chapter 33, "Metastasis and Recurrence"). In this section the discussion is limited to primary cancer of the adrenal glands (that is, cancer that begins in the glands).

One type of adrenal tumor, called *pheochromocytoma* (see "Types," later), is usually benign and curable (only 10 percent are malignant). This type of cancer may be inherited as part of a syndrome called *multiple endocrine neoplasia* (MEN) type II. Pheochromocytomas are also associated with other syndromes that may have a genetic link, such as neurofibromatosis, von Hippel-Landau disease, and Sturge-Weber's syndrome. The cause of other types of adrenal cancer is unknown.

The adrenal glands are part of the hormone-secreting *endocrine system*. A triangular-shaped adrenal gland covers the top of each kidney and has two parts, the inner *medulla* and the outer covering, or *cortex*. The adrenal medulla stores and secretes the hormones *norepinephrine (noradrenaline)*, which constricts blood vessels, raises blood pressure, and slows the heart; and *epinephrine (adrenaline)*, which has a variety of effects when released, including increasing heart rate, widening the airways, stimulating sugar production in the liver, and slowing digestion.

The adrenal cortex secretes three steroid hormones: the *glucocorticoids* (such as *hydrocortisone*), which change carbohydrates into glycogen

in the liver for later conversion to glucose to supply the body's energy needs; the *mineralocorticoids* (such as *aldosterone*), which help maintain the balance of sodium, potassium, and fluid in the body; and the sex hormones (such as *progesterone*, *androgen*, and *estrogen*), which affect the reproductive cycle and sex characteristics.

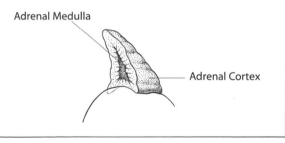

Adrenal Medulla

Adrenal Cortex

Who Is at Risk?

Pheochromocytoma

- People with von Hippel-Landau syndrome, neurofibromatosis, MEN type II, and Sturge-Weber's syndrome;

- People between 30 and 50;

- People with a family history of pheochromocytoma (10 to 15 percent of pheochromocytomas are hereditary).

Adrenocortical Carcinoma

- People between 40 and 50;

- People with a history of abnormal hormone production by the adrenal cortex.

Screening Tests

No tests are available.

Types of Adrenal Cancer

Pheochromocytoma

Ten percent of pheochromocytomas are malignant. This extremely rare cancer affects only about 100 people in the United States each year. Ninety percent of the time, a pheochromocytoma occurs within the tissue of the adrenal medulla and is surrounded by a capsule or covering. Although the cells appear malignant under the microscope, the tumor is considered benign unless it has invaded the capsule or spread to other parts of the body, such as the liver, lungs, or bones. In either case, this type of tumor may produce dangerously high blood pressure by releasing abnormally large amounts of the hormones epinephrine and norepinephrine into the blood.

About one in 10 pheochromocytomas occur outside of the adrenals in similar kinds of tissues in the liver, genitourinary tract, heart, or nervous system. They are more frequently malignant and have a poor prognosis.

Adrenocortical Carcinoma

Adrenocortical carcinoma involves the adrenal cortex. It is also very rare, affecting only one or two people in a million. Adrenocortical cancer is most often discovered at an advanced stage (stage III or IV) because so many are nonfunctioning tumors and produce no early symptoms to signal trouble. Approximately 1 percent of patients who are having a CT or MRI scan for another reason are found to have an adrenal tumor, most of which are benign. However, those more than 5 to 6 centimeters at their largest dimension are more likely to be cancerous. These so-called functioning tumors can cause diabetes, high blood pressure, bone weakening, swelling of the breasts or sex organs, facial hair growth, voice change, or Cushing's syndrome, which involves changes in body fat deposits, abnormal hair growth, and skin fragility. About 60 percent of the time, they produce too much of one or more hormones.

Malignant pheochromocytomas and adrenocortical carcinomas may spread to other parts of the body, including the liver, lungs, lymph nodes, bone, pancreas, spleen, diaphragm, brain, peritoneum, skin, and palate.

Signs and Symptoms

Pheochromocytoma

- Severe headache;

- Weight loss;

- Heavy sweating;

- Heart palpitations;

- Dizziness;

- Blurring of vision;

- Paleness;

- Abdominal pain;

- Increased appetite;

- Nervousness and irritability;

- Faintness;

- Chest pain;

- Variable or constant high blood pressure (may be severe and/or may occur in stressful situations such as during surgery);

- Rapid heart rate with below normal blood pressure.

Adrenocortical Cancer

- Abdominal pain;
- Weight loss;
- Weakness;
- Excessive thirst;
- Frequent urination;
- Dizziness;
- Headache;
- Fatigue.

Functioning adrenal tumors produce hormone-related symptoms such as:
- Back pain;
- Weight gain;
- Muscle wasting;
- Fat buildup on the upper back;
- Round face;
- Abnormal hair growth;
- Skin that is easily broken;
- Deepening of the voice;
- Facial hair;
- Swelling of the sex organs;
- Swelling of the breasts;
- Baldness (in women);
- Muscle spasms;
- Tingling in arms, legs, and feet;
- Temporary paralysis.

The first signs of a nonfunctioning tumor are usually related to its size and the resulting pressure on surrounding tissue. These symptoms include:
- Fever;
- Anemia;
- Pain in the abdomen;
- Feeling of pressure.

Diagnostic and Staging Tests

For more information regarding these tests, see Chapter 8, "Diagnostic Tests."

Pheochromocytoma

- Twenty-four-hour urine analysis to measure levels of epinephrine, norepinephrine, and their metabolites metanephrine, normetanephrine, and vanillylmandelic acid (VMA);
- Blood tests to measure levels of epinephrine, norepinephrine, and their metabolites, including VMA;
- CT or MRI scan.

Tests Unique to Pheochromocytoma

- *Clonidine suppression test.* During this procedure, the person has a catheter inserted into a vein and lies in a quiet room. After 30 minutes, blood is drawn and analyzed for hormone levels. Then the antihypertension drug clonidine is given orally. After three hours, hormone levels are measured again. A high level indicates the presence of a pheochromocytoma.
- The iodine-123 (or 131-I-labeled metalodobenzyl-guanidine) test, or I-MIBG test. This test is used to locate a pheochromocytoma. Radioactive isotopes are injected and are absorbed by the tumor, if one is present.

Adrenocortical Carcinoma

- Urine analysis for cortisol;
- Blood test for high levels of adrenocorticotropic hormone (ACTH);
- CT or MRI scans;
- Needle biopsy;
- Aortography to differentiate an adrenal tumor from a tumor of the kidney.

Staging

Pheochromocytoma

There is no established staging for pheochromocytomas.

Adrenocortical Carcinoma

- Stage I: The tumor size is less than 5 centimeters at its greatest diameter, no lymph nodes are involved, and there is no spread to nearby organs or tissues. No metastasis is present.

- Stage II: The tumor is larger than 5 centimeters at its greatest dimension. No lymph nodes are involved, and there is no spread to nearby organs or tissues. No metastasis is present.

- Stage III: A tumor of any size with invasion of adjacent tissues, or node involvement but no spread to nearby organs. No distant metastasis is present.

- Stage IV: A tumor of any size with involvement of lymph nodes and nearby organs or tissues and distant metastasis.

Treatment

Pheochromocytoma

The standard treatment for a pheochromocytoma, whether it is malignant or not, is surgery to remove the tumor (see Chapter 15, "Surgery"). Patients are given drugs to prevent dangerously high blood pressure that results from the release of hormones during the operation, a situation that can cause such complications as heart attack, shock, and kidney failure. In appropriately prepared patients, the survival rate for this procedure is high. Hormone levels are evaluated one or two weeks after surgery to ensure that the tumor has been completely removed. Annual scans using the radioactive isotope I-MIBG may be done to detect recurring or metastatic tumors. (MIBG is not available everywhere, and it is expensive.)

If the tumor cannot be removed, the doctor prescribes medication to block the action of the adrenal hormones, which helps to maintain the blood pressure at safe levels.

Therapy for advanced or metastatic disease can be provided by combination chemotherapy (see Chapter 17, "Chemotherapy," and Chapter 20, "Combination Treatments") and/or high doses of radioactive I-131 MIBG. I-131 MIBG is available primarily at university medical centers.

Adrenocortical Carcinoma

The primary treatment is removal of the tumor or the entire adrenal gland. If the tumor is less than 3 centimeters at its largest dimension and is not producing hormones, the doctor may advise doing nothing for six months and then look for a change in tumor size. A small (less than 5 centimeters) nonfunctioning tumor is usually benign, which doesn't need removal as long as hormone production remains normal and the tumor is not growing larger.

When the tumor is between 3 and 6 centimeters at its greatest dimension and is nonfunctioning, the usual procedure is also to follow it closely with CT or MRI scans. Sometimes a fine-needle aspiration of the tumor is done to retrieve the cells for analysis (see Chapter 8, "Diagnostic Tests"). If cancer cells are present, the tumor is removed.

Injections of corticosteroids are given to patients just before functioning tumors are removed, because the remaining normal adrenal gland may have shrunk and not be producing enough hormones. These levels are monitored following surgery and lower oral doses of hormone are given daily, if needed, for long-term therapy.

When a tumor measures between 6 and 10 centimeters at its greatest dimension, exploratory surgery is usually recommended, so the surgeon can determine if any spread to nearby areas has occurred. Invasion of adjacent structures is common with the larger tumors. In this case, surgery may involve not only the complete removal of the adrenal gland, but also parts of the liver, kidneys, and lymph nodes.

Stage IV cancers are treated with surgery to remove the local disease and possibly distant tumors. Chemotherapy with mitotane (Lysodren) results in partial remissions of the disease in up to 34 percent of cases, and excellent palliation, or the relief of symptoms without cure, is common.

Survival

The prognosis for patients with benign pheochromocytoma is excellent. The five-year survival rate is about 95 percent. The five-year survival rate for people with inoperable malignant metastatic pheochromocytoma is about 40 percent. No figures are available for those with limited disease, but if the tumor and any other evidence of cancer are removed, long-term survival is possible.

For adrenocortical carcinoma, the survival rates are:

- Five-year survival for stage I cancer is 80 percent.

- Five-year survival for stage II cancer is 50 percent.

- Five-year survival for stage III cancer is 20 to 30 percent.

- Five-year survival for stage IV cancer is 1 to 10 percent.

Special Needs

Patients who have had surgery to cure adrenocortical carcinoma must have frequent check-ups for years, because tumors can recur in the area of the original tumor. Surgery to remove these recurrent tumors as well as distant metastases is often successful. Frequent checkups are necessary to detect pheochromocytoma recurrence, because it may not produce symptoms.

Careful follow-up after treatment is also necessary to manage hormone replacement therapy.

For example, cortisol supplements may be required. Too much aldosterone is rare, but when it is produced by adrenal cancer it may lead to high blood pressure, muscle weakness or paralysis, low potassium levels, and muscle spasms. These symptoms may pass after surgery and, possibly, hormone replacement therapy. If no surgery is planned, the aldosterone effect can be decreased with the drug spironolactone (Aldactone).

In both types of adrenal cancers, a team effort by the endocrinologist, surgeon, and anesthesiologist is needed. The role of the anesthesiologist is very important in controlling symptoms brought on by an outpouring of hormones as the tumor is removed.

Ask About

If you have adrenocortical cancer, particularly stage II or IV, there are several clinical trials you may want to investigate (see Chapter 21, "Investigational Treatments"). For example, in inoperable stage III adrenocortical carcinoma, studies evaluating radiation therapy are under way. Another clinical trial is evaluating treatment with chemotherapy using high doses of mitotane.

For stage IV or recurrent or metastatic adrenocortical carcinomas, other chemotherapy regimens are currently being evaluated.

THYROID AND PARATHYROID

Despite the fact that thyroid cancer is responsible for about 90 percent of all cancers of the endocrine system, it is very uncommon, accounting for about 1 percent of all cancers. Nearly 90 percent of thyroid cancers are the slow-growing *papillary* and *follicular* types or a mix of the two. About 5 to 10 percent are *medullary carcinomas*. Most are slow growing, but some people develop a fast-growing form. The incidence of the far more aggressive *anaplastic* type, which usually occurs in the elderly, is decreasing (see "Types," later).

Radiation to the head and neck region, or ingestion of radioactive iodine, particularly in infancy or early childhood, have been associated with thyroid cancer. In the past, a lack of iodine in the diet was implicated. This problem has been solved because iodine is now added to salt. About 20 percent of cases of thyroid cancer are inherited. These include *familial medullary thyroid carcinoma* and *multiple endocrine neoplasia* (MEN) syndromes, in which tumors are also found in other endocrine glands.

The thyroid is a butterfly-shaped gland of the hormone-secreting endocrine system. It consists of two lobes connected by a narrow band, the *isthmus*, that overlies the *trachea*, or windpipe. It is in the front of the neck, just below the Adam's apple. The average thyroid gland is less than 2 inches high and 2 inches wide. In adults the gland usually weighs about an ounce, although an enlarged gland, or *goiter*, can weigh 20 ounces or more.

The cells of the thyroid gland secrete the hormones thyroxine, or T4, and triiodothyronine, or T3. These hormones regulate a wide range of the body's activities, including the rate at which the body uses protein, fat, and carbohydrates; the rate and force of the heart's contractions; the maintenance of good muscle tone; and the secretion of growth hormone, which is important for normal development in childhood. Closely behind each thyroid lobe are four small *parathyroid* glands, whose job is to secrete parathyroid hormone (PTH). This hormone regulates the amount of calcium in the blood and ensures that nerves and muscles work properly and that bones contain enough calcium. Occasionally, one or more parathyroid glands will be located at a distance from the thyroid in the neck or upper chest.

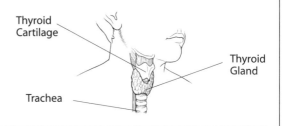

Who Is at Risk?

- People between the ages of 25 and 65;

- People exposed to radiation to the head and neck early in life;

- Those who consume too much or too little iodine in their diets;

- People with a family history, particularly of the medullary type with MEN.

Screening Tests

- *Blood test for calcitonin.* Adults and children who are at risk for the inherited medullary thyroid cancer can have an annual test for a tumor marker—a high level of the hormone *calcitonin*. When the results are unclear, a calcitonin stimulation test is done. It involves an intravenous infusion of a hormone, pentagastrin, with or without calcium, after an overnight fast, to test the reaction of the thyroid.

Testing should begin about age 3 for the inherited syndromes and repeated annually. The test itself may have unpleasant side effects, including a burning sensation in the chest and abdomen, nausea, vomiting, and numbness. Recently, the gene for this inherited variety of cancer has been identified, and some centers are beginning to screen family members using a chromosome analysis of their blood.

- A new genetic test for inherited medullary thyroid cancer (MEN) is available that detects a defective gene on chromosome 10. This blood test is being used in some centers for newborns at risk of developing the disease, and it is being employed with family members.

Types of Thyroid Cancer

Thyroid cancer often starts in a single nodule inside the thyroid. *Papillary cancer* can spread into adjacent normal thyroid tissue and to nearby tissues beyond the gland or to lymph nodes in the neck. In later stages there may be lung or bone metastases. *Follicular cancers* typically spread through the bloodstream to the lung and bones. *Medullary cancer* can spread locally by way of the lymph nodes as well as the bloodstream.

Signs and Symptoms

- Lump in the neck;
- Enlarged lymph nodes in the neck;
- A sudden swelling in the front of the neck;
- Difficulty swallowing, or *dysphagia*;
- Pain in the neck over the thyroid;
- Occasionally, hoarseness and difficult breathing, which occur late in the illness.

Diagnostic and Staging Tests

For more information regarding these tests, see Chapter 8, "Diagnostic Tests."

- Physical examination, including palpation of the neck;
- Calcitonin stimulation test;
- Chromosome analysis;
- CT or MRI scan of people with goiters to see if their glands contain any nodules that might indicate malignant changes;
- Ultrasound, which can determine whether a lump in the neck is a cyst or a solid lump and can detect lymph node enlargement (solid lumps are more likely to be malignant);
- Needle biopsy of suspicious lumps;
- Excisional biopsy, usually in the form of a thyroidectomy.

Tests Unique to Thyroid Cancer

- *Thyroid scan.* A very small dose of radioactive substance such as radioactive iodine or thallium is injected into a vein, and an image is obtained that shows how much of the material is absorbed by the thyroid. Thyroid cancers usually don't absorb as much of the radioactive substance as non-

cancerous nodules do. This is sometimes referred to as a *cold nodule*. Thyroid scans are not a definitive diagnostic test, because other conditions can create an image similar to that of cancer.

Staging

None of the staging systems has been universally accepted, but one commonly referred to is that of the American Joint Committee on Cancer.

Papillary or Follicular Thyroid Cancer

In people under 45:
- Stage I: any cancer in the thyroid or regional lymph nodes;
- Stage II: spread beyond the thyroid and lymph nodes to distant sites.

In people over 45:
- Stage I: a tumor 1 centimeter or less in the thyroid only;
- Stage II: a tumor 1 to 4 centimeters or greater but limited to the thyroid;
- Stage III: a tumor of any size that extends beyond the thyroid gland and that may involve the lymph nodes;
- Stage IV: metastasis to the lymph nodes and distant sites, such as the lung and bones.

Medullary Thyroid Cancer

- Stage I: A tumor is less than 1 centimeter.
- Stage II: A tumor 1 to 4 centimeters.
- Stage III: The cancer has spread to the lymph nodes.
- Stage IV: The cancer has spread to the lymph nodes and other parts of the body.

Anaplastic Thyroid Cancers

All are considered stage IV. The cancer cells revert to a primitive type, grow rapidly, and spread widely.

Treatment

Treatment depends on the type and stage of the disease as well as on the person's age, which is an important prognostic factor. In most cases surgery to remove the lobe containing the tumor, a procedure called *lobectomy* or *subtotal thyroidectomy*, is the treatment of choice (see Chapter 15, "Surgery"). If the cancer has not spread, it is cured by surgery. *Total thyroidectomy*, removal of the entire thyroid, may be necessary if both lobes are involved, the person is over 50, tumors are large (more than 5 centimeters), or there is a high risk of recurrence or metastasis. Any palpable lymph nodes are removed also. After surgery the person takes thyroid hormone supplements.

Some oncologists may suggest radiation therapy following surgery to remove papillary or follicular thyroid cancer if there is a risk of recurrence or when cancer cells may remain behind. Radiation therapy is sometimes also advised for patients over 45 (see Chapter 16, "Radiation").

A common method of treatment is *ablation*, or destruction, of thyroid tissue with radioactive iodine in a form called I-131. Hospitalization is required because of the special precautions needed in handling both the radioactive material and the person being treated with it. The patient must stay in a special room after taking the radioactive iodine solution (I-131) or capsules until the isotope is completely eliminated from his or her body, usually 48 to 72 hours.

A large amount of I-131 is trapped by thyroid cells, which are then destroyed by the substance's radioactivity. Side effects of treatment are mild but may include nausea and vomiting, inflammation of the salivary glands, and sometimes damage to the bone marrow. If necessary, the treatment may be repeated at four- to six-month intervals. Because the whole body is exposed to radioactivity, there is some debate about whether the risks of "iodine ablation" are worth the benefit for initial treatment of disease. Therapy may decrease the chances of recurrence, but there is no evidence it increases survival time.

If ablation fails and cancer cells remain, external beam radiation therapy and chemotherapy may be recommended (see Chapter 20, "Combination Treatments"). Occasionally, both types of therapy are suggested, particularly when the cancer is inoperable. Doxorubicin (Adriamycin) alone or with cisplatin (Platinol) may help some patients. Another treatment combination—involving doxorubicin, bleomycin (Blenoxane), vincristine (Oncovin), and melphalan (Alkeran)—can shrink some cancers in people with advanced disease (see Chapter 17, "Chemotherapy").

There is no preferred treatment for anaplastic thyroid cancer, and a thyroidectomy is frequently difficult or impossible. Because this type grows so rapidly, the tumor can exert so much pressure on the windpipe that it is necessary for the surgeon to create a permanent tracheostomy (a hole in the windpipe that relieves breathing difficulties). People with anaplastic cancers may need both chemotherapy and external-beam radiation therapy to slow tumor growth and relieve symptoms, but these cancers are not curable.

Survival

Survival depends on the age of the person when the diagnosis is made. Very young children and older adults tend to do less well than 20- to 50-year-olds. The possibility of long-term survival after treatment for papillary cancer is excellent in young adults (20- to 30-year-olds), even in the presence of lung metastasis.

- Five-year survival for stage I and stage II papillary thyroid cancer is 95 percent.

- Five-year survival for stage III papillary thyroid cancer is 60 percent.

- Five-year survival for stage I follicular thyroid cancer is 70 to 90 percent.

- Five-year survival for stage II follicular thyroid cancer is 50 to 70 percent.

- Five-year survival for stage III follicular thyroid cancer is 20 to 60 percent.

- Five-year survival for anaplastic thyroid carcinoma is less than 5 percent, with survival measured in months for most patients.

- Five-year survival for medullary thyroid cancer is 40 to 60 percent.

Special Needs

Replacement thyroid hormone therapy is needed after thyroidectomy. Those at risk of osteoporosis also may need to take supplemental calcium and vitamin D, or possibly estrogen/progesterone therapy after menopause, to prevent fractures. Replacement doses of thyroid hormone to suppress normal TSH (thyroid stimulating hormone) and prevent stimulation of any remaining thyroid cancer cells may be considered part of cancer treatment as well.

Ask About

Because there is disagreement about whether the entire thyroid gland should be removed, you may want to seek a second opinion (see Chapter 12, "How Many Opinions Do You Need?"). Some surgeons feel that men over 40 and women over 50 are more likely to benefit from total thyroidectomy regardless of the type of thyroid cancer. However, those who argue for limiting removal of the thyroid gland note that a lobectomy reduces the chances of complications such as nerve damage that causes vocal cord paralysis, as well as hypoparathyroidism and the resulting low calcium.

If you have stage IV thyroid cancer or recurrent disease, you may want to discuss participating in a clinical trial with your oncologist. Studies comparing chemotherapy to standard treatments have shown some good and long-lasting responses (see Chapter 21, "Investigational Treatments").

Parathyroid Cancer

Cancer in one of the four tiny parathyroid glands under the thyroid gland is quite rare, affecting one person in 100,000, mostly older women. The cause is unknown, but it appears there is a genetic susceptibility.

A condition called hyperparathyroidism associated with benign tumors is quite common, affecting about one person in 1,000. However, occasionally it is associated with MEN type I, and the symptoms it causes may be what brings the person to the doctor in the first place.

The growth rate of parathyroid cancer is variable. Eventually, the tumor can extend into the surrounding thyroid and neck tissue and spread to nearby lymph nodes. Because the parathyroid gland makes parathyroid hormone (PTH), which helps to regulate the amount of calcium in the bloodstream, cancer in the gland results in an excessive amount of calcium in the blood. The problems this calcium imbalance causes—such as fatigue, muscular weakness, nausea and vomiting, bone pain, and kidney stones or other kidney disorders—may be the first symptoms of cancer. Local symptoms, such as a lump in the neck and hoarseness, may also occur.

The cancer can be cured by removing the affected parathyroid gland and other involved tissues. However, regular checkups of calcium levels in the blood are important, because recurrences are common. The five-year survival rate after surgery is approximately 50 percent.

Studies are being done to determine if radiation therapy after surgery improves the chances for cure.

PANCREAS

Pancreatic cancer is the ninth most common cancer, affecting about eight people in 100,000 each year. It is the second most common cancer of the gastrointestinal tract. Because the early symptoms are vague, and there are no screening tests to detect it, early diagnosis is difficult. At the time of diagnosis, only about 10 percent of cancers can be removed. If the cancer has spread to local vital structures and blood vessels, the tumor is usually not removed.

No specific cause has been identified, but carcinogens and inherited factors that make people less able to detoxify them may play a role. There also appears to be an association with a high-fat diet. Studies are now under way to see why pancreatic cancer seems to occur in certain families.

The pancreas is about 6 inches long and is shaped something like a thin pear. It has three parts: the *head*, which is tucked into the curve of the duodenum; the *body*, the mid-portion that lies astride the backbone; and the *tail*, the thinnest part, which lies in front of the left kidney, just touching the spleen.

The pancreas is an organ of the endocrine and the digestive systems. The *endocrine* portion contains *islet* cells that produce the hormones insulin and glucagon, which regulate the amount of sugar in the blood. The *exocrine* portion of the pancreas makes and secretes enzymes into the duodenum that help digest protein, starches, and fat.

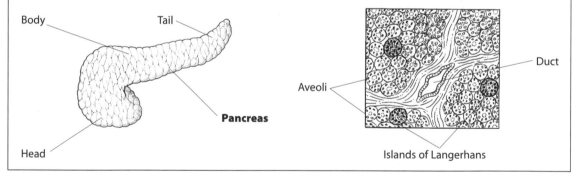

Body   Tail

Pancreas

Head

Aveoli

Duct

Islands of Langerhans

Who Is at Risk?

- People between 60 and 80 years of age;

- Men (slightly more common than in women);

- African-Americans (slightly more common than in Caucasians);

- People who smoke;

- Workers exposed to solvents and petroleum compounds;

- People with a history of pancreatic cancer in a close family member.

Screening Tests

There are no screening tests.

Types of Pancreatic Cancer

At least 90 percent of pancreatic cancers occur in the exocrine part of the gland, and most of these are called *ductal adenocarcinomas*.

About 5 percent of pancreatic cancers occur in the endocrine part of the gland. They are *islet cell carcinomas*.

Cancer may start at a single site or at several locations within the pancreas. Usually, ductal adenocarcinoma occurs in the head of the pancreas, but it may be diffuse, arising throughout the organ.

Cancer may spread within the pancreas and to other sites such as the liver and surrounding lymph nodes, the duodenum, the uppermost part of the small bowel just adjacent to the stomach, the base of the transverse colon, and lungs. Diffuse spreading of the cancer may be present throughout the abdominal cavity, affecting various organs, including the stomach, spleen, and colon.

Signs and Symptoms

Early signs of exocrine pancreatic cancer are vague and easily ignored. They include:

- Nausea and vomiting;

- Loss of appetite;

- Eating a small amount but feeling full;

- Alterations in bowel habits, including diarrhea, constipation, bloating, and gas;

- Difficulty digesting fatty foods;

- Gradual loss of more than 10 percent of body weight;

- *Jaundice*, a yellowing of the skin and eyes, sometimes accompanied by intense itching;

- Swollen legs;

- Sudden attack of *pancreatitis*, an inflammation of the pancreas.

Signs of progressive exocrine pancreatic cancer include:

- Pain in the back or abdomen, which may be localized more to stomach or back, but later is often described as "going through to the middle of the back";

- Pain that is aggravated by lying flat and relieved by lying in fetal position or sitting up and bending forward;

- Steady pain, sometimes described as "boring";

- Pain that worsens at night;

- Continuing weight loss;

- Urine so dark it resembles cola (accompanies jaundice);

- Clay-colored stool;

- Fatigue;

- Depression;

- Glucose intolerance (diabetes may precede pancreatic cancer in some individuals).

Signs of the following types of endocrine pancreatic cancer vary according to which hormone the tumor produces in excess. The symptoms may be dramatic so that early diagnosis and treatment are likely.

Insulinoma

(Ninety percent are benign, and there may be multiple tumors.)

- Extreme *hypoglycemia*, low blood sugar;

- Apathy;

- Sluggishness;

- Somnolence;

- Slowed thinking;

- Sudden behavior changes, bizarre behavior;

- Seizures;

- Coma;

- Hunger, epigastric pain.

Gastrinoma

- High stomach acidity;

- Stomach ulcers, accompanied by abdominal pain;

- Diarrhea.

Glucagonoma

- Sudden development or worsening of diabetes;

- Skin rashes, itching, skin ulceration;

- Anemia;

- Diarrhea;

- Weight loss;

- Depression.

Vipomas

- Copious watery diarrhea (10 to 15 stools a day);

- Copious urine;

- Muscle weakness, as a result of potassium loss in the stool.

Somatostatin-Secreting Tumors

- Diabetes;

- Stones in the gallbladder or bile ducts;

- Fatty stools;

- Muscle weakness.

Carcinoid or Islet Cell Tumors

- Flushing of the face;

- Diarrhea;

- Wheezing;

- Abdominal cramps.

Diagnostic and Staging Tests

For more information regarding these tests, see Chapter 8, "Diagnostic Tests."

- CT scan;

- Transabdominal ultrasonography;

- Fine-needle aspiration biopsy;

- Laparotomy;

- Laparoscopy;

- Angiography;

- Blood Tests;

- Endoscopic retrograde cholangiopancreatography (ERCP) involves insertion of a thin, flexible tube through the mouth, esophagus, and stomach into the duodenum to allow visualization of the opening of the pancreatic duct. Dye may be injected, so that if a cancer is pressing on or blocking the bile ducts or pancreatic duct it will be visible on an x-ray of the pancreas (there is a risk of pancreatitis, which can be serious). Intravenous sedation is usually adequate to ease discomfort during the test.

Tests Unique to Pancreatic Cancer

No tests are available.

Staging

Exocrine Pancreatic Cancers

- Stage I: Cancer is only found in the pancreas itself or limited to nearby tissues such as the small intestine, stomach, and bile duct.

- Stage II: Cancer has spread to nearby organs such as the stomach, spleen, or colon to the extent that surgical removal of the tumor is usually impossible.

- Stage III: Cancer has spread to lymph nodes near the pancreas. The cancer may have spread to nearby organs.

- Stage IV: Cancer has spread to distant sites such as the lungs or liver.

Treatment

Surgery offers the best hope of cure. Exocrine tumors can be surgically removed by a *Whipple resection (pancreaticoduodenectomy)*, in which the surgeon excises the head of the pancreas, the duodenum, a portion of the stomach, the gallbladder and common bile duct, adjacent tissues and lymph nodes.

Removal of the entire pancreas, *total pancreatectomy*, does not appear to increase survival time (see Chapter 15, "Surgery").

More recently, the surgery has been modified to preserve the stomach. This is called *pyloric-sparing Whipple resection* or the *pylorus-preserving pancreaticoduodenectomy (PPPD)*. It appears to result in less weight loss after surgery than occurs with a conventional Whipple operation.

The incidence of postoperative complications ranges from 25 to 50 percent. Typical complications include infection, bleeding, and formation of a *fistula*, or an abnormal opening.

When a tumor cannot be removed, treatment is directed toward symptom relief. For instance, parts of the digestive tract that are obstructed by the cancer can be surgically bypassed so that the person can digest food more normally and have relief from pain. A surgical connection can be made from the gallbladder to the intestine, allowing bile to get from the liver to the intestine, bypassing the tumor in between. Also, tumor blockages of the bile duct can be opened with a *stent*, or tube, which may be inserted through an endoscope. This procedure avoids major surgery.

Radiation therapy may be used to shrink or slow tumor growth as well as relieve pain (see Chapter 16, "Radiation").

Chemotherapy alone has been tried, but the drugs appear to have only a partial effect. The drug most commonly used is fluorouracil (5-FU). About 20 percent of patients respond with some shrinkage of the tumor, but there is little or no increase in survival time (see Chapter 17, "Chemotherapy").

A combination of fluorouracil (5-FU) and radiation therapy may may be recommended when surgery has successfully removed the tumor (see Chapter 20, "Combination Treatments"). Some studies have shown this combination raises the survival to 40 percent at two years. Combination chemotherapy with various drugs such as actinomycin-C, streptozocin (Zanosar), doxorubicin (Adriamycin), and methyl CCNU has produced some improvement in response rates. Clinical trials are evaluating drug combinations that may produce a better response.

Survival

- Three-year survival rate for stage I after tumor removal is 15 percent.

- Three-year survival rate for stage II is 2 percent.

- Three-year survival rate for stage III is less than 2 percent.

- Three-year survival rate for stage IV is less than 1 percent.

When a tumor is confined to the head of the pancreas and is small (less than 2 centimeters), with no lymph node involvement or metastasis, the two-year survival rate after that portion of the pancreas is removed is about 20 percent.

Median survival time for individuals who cannot have surgery but are treated with chemotherapy and radiation is less than one year.

Special Needs

Avoiding fatty foods makes some people feel more comfortable. Pancreatic enzyme tablets taken after meals sometimes help to improve digestion. Also, low-fat foods or supplements provide necessary protein and calories. Some people may require feeding through a tube inserted through the mouth to the stomach.

Symptom relief will be a priority, particularly when the tumor cannot be removed. Consultation with a pain specialist may be helpful, because managing any discomfort will greatly improve the quality of life.

After treatment, blood tests for the tumor markers CEA and CA-19 may be useful for detecting a recurrence.

Ask About

Because treatment results are modest so far, it's wise to seek treatment where oncologists have experience treating this particular cancer. You may want to discuss participating in a clinical trial with your doctor regardless of the stage of your cancer (see Chapter 21, "Investigational Treatments"). If you are considering volunteering, it's important to talk about all your options as soon after diagnosis as possible because some choices will affect your primary treatment. For example, radiation therapy and chemotherapy are being used before surgery to shrink tumors so they can be removed more easily. And some adjuvant therapies are actually administered during surgery. For instance, direct exposure to radiation when the abdomen is opened for surgery, as well as implanting radioactive materials directly into the tumor, is being compared to standard treatments.

Because the cure rate is low, several investigations are attempting to determine how pain can best be controlled to enhance the quality of life. For instance, a technique of injecting nerves in the area of the pancreas with alcohol, called percutaneous celiac axis nerve block or intrapleural block, is being evaluated.

Several new chemotherapeutic agents and biological therapies (see Chapter 18, "Biological Therapies") are also under study, particularly for people with stage III and IV disease.

PITUITARY

Tumors of the pituitary gland are relatively common, but less than 1 percent of them are malignant. It is estimated that from one to 15 people in 100,000 develop some type of tumor of the pituitary. Although many of these growths are harmless, they do have the potential for causing serious problems. Benign tumors called *adenomas*, for example, may form and never cause any symptoms, but because an adenoma can destroy the bone surrounding it (the *sella turcica*) and invade nearby structures, it is sometimes thought of as malignant and is treated similarly.

Pituitary tumors are unique in that malignant and benign cells look similar under the microscope. (Note: the term *pituitary cancer* is often not used for this reason.) It is also impossible to determine that a tumor is cancerous just because it extends to adjacent tissues, because up to 85 percent of benign pituitary tumors also spread in a similar way. One confirmation that a pituitary tumor is malignant is if it spreads to the nervous system or throughout the body (see "Types").

About 4 percent of cases are linked to multiple endocrine neoplasia (MEN) type I, but other than that, there are few known genetic or environmental associations.

The pituitary gland is an organ of the hormone-secreting *endocrine* system.

The pea-sized pituitary gland is attached to the base of the brain. It sits in the sella turcica, a bony depression in the base of the skull behind the bridge of the nose, behind and between the eyes. The two parts of the pituitary gland are the larger *anterior* lobe and the *posterior* lobe, or *neurohypophysis*, which is an extension of the central nervous system.

Because the pituitary gland secretes several hormones that stimulate other endocrine glands, it is often called the "master gland." Its anterior lobe contains five different types of cells, each of which produces a specific hormone. They include *prolactin* (PRL), which stimulates milk production in nursing mothers but can also promote nipple discharge in women who are not nursing; *adrenocorticotropic hormone* (ACTH), which stimulates the adrenal glands; *thyroid stimulating hormone* (TSH), which stimulates the synthesis and secretion of hormones from the thyroid gland; the gonadotropins, *follicle-stimulating hormone* (FSH) and *luteinizing hormone* (LH), which affect the ovaries and the testes; and growth hormone (GH), which stimulates growth in most tissues and is one of the major regulators of metabolism.

The posterior lobe produces *oxytocin*, which stimulates the uterus to contract during childbirth, and vasopressin (antidiuretic hormone, or ADH), which acts on the kidneys to control the amount and concentration of urine. Vasopressin also elevates blood pressure by causing the capillaries and arteries to contract.

Who Is at Risk?

- People between 30 and 60;

- People with multiple endocrine neoplasia type I syndrome (MEN I) often have pituitary tumors;

- People who have had a benign pituitary adenoma.

Screening Tests

No screening tests are available.

Types of Pituitary Tumors

Most primary pituitary tumors develop in the anterior lobe of the gland. Metastatic or *secondary* pituitary cancers tend to affect the posterior lobe and usually have spread from tumors arising in breast, lung, kidney, colon, or other organs.

Cancer of the pituitary gland encroaches on surrounding tissue and can extend to the brain or the spinal column via the cerebrospinal fluid. If the tumor enters the spaces around the pituitary gland, cancer cells may enter the bloodstream supplying the gland and spread to the liver, kidneys, heart, lymph nodes, or bone. The disease may progress slowly or develop rapidly.

If the tumor penetrates the base of the skull, it may also enter the lymphatic system and surrounding tissues beyond the skull, including the muscles and other structures.

Depending on which pituitary cells are involved, some tumors secrete excessive amounts of ACTH, prolactin, or growth hormone, causing symptoms and sometimes specific disorders. For example, too much ACTH (adrenocorticotropic hormone) from the pituitary gland stimulates the adrenal glands to overproduce glucocorticoids, which may cause *Cushing's disease*, a disorder that involves changes in body fat deposits, abnormal hair growth, and skin fragility. In women, too much prolactin can cause menstruation to stop and nipple discharge; in men, impotence may result. Excess growth hormone can result in *acromegaly*, or gigantism, a condition characterized by abnormal bone growth and coarse facial features.

Signs and Symptoms

Indications of a tumor vary enormously, depending on whether there is a hormone imbalance. *Silent tumors*, those that don't affect hormone-producing cells, may not create any symptoms until they grow large enough to press on nearby structures in the brain or eyes. These general symptoms include:

- Headache;
- Vision loss (usually peripheral vision is affected first);
- Fatigue;
- Widening of one pupil;

- Drooping eyelid;
- A loss of feeling in the face.

Cushing's Disease

- Distinctive rounding and flushing of the face;
- Increased body fat, including a round fat deposit—the so-called buffalo hump—on the upper back;
- Obesity in the trunk and abdomen, and thinning and weakening of the legs and arms;
- Skin changes, including purple lines on the abdomen and increased pigmentation;
- Generalized weakness.

Prolactin-Secreting Tumors

- Cessation of menstruation;
- Secretion of breast milk;
- Impotence and infertility in men.

Acromegaly

- A gradual thickening of the soft tissues and bones of the hands, feet, and face;
- Slow enlargement of body structures and organs, such as the heart;
- Headache;
- Nausea and vomiting.

Diabetes Insipidus (Posterior Pituitary Involvement)

- Very frequent urination;
- Excessive thirst;
- Constipation;
- Dry hands.

Diagnostic and Staging Tests

For more information regarding these tests, see Chapter 8, "Diagnostic Tests."

- Blood and urine tests to detect abnormal hormone levels;
- Eye examination;
- MRI or CT scan;
- Cerebral angiography (rarely indicated).

Tests Unique to Pituitary Tumors

No tests are available.

Staging

None.

Treatment

The initial treatment of choice for any pituitary tumor is surgery to remove the growth (see Chapter 15, "Surgery"). In most cases, the surgeon can make the incision inside the nose, a *transsphenoidal* approach, because the pituitary sits close to the upper nasal passages. Complications are rare, though the incidence of problems increases with the size of the tumor and the extent of its invasion into surrounding tissue. In the rare case where the tumor extends outside the bony cavity in which the pituitary gland sits, a *craniotomy*, an incision through the front of the skull, may be required. This is a far more complex surgery and complications are more likely than with the transsphenoidal approach.

Radiation therapy frequently follows surgery when a tumor cannot be removed completely, when tumors recur, or when local spread has occurred or is suspected (see Chapter 16, "Radiation").

Drug therapy for hormone-secreting tumors that cannot be completely removed may be necessary. For ACTH-producing tumors, the drugs mitotane (Lysodren) or ketoconazole (Nizoral) may be used. For tumors producing prolactin, bromocriptine (Parlodel) may be prescribed. For tumors that produce growth hormone, bromocriptine (Parlodel) or somatostatin or octreotide (Sandostatin) may be used. These drugs modulate, decrease, or otherwise interfere with hormone production. Hormone replacement therapy may be needed after surgery, depending on how much pituitary tissue has been removed.

Chemotherapy with fluorouracil (5-FU) and methotrexate has been used for malignant primary tumors and metastases, but its effectiveness has not been proven (see Chapter 17, "Chemotherapy").

Survival

Successful therapy to pituitary adenomas results in excellent (greater than 90 percent) long-term survival. If untreated, Cushing's disease is life-threatening, with a five-year survival rate of 50 percent. Untreated acromegaly also shortens life. When metastases exist, survival is usually less than three years. Death usually results from disease within the brain.

Special Needs

Because the rare malignant tumors of the pituitary are usually found at an advanced stage, patients may need to receive palliative treatment, including therapy to control pain (see Chapter 34, "Supportive Care").

Ask About

After surgery, you will want to consult an endocrinologist regarding whether hormone replacement therapy is needed. Focused radiosurgery (gamma knife) is being more frequently used when radiation therapy is indicated.

Experimental therapies include the use of heavy-particle radiation therapy (see Chapter 16, "Radiation") for ACTH- and prolactin-producing tumors. This treatment is only available at a few centers.

If you have a recurrent pituitary tumor, you may want to discuss volunteering for a clinical trial with your physician (see Chapter 21, "Investigational Treatments"). Long-term control has been achieved with repeated use of radiation therapy.

EYE

Eye cancers are very rare, accounting for less than 1 percent of all cancers. Of these, the most common is melanoma, which accounts for 70 percent of all primary eye cancers. *Retinoblastoma*, the next most common eye malignancy, occurs only in children and is highly curable. About 200 cases are diagnosed each year. Cancers arising from the eyelids are primarily skin cancers. Other types of eye cancer, such as malignant tumors that arise in or around the muscles of the orbit or eye socket (a form of childhood *rhabdomyosarcoma*), cancers of the *lacrimal* (tear-producing) gland, or lymphomas of the orbit are extremely rare and so will not be discussed in this section.

The cause of eye cancer is unknown. Environmental factors may be involved in the initiation of retinoblastoma, but no direct link has been proved. About 40 percent of the cases of retinoblastoma are caused by inherited defective chromosomes. Many people with this type of tumor develop it in both eyes.

The eyeball is a fluid-filled globe housed within a bony cavity called the *orbit*. The *conjunctiva* is a membrane that lines the inside surface of the eyelids. The *sclera*, the white of the eye, forms most of the outermost part of the eyeball and helps maintain its shape. It also protects the fragile inner structures of the eye. The *cornea*, the transparent covering of the front of the eye, permits light to enter and is part of the focusing system. Directly behind the cornea is the anterior chamber, a raised space between the cornea and the *iris*. The iris is the colored part of the eye, and the black circle in this area is the *pupil*. By dilating and contracting, the iris controls the amount of light that reaches the *lens*. The lens focuses light, which travels through thick fluid (called *vitreous*) within the eyeball to the back of the eye and is conveyed to the brain. The area where light reaches the back of the eye is the retina. The *optic nerve* transmits images from the retina to the brain. Surrounding the retina is tissue called the *choroid*, a layer that extends forward to the *iris*, a region in front of the eye. The *ciliary body* connects the choroid to the iris.

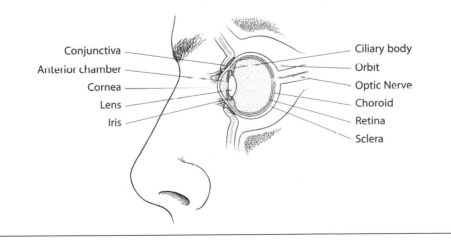

Conjunctiva
Anterior chamber
Cornea
Lens
Iris

Ciliary body
Orbit
Optic Nerve
Choroid
Retina
Sclera

Who Gets It

Ocular Melanoma

- Generally older people aged 70 to 80;

- Caucasians, who have eight times the incidence of ocular melanoma that African-Americans do, and three times the incidence of some Asian populations;

- People with a history of *ocular melanocytosis*, an overabundance of cells that produce the pigment *melanin* within the eye;

- People with a light iris color.

Screening Tests

Ocular melanoma is sometimes detected during a routine eye examination. There are no formal guidelines established by the American Cancer Society for screening eye exams because cancer of the eye is so rare.

Types of Eye Cancer

Ocular Melanoma

Ocular melanomas occur most often in the choroid, ciliary body, or iris. They can begin in the conjunctiva, but this is extremely rare. A small fraction of ocular melanomas occur in the iris adjacent to the pupil. Fortunately, they are likely to be detected early, because they are visible to someone looking at the eye. Melanomas in this site are virtually all curable.

Tumors of the choroid and ciliary body are more common than those in the iris, contain more aggressively malignant cells, and are more capable of spreading. They also tend to be diagnosed in a later stage, because they start inside the eyeball and are not visible except by specialized eye examination. Choroidal melanoma, which is more common than ciliary body melanoma, is the most likely type to spread through the bloodstream, often to the liver.

As a tumor grows in the eye, it can disrupt the retina, creating a condition known as *retinal detachment*. The cancer may spread locally to other parts of the orbit or adjacent brain, but diagnosis generally is established and treatment is initiated before this occurs. There can be metastasis to other areas, such as the lungs, bones, or distant sites under the skin. The liver is usually involved when distant spread occurs.

Retinoblastoma

Retinoblastoma is a cancer that occurs in infancy and childhood, usually before age 5 (see Chapter 35, "Cancer in Children"). It affects the retina of one or both eyes, the latter often occurring in the inherited type. If the disease affects both eyes, it is usually more advanced in one eye than in the other.

Most children with retinoblastoma have disease that is confined to the eye and orbit. It may progress forward from the retina into the vitreous-containing fluid in the cavity of the eyeball or grow outward from the retina to the choroid and other tissues that surround the retina. The disease may also spread evenly throughout the surface of the entire retina.

If untreated, retinoblastoma is most likely to extend to the brain via the optic nerve, or spread via the bloodstream to the bones, bone marrow, and lymph nodes.

Signs and Symptoms

Melanoma

- Dark spot on the iris;

- Protrusion of the eyeball;

- Changes in vision, including double or blurry vision, loss of visual acuity, and/or the presence of floating spots;

- Painful eyes;

- Numbness in the eye region;

- Headaches.

Retinoblastoma

- White area in the center of the pupil;

- Uncontrollable squinting ("cat's eye" reflex);

- Protrusion of the eyeball;

- Difference of color between the irises, or two or more separate colors within one iris;

- Eyes that suddenly become bloodshot;

- Painful, inflamed eye(s);
- Changes in vision, including blurry vision and loss of visual acuity in older children.

Diagnostic and Staging Tests

For more detailed information regarding these tests, see Chapter 8, "Diagnostic Tests."

With the exception of ultrasound, the following tests are used to detect metastasis of eye cancer.

- Ultrasound scan, which can calculate tumor thickness;
- MRI and CT scan;
- Chest and skeletal x-rays;
- Liver function studies;
- Bone scan;
- Bone marrow aspiration and biopsy;
- Lumbar puncture for retinoblastoma.

Tests Unique to Eye Cancer

- *Ophthalmoscopy* allows the doctor to see inside the eye. Usually, the pupils are dilated with special eye drops before the exam. Direct ophthalmoscopy uses an small hand-held instrument called an *ophthalmoscope* that provides illumination and magnification. Your retina and the end of the optic nerve will be examined thoroughly with this instrument.

- A genetic test called *karyotype analysis* is used in people with retinoblastoma to identify those at risk for other problems, including second cancers.

Staging

Ocular Melanoma

Ocular melanoma is staged according to the TNM system established by the American Joint Committee on Cancer.

The staging process, in terms of the primary tumor (T) differs somewhat for melanoma of each of these anatomic sites in the eye. For the conjunctiva, T1–3 is a measure of the size and physical extent of the melanoma, whereas T4 indicates additional involvement of the eyelid, cornea, or other orbital structures. The T classification is quite similar to this for melanomas of the iris. T stage for the deeper and less visible choroidal melanomas is determined by the actual size and elevation of the melanoma. As with other ocular sites, T4 for choroidal sites represents extension of the melanoma to other structures.

The TNM stage groupings for all sites are primarily determined by the T classification, because node involvement (N1) or metastasis (M1) lead to stage IV classification for both iris and choroidal melanoma.

Retinoblastoma

There is no universally used staging system for retinoblastoma. Both the TNM system and the Reese-Ellsworth classification are used. When both eyes are affected with this cancer, each is staged separately. Also, because there are no lymph vessels in the eyeball itself, regional lymph nodes refer to the parotid, preauricular, submandibular, and cervical nodes.

According to the TNM system, stage I describes a tumor that involves up to 50 percent of the retina but with no lymph node involvement or metastasis. Stage II retinoblastoma involves more than 50 percent of the retina and/or invades beyond the retina but still remains within the eye. Again, there is no lymph node involvement or metastasis. Stage III describes a tumor that extends beyond the eye without regional lymph node involvement or other metastasis. Stage IV tumors have either regional lymph node involvement or distant metastasis.

The Reese-Ellsworth classification is for stage definition of intraocular tumors only. It has some similarities to the T classification of the TNM system.

- Group I: Solitary or multiple tumors, less than 4 disc (disc refers to the width of the optic nerve when viewed through the ophthalmoscope) diameters in size, at or behind the equator of the eye. It is a very favorable situation for the maintenance of sight;

- Group II: Solitary or multiple lesions, between 4 and 10 disc diameters in size, at or behind the equator. It is favorable for the maintenance of sight;

- Group III: Any lesions in front of the equator of the eye, or lesions greater than 10 disc diameters behind the equator. There is a possibility for the maintenance of sight;

- Group IV: Multiple tumors, some larger than 10 disc diameters, or any lesion extending to the edge of the retina. Maintenance of sight is unfavorable;

- Group V: Massive tumors invading more than half the retina, or spread into the interior of the eye. Maintenance of sight is very unfavorable.

Treatment

Iris Melanoma

Iris melanoma can be present for a long time without causing symptoms. Your doctor may recommend only that he examine you every three months, closely observing the melanoma for signs of change if it is small or completely removed by the biopsy, because it grows so slowly and is usually curable. Depending on the size or the extent of involvement, you may have an *iridectomy*, a local operation that removes part of the iris; *iridotrabeculectomy*, which removes parts of the iris as well as some supporting tissues around the cornea; or *iridocyclectomy*, which removes parts of the iris and the adjacent ciliary body. The extent of visual impairment resulting from surgery depends, of course, on the extent of the resection. If the cancer cannot be removed with these surgeries, an *enucleation*, or removal of the eyeball, is necessary. However, this surgery would be quite uncommon for a melanoma arising from the iris.

Choroidal and Ciliary Body Melanomas

Treatment methods for choroidal and ciliary body melanomas depend on their size and growth rate. Observation without further treatment might be appropriate, if your tumor is small, is not growing, and causes no symptoms. But most melanomas in this site are treated.

Small melanomas may respond to *photocoagulation*, which uses a laser to destroy the blood vessels that feed the tumor. Most choroidal melanomas are treated by some form of radiation therapy or surgery.

In some centers, small to medium-sized tumors have been successfully removed with eye-preserving surgery, but the procedure is difficult. Iridocyclectomy, as described for more extensive iris melanomas, is a widely accepted treatment for some melanomas arising in the ciliary body, but the standard treatment for both choroidal and ciliary body melanoma has been either enucleation of the eye or some form of radiation therapy, which has the obvious advantage of preserving vision.

Radiation therapy for melanoma may be administered from an external beam or from tiny radioactive implants set at appropriate intervals in a flat appliance called a *plaque*. This is placed surgically and sutured to the outside surface of the eye. Typically, the plaque, with its radioactive seeds, remains on the eye for one or two weeks and is removed (see Chapters 16, "Radiation," and 20, "Combination Treatments").

If the diseased eye must be removed, you may receive radiation therapy before surgery to shrink the tumor. It may reduce the chance of "seeding" cancer cells into the area during surgery.

Enucleation remains the standard treatment for truly large eye melanomas, regardless of their location, but doctors disagree on the best treatment for ocular melanoma that has spread beyond the eye. *Exenteration* of the orbit, removal of both the eye and surrounding muscle and fatty tissues, may be required. If the tumor is this advanced, you may be given radiation therapy before or after surgery.

Retinoblastoma

The goal of treatment for retinoblastoma is to cure the cancer without jeopardizing the child's ability to see if possible. The treatment choices depend on how advanced the disease is in the affected eye, the state of the other eye (affected or not), and whether the cancer has spread outside the eye to the brain or other parts of the body.

Retinoblastoma can often be cured with radiation therapy if it is diagnosed at an early stage. The radiation may be administered from an external beam, or with brachytherapy, using radioactive implants on plaques that can be applied to the surface of the eye (see earlier).

Cryotherapy (freezing the cancer with specially designed probes) may be employed in addition to radiation therapy. These two treatments together offer the best chance of cure while preserving vision in children with small tumors.

Photocoagulation, treating the cancer with a high-powered beam of laser light, is occasionally used alone or in combination with radiation therapy to treat small lesions.

If cancer is extensive or has spread outside the eye, chemotherapy may be given in addition to radiation therapy (see Chapter 17, "Chemotherapy") in the hope of preventing or curbing metastasis to other sites. When the disease has advanced to this extent, the eyeball may have to be removed. If the cancer has already spread to the optic nerve and other tissues in the eye socket at the time of diagnosis, removal of the eye, the surrounding muscles, and the optic nerve may be required.

Treatment of retinoblastoma varies, depending on whether one or both eyes are involved. If both eyes are affected, the more affected one may be removed and the other treated with radiation therapy, or both eyes may be treated with radiation therapy. Choices depend on the extent of the disease.

Survival

Ocular Melanoma

- Five-year survival rate for iris melanoma is 96 percent.

- Five-year survival rate for choroidal melanomas is 60 percent.

Retinoblastoma

- The overall cure rate is about 85 percent.

- If the disease is confined to the eye, the five-year survival rate is more than 90 percent.

- If disease extends beyond the eye, the five-year survival rate is about 50 percent with optic nerve involvement and about 25 percent when the cancer extends to other tissues surrounding the eye.

- Survival of those with bilateral retinoblastoma is significantly lower than unilateral disease, mostly because of second cancers in other organs.

Special Needs

Radiation therapy for ocular melanoma or retinoblastoma can damage the lens and eventually cause cataracts that require treatment.

Those who have had their eye removed are candidates for a prosthesis, which can preserve the appearance of the eye but cannot restore sight.

Children with a history of retinoblastoma should be examined by an ophthalmologist several times a year for four to six years to detect recurrence at an early stage. Those with this disease, especially the hereditary type, have a greater chance of developing second malignancies, usually in the bones. These secondary tumors can often be cured, so surveillance is important. People with retinoblastoma are at risk of developing glaucoma and should have routine testing of intraocular pressure at intervals.

Siblings of children with the disease and their parents should be offered genetic counseling, and an ophthalmologist should examine the children regularly.

Of course, anytime a child has cancer, there are special needs.

Ask About

If standard treatment has failed to control your ocular melanoma or if it is advanced when it is diagnosed, you may want to discuss with your doctor one of the experimental therapies currently being studied (see Chapter 21, "Investigational Treatments").

Retinoblastoma

If the cancer has spread to tissue around the eye or has recurred, you may want to consider entering your child in a clinical trial. Several chemotherapy drugs are being evaluated for advanced disease.

VAGINA

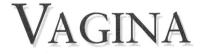

Primary vaginal cancer is a relatively uncommon disease, accounting for about 1 to 2 percent of all gynecologic cancers. An estimated 2,000 American women are diagnosed with it each year. About 90 percent of them have *squamous cell carcinoma*, which usually occurs in the surface cells lining the vagina (see "Types," later).

Most vaginal cancers are secondary; that is, the cancer has spread there from a malignancy in another part of the body, usually the colon, uterus, or stomach. This section will discuss primary cancer only.

The vagina is a 4- to 6-inch-long flexible, muscular tube through which menstrual fluid from the uterus leaves the body. It is also called the birth canal. The vagina connects the *cervix* (the lower portion or "neck" of the uterus) to the *vulva* (the folds of skin around the opening to the vagina).

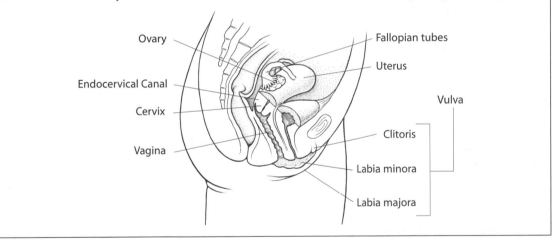

Who Is at Risk?

- Women with a history of genital human papilloma virus (HPV) of certain types (particularly 16, 18, 31, and 33);

- Daughters of women who took synthetic estrogen (diethylstilbestrol [DES]);

- Women with prior radiation therapy to the genital tract;

- Women with a history of any cancer of the genital tract, such as endometrial, cervical, or vulvar cancer.

Those at risk of particular cancers of the vagina follow.

- Squamous cell carcinoma is usually found in women more than 60 years old.

- Primary adenocarcinoma (see "Types," later) occurs most often in women 12 to 30 years old.

- Clear cell adenocarcinoma usually occurs in women 17 to 21 years old whose mothers took diethylstilbestrol (DES) during pregnancy. (DES was given to some pregnant women between 1945 and 1970 to help prevent miscarriage. It affects about one in 10,000 women exposed to DES in utero.)

- Melanoma tends to occur in women over the age of 50.

Screening Tests

- Pelvic examination (see Chapter 4, "The Cancer Checkup");

- Papanicolaou test (Pap smear; see Chapter 6, "Routine Tests").

Types

Squamous Cell Carcinoma

Squamous cell carcinoma is usually diagnosed by Pap smear in its early stages, when it remains confined to the cells lining the vagina. This is known as *vaginal dysplasia, vaginal intraepithelial neoplasia (VAIN)*, or *vaginal carcinoma in situ*. It may remain at this stage for several years and is curable.

Research suggests a strong association between squamous cell carcinoma of the vagina and human papilloma viruses (HPV) that can be sexually transmitted. Malignancies usually arise five to 10 years after initial infection.

About 10 percent of women with squamous cell carcinoma of the vagina have been treated previously with vaginal radiation therapy, usually for cervical cancer.

Squamous cell carcinoma most commonly arises in the upper third of the vagina near the cervix. Although it is slow growing, squamous cell carcinoma eventually can invade the vaginal wall. It can spread directly into surrounding tissue, including the pelvic wall, bones, bladder, and rectum, or it can spread through the lymphatic system to other parts of the body, most commonly to the lungs and liver.

Adenocarcinoma

Adenocarcinoma, which develops in glandular tissues, accounts for about 5 percent of primary vaginal cancers and most vaginal metastases

---

DES-Exposed Women

Women who were exposed to DES before birth should be followed carefully for vaginal cancer. Some experts recommend that these women have semiannual checkups, including a pelvic examination, Pap smears of the cervix and vaginal wall, and colposcopy (see page 44).

---

from elsewhere in the body.

Primary adenocarcinomas metastasize in a way similar to squamous cell carcinoma but may be more apt to spread to the pelvic lymph nodes and lungs.

Melanoma

Vaginal melanoma, which is a very aggressive cancer, accounts for 3 to 5 percent of primary vaginal cancers.

Signs and Symptoms

- Abnormal vaginal bleeding;

- Vaginal discharge, which may be foul-smelling;

- Pain in the pelvis, back, or legs.

Diagnostic and Staging Tests

For more detailed information regarding these tests, see Chapter 8, "Diagnostic Tests."

- Colposcopy (see "Cervix" in the Encyclopedia);

- Biopsy (including cervical biopsy to rule out cancer of the cervix);

- Intravenous pyelogram (IVP), cystoscopy, and sigmoidoscopy, which may be done to determine if the cancer has spread beyond the reproductive organs;

- Chest and skeletal x-rays, CT scan, liver and lymph node scans, and urinary tract scans, which may be done if metastasis is suspected.

Tests Unique to Vaginal Cancer

No tests are available.

Staging

- Stage 0, or carcinoma in situ: This is very early cancer, found only in the first layer of cells on the surface of the vaginal wall.

- Stage I: Cancer is found in the vaginal wall but not outside of it.

- Stage II: Cancer has spread to tissues just outside the vaginal wall but has not spread to the pelvic bones.

- Stage III: Cancer has spread from the vagina to the bones of the pelvis. It also may have metastasized to the pelvic lymph nodes and nearby organs.

- Stage IV: Cancer has spread to other parts of the body. In stage IVA, cancer is found in the bladder or rectum. In stage IVB, it is found in more distant organs, such as the lungs or liver.

Treatment

Stage 0 vaginal intraepithelial neoplasia (VAIN) is usually easily cured with any one of several treatment methods, which have equal success rates. The method chosen will depend on the physician expertise and the extent and location of the dysplasia. Topical chemotherapy with fluorouracil (5-FU) cream involves inserting the cream into the vagina at prescribed intervals (see Chapter 17, "Chemotherapy"). There will be some vaginal discharge and possibly some local irritation during the treatment period.

Abnormal cells can be vaporized by laser therapy, a brief procedure, but one usually requiring general anesthesia. (This is different from cervical laser surgery, which does not require general anesthesia.) This treatment causes some discomfort but no severe pain (see "Cervix" in the Encyclopedia).

Radiation therapy can be delivered directly into the vagina via intracavitary radiation (see Chapter 16, "Radiation"). A radioactive isotope held in a container is placed in the vagina and kept in place with gauze packing. It feels like a very large tampon and remains in place for 24 to 48 hours while you remain in the hos-

pital in bed. Painkillers may be given for mild to moderate discomfort.

Abnormal cells can also be excised with minor surgery. Although this is done in the hospital with general anesthesia, it is usually a one-day outpatient procedure (see Chapter 15, "Surgery").

For more extensive disease, partial or total vaginectomy (surgical removal of the vagina) may be recommended. Total vaginectomy may be accompanied by taking a skin graft from the buttocks or thigh to create a new vagina.

For stage I squamous cell carcinoma, the cure rates in women who have not had any prior radiation therapy (such as for earlier cervical cancer) are similar with either surgery or radiation therapy. Depending on the extent of the cancer, surgery may entail partial or total vaginectomy, with or without removal of the pelvic lymph nodes and/or the uterus by hysterectomy. Radiation therapy may be intracavitary, external beam, or both.

For stage I adenocarcinoma, more aggressive surgical therapy is indicated. Total vaginectomy, hysterectomy, and removal of local lymph nodes may be recommended for cancers of the upper vagina. Vaginectomy and/or vulvectomy may be necessary for early cancers of the lower vagina. Another option is radiation therapy similar to that used for squamous cell carcinoma.

For stage II to IVA vaginal cancer, whether squamous cell or adenocarcinoma, the usual therapy is a combination of intracavitary and external beam radiation instead of surgery. In more advanced cases, a combination of surgery, radiation, and chemotherapy may be recommended (see Chapter 20, "Combination Treatments").

There is no standard treatment regimen for treatment of Stage IVB squamous cell or adenocarcinoma, and no current techniques can cure these malignancies. Radiation or chemotherapy with drugs such as cisplatin (Platinol) or ifosfamide (IFEX) can be given to alleviate symptoms of the disease.

If squamous cell or adenocarcinoma recurs, total pelvic exenteration—removal of the lower colon, rectum, and bladder, together with hysterectomy and total vaginectomy—may be necessary (see Chapter 30, "Sexuality").

Because vaginal melanoma has a high rate of recurrence after conservative treatment, doctors now recommend total vaginectomy, radical hysterectomy (removal of the uterus, about one-third of the upper vagina, and the lymph nodes around the groin), or pelvic exenteration for locally advanced disease. Combination chemotherapy also may be recommended to prevent or control metastasis.

Survival

When diagnosed early, vaginal cancer is nearly 100 percent curable.

- Five-year survival for stage 0 carcinoma in situ is nearly 100 percent.

- Five-year survival for stage I vaginal cancer is up to 94 percent.

- Five-year survival for stage II vaginal cancer is up to 80 percent.

- Five-year survival for stage III vaginal cancer is 50 percent.

- Five-year survival for stage IVA vaginal cancer is up to 18 percent; that for stage IVB is 10 percent.

- Five-year survival for malignant melanoma is less than 15 percent.

Special Needs

Although partial vaginectomy usually does not interfere with sexual intercourse, total vaginectomy, obviously, does. In addition, radiation therapy may leave the vagina less accommodating for sexual activity. Counseling may be helpful (see Chapter 30, "Sexuality").

If vaginal reconstruction is done after total vaginectomy, a *dilator*, a lightweight plastic stent, is inserted after surgery to help prevent the development of scar tissue and maintain the caliber of the new vagina. It is worn all the time for the first year, except when having intercourse, which may begin six weeks after the operation. Thereafter, the stent is worn only during sleep.

Most recurrences of vaginal cancer arise within two years after initial treatment. Therefore, follow-up visits, as recommended by your doctor, should be frequent and may include a pelvic examination, Pap smear, chest x-ray, IVP, and CT scans of the abdomen and pelvis.

Ask About

If you have advanced disease, and a total vaginectomy is necessary, talk to your surgeon before the operation about vaginal reconstruction. It is not standard practice, although it is becoming more widely available.

Clinical trials are available using chemotherapy with such single drugs as mitomycin (Mutamycin), fluorouracil (5-FU), and cisplatin (Platinol), carboplatin (Paraplatin), vincristine (Oncovin), bleomycin (Blenoxane), ifosfamide (IFEX), and etoposide (VePesid)—and various combinations for every stage of vaginal cancer. Radiation therapy, including radiation therapy with heat (hyperthermia), alone or in combination with chemotherapy, is also being evaluated.

Because this cancer is so rare, talk to your doctor about the variety of investigational treatments and ask which trials might be best to consider in view of your particular type of vaginal cancer and its stage (see Chapter 21, "Investigational Treatments").

VULVA

Vulvar cancer is relatively uncommon, accounting for 3 to 5 percent of all female malignancies. As in cervical cancer, premalignant changes occur, which if removed early, can prevent the disease (see the box "Vulvar Self-Examination").

Another similarity to cervical cancer is the strong association between one type of vulvar cancer and the human papilloma virus (HPV), which causes genital warts and is sexually transmitted. Five to 10 percent of women with invasive squamous cell carcinoma of the vulva have a history of genital warts, 80 percent of which are associated with HPV types 16 or 18. Squamous cell carcinoma is becoming increasingly common in women under age 40.

The vulva is the external female genitalia: folds of skin around the opening to the vagina, or birth canal, which include the *labia majora* (the large lips) and the *labia minora* (the small lips). Two *Bartholin's glands*, which secrete lubricating fluid, are located at the base of the labia majora, one on each side wall of the vestibule, the entrance to the vagina. The hooded *clitoris*, the organ of female sexual pleasure, is in the front of the vestibule where the labia minora meet.

Who Is at Risk?

- Women over 50, especially those over 60;

- Women with a history of genital warts caused by human papilloma virus (HPV) of certain types (particularly 16 and 18);

- Women with a history of other sexually transmitted diseases, including syphilis, herpes simplex II, and lymphogranuloma venereum;

- Women with multiple sexual partners;

- Women with a history of infectious vulvitis (skin inflammation), vulvar dysplasia (a proliferation of abnormally developed cells), or vulvar dystrophy (abnormal but benign skin changes);

- Women with a history of cervical cancer.

Screening Tests

- Visual inspection of the vulva and pelvic examination (see Chapter 4, "The Cancer Checkup");

- Vulvar self-examination.

Types of Vulvar Cancer

Vulvar dysplasia, the proliferation of abnormally developed cells, is a first step toward the development of vulvar cancer and is found along the edges of 50 percent of invasive cancers.

Squamous Cell Carcinomas

Most vulvar cancers (86 percent) are squamous cell carcinomas. This type of cancer usually remains confined to the skin for one to 10 years, when it is called *carcinoma in situ* or *vulvar intraepithelial neoplasia (VIN)*. Eventually, it becomes invasive.

Most squamous cell cancers arise in the labia, clitoris, and perineum and can spread locally to the vagina, urethra, and anus. Even at this stage this cancer may be highly curable for several years. The cancer cells can invade the lymph nodes in the groin and pelvis, but they rarely enter the bloodstream or spread to distant sites.

Melanoma

Melanoma of the vulva is rare, accounting for about 6 percent of all vulvar cancers. When it does occur, it usually affects the labia minora and clitoris. The most common type, accounting for two-thirds of cases, is superficially spreading melanoma, which grows relatively slowly (see "Melanoma" in the Encyclopedia). Patterns of spread are similar to squamous cell carcinoma.

Adenocarcinoma

About 4 percent of cancers of the vulva are adenocarcinomas. They usually develop from one of the Bartholin's glands. Because this type of cancer tends to be advanced at the time of diagnosis, aggressive treatment is often required.

Basal Cell Carcinoma

Basal cell carcinoma is a relatively slow-growing cancer that usually affects the labia majora. It is very rare.

Sarcoma

Sarcoma is quite rare. It may grow slowly or very rapidly, depending on the characteristics of the cancer cells.

Paget's Disease

This is the third most common malignancy of the vulva. It appears as a red, sometimes violescent discoloration of the skin. About 10 percent of cases are associated with an underlying adenocarcinoma. The remainder are limited to the skin, such as vulvar dysplasia.

Signs and Symptoms

Two out of three women diagnosed with vulvar cancer have had symptoms for more than six months, and one out of three has had one or more of the following symptoms for more than a year.
- Vulval itching, burning, or pain;

- A lump in vulval tissue;

- Change in color or appearance of the vulva;

- Pigmented mole on the vulva that changes in size or color;

- Nonmenstrual vaginal bleeding or discharge.

Diagnostic and Staging Tests

For more detailed information regarding these

Vulvar Self-Examination

Some gynecologists suggest that women over 18, sexually active or not, visually examine their external genitalia once a month to look for such abnormalities as growths, sores, and new areas of white, red, or darkening pigmentation (see "Signs and Symptoms"). This self-examination includes visually examining the external genitalia with a hand-held mirror and feeling the area above the pubic bone, the clitoris, the labia majora and minora, the *perineum* (the area of skin between the vagina and the rectum), and the anal opening for lumps or any other irregularity.

---

tests, see Chapter 8, "Diagnostic Tests."
- Punch biopsy, sometimes done with the aid of a colposcope to magnify small lesions (see "Cervix" in the Encyclopedia);

- Intravenous pyelogram (IVP), cystoscopy, and sigmoidoscopy, done to determine if the cancer has spread beyond the reproductive organs;

- Chest x-rays, CT, or MRI scans of the pelvis and abdomen, blood tests, and liver and kidney function tests, done if metastasis is suspected.

Tests Unique to Vulvar Cancer

No tests are available.

Staging

- Stage 0, or carcinoma in situ: This is a very early cancer, found only in the surface skin of the vulva.

- Stage I: Cancer of 2 cm or less at its widest part is found only on the vulva and/or the perineum.

- Stage II: Cancer of more than 2 cm is found, but only on the vulva and/or the perineum.

- Stage III: Cancer is found in the vulva, perineum, or both and has spread to nearby structures, such as the lower part of the vagina, urethra, or anus, or to nearby lymph nodes.

- Stage IV: Cancer has spread beyond the vagina, urethra, and anus. In stage IVA, cancer is found in the lining of the bladder and the bowel or local lymph nodes. In stage IVB, cancer is found in pelvic lymph nodes or in other parts of the body.

Treatment

Depending on the depth and extent of the tumor, the most common treatment for vulvar cancer is surgery (see Chapter 15, "Surgery"). The operations include:

- *Radical local incision* (sometimes called wide local incision), in which the tumor and a margin of tissue surrounding it are removed;

- *Partial or simple vulvectomy*, in which one side of the vulva or the central portion of the labia majora is removed;

- *Skinning vulvectomy*, in which the surface skin of the vulva is removed and replaced with a tissue-paper-thin layer of skin grafted from the inner thigh or buttocks (in some cases, local lymph nodes are also removed);

- *Radical vulvectomy* for advanced vulvar cancer, involving surgical removal of all the external skin and appendages, including the labia major and minora, clitoris, entrance to the vagina, and lymph nodes in the groin;

- *Pelvic exenteration* for advanced disease, involving removal of all the pelvic organs—the uterus, ovaries, bladder, rectum, and vagina—along with vulvectomy.

Oncologists may recommend combining surgery with chemotherapy and/or radiation therapy, depending on the stage of the disease (see Chapter 20, "Combination Treatments").

- Stage 0 vulvar intraepithelial neoplasia (VIN) can be cured with any of several treatment methods. The abnormal cells can be vaporized by laser therapy, which may be done in a doctor's office using local anesthetic. Surgery is more likely to be necessary when the cancer arises on the hairy sites of the labia majora. The abnormal area can be removed, either with a wide local incision in the doctor's office or, in the hospital, by skinning vulvectomy, with or without grafting, depending on the size of the cancer and the extent of the surgery. Less commonly, topical chemotherapy with fluorouracil (5-FU) cream may be recommended, but this is not considered a reliable first choice for treatment. It's most often used when laser therapy fails or when surgery is refused.

- For stage I vulvar cancer, wide local excision or vulvectomy (simple or radical) may be performed, depending on the extent of the tumor. A biopsy of nearby lymph nodes on one or both sides of the vulva will determine if postoperative radiation therapy is necessary (see Chapter 16, "Radiation").

- For stage II vulvar cancer, radical vulvectomy with removal of the lymph nodes on both sides of the vulva is indicated, again with postoperative radiation therapy if the nodes contain cancer cells.

- For stage III vulvar cancer, radical vulvectomy with removal of the lymph nodes on both sides of the vulva is the standard therapy, followed by radiation therapy if the nodes are involved or if the vulvar tumor is extensive. Preoperative radiation therapy may reduce the size of large tumors and facilitate less extensive surgery.

- For stage IV vulvar cancer, radical vulvectomy and pelvic exenteration are usually necessary. This may involve removal of the vagina, cervix, uterus, lower colon, rectum, and bladder. Radiation therapy may follow.

Extensive radiation therapy is rarely the treatment of choice for any stage of vulvar cancer, except in women who are not healthy enough to tolerate the stress of surgery.

Survival

- Five-year survival for stage 0 carcinoma in situ is nearly 100 percent.

- Five-year survival for stage I vulvar cancer is 95 percent.

- Five-year survival for stage II vulvar cancer is 75 to 85 percent.

- Five-year survival for stage III vulvar cancer is 55 percent.

- Five-year survival for stage IVA vulvar cancer is 20 percent, that for stage IVB is 5 percent.

Special Needs

Wide local excision or even partial vulvectomy usually does not interfere with sexual pleasure if the clitoris is left intact. However, if surgery must be more extensive, reconstructive surgery may be necessary to make an artificial vulva or vagina (see "Vagina").

If the clitoris is removed because of invasive cancer, sexual pleasure will be markedly reduced (see Chapter 30, "Sexuality").

A significant number of patients with VIN develop recurrences, most commonly on the clitoris and the skin around the anus. Therefore, frequent follow-up visits are necessary and may include a pelvic examination and Pap smear. Chest x-rays, IVP, and CT scan of the abdomen and pelvis are usually suggested every six months to detect recurrences.

Ask About

If you have early-stage vulvar cancer you will want to discuss the extent of surgery necessary very carefully with your oncologist and/or surgeon. Many specialists are now suggesting conservative surgery in order to leave most of the vulva intact, especially the clitoris. The main reason is to preserve the ability to experience sexual pleasure. Another is to avoid the high rate of complications that accompany radical vulvectomy and bilateral groin lymphadenectomy, such as infection, chronic edema (fluid retention) in the legs, lymph gland problems, and stress urinary incontinence (involuntary release of urine).

If you have advanced vulvar cancer, talk with your oncologist about local radiation therapy in combination with chemotherapy before surgery. This is sometimes suggested to reduce the extent of surgery needed or to improve the odds that malignant cells can be completely removed. You might also consider participating in a clinical trial in which chemotherapy and radiation therapy are given simultaneously, either before, after, or instead of surgery (see Chapter 21, "Investigational Treatments"). Because there is no standard chemotherapy regimen, you may want to ask your doctor about various clinical trials involving such drugs as fluorouracil (5-FU), mitomycin (Mutamycin), and cisplatin (Platinol).

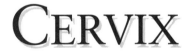

CERVIX

Cervical cancer is the seventh most common cancer among women, accounting for about 6 percent of all female malignancies and affecting 2.4 percent of women by the age of 80. Since Pap smear screening was introduced in the 1950s, cervical cancer is more likely to be detected in its early and curable stage. In fact, most women with advanced, invasive cancer of the cervix have not had a Pap smear in five years.

Because the incidence of cervical cancer is so low among celibate and monogamous women and so high among women who have had numerous sex partners, there appears to be a link to sexual behavior. Research suggests a strong association with human papilloma viruses (HPV) that can be sexually transmitted. Ninety percent of tumors contain genetic material from HPV. Some researchers also believe the herpes virus may contribute to the transformation of normal cells into malignant ones. Smoking may be another cofactor.

The cervix is the lower portion, or "neck," of the uterus, the hollow muscle organ in which a fetus develops. Ranging in diameter from the size of a quarter to that of a silver dollar, the cervix is a cylindrical protrusion about 1 inch into the *vagina*, or birth canal, that joins it to the uterus at a right angle.

The opening in the center of the cervix, the *endocervical canal*, serves as a valve through which menstrual blood and other tissue leave the uterus and sperm enters it to achieve fertilization. The cervix defends the uterus from penetration by foreign objects, fluid, and infectious agents. In pregnancy, it protects the fetus until birth begins.

Who Is at Risk?

- African-Americans, Latin Americans, and Native Americans are at higher risk;

- Women with a history of genital HPV of certain types (particularly 16, 18, 31, and 33) (this outweighs all other risk factors);

- Those in the 40 to 49 age group;

- Daughters of women who took the synthetic estrogen diethylstilbestrol (DES) during pregnancy;

- Women engaging in intercourse before age 18;

- Women who smoke;

- Women with multiple sexual partners;

- Women who have been pregnant more than five times, starting at an early age;

- Women taking immunosuppressant drugs or who have HIV infection or AIDS;

- Women who are deficient in beta carotene, vitamin C, or folic acid.

In addition, it should be noted that carcinoma in situ is more common in 30- to 40-year-olds and that invasive carcinoma occurs most often in those between 45 and 55.

Screening Tests

- Pelvic examination (see Chapter 4, "The Cancer Checkup");

- Papanicolaou test (Pap smear; see Chapter 6, "Routine Tests").

In the late 1980s, considerable attention was focused on mishandling slides and misreading results at so-called Pap smear mills, yielding a higher than expected number of false-negative reports. Tightened standards have largely remedied these problems. Indeed, when in doubt, many pathologists now choose to err on the side of safety, leading to more false-positive or questionable reports requiring further follow-up (see Chapter 5, "Screening for Cancer").

Many laboratories now use The Bethesda System (TBS) of classifying results. TBS also indicates other conditions such as yeast infections and describes low- and high-grade lesions. If a cell sample is inadequate, the report may specify the problem and suggest how it might be avoided on a repeat test.

There is some controversy about how often Pap smears should be done. The American Cancer Society recommends an annual Pap smear for sexually active women or for any woman who has reached the age of 18. After three or more consecutive annual normal tests, the physician may recommend less frequent testing. For women who have had two normal smears since turning 60, further Pap smears are no longer required. The American College of Obstetricians and Gynecologists recommends annual tests from age 18 or the onset of sexual activity throughout life.

Types of Cervical Cancer

A cervical cancer may be a squamous cell carcinoma or an adenocarcinoma.

Dysplasia, the proliferation of abnormally developed cells, is the first step toward cervical cancer, although it may never lead to cancer and may even reverse itself. Typically, mildly abnormal cells gradually become more prevalent. When they cover the entire surface of the cervix, they are considered cancerous and called carcinoma in situ. At this stage, the disease is likely to be completely curable.

If treatment of carcinoma in situ is not prompt, the malignant cells can proliferate and extend into surrounding tissue. Cervical cancer typically moves into the endocervical canal, but it may spread into the pelvic wall, vagina, large bowel, bladder, and pelvic bones. Once it enters lymph channels and blood vessels, it can travel to distant organs.

Cervical cancer is a slow-growing malignancy and can remain limited to the surface cells for as long as 10 years. However, sometimes it becomes invasive in less than a year. Once the cancer spreads beyond the surface cells, it develops quickly and, if uncurtailed, can cause death in two to three years.

At the time of diagnosis, about 45 percent of cases are localized, 34 percent have already spread to the surrounding region, and 10 percent have metastasized to distant organs.

Signs and Symptoms

- Rarely causes symptoms in early stages;

- Bleeding after intercourse;

- Painful intercourse;

- Bleeding between menstrual periods;

- Heavy menstrual flow;

- Watery, foul-smelling discharge.

Diagnostic and Staging Tests

For more detailed information regarding these tests see Chapter 8, "Diagnostic Tests."

- *Colposcopy* is a painless method for examining the surface of the cervix and the walls of the vagina, with a colposcope, a viewing instrument that looks like binoculars on a camera tripod. A bright light illuminates the genital area, and the examiner uses the colposcope to view the vaginal walls and cervix. The gynecologist may remove a tissue sample for biopsy (see later).

- CT scan, intravenous pyelography (IVP), cystoscopy, and sigmoidoscopy may be used to determine whether the cancer has spread beyond the reproductive organs.

- Chest and skeletal x-rays may be done if metastasis is suspected.

- Blood test for HIV infection since it increases the risk of cervical lesions.

Tests Unique to Cervical Cancer

- *Endocervical curettage* is the retrieval of a tissue sample from the center of the cervical opening. The doctor obtains a sample of tissue from the cervix with a curette. The discomfort is mild to moderate, similar to a severe menstrual cramp, and can be alleviated by taking a nonsteroidal anti-inflammatory drug such as ibuprofen an hour before the procedure. Minimal bleeding may last for a day and can be absorbed with a tampon or minipad. Although the tissue fragments obtained by this method may suggest the possibility of malignancy, the larger sample available by loop electrode excision procedure (LEEP) or cone biopsy (see later) is necessary to confirm malignancy.

- Cone biopsy, or *conization*, is the removal of a cone-shaped piece of tissue from the cervix for laboratory examination. Sometimes it completely removes the cancerous area, particularly in cases of early cervical carcinoma in situ. Because this procedure requires general anesthesia, it is performed in a hospital, but no overnight stay is necessary. Closing the wound and stemming the bleeding may require several stitches.

- *LEEP biopsy* (also known as large loop excision of transformation zone or LEEP biopsy staging) is a conization done with a hot wire rather than a scalpel. An electrical current makes the wire hot enough to pass through cervical tissue in seconds. Because it is so quick and relatively bloodless, it can be done in the office with a local anesthetic. From the moment a local anesthetic is injected into the cervix to completion, the procedure takes less than 10 minutes, with minimal if any discomfort, although uterine cramps may occur and can persist for a day or two. There is mild to moderate bleeding for up to six weeks. During the healing period nothing should be placed in the vagina.

When advanced cancer is present, direct examination of the internal organs may be necessary to check for cancer cells in the pelvis and evaluate the lymph nodes, which may be removed during the procedure. This is a major abdominal operation.

Staging

- Stage 0 or carcinoma in situ: This is very early cancer, found only in the first layer of cells on the surface of the cervix.

- Stage I: Cancer is found throughout the cervix. In stage IA, minimal penetration occurs into the deeper tissues of the cervix; stage IB involves greater penetration into deeper cervical tissue.

- Stage II: Cancer has spread beyond the uterus but not to the pelvic wall.

- Stage III: Cancer extends to the pelvic wall and/or involves the lower part of the vagina, and/or affects kidney function. Regional lymph nodes may be involved.

- Stage IV: Cancer is found in the bladder or rectum and may extend beyond the pelvis. Regional nodes are affected and, in stage IVB, cancer is found in more distant organs, such as the lungs.

Treatment

Carcinoma in situ is easily treated by surgically removing or destroying the abnormal cells and a margin of surrounding healthy tissue. This may be accomplished by LEEP or cone biopsy during the diagnostic process, or destruction may be done by cryotherapy or laser surgery. Both of the latter procedures can be performed in the doctor's office. There is some discomfort but no severe pain.

In *cryotherapy* (also known as cold cautery), abnormal cells are destroyed by freezing with liquid nitrogen, delivered to the cervix with a metal probe. Over the next few weeks there may be a brownish watery discharge as the destroyed cells slough off. Tampons and intercourse should be avoided for about a month.

Laser therapy uses a highly focused beam of light to vaporize the abnormal cells. This is the most precise technique for removing surface lesions. The experience for the patient is similar to that with cryotherapy, except there is much less damage.

The choice of treatment methods depends on diverse factors. If cost is a concern, cryotherapy is the least expensive. Healing time is fastest with the laser. A significant tissue sample for laboratory evaluation is available only with LEEP or cone biopsy. If the doctor suspects that malignancy extends into the endocervical canal, cone biopsy is preferred to obtain a deep tissue sample and completely remove all malignant cells.

Getting an Accurate Cancer Test

Do not have a Pap smear during menstruation. For 24 hours prior to a Pap smear, colposcopy, or any other procedure to evaluate or biopsy the cervix, avoid intercourse, any vaginal medications, spermicidal creams, douching, and tampons.

Give the examiner any information that could affect the specimen, such as whether you are taking oral contraceptives or estrogen replacement therapy, whether you have a known or suspected infection, or whether you have previously received radiation or chemotherapy.

Rarely, hysterectomy may be recommended for carcinoma in situ. However, it may be suggested to a woman who has completed childbearing, if she is extraordinarily fearful of recurrence or if other gynecological problems, such as fibroids or heavy bleeding, which might be alleviated by the procedure (see Chapter 15, "Surgery").

However, even in stage IA cervical cancer, when the depth of the cancer is minimal, conization may be appropriate in those who want to have children.

Surgery and radiation therapy are equally effective for treating small stage IA cancers (see Chapter 20, "Combination Treatments"). Depending on the extent of the tumor, surgery may mean total hysterectomy (removing the cervix and uterus), vaginal hysterectomy (removing the vagina, cervix, and uterus), or radical hysterectomy (removing the cervix, uterus, and part of the vagina). Radiation therapy is delivered by external beam and intracavitary radiation (see Chapter 16, "Radiation").

For stage IB and IIA cancers, radical hysterectomy with pelvic lymphadenectomy (removal of the lymph nodes) or intracavitary and external beam radiation are equally effective. In some cases, the ovaries and fallopian tubes also are removed in an operation called *bilateral salpingo-oophorectomy*.

Because radiation therapy can cause vaginal dryness and shrinkage, and may damage the ovaries and bring on menopause, younger women often prefer surgical treatment (see Chapter 30, "Sexuality"). However, in some cases, postsurgical radiotherapy may be recommended as well, especially if metastasis to the lymph nodes has occurred. Radiation therapy may be preferred when the woman is elderly and/or not healthy enough to withstand the trauma of surgery.

Stage IIB to IVA advanced cervical cancers are routinely treated with a combination of intracavitary and external beam radiation. In addition, chemotherapy may be given to help sensitize the cancer cells to the radiation. The drugs used may include hydroxyurea (Hydrea), cisplatin (Platinol), or ifosfamide (IFEX). In some cases, surgery is also necessary and is performed after radiation therapy has reduced the size of the tumor as much as possible. If the cancer has spread to nonreproductive organs, removal of the lower colon, rectum, or bladder in an operation called *pelvic exenteration* may be necessary together with hysterectomy.

There is no standard treatment regimen for stage IVB cervical cancer. Radiation or chemotherapy (with such drugs as cisplatin or ifosfamide) may alleviate symptoms.

Survival

- Five-year survival for stage 0 cancer is nearly 100 percent.

- Five-year survival for stage I cancer is 65 to 90 percent for squamous cell carcinoma and 70 to 75 percent for adenocarcinoma.

- Five-year survival for stage II cancer is 45 to 80 percent for squamous cell carcinoma and 30 to 40 percent for adenocarcinoma.

- Five-year survival for stage III cancer is up to 61 percent for squamous cell carcinoma and 20 to 30 percent for adenocarcinoma.

- Five-year survival for stage IV cancer is less than 15 percent.

Special Needs

Most recurrences of cervical cancer arise within two to three years after initial treatment. Therefore, frequent follow-up visits, as recommended by your doctor, should be undertaken during that time. Follow-up visits may include a pelvic examination, Pap smear, chest x-ray, IVP, and CT scan of the abdomen and pelvis.

Ask About

If you doctor suggests surgical conization to determine if cancer cells are present or suspects you have carcinoma in situ, ask about the LEEP procedure (see "Tests Unique to Cervical Cancer"). It is now widely available and, because it is done with local anesthesia, is replacing other types of surgery.

If your cancer is in an advanced stage, you may want to discuss *induction chemotherapy* to shrink the tumor before surgery with your oncologist. Sometimes the improvement is significant enough to allow safe radical hysterectomy, rather than radiation therapy alone (see Chapter 20, "Combination Treatments").

If you are pregnant, your doctor may suggest no therapy until after your child is born if you have carcinoma in situ, as long as colposcopy has ruled out invasive cancer. Treatment of invasive cancer during pregnancy depends on the extent of disease, the stage of your pregnancy, and your desires. In the past, therapy was delayed only if cancer was detected in the final trimester, to help assure the safety of the fetus.

In the first and second trimesters, immediate therapy appropriate for the disease stage was recommended. Unfortunately, this usually results in death of the fetus. However, it now appears that delaying treatment may be a reasonable option for women with early stage I cervical cancer diagnosed early in pregnancy.

Because the value of chemotherapy in addition to radiation therapy is uncertain in treating more advanced disease (stage III or IV disease), you may want to discuss entering a clinical trial exploring various combinations of these two treatments (see Chapter 21, "Investigational Treatments").

UTERUS

Endometrial carcinoma, cancer of the lining of the uterus, is the most common female genital cancer, affecting about one woman in 1,000 each year. It accounts for 13 percent of all cancers in women. Fortunately, if diagnosis occurs early, the cure rate is about 95 percent. Uterine sarcoma, which arises in the muscle or other supporting tissues of the uterus, accounts for less than 1 percent of gynecologic malignancies (see "Types," later).

The cause of uterine cancer remains unknown. However, it is more common in women who have had prolonged periods of estrogen exposure without progesterone to balance its effects. This includes women who have not had children (pregnancy produces a flow of progesterone), who took estrogen replacement therapy without supplemental progestin, who went through menopause after the age of 52, and who have not menstruated for extended periods, such as obese women. Although there have been reports of an association between uterine cancer and hypertension and diabetes mellitus, some experts believe the association is related to the underlying obesity that often accompanies these conditions.

Some types of uterine sarcoma appear to be more common in women who received pelvic radiation for other gynecologic conditions 15 to 20 years earlier.

The *uterus*, or womb, is the hollow organ in a woman's pelvis where a fetus develops. Its thick, muscular walls help expel the baby during delivery. The uterus is normally about the size and shape of a medium-sized pear, except during pregnancy.

Extending from each side of the top of the uterus are the *fallopian tubes*. Eggs released from the *ovaries* pass through these tubes into the uterus for fertilization. The base of the uterus ends in the *cervix*, which connects it to the vagina, or birth canal. The lining of the uterus, called the *endometrium*, is constantly changing throughout the menstrual cycle. It is embedded with tiny glands that develop each month in preparation for pregnancy, when they will secrete embryo-nourishing substances. The top layer of the endometrium sloughs off each month in a process called *menstruation* if pregnancy does not occur.

Who Is at Risk?

- Obese women;

- Women over age 50;

- Women with a history of pelvic radiation therapy;

- Women who have menopause after age 52;

- Women who have not had children;

- Women who have taken estrogen replacement therapy without supplemental progesterone;

- Women who have had tamoxifen therapy.

Endometrial cancer affects mostly post-menopausal women; 25 percent of cases occur in premenopausal women.

Uterine adenocarcinoma (see "Types," later) usually affects middle-aged women. Incidence peaks between the ages of 50 and 64. (The lifetime risk for Caucasians is 2.4 percent; it is 1.3 percent for African-Americans.)

Screening Tests

- Pelvic examination (see Chapter 4, "The Cancer Checkup");

- Papanicolaou test (Pap smear; see Chapter 6, "Routine Tests"). Because uterine cancer begins inside the uterus, it is not usually diagnosed by a Pap smear until it has spread to the cervix.

Types of Uterine Cancer

Endometrial *hyperplasia*, an overgrowth of normal cells lining the uterus, is the first step toward development of cancer. However, the condition (also known as *cystic* or *adenomatous hyperplasia*) may never lead to cancer and can even reverse itself without treatment.

If uterine cancer is not detected at an early stage, it may eventually spread from the inside of the uterus to the cervix. It can also extend through the uterine wall and spread through the fallopian tubes. Common sites of metastasis are the ovaries, cervix, vagina, rectum, and bladder.

Cancer cells can also enter the lymphatic system underneath the endometrium and eventually flow into lymph vessels outside the uterus. From the lymph and blood vessels, the cancer cells can spread to the abdominal cavity, liver, lungs, bone, and brain.

Endometrial Carcinoma

About 75 percent of endometrial carcinomas arise from the glands in the lining of the uterus and so are called endometrial adenocarcinomas. Less common but more threatening are three types of cancer: *adenosquamous carcinoma*, in which cancer arises from both gland cells and squamous cells; *papillary carcinoma*, which appears as mushroomlike growths extending from the endometrium; and *clear cell carcinoma*, which is rare.

Uterine Sarcoma

Tumors with only one type of cell are known as *pure sarcomas*. Those that arise from the smooth muscle layer of the uterus are called *leiomyosarcoma*. They account for about 30 percent of all uterine sarcomas. About 15 percent of uterine sarcomas are called *endometrial stromal sarcomas*, tumors that arise from the cells that surround and support the glands within the endometrium. About half of all uterine sarcomas arise from both the endometrial glands and the supporting cells of the endometrium and are called *mixed mesodermal sarcomas*.

Signs and Symptoms

- Most commonly, abnormal uterine bleeding, ranging from minor spotting to heavy hemorrhage;

- About 15 percent of women with postmenopausal bleeding have endometrial carcinoma;

- Pain in the pelvis, back, or legs;

- Changes in bowel or bladder patterns;

- Weight loss;

- General weakness.

Diagnostic and Staging Tests

For more details, see Chapter 8, "Diagnostic Tests."

- Transvaginal ultrasound;

- Tumor markers: Elevated levels of CA-125 often indicate that malignancy has spread beyond the uterus;

- Blood tests: Complete blood count and tests of liver and kidney function;

- CT and MRI scans of the pelvis and abdomen;

- Intravenous pyelogram (IVP), barium enema, cystoscopy, and sigmoidoscopy, to determine if the cancer has spread beyond the uterus;

- Lymphangiography;

- Chest and skeletal x-rays if metastasis is suspected.

Tests Unique to Uterine Cancer

Laboratory examination of uterine tissue is essential for definitive diagnosis. This tissue may be obtained in one of two ways: endometrial biopsy or dilation and curettage (D&C).

Endometrial Biopsy. An endometrial biopsy is an office procedure in which a sample of endometrial tissue is obtained through a very thin flexible tube inserted into the uterus through the cervix. The tube is attached to a suction device that vacuums out a small amount of endometrium. The suctioning takes about a minute or less. The discomfort is similar to a severe menstrual cramp and can be alleviated by taking a nonsteroidal anti-inflammatory drug such as ibuprofen an hour before the test.

Dilation and Curettage. If endometrial biopsy provides an inadequate amount of tissue or suggests a malignancy, a D&C must be done. In this outpatient procedure, the cervix is dilated and a small curved knife is used to scrape tissue from inside the uterus. The procedure takes about an hour and usually requires general anesthesia.

The tissue sample obtained during the D&C will be evaluated for both progesterone and estrogen receptors. Studies have shown that these receptors (which bind to the hormones) are associated with increased survival time in women with endometrial cancer.

Staging

The following staging descriptions are for all types of uterine cancer, except when otherwise noted.

- Stage 0 or carcinoma *in situ*: This is very early cancer found only on the surface layer of endometrium.

- Stage I: Cancer is found only inside the uterus. In stage IA the tumor is limited to the endometrium. Stage IB involves invasion to less than half of the myometrium, the muscular layer underlying the endometrium. Invasion in stage IC involves more than half of the myometrium.

- Stage II: Cancer has spread to the cervix. In stage IIA, only endocervical glandular involvement. In stage IIB, cervical stromal invasion exists.

- Stage III: Cancer has spread outside the uterus but remains within the pelvis. In stage IIIA, local membranes, such as the peritoneum, which lines the abdominal cavity and covers local organs, are invaded. In stage IIIB in endometrial cancer, cancer has spread to the vagina. In stage IIIB in uterine sarcoma and IIIC in endometrial carcinoma, cancer has spread to regional lymph nodes.

- Stage IV: Cancer has spread to the bladder or rectum or other parts of the body, including regional lymph nodes. In stage IVA, tumor has invaded the bladder and/or bowel. In stage IVB, cancer has metastasized to distant sites.

Treatment

The main treatment for uterine cancer is hysterectomy (surgical removal of the uterus) and bilateral salpingo-oophorectomy (removal of the fallopian tubes and ovaries, because they are often a site of early spread of disease). The ovaries are sometimes left in place in younger women with early-stage disease, to avoid premature menopause. Lymph nodes are a frequent site of metastasis, so many surgeons recommend removing them at the time of surgery.

A hysterectomy is major abdominal surgery, requiring general anesthesia and a hospital stay of several days. Complete recovery takes about a month or longer. If the cancer is beyond stage I, the cervix and part or all of the vagina also may need to be removed (see Chapters 15, "Surgery," and 30, "Sexuality").

If cancer cells are in the lymph nodes, radiation therapy may follow surgery (see Chapters 16, "Radiation," and 20, "Combination Treatments"). A five-week course of radiation therapy is typical and can destroy any cancer cells remaining in the pelvis. Rarely, when the individual cannot tolerate the stress of hysterectomy, treatment may consist of radiation therapy alone.

In some cases, when cancer has spread beyond the uterus, adjuvant chemotherapy, often with doxorubicin (Adriamycin) is recommended. Combinations of doxorubicin, cyclophosphamide (Cytoxan), fluorouracil (5-FU), and vincristine (Oncovin) may also be used (see Chapter 17, "Chemotherapy").

When stage 0 endometrial hyperplasia is diagnosed in a premenopausal woman who wants to have children, some doctors recommend a D&C followed by hormonal therapy with progestins.

In stage IIB and stage III endometrial carcinoma, a radical hysterectomy removes the uterus, fallopian tubes, ovaries, supporting ligaments of the cervix and uterus, and the pelvic lymph nodes. Preoperative radiation therapy may reduce the size of the tumor, and then it may be necessary to remove only the uterus, ovaries, and fallopian tubes.

Stage III endometrial carcinoma with a tumor extending into the pelvic wall is usually inoperable. Treatment consists of intracavitary and external beam radiation therapy.

Treatment for stage IV endometrial carcinoma depends on the site(s) of the metastases. Those that are limited to the pelvis are treated with radiation therapy, whereas distant metastases are often treated with hormonal therapy (progesterone) or chemotherapy.

Most stages of uterine sarcoma are treated with hysterectomy, with or without removal of the fallopian tubes and ovaries, depending on the woman's age and the extent of the disease, plus removal of local lymph nodes. Some oncologists suggest postoperative radiation therapy and/or chemotherapy.

There is currently no standard therapy for women with stage IV uterine sarcoma, although symptoms may be alleviated with hormonal therapy or chemotherapy.

Survival

When diagnosed early, endometrial cancer is nearly 100 percent curable.

- Five-year survival for stage 0 cancer is nearly 100 percent.
- Five-year survival for stage I cancer is 75 to 100 percent.
- Five-year survival for stage II cancer is up to 60 percent.
- Five-year survival for stage III cancer is up to 30 percent.
- Five-year survival for stage IV cancer is up to 5 percent.

Uterine sarcoma is not as amenable to successful therapy.

- Five-year survival for stage I cancer is 50 percent.
- Five-year survival for stage II cancer is up to 20 percent.
- Five-year survival for stage III cancer is up to 10 percent.
- Five-year survival for stage IV cancer is up to 5 percent.

Special Needs

Most recurrences arise within three years, so follow-up tests are important. Most doctors recommend a physical examination and Pap smear every three months for the first two years, then every six months for another three years. If blood levels of CA-125 were elevated before treatment, they should be monitored.

Women who have had their ovaries removed will immediately enter menopause, because their natural source of estrogen has been removed. Because the hormonal flow ceases suddenly, rather than gradually, as in normal menopause, symptoms such as hot flashes tend to be more severe. The estrogen replacement therapy often prescribed for women going through normal menopause is usually not recommended for women with endometrial or breast cancers. (Studies are under way to determine whether estrogen replacement therapy is truly contraindicated for this group of women.) However, other options, including progesterone, for treating hot flashes may be explored.

Ask About

Because a significant number of women with uterine cancer have cancer cells in the lymph nodes, surgeons often remove local nodes during hysterectomy. Whether or not the lymph nodes are involved will be important information that affects the need for adjuvant radiation therapy.

Before your surgery, ask your doctor if the tissue retrieved will be evaluated for hormone receptors. This may become important later when you are deciding about adjuvant treatment or if the cancer recurs.

If you have stage III or IV endometrial cancer, ask your oncologists about participating in one of the several clinical trials evaluating hormonal and chemotherapy regimens with new drugs and/or new combinations of common agents (see Chapter 21, "Investigational Treatments").

Many oncologists recommend that women with uterine sarcomas join an ongoing trial of adjuvant therapy, because the risk of recurrence is high. Ask your doctor about chemotherapy or radiation therapy following surgery to remove the tumor. Several clinical trials are being conducted by the Gynecologic Oncology Group (GOG) to evaluate these combination therapy options.

OVARY

Ovarian cancer is the fifth most common cancer in women and the second most common gynecologic cancer. It has been estimated that one in 65 women will develop ovarian cancer by age 85. Ovarian cancer has the highest mortality rate of all the female cancers, primarily because it produces few early-warning signs and is, therefore, often detected late. About 70 percent of women have advanced disease at the time of diagnosis.

The cause is unknown but the most important risk factor is family history of a first-degree relative (mother, daughter, or sister; see the box "Preventing Familial Ovarian Cancer," page 570). Other influencing factors may be in the environment, because the incidence is highest in industrialized countries, with the exception of Japan. Occupational exposure to asbestos and long-term use of talc for personal hygiene in the genital area also appear to increase risk.

Prior use of oral contraceptives or having a child, which interrupts ovulation, lowers estrogen output and decreases the risk of ovarian epithelial cancer (see "Types," later) by 30 to 60 percent. Each successive child further reduces a mother's ovarian cancer risk by about 14 percent. Even pregnancies that end in miscarriage, elective abortion, or stillbirth reduce the risk proportionate to the months of gestation. Recent studies also suggest that tubal ligation, and perhaps hysterectomy, may substantially reduce the risk of this type of ovarian cancer.

The two *ovaries* are each about 1.5 inches long and less than 1 inch wide before menopause. Afterward, they become somewhat smaller. One ovary is located on either side of the *uterus*, the hollow muscular organ in which a fetus develops. The *fallopian tubes* convey eggs from the ovaries to the uterus. During each monthly menstrual cycle, one ovary releases an egg, which travels through a fallopian tube to the uterus.

The ovaries secrete *estrogen* and *progesterone*, the female hormones that control the development of the breasts and other female body characteristics as well as regulate the menstrual cycle and pregnancy.

Who Is at Risk?

- Women between the ages of 50 and 54;

- Those whose first-degree (mother, sister, or daughter) or second-degree relatives (grandmother or aunt) have had ovarian cancer (three hereditary syndromes have been identified: site-specific ovarian cancer, also known as *familial ovarian carcinoma*, the most common type in which only ovarian cancer occurs; *breast/ovarian cancer syndrome*, in which there is a clustering of both types of cancer in the extended family; and Lynch II syndrome, in which the family history includes cancers of the colon, lung, and uterus). In contrast to a lifetime ovarian cancer risk of only 1.5 percent in the general population, the risk is 40 to 50 percent among families with familial ovarian carcinoma, which accounts for less than 5 percent of ovarian cancers;

- Women with a family history of breast or colon cancer;

- Older women;

- Women with few or no children;

- Women who delayed childbirth until after 35;

- Women who have undergone treatment of infertility with drugs such as clomiphene that trigger ovulation;

- Women with a history of breast or endometrial cancer;

- Women who have used talc in the genital area for many years;

- Caucasians, who are at higher risk than African-Americans.

Epithelial carcinoma affects most women after menopause. Average age at diagnosis is 61. Average age at diagnosis of the inherited type, familial ovarian carcinoma (see "Types," later), is 48.

Germ cell tumors primarily afflict young women; 60 percent are under 20 at the time of diagnosis.

Screening Tests

Screening for ovarian cancer is controversial. No screening tests are currently recommended for the general population because current methods (such as transvaginal ultrasound and blood tests for CA-125) have a high rate of false-positive results (see Chapter 8, "Diagnostic Tests"), requiring costly follow-up. Because ovarian cancer is uncommon, many health care specialists do not believe the cost of these follow-up evaluations to the health care system is worth the relatively few malignancies that are detected early.

However, if you are at higher risk of ovarian cancer because one or more first-degree relatives have had the disease, many doctors recommend the following tests every six months after 35.

- Pelvic examination (see Chapter 4, "The Cancer Checkup");

- *Transvaginal ultrasound*, in which a probe that projects sound waves in placed inside the vagina (the echoes from the sound waves are translated by a computer into a picture of the reproductive organs; this painless procedure may detect ovarian tumors that are still small and in an early stage);

- CA-125 blood test (elevated CA-125 levels may indicate ovarian cancer but may also accompany endometriosis, pregnancy, and nongynecologic conditions; see Chapter 6, "Routine Tests").

Types of Ovarian Cancer

About 90 percent of ovarian cancers arise in the covering of the ovary, called the *epithelium*. Of these, 15 percent are *borderline tumors* of low malignant potential, which tend not to become invasive, and 65 percent are called *ovarian epithelial carcinoma*. About 5 percent of ovarian cancers are *germ cell tumors*, which are found in the egg-making cells of the ovary. Another 5 percent are *stromal tumors*, which arise from the *stroma*, the fibrous tissue that forms the framework of the ovary.

Ovarian malignancies tend to grow rapidly and rarely cause pain or other symptoms that might lead to early detection. The cancer usually spreads directly by shedding malignant cells into the abdominal cavity. Adjacent tissues and organs such as the liver, stomach, intestines, *omentum* (the fatty tissue attached to the intestines), and diaphragm are likely areas of invasion. Ovarian cancer can also spread through the blood or lymph glands to other parts of the body, such as the lungs and brain.

When the diaphragm is affected, normal drainage of fluid from the abdominal cavity may be impaired, resulting in *ascites*, the accumulation of fluid that distends the abdomen.

Signs and Symptoms

In the early stages there are usually no symptoms. Later, the following signs and symptoms may appear:

- Abdominal pain;
- Abdominal swelling due to ascites;
- Bloating, indigestion, gas;
- Pelvic pressure;
- Feeling full before finishing even a light meal;
- Loss of appetite;
- Weight gain;
- Fatigue;
- Frequent urination;
- Constipation;
- Nausea and vomiting;
- Shortness of breath.

Diagnostic and Staging Tests

For more information about these tests, consult Chapters 6, "Routine Tests," and 8, "Diagnostic Tests."

- Pelvic examination;
- Blood tests, including assessment of tumor markers, such as CA-125 for suspected ovarian epithelial carcinoma, and LDH (the enzyme, lactate dehydrogenase), HCG (human chorionic gonadotropin), and AFP (alpha-fetoprotein) if germ cell tumors are suspected;
- Transvaginal ultrasound;
- Exploratory laparotomy to obtain tissue for pathological evaluation, which is the only way to diagnose this cancer accurately (lymph nodes and tissue samples from various areas within the abdomen are also retrieved for analysis);
- Pap smear;
- Urine test;
- CT and MRI scans of the pelvis and abdomen;
- Intravenous pyelogram (IVP), cystoscopy, and sigmoidoscopy, to determine if the cancer has spread beyond the ovaries;
- Chest and skeletal x-rays, liver and lymph node scans, and urinary tract scans if metastasis is suspected.

Tests Unique to Ovarian Cancer

No tests are available.

Preventing Familial Ovarian Cancer

If you have two or more first- or second-degree relatives who have had ovarian cancer, it may be appropriate to have genetic counseling to determine if you have a rare hereditary syndrome that markedly increases your risk. In such cases, if you know you want to have children, it may be best not to postpone childbearing, because some doctors recommend *prophylactic oophorectomy* (surgical removal of the ovaries to prevent the disease) after 35.

However, *prophylactic* or preventive oophorectomy may not entirely eliminate the risk of malignancy. There may be an inherited susceptibility to cancer in tissue that shares the same origin as the ovary. Thus, development of carcinoma of the nearby *peritoneum*, the membrane covering the abdominal organs, has been reported after prophylactic oophorectomy.

Women who have any family history of ovarian cancer might consider joining a cancer registry, such as the Gilda Radner Familial Ovarian Cancer Registry, reachable at 1-800-OVARIAN.

Staging

- Stage I: Cancer is found only in one or both ovaries. In stage IA, the tumor is limited to the inside of one ovary; the ovarian capsule, which covers the organ, is intact; and ascites is not present. At stage IB the tumor is limited to the inside of both ovaries, the ovarian capsule is intact, and ascites is not present. In stage IC, the tumor also is found on the surface of one or both ovaries, the capsule has ruptured, or ascites is present and malignant cells are found in the fluid.

- Stage II: Cancer is found in one or both ovaries and has spread elsewhere in the pelvis. In stage IIA, the tumor is found in the uterus, fallopian tubes, or both. In stage IIB, the tumor involves other pelvic tissues. At stage IIC, stage IIA or IIB cancer is present, and tumor cells occur on the surface of one or both ovaries, the capsule

has ruptured, or ascites is present and malignant cells are found in the fluid.

- Stage III: Cancer is found in one or both ovaries and has spread to lymph nodes or to other body parts inside the abdomen, such as the surface of the liver or intestine. In stage IIIA, there is microscopic invasion of abdominal peritoneal surfaces. In stage IIIB, abdominal peritoneal surfaces are invaded and no tumor exceeds 2 centimeters in diameter. In stage IIIC, there are abdominal tumors that are greater than 2 centimeters in diameter or that have spread to regional lymph nodes.

- Stage IV: Cancer involves one or both ovaries, regional lymph nodes are involved, and there is spread beyond the abdomen to distant sites, such as the lungs or liver.

Treatment

Borderline tumors of low malignant potential that can be completely removed surgically may require no further treatment, although chemotherapy may be recommended to reduce the risk of recurrence (see Chapter 14, "Principles of Treatment"). When the tumor is in only one ovary and the woman hopes to become pregnant, only the affected ovary and its adjacent fallopian tube are removed in a procedure called unilateral salpingo-oophorectomy (see Chapter 15, "Surgery"). If cystic tumors are present in both ovaries and the ability to have children is a concern, sometimes only the tumors and a margin of tissue surrounding them are removed, leaving ovarian function intact. If childbearing is not an issue, removal of both ovaries and fallopian tubes, called bilateral salpingo-oophorectomy, and hysterectomy are recommended. Whatever approach is taken, five-year survival is nearly 100 percent in borderline tumors, even when diagnosed in stage II or III. Surgery in the later stages is likely to include omentectomy, the removal of the fatty tissue attached to the intestines, removal of nearby lymph nodes, and chemotherapy.

Ovarian cancer is highly curable in stage I with surgery, followed by chemotherapy, radiation therapy, or both (see Chapter 20, "Combination Treatments"). The effectiveness of therapy decreases markedly in later stages, although further treatment often can bring long remissions. Chemotherapy regimens usually include two or more drugs, one being a platinum-based drug such as cisplatin (Platinol). Other drugs used include fluorouracil (5-FU), cytarabine (Cytosar-U), etoposide (VePesid), melphalan (Alkeran), doxorubicin (Adriamycin), hexamthylmelamine, and carboplatin (Paraplatin) (see Chapter 17, "Chemotherapy").

Standard treatment for stage I ovarian cancer is bilateral salpingo-oophorectomy with total abdominal hysterectomy and omentectomy and removal of local lymph nodes. Again, however, conservative surgery in selected patients who desire further childbearing may be possible, especially for those with germ cell tumors. For cancers beyond stage IA, systemic chemotherapy usually begins a week or two after surgery and consists of six to 12 monthly cycles with combination chemotherapy. If there is no visible cancer remaining after surgery, radiation therapy to the pelvis may be an alternative to chemotherapy.

In stages II and III ovarian cancers that have spread in the pelvis, surgery such as that described for stage I is performed with excision of as much of the tumor as possible. In addition, samples of adjacent tissues are taken for biopsy. The remaining tumor cells are treated with chemotherapy to shrink the cancer. This may increase disease-free periods and overall survival time.

"Second-look" laparotomy (see Chapter 15, "Surgery") is often recommended for stage II and III cancers after the completion of six cycles of chemotherapy. Even women who have a negative CT scan and normal CA-125 levels six months after surgery have been found to have minimal residual disease upon second-look surgery.

Intraperitoneal chemotherapy, delivering drugs directly into the abdominal cavity, or *peritoneum* (see Chapter 17, "Chemotherapy") may be recommended for women who had an initially positive response to systemic chemotherapy but who are found to have a small amount of cancer at second-look surgery. This approach also may be used to shrink stage III tumors, as secondary treatment after debulking surgery, or as an initial treatment in advanced disease.

Stage IV cancers are primarily treated with chemotherapy, although surgery is sometimes performed to relieve intestinal obstruction or to remove as much of the tumor as possible. This is called cytoreductive or debulking surgery (see Chapter 15, "Surgery").

Survival

When diagnosed early, ovarian cancer is highly curable. Cure rates are highest in those with borderline tumors of low malignant potential.

- Five-year survival for stage I cancer is 90 percent.

- Five-year survival for stage II cancer is 70 percent.

- Five-year survival for stage III cancer is 25 percent.

- Five-year survival for stage IV cancer is 10 percent.

Special Needs

When both ovaries are removed, a woman's natural source of estrogen is interrupted and menopause begins immediately. Because the hormonal flow ceases suddenly, rather than gradually as in normal menopause, symptoms such as hot flashes tend to be more severe. The estrogen replacement therapy often prescribed for women going through normal menopause can be recommended for women with ovarian cancer. However, other options for treating hot flashes may be explored, including progesterone. (See Chapter 30, "Sexuality.")

In the past, patients with advanced metastatic disease that was not in control often spent weeks or months in the hospital receiving intravenous pain medication, antibiotics, nutrition, and other therapies. With the increasingly widespread availability of home health care, intravenous therapy can be provided in the home, giving patients greater comfort and the support of family and friends (see Chapter 34, "Supportive Care").

Ask About

Regardless of the stage of your cancer, you are probably eligible for participation in a clinical trial. The treatment possibilities are changing so rapidly that there are many options to discuss with your oncologist, should you choose to enter a study (see Chapter 21, "Investigational Treatments"). Some of these investigations involve fine-tuning existing therapies, some are testing new combinations and delivery systems as well as high-dose chemotherapy with autologous bone marrow transplant (see Chapter 19, "Bone Marrow Transplant") and hormone therapy.

You may want to ask about clinical trials evaluating the new drug paclitaxel (Taxol), the use of which is becoming more widespread as a first-line therapy rather than a treatment solely for recurrent disease.

ESOPHAGUS

Esophageal cancer accounts for less than 2 percent of all cancers and only 5 percent of gastrointestinal cancers. Considered a rare cancer in the United States, it affects fewer than eight people in 100,000, but the incidence has increased slightly in the last two decades. Cancer of the esophagus has a high prevalence in the Far East, Iran, Africa, and Finland, where such habits as chewing betel nuts and bidi smoking (India) are common, where exposure to environmental carcinogens is possible, and where diets are deficient in certain vitamins and minerals.

Most cases of esophageal cancer in this country are associated with long-term smoking and excessive drinking of alcohol. The primary chemicals of each, nicotine and ethanol, appear to act synergistically, increasing the likelihood of esophageal cancer in those who both smoke and drink. Frequently eating foods that contain nitrates and nitrites, such as cured ham and bacon, is a risk for this type of cancer, because these chemicals can turn into the carcinogen nitrosamine in the body (see Chapter 10, "Cancer Causes and Risks").

The esophagus is a 10-inch-long, hollow, muscular tube that carries food and liquids from the throat to the stomach. It begins at the pharynx (throat) and enters the stomach through an opening in the diaphragm.

The esophagus resembles other organs of the digestive tract: It consists of an inner mucosa layer, containing numerous mucus-secreting glands. Its thick, muscular wall is made of an outer layer of muscle fibers that run lengthwise, and an inner layer of muscle fibers that encircle the tube. Sphincters at its upper and lower ends regulate movement of food and liquid into and out of it.

Esophagus

Liver

Stomach

Gall Bladder

Transverse colon

Descending colon

Sigmoid colon

Rectum

Ascending colon

Cecum

Who Is at Risk?

- Long-term smokers or drinkers or both;

- Men, who are three times more likely to get esophageal cancer than women;

- People over 60;

- African-Americans, who are three times more likely to get this type of cancer than Caucasians;

- People with a history of some precancerous conditions, including Barrett's esophagus (inflammation or ulcer of the esophagus or ulcer related to reflux, backup of stomach acid into the esophagus), *achalasia* (a chronically spastic muscle at the lower end of the esophagus), and chronic stricture of the esophagus, resulting from accidental swallowing of caustic substances, usually in childhood.

Screening Tests

- No tests are available. If you have one of the conditions that put you at increased risk, such as Barrett's esophagus, your doctor may suggest endoscopy with appropriate biopsies (see "Tests Unique to Esophageal Cancer") every three to 12 months.

Types of Esophageal Cancer

About 60 percent of esophageal cancers are *squamous cell carcinomas*, which arise most often from the surface cells of the esophagus. As the cancer grows, it spreads through the muscle wall and into the surrounding tissue. As it narrows the opening of the esophagus, it causes difficulty in swallowing.

An estimated 40 percent of esophageal cancers are *adenocarcinomas*, which develop in the glands of the mucosa.

A very few esophageal cancers have a different microscopic structure from that of the two major types. They are adenoid cystic carcinoma, mucoepidermoid carcinoma, adenosquamous carcinoma, sarcoma, melanoma, plasmacytoma, verrucous carcinoma, and oat cell or small cell carcinoma. These variants behave in a fashion similar to the more common types.

Unlike other organs of the gastrointestinal system, the esophagus lacks a *serosa*, or outer membrane, which normally acts as a protective barrier against the spread of cancer cells. For this reason, and because the esophagus has a rich supply of blood and lymphatic vessels, esophageal cancer can metastasize early. The most common sites of cancer spread are the lungs, liver, brain, adrenal glands, and bones.

Signs and Symptoms

Symptoms do not occur until the esophagus is narrowed so much that even the natural elasticity of the organ cannot accommodate the growth. At this relatively advanced stage, the following signs and symptoms may appear.

- Difficulty in swallowing or *dysphagia*;

- Pain on swallowing;

- Severe weight loss or cachexia.

When the disease progresses, there may be

- Hoarseness;

- Chronic cough;

- Pain in throat or back;

- Pneumonia;

- Coughed-up blood;

- Enlarged lymph nodes, especially over the left collarbone;

- Pain when the spinal cord is tapped;

- Thickening and scaling of the palms of the hands and soles of feet.

Diagnostic and Staging Tests

For more information regarding these tests, see Chapter 8, "Diagnostic Tests."

- Blood tests: complete blood count (elevated levels of LDH [lactate dehydrogenase] and alkaline phosphatase may indicate metastases to the liver or bone; elevated CEA [carcinoembryonic antigen] may indicate metastasis);

- CT and MRI scans.

Tests Unique to Esophageal Cancer

- X-rays of the esophagus, in which the person swallows a drink containing barium just before the x-ray to outline the organ;

- Exfoliative cytology, which involves gathering cells from the lining of the esophagus for laboratory analysis under a microscope. Cells are obtained by passing a special brush through an *endoscope*, a small viewing instrument, into the esophagus or with a technique called *balloon mesh cytology*, which involves inserting a catheter with a nylon-mesh balloon on the end into the esophagus to collect cells;

- Esophagoscopy, which involves passing a rigid or flexible endoscope through the mouth into the esophagus, allowing both visualization of internal abnormalities and tissue collection for microscopic analysis;

- Endoscopic ultrasound, which is performed through an endoscope, to estimate the depth of invasion of the cancer;

- DNA analysis of tumor cells with abnormal chromosomes , which may provide an early indication that benign Barrett's esophagus is becoming malignant.

Staging

- Stage 0 cancer, or carcinoma in situ, includes tumors that are usually small, self-contained, on the surface lining and not invading the wall of the esophagus itself. Diagnosis at this stage is very unusual. The cancer may be detected inadvertently, perhaps during an examination of the esophagus for some other reason. This is not a true cancer, because it does not invade; it might more properly be considered precancerous.

- Stage I indicates the tumor has invaded the mucosa but not the muscular wall and does not block or encircle the esophagus. It is considered an early stage of the disease, with no spread to other organs or lymph nodes.

- Stage II cancer is divided into two types. Stage IIA indicates the tumor has invaded the muscle, but there is no involvement of lymph nodes and no distant metastasis. In stage IIB, cancer cells have spread to the local lymph nodes .

- Stage III cancer means the tumor has invaded all the way through the muscle of the esophagus and may have invaded adjacent structures. There is lymph node involvement.

- Stage IV indicates the tumor has metastasized or spread beyond the local lymph nodes.

Treatment

By the time the most common symptom, difficulty in swallowing, occurs, most esophageal cancers have invaded adjacent structures. Even though surgery is unlikely to cure many of these cases, it can accomplish a great deal by relieving symptoms, such as difficulty swallowing (see Chapter 15, "Surgery").

Location of the tumor is critical when considering the choice of treatment. If the cancer is in the lower two-thirds of the esophagus (*intrathoracic esophagus*), surgery is usually performed. When the lowest thoracic portion is involved, a part of the stomach may also require removal; the remaining upper section of the esophagus and the stomach are then reconnected.

Tumors in the upper third of the chest or in the neck (*cervical esophagus*) present greater challenges, especially if the cancer has invaded nearby structures, such as the trachea or larynx. The surgeon must reconstruct that portion of the esophagus that has been removed, which entails a high risk of complications. If the entire esophagus is removed, the stomach may be pulled all the way up to the neck to reconstruct an esophageal passage. A part of the colon can also be used as a "transplant" to reconstruct the defect produced by removal of the esophagus.

You need to be aware that there is some controversy about which type of operation is the most effective and carries the least risk. Also cancers in the middle and upper third of the chest, or neck, are often treated by radiation therapy rather than surgery. Therefore, you may want to get a second or even a third opinion about which treatment is best in your case.

Because the survival rate is low for locally advanced esophageal cancer, combination therapy is often recommended in an attempt to slow the cancer's progress. The chemotherapy and radiation therapy may precede or replace surgery (see Chapters 17, "Chemotherapy"; 16, "Radiation"; and 20, "Combination Treatments"). For example, chemotherapy with fluorouracil (5-FU) and cisplatin (Platinol) plus radiation may be suggested as an initial treatment for stage I or II cancer. (Squamous cell carcinomas are considered more sensitive to the chemotherapy–radiation therapy combination than adenocarcinomas, but both types do respond.)

Stage III cancers are treated in several ways. To slow cancer spread and prolong survival, radiotherapy is used in conjunction with various combinations of chemotherapeutic agents (fluorouracil [5-FU] plus cisplatin [Platinol]; fluorouracil [5-FU] plus cisplatin [Platinol] plus doxorubicin [Adriamycin]; or fluorouracil [5-FU] plus mitomycin [Mutamycin]). This approach to combination therapy has shown greater initial benefit than using radiotherapy alone for shrinking the tumor and preventing cancer spread. However, the long-term benefit is still unclear.

If the tumor has blocked the esophagus and prevents swallowing, and resection is impossible because of the local extent of the tumor, the obstruction may be relieved in a number of ways. The surgeon may insert a tube from above, through the cancer, allowing liquids to pass through to the stomach. Endoscopic laser surgery may vaporize the blockage, or a portion of it, and temporarily relieve the swallowing difficulty. The procedure usually has to be repeated every four to six weeks, as the cancer grows back, and it does carry a risk of perfora-

tion of the esophagus. If other methods are inappropriate, the surgeon may create an opening in the abdomen through which a feeding tube is inserted into the stomach.

Stage IV and recurrent esophageal cancer are considered inoperable because there is extensive local spread or distant organs are involved. A variety of treatments—radiation and chemotherapy, for instance—may be used to ease symptoms during the short expected survival time.

Survival

- Five-year survival for stage I cancer is less than 50 percent.

- Five-year survival for stage IIA cancer is 15 percent.

- Five-year survival for stage IIB cancer is 10 percent.

- Five-year survival for stage III cancer is less than 10 percent.

- Prolonged survival is rare for those with stage IV disease.

Special Needs

Anyone with esophageal cancer requires special nutritional support, particularly when disease is advanced and difficulty in swallowing becomes a major problem. Liquid diets and nutrition supplementation delivered through a tube may become necessary (see Chapters 26, "Food and Nutrition," and 34, "Supportive Care").

Ask About

Almost everyone diagnosed with esophageal cancer is a candidate for a clinical trial. You may want to discuss volunteering for one before you undergo surgery, because some trials are evaluating different types of therapy and combinations of therapies to shrink the tumor before it is removed.

Clinical trials of other types of therapy are

also under way. For example, photodynamic therapy, in which chemicals are used to make cancer cells more sensitive to the light of a laser, is being studied in people with stage III cancer.

STOMACH

In the past half century, the incidence of stomach cancer has plummeted to the point where it accounts for only about 2 percent of all new cancers, affecting about one person in 10,000 each year. Improved methods of food handling and preservation, such as freezing, and increased vitamin C intake are believed to be responsible for its decline.

Although researchers cannot point to any single cause of stomach cancer, some experts believe one factor is prolonged exposure to foods that have nitrates (such as smoked foods), that contain a high amount of salt, and that have been pickled. This theory is, however, quite controversial. Such prior conditions as gastritis, *Helicobacter pylori infection* (which is also associated with peptic ulcers), and certain types of anemia, which decrease stomach acid production, may predispose a person to gastric cancer.

About 90 percent of gastric cancers originate in the *mucosa* layers of the stomach. They are called *adenocarcinomas* because they begin in the glands that secrete stomach acid and digestive enzymes.

Nearly half of adenocarcinomas form in the lower third of the stomach, especially in the lower curvature, which is the inside portion of the organ's J-shape. The remaining half appear within the middle portion and the upper third of the stomach.

The stomach is a J-shaped expandable organ of the digestive tract that varies in size from one person to another, and according to whether it is full or empty. It is suspended in the upper abdomen, behind the liver, and to the right of the spleen. The stomach joins the *esophagus*, the tube through which food enters from the mouth, at its upper, or *proximal*, end and the *duodenum*, the first portion of the small intestine, at its lower, or distal, end.

The stomach acts as a food reservoir that regulates the passage of food to the rest of the intestinal tract. Acids and enzymes secreted by glands of the stomach *mucosa*, the mucous membrane lining the inside of the stomach, initiate digestion by chemically breaking down food. Contractions of the smooth muscular walls of the stomach move partially digested food into the small intestine.

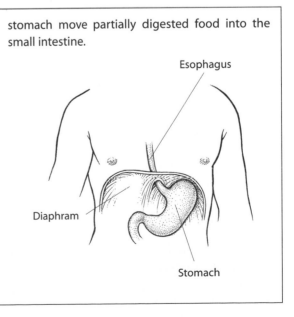

Esophagus

Diaphram

Stomach

Who Is at Risk?

- People between the ages of 50 and 70;

- Men, who are twice as likely to get stomach cancer as women;

- People who have had prior stomach surgery (increases risk 20 years later);

- People with pernicious anemia;

- People who frequently eat uncooked pickled foods and/or dried, salted, smoked fish;

- People with any condition that reduces the amount of stomach acids that break down bacteria;

- People who have had *Helicobacter pylori* infection.

Screening Tests

No tests are available.

Types

Adenocarcinomas are divided into subtypes: *fungating*, also called *polypoid*, meaning the tumor cells are well developed; *ulcerating*, or having the appearance of an ulcer with distinct borders and a diameter larger than 2 centimeters; *superficial spreading*, with sheetlike collections of cancer cells replacing the normal stomach lining; and *diffusely spreading*, in which the tumor cells cause the stomach wall to thicken and become stiff. This condition is also known as *linitis plastica*, or "leather stomach."

The second most common stomach cancer, called *malignant lymphoma*, accounts for about 8 percent of all gastric cancers. It can be a primary cancer site or a local sign of a more systemic cancer. Much less common are the leiomyosarcomas (1 to 3 percent of all gastric cancers), which begin in the muscular layer of stomach tissue, and others, including types called *liposarcomas, fibrosarcomas,* and *carcinosarcomas. Carcinoids* are small, firm, yellow lesions in the stomach lining and are very rare.

Cancer located in the upper part of the stomach carries the worst prognosis. Ten to 20 percent of gastric cancers occur in the lower portion of the stomach. It is estimated that more than half are curable.

The stomach is supplied by many blood and lymph vessels, so the possibility of metastasis to distant sites is great. The most common route of spread, which occurs in two-thirds of those with gastric cancer, is through the lymphatic system. The cancer extends to regional lymph nodes around the stomach or to distant ones, such as those near the base of the neck. The tumor may also penetrate the stomach wall and extend to adjoining organs of the digestive tract. Cancer cells may also enter the bloodstream and spread to distant sites.

Signs and Symptoms

Early signs of gastric cancer are nonspecific and mimic symptoms of other conditions such as an ulcer. Some people may complain of stomach discomfort or indigestion, occasional belching, or a feeling of fullness after even a small meal. A few may experience anemia, weakness, and weight loss.

Signs of advanced cancer include:

- Acute upper abdominal pain;

- Blood in the stool;

- Vomiting;

- Extreme weight loss;

- A palpable abdominal mass;

- Ascites, or accumulation of fluid in the abdomen;

- Jaundice, or yellowish appearance of the skin;

- Cachexia, or extreme malnutrition.

Diagnostic and Staging Tests

For more information regarding these tests, see Chapter 8, "Diagnostic Tests."

Because the symptoms of early gastric cancer are so vague, physicians recommend a complete evaluation of people who complain of persistent gastrointestinal (GI) symptoms.

- History and physical examination, including feeling for evidence of enlarged lymph nodes, an indication of metastasis;

- X-rays of the upper gastrointestinal tract (an upper GI series), in which the person swallows a barium drink that makes the organ visible on the x-ray;

- Endoscopic ultrasound, a new technique using ultrasound inside the esophagus and stomach and performed through an endoscope, permitting viewing of all the stomach's internal layers, increasingly used for staging cancer;

- CT scan;

- Laparotomy, which provides a definitive diagnosis, often established only after surgery (curative surgery may also be performed at the same time).

Tests Unique to Stomach Cancer

- Upper GI endoscopy, in which an *endoscope*, a small fiberoptic viewing instrument, is passed through the mouth and esophagus into the stomach. The doctor can visually examine the stomach lining and obtain a tissue sample through the endoscope.

Staging

- Stage 0, or in situ, cancer indicates that the tumor is confined to the mucosa. There is no lymph node involvement and no metastasis.

- Stage I is divided into two groups, IA and IB. In stage IA, the tumor is limited to the mucosa and submucosa, the layer immediately beneath the mucosa. In stage IB the tumor is limited to the mucosa and submucosa, having spread to nodes around the stomach within 3 centimeters of the tumor, or the tumor has advanced *to* but not *through* the serosa.

- Stage II may mean that lymph nodes farther than 3 centimeters from the tumor are involved or the tumor has penetrated the serosa but not adjacent organs.

- In stage III, the tumor has penetrated the serosa and may involve nearby organs by direct extension, or it has penetrated the serosa and involves the liver, diaphragm, pancreas, abdominal wall, retroperitoneum, small bowel, or duodenum. There is often local lymph node involvement.

- Stage IV means the tumor has metastasized to distant organs, tissues, or lymph nodes.

Treatment

Surgery to remove part of the stomach or, in some cases, the entire stomach, is the treatment of choice (see Chapter 15, "Surgery"). The extent of the surgery will depend upon the stage of the cancer. In general, stages I through III are considered to be operable for cure; stage IV cancers generally are not. Chemotherapy alone or in combination with radiation therapy is also an option, before or after surgery, or in place of it.

Two main types of stomach surgery are designed to remove the cancer and/or slow its spread: *subtotal* and *total gastrectomy*.

Subtotal gastrectomy removes the part of the stomach containing the primary tumor and portions of nearby tissue. If the upper end of the stomach is removed, the operation is called a *proximal subtotal gastrectomy*. Removal of the lower end of the stomach is called a *distal subtotal gastrectomy*. To restore normal digestive functioning, the remainder of the stomach is attached to either the esophagus (as with the proximal gastrectomy) or the small intestine (after distal gastrectomy).

Total gastrectomy removes the whole stomach and parts of the esophagus, small intestine, and other tissues near the tumor. Lymph nodes in the region and possibly the spleen are removed. Digestive function is restored by joining the small intestine directly to the esophagus (*esophagojejunostomy*). A pouch may be created out of healthy tissue to serve as a reservoir for food.

In more than 60 percent of people with gastric cancer who undergo surgery, metastasis is present, which makes complete excision of the cancer impractical. Nevertheless, the surgeon may remove a large part of the tumor to relieve pain and prevent blockage. In some cases of obstruction, total gastrectomy may be performed as a palliative measure.

Radiation therapy may also be used to shrink tumors, or to treat cancers that are causing chronic bleeding and cannot be removed (see Chapter 16, "Radiation").

Chemotherapy, in most cases, is used as an adjunct to surgery in advanced gastric cancer and may provide some temporary benefit, such as slowing tumor growth. However, there is no strong evidence that it prolongs life (see Chapter 17, "Chemotherapy").

Most commonly, adjuvant chemotherapy is used when the excised tumor has completely penetrated the stomach wall and no residual tumor is present. Fluorouracil (5-FU) is the most frequently used drug. When given in combination with doxorubicin (Adriamycin) and mitomycin (Mutamycin) or methyl CCNU, fluorouracil (5-FU) has been associated with good response to therapy in 40 percent of cases.

Survival

Because gastric cancer usually goes undetected in its early stages, the prognosis for almost two-thirds of those presenting with symptoms is discouraging. However, much depends upon location of the cancer and the type of surgery the surgeon can perform.

- Five-year survival rate for stage I gastric cancer was 43 percent.

- Cancers in the lower portion of the stomach have a better five-year survival than those arising nearer to the esophagus.

- Regrowth of a cancer following gastric surgery usually occurs within three years. Among people who reach the five-year mark after surgery, about 95 percent can expect to remain well.

Special Needs

Following stomach surgery, most people need to alter the size and content of their meals. Eating a big meal can lead to the so-called dumping syndrome, when all the food goes immediately to the small intestine, causing nausea and vomiting, dizziness and sweating, and a generalized feeling of weakness. To avoid this syndrome, a person can reduce discomfort by eating six smaller meals per day that are high in protein and low in carbohydrate (see Chapter 26, "Food and Nutrition"). If only part of the stomach has been removed, a person can expect to eat fairly normally.

Ask About

If you have stage II cancer involving more than three lymph nodes, your oncologist may advise you to participate in a clinical trial evaluating adjuvant chemotherapy and/or radiation therapy (see Chapter 21, "Investigational Treatments"). Various chemotherapy trials are also under way for patients with stage III and IV disease.

COLON AND RECTUM

Although colorectal cancer is the third most common cancer—affecting about 58 men out of 100,000 and 40 women out of 100,000 each year—its incidence among Americans is decreasing. The mortality rate is also decreasing, which may reflect advances in detection and screening as well as the increasing use of combination therapies (see Chapter 20, "Combination Treatments"). Nevertheless, recurrence continues to be a serious problem.

Cancer can affect the colon (the last part of the large intestine) or the *rectum*, the last 8 to 10 inches of the colon. Because cancer often affects both areas, it is frequently referred to as *colorectal cancer*.

Americans have about a one in 20 lifetime risk of developing colorectal cancer. It affects primarily those over 65, but risk starts increasing at age 40. Only about 3 percent of these malignancies occur in those under 40, when it is often due to an inherited condition.

The exact cause of colorectal cancer is unknown, but at least eight different genes involved with the origin of this cancer have been identified. Most researchers agree that there is a link to dietary fat, particularly animal fat. During fat metabolism, bacteria in the bowel form carcinogens (cancer-causing agents) that irritate the intestinal lining. It is believed that polyps form in response to this irritation, and they are often a precursor of cancer.

A high-fiber diet is thought to be somewhat protective, because it helps accelerate the rate at which fats pass through the bowel, and/or dilutes the concentration of fats, reducing the exposure of the large intestine to carcinogens. This supposition is based on various epidemiologic studies. However, clinical trials are under way that are designed to demonstrate whether there is any benefit, such as preventing polyps, from increasing the fiber content of the diet.

Together, the colon and rectum form the *large intestine* or *large bowel*, which is the lowermost portion of the digestive system. During the 18 to 24 hours it takes for material to pass to the colon, *chyme*, the semifluid mix of stomach secretions and food, becomes feces. This waste is stored in the large bowel until it passes through the rectum and out of the body.

The colon is 3 to 4 feet long and is looped around the organs of the lower abdominal cavity. It consists of five sections: the *cecum*, which is joined to the small intestine; the *ascending*, or right, colon; the *transverse* colon, which travels across the abdominal cavity just under the ribs; the *descending*, or left-sided, colon; and the *sigmoid* colon, the S-shaped section that joins the rectum. The *rectum* is about 8 to 10 inches long and terminates at the *anal* opening.

The innermost lining of the colon is the *mucosa*, which is composed of loose, connective tissue and epithelial lining containing tube-shaped glands. Above the mucosa are layers of muscles, which move waste along. Outside of the muscle is the *serosa*, the thin, shiny surface lining the outside of the colon.

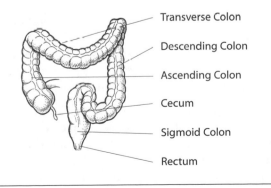

- Transverse Colon
- Descending Colon
- Ascending Colon
- Cecum
- Sigmoid Colon
- Rectum

Who Is at Risk?

- People over 65;

- People who eat a high-fat (particularly one high in saturated fat), low-fiber diet;

- People with Crohn's disease;

- Women with a history of breast or ovarian cancer;

- Sedentary people;

- People with intestinal polyps (see "Types," later).

Approximately 15 percent of people who develop colorectal cancer have a family history of the cancer in a first-degree relative.

About 1 percent of those with colorectal cancer have familial adenomatous polyposis (FAP), or Gardner's syndrome, a condition that causes them to develop hundreds of polyps or growths in the colon, usually by young adulthood. If left untreated, this condition leads to cancer by age 40. There are now genetic markers to identify those at risk for this condition.

About 1 percent of people with colorectal cancer have chronic ulcerative colitis.

Screening Tests

For more detailsabout these tests, see Chapter 6, "Routine Tests."

- Annual stool examination for occult blood in those over 40 without symptoms;

- Annual digital rectal exam in those over age 40;

- Flexible sigmoidoscopy at age 50 and every three to five years thereafter;

- Colonoscopy or double-contrast barium enema x-ray examination at age 35 to 40 in persons whose first-degree relative was diagnosed with colorectal cancer before age 55; and then every three to five years.

All siblings and children of people known to have familial polyposis should have a colon evaluation in adolescence to determine if they have inherited the problem. (All people with familial polyposis need their colon removed—usually as young adults—because they all will develop colorectal cancer.)

Types of Colorectal Cancer

Adenocarcinomas account for 90 to 95 percent of all large bowel tumors. They typically originate in the mucosa from a benign growth or *adenoma*. (Note that not all adenomas become malignant.) Adenomatous polyps look like grapes on the surface of the bowel's inner wall. The larger their size and the greater the degree of *dysplasia* (abnormally developed cells), the more likely the polyps are to progress to cancer.

On the right side of the colon near the cecum, cancers usually grow into the space within the colon. They can become large enough to be painful and are likely to cause bleeding. That is why anemia from chronic blood loss is often the first sign and why the stool test for *occult*, or hidden, blood is important (see Chapter 5, "Screening for Cancer").

Most polyps and cancers appear on the left side of the colon. In the left or descending colon, where the channel is narrow, the cancer usually grows around the colon wall and encircles it. Left-sided colon cancer typically constricts the bowel channel, causing partial blockage. One typical symptom is constipation; others are changes in bowel habits and, when a cancer is low in the rectum, narrow, ribbon-shaped stool.

In general, colorectal cancers tend to be slow growing, gradually enlarging and eventually penetrating the bowel wall. When they do spread, it is usually a result of invasion of nearby lymph nodes. In fact, cancer cells may enter a lymph node even before the tumor penetrates through the intestinal wall. The most common sites of distant metastasis are the liver, lungs, and brain.

Rectal cancer can spread to adjacent organs in the pelvic region, such as the ovaries or the prostate. Bone metastases can occur in the pelvis or other bones.

Signs and Symptoms

The early signs of colorectal cancer can mimic symptoms caused by other gastrointestinal illnesses, such as the flu, ulcers, and colitis, an inflammation of the colon. If any of the symptoms last more than two weeks, however, it is important to see a physician for an evaluation.

- Unexplained persistent diarrhea or constipation;

- Blood in or on the stool (can be bright red or very dark);

- Narrower stools than usual;

- Unexplained iron deficiency anemia;

- Bloating and distension of the abdomen;

- Intermittent abdominal pain.

Rectal Cancer

- Blood in the stool;

- Diarrhea;

- A sense of bowel movement urgency;

- Feeling of inadequate emptying of bowel;

- Excessive straining to have a bowel movement without passing of stools.

Diagnostic and Staging Tests

- CT scan.

Tests Unique to Colorectal Cancer

For more details about these tests, see Chapter 8, "Diagnostic Tests."

- *Sigmoidoscopy*, in which an *endoscope*, a hollow flexible tube 10 inches long, is gently inserted into the rectum and passed upward into the recto-sigmoid colon to look for growths. Flexible versions of the sigmoidoscope are longer, about 24 inches. Removal of polyps can also be accomplished with an instrument inserted through either type of endoscope.

- *Colonoscopy*, performed by inserting a long, flexible tube that allows examination of the entire colon as far as the cecum.

- *Barium enema air-contrast* x-ray, in which a person has an enema with a barium-containing solution to outline the inside of the colon and identify suspicious growths on an x-ray;

Staging

Most oncologists categorize colorectal cancers using either the TNM (tumor-nodes-metastasis) staging system of the American Joint Committee on Cancer (AJCC), or the Dukes classifications, named after a pioneering English oncologist, Cuthbert Dukes, who established the system in the 1930s. The Dukes system rates tumors "A" through "C," depending on the size of the tumor and depth of tissue penetration, as well as on whether the cancer affects lymph nodes. It is quite similar to the TNM system.

Dukes Classification

The classification is determined on the pathology specimen after the colon or rectum containing the cancer is removed. It is simple but the categorization is effective in predicting the outlook for people with colorectal cancer:

- A: The cancer may or may not invade from the mucosal lining into the muscle of the bowel wall, but it does not go through the entire muscle layer.

- B: The cancer extends through the entire muscle and involves the serosal surface.

- C: Cancer has spread to the local (or regional) lymph nodes. Modifications of this system break down the categories in a slightly different way, such as the Astler-Coller system, which uses A, B1, B2, C1, and C2. However, the concept is the same, and no advantage has been demonstrated for increasing the number of groups.

TNM System

The TNM system is similar to Dukes classification. It is usually based on pathology of the tissue removed at the operation and has the advantage over Dukes classification of using the same staging "language" as that used for other sites.

- Stage 0 colorectal cancer signifies Tis, or tumor in situ, which is a self-contained and noninvasive tumor that has not spread below the surface lining. The chance for complete cure when the cancer is detected this early is more than 95 percent, because it might well be considered precancerous.

- Stage I can mean that the tumor has spread beyond the inner lining to the second layer (submucosa) or third layer (muscular) of the bowel. Stage I is the same as Dukes A colon cancer.

- Stage II correlates with Dukes B. The cancer has penetrated the serosa.

- Stage III, also called Dukes C, includes three different types of tumor. The defining factor is that there is spread to the regional lymph nodes.

- Finally, stage IV, or late colorectal cancer, has a primary tumor of any size or extent with or without node involvement, but metastasis is evident at a distant site.

Treatment

Surgery to remove the tumor, a section of the colon on either side of it, and the local lymph nodes remains the treatment of choice, regardless of the tumor's location. There is a trend to follow such surgery with radiation therapy or chemotherapy or both for selected patients (see Chapter 20, "Combination Treatments"). Treatment plans vary according to the stage of disease and the area of the colon or rectum involved.

Colon Cancer

A stage 0 cancerous polyp in the colon often can be removed through a sigmoidoscope or colonoscope (a polypectomy), depending on the location. The physician inserts an instrument through the endoscope and frees the polyp from its attachment to the bowel lining.

With stage I colon cancer, the surgeon removes the tumor through an abdominal incision. The two free ends of the colon are attached to each other by a process called anastomosis (see Chapter 15, "Surgery"). Because of advances in operative techniques for reattaching sections of the colon, a colostomy is almost always unnecessary, unless the cancer is low in the rectum itself (see Chapter 28, "Managing Disabilities and Limitations").

Stage II colon cancer cases are also treated primarily with surgery. Many oncologists recommend adjuvant chemotherapy for stage II cancer, but its effectiveness has not been demonstrated.

Stage III (Dukes C) colon cancer carries a greater chance of recurrence because one or more lymph nodes are involved. Therefore, adjuvant chemotherapy, usually a combination of 5-FU and leucovorin or levamisole, follows surgery. Adjuvant chemotherapy has been shown to delay recurrence and increase the likelihood of cure of this stage of colon cancer (see Chapter 17, "Chemotherapy").

A stage IV tumor in the colon usually requires surgery to remove the involved segment even though metastasis has occurred. The aim is to prevent obstruction and anemia from bleeding. In the case of spread to the liver, affected portions of the organ often can be removed, resulting in a longer survival time. More extensive liver metastases may be treated directly with *intra-arterial chemotherapy*, in which an anticancer drug is injected directly though an artery supplying the liver or by the more standard systemic chemotherapy (see Chapter 17, "Chemotherapy"). There is no standard recommended adjuvant therapy for colon cancer metastasis.

Rectal Cancer

As with colon cancer, rectal cancer can be cured by surgically removing the tumor and nearby lymph nodes.

Chemotherapy recommendations are based on the stage of the disease in much the same way as described for colon cancer. Because of the possibility of localized recurrence, radiation therapy is often used also to destroy any cancer cells that may be in adjacent pelvis tissue at the site of removal of the rectum.

In the case of a large rectal tumor, some oncologists recommend radiation therapy before surgery to shrink the growth so it may be more easily removed. Radiation therapy also may be delivered intraoperatively with an external beam aimed at the pelvic region or through a tube directly to the tumor. Internal radiation involves delivering radioactive isotopes through implanted catheters to the tumor (see Chapter 16, "Radiation").

- Stage 0 rectal cancer often requires only a simple polypectomy to cure it, as with colon cancer.

- Stage I rectal cancer may be treated in a number of ways, depending upon the location of the tumor. If the tumor is in the mid- or upper rectum, closer to the colon, surgical removal with anastomosis and no added treatments may be sufficient. If the tumor is located in the lower rectum, closer to the anal opening, surgery may include removal of the tissues around the anus along with the rectum and lower colon and placement of a colostomy opening on the abdominal wall. A small, stage I tumor in the lower rectum may be removed by local surgical means or by electrocautery, but this is usually supplemented with radiation therapy.

- Stage II or III (Dukes B or C) rectal cancer, regardless of the location of the tumor, is treated similarly to stage I and nearly always includes adjuvant radiation therapy. Researchers have found that using chemotherapy (fluorouracil [5-FU]) in conjunction with radiation therapy enhances its effectiveness. Local surgery or electrocautery is unsuitable for cancer at this stage.

- In stage IV rectal cancer, surgery may be performed in selected cases to remove the cancer, but it is not curative. Surgery may also be performed to remove isolated metastases in the liver, lung, or ovaries. Both radiation and chemotherapy may be given for palliation to slow growth and relieve symptoms in people with stage IV rectal cancer and recurrent rectal cancer.

Survival

More than 80 percent of people with colorectal cancer are curable at the time of their diagnosis, if the tumor has not penetrated the colon wall or spread to lymph nodes.

- Stage 0 has a cure rate better than 95 percent.

- Stage I disease has a 90 percent cure rate.

- Survivability is still a relatively high 65 to 75 percent for those with stage II colorectal cancer. The prognosis shifts, however, when lymph nodes become involved, because this indicates that the cancer may have spread more extensively.

- For stage III disease, depending on the number of lymph nodes involved, the cure rate is 35 to 65 percent.

- Stage IV colorectal cancer survivability depends on the cancer's growth rate and spread at time of detection. The median survival time for people with stage IV disease is approximately 18 months.

Special Needs

When removing a cancer in the rectum, the surgeon usually tries to preserve the anal sphincter so that the person is able to have reasonably normal bowel movements after recovery from surgery. However, if the entire lower rectum must be removed, the surgeon will create a *colostomy*, an opening, or *stoma*, in the abdomen through which the waste from the bowel can exit. An enterostomal therapist can help you learn how to care for the colostomy. (See "Living with an Ostomy," pages 342–43.) Postoperative support groups are helpful in adjusting to this change. (See Chapters 13, "Your Support Network"; 28, "Managing Disabilities and Limitations"; and 29, "Body Image and Self-Esteem.")

After treatment, your physician may suggest a variety of follow-up tests, including periodic sigmoidoscopy, colonoscopy, barium enema, and a blood test for the tumor marker CEA (carcinoembryonic antigen; see page 64) at prescribed intervals. Which tests should be done at which times is a controversial subject. Many doctors individualize their follow-up plan, depending on their patients' general health, extent of disease, and treatment needs.

Ask About

Many chemotherapy regimens are currently under investigation for both adjuvant therapy and palliative therapies for colorectal cancer. Current attention focuses on using various chemotherapy agents and on biological response modifiers in combination with the standard agent, fluorouracil (5-FU). If you have stage II, III, or IV colorectal cancer, you may want to discuss with your doctor the possibility of participating in a clinical trial (see Chapter 21, "Investigational Treatments"). Adjuvant chemotherapy has been beneficial in extending disease-free survival time for a number of people with these cancers. Radiation therapy has shown improvement in achieving local control of rectal cancer. Various combinations of radiation therapy are also under investigation, including radiation therapy in combination with pre- or postoperative chemotherapy.

LIVER

The liver is one of the largest organs of the body and serves the vital function of filtering all the circulating blood. Wayward cancer cells adrift in the bloodstream are likely to end up in one of the liver's thousands of blood-straining lobules, making this organ one of the most frequent sites of metastatic cancer. However, *primary* liver cancer (that is, cancer that originates in the liver) is very rare in the United States, accounting for less than 2 percent of all cancers. It occurs much more frequently in some parts of Asia. This section will discuss primary liver cancer only, though many aspects of the disease are the same in secondary, or metastatic, liver cancer.

The liver is a 3-pound, dark-red gland that resembles a rounded mound. It is tucked just beneath the diaphragm and heart, fills the upper right side of the abdomen, and is protected by the rib cage.

The liver consists of thousands of tiny blood-filtering lobes that together form two major lobes—the right and left lobes—each of which consists of several segments. On the underside of the liver are the major blood vessels that supply the organ, including the portal vein and the hepatic artery, the lymphatic vessels, the ducts that carry bile, and the gallbladder that stores it.

In addition to its filtering functions, the liver produces bile, cholesterol, digestive enzymes, and complex proteins; it detoxifies harmful chemicals and alcohol; and it stores vitamins A and D.

The liver has an amazing ability to regenerate: Up to 80 percent of the liver can be removed without adverse consequences. The organ will begin to regenerate within a few days and can completely replace its original volume within a period of months to a year.

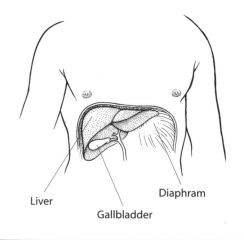

Liver

Gallbladder

Diaphram

A primary cancer of the liver most often occurs in a person whose liver is damaged and "cirrhotic" because of chronic infection, particularly chronic hepatitis B and hepatitis C infections; alcoholism; or, rarely, exposure to cancer-producing substances. It has been linked also to estrogen-like hormones in birth control pills and anabolic steroids that are sometimes taken by athletes. Finally, a number of chemical compounds are believed to play a role in causing liver cancer, the most common one being aflatoxin, a mold found in nuts, grains, or foods grown in contaminated soils. An extremely rare type of liver cancer is associated with exposure to polyvinyl chloride (PVCs) and other industrial toxins.

Who Is at Risk?

- People with a history of chronic liver disease, particularly cirrhosis that results from chronic hepatitis B or C infections or alcoholism;

- Workers exposed to industrial chemicals such as vinyl chloride, used in plastics manufacturing;

- People who have ingested plant toxins, such as aflatoxin;

- People in late middle age or older;

- People who have taken anabolic steroids, Throtrast (an x-ray contrast agent that has now been discontinued), and immunosuppressive agents;

- People with nutritional deficiencies, or hemochromatosis (excessive iron deposits in the body's tissues);

- Workers exposed to pesticides, chlorinated hydrocarbons, aromatic amines, and chlorophenols.

Screening Tests

No tests are done routinely in the U.S.

Types of Liver Cancer

Approximately 75 percent of all primary liver cancers are the *hepatocellular carcinomas* (*HCC*), which originate from *parenchymal* cells, the cells that perform most of the blood-filtering functions. HCC varies from small to large, solitary nodular masses (though there are sometimes more than one) that invade the adjacent diaphragm and gallbladder or the stomach. They tend to be soft and occasionally may rupture into the abdominal cavity. Cells that enter the major veins draining the liver can lead to metastatic cancer in other parts of the body. One rare subtype of HCC is *fibrolamellar*, which in contrast to the others is fibrous and slow growing, and thus more responsive to treatment and therefore more curable. It occurs more often in young women.

Seven percent of primary liver cancers actually begin in the bile duct cells within the liver (*cholangiocarcinomas*) rather than in the liver cells. The remaining cases—and more rare ones—are categorized as angiosarcomas, hepatoblastomas, and sarcomas, all diagnoses being based on the appearance of the tumor cells when viewed through the microscope. Hepatoblastoma is a highly curable form of liver cancer that occurs in children.

Primary liver cancer spreads most often to the regional, or local, lymph nodes; the lungs; bones; adrenal glands; or brain.

Signs and Symptoms

Symptoms of primary liver cancer, which are vague and are usually produced by an enlarging abdominal mass, resemble those of benign liver tumors, such as adenomas. Abdominal bulging and discomfort are common with both benign and malignant liver tumors.

- Weakness;

- Discomfort on right side of upper abdomen;

- A lump below the ribs on the right side;

- Pain around the right shoulder blade;

- Lack of appetite;

- Abdominal swelling;

- Generalized abdominal pain;

- Bloated feeling;

- Unexplained fever and nausea;

- Weight loss;

- Jaundice, or yellowing of the skin;

- Ascites, accumulation of fluid in the abdomen.

Diagnostic and Staging Tests

For more information regarding these tests, see Chapter 8, "Diagnostic Tests."

- History and physical examination;

- X-rays of chest and abdomen;

- Liver function tests;

- AFP (alpha-fetoprotein) blood test (blood levels of AFP are elevated in 50 to 70 percent of those with HCC);

- CT or MRI scan;

- Ultrasound;

- Angiography;

- *Percutaneous* (meaning "through the skin") needle biopsy or open biopsy (if it is suspected that the tumor is richly supplied with blood, needle biopsy can cause hemorrhage).

Tests Unique to Liver Cancer

- Liver imaging.

Staging

- Stage I liver cancer involves a solitary tumor less than 2 centimeters at its greatest dimension without evidence of growth into adjacent blood vessels.

- Stage II may be the same as stage I but with some variations: the tumor of 2 centimeters or less may have growth into blood vessels; the tumor may be larger than 2 centimeters but without a lot of blood vessel involvement; or there may be several tumors that are 2 centimeters or smaller, without invasion of blood vessels and confined to one of the two major lobes.

- A stage III tumor may be larger and invade the blood vessels. Or there may be several tumors with or without blood vessel invasion. They are, however, limited to one lobe. Regional lymph node involvement is possible but not necessary.

- Stage IVA indicates multiple tumors in more than one lobe of the liver, or involvement of the major branches of the main veins entering or leaving the liver.

- Stage IVB denotes any tumor with distant metastasis, usually to the lungs and/or bone.

Treatment

For treatment purposes, tumors are classified as localized and resectable, meaning the cancer is found in one place and can be removed; localized unresectable, indicating the cancer is in one area but cannot safely be totally excised; advanced, meaning the cancer has spread through the liver and/or to other parts of the body; and recurrent, indicating that the treated cancer has returned to the liver or another part of the body.

Localized Resectable Tumor

Excising the tumor and a margin of healthy tissue surrounding it is the treatment of choice for localized liver cancer. Typically, at least one segment (*partial hepatectomy*) or one lobe (*lobectomy*) of the liver is removed. A *trisegmental resection* involves removal of one lobe and a segment of another lobe. This comprises 75 to 80 percent of the liver. The extent of the resection depends on the size and location of the liver cancer. Liver function tests done before surgery are important in assessing the organ's ability to tolerate the operation. Unfortunately, surgery for people with chronic hepatitis or cirrhosis is a high-risk operation because of the limited function of liver remaining after resection (see Chapter 15, "Surgery").

Localized Unresectable Tumor

Although localized unresectable liver cancer is confined to the liver, it is not anatomically possible to remove the entire tumor by standard resections that leave some functioning liver tissue behind.

Although there is no standard therapy for unresectable disease, systemic or regional chemotherapy (see Chapter 17, "Chemotherapy"), external radiation therapy (see Chapter 16, "Radiation"), and chemotherapy combined with other agents or modalities (see Chapter 20, "Combination Treatments"), and radiolabeled antibodies (see "Ask About," later) have achieved remission.

Combination chemotherapy is commonly used, by administering fluorouracil (5-FU) with one of several drugs: carmustine (BiCNU), doxorubicin (Adriamycin), mitomycin (Muta-mycin), streptozocin (Zanosar), or methyl-CCNU.

Some people who are in good health except for their unresectable cancer may be candidates for total removal of the liver with liver transplantation. However, many oncologists and surgeons question the advisability of this approach, except for fibrolamellar cancer.

Advanced Metastatic Hepatoma

No standard therapy is currently being prescribed for advanced metastatic hepatoma, but several different approaches may alleviate symptoms and slow the progress of the disease.

Survival

For localized, resectable cancer (see "Treatment" for an explanation of these categories), the five-year survival rate is 10 to 30 percent. Those with the relatively rare fibrolamellar type of HCC are the most likely to be completely cured by surgery. For localized unresectable cancer, the five-year survival rate is less than 1 percent. When liver cancer is advanced, the average survival time is two to four months.

Special Needs

Toxicity from chemotherapy may be managed with antinausea medication. Those few individuals who have received a liver transplant will be given immunosuppressants to fight rejection of the new liver. As with all transplant surgery, convalescence after the surgery takes time and entails skilled care and monitoring.

Ask About

If you have unresectable liver cancer, it may be helpful to speak to your oncologist about entering a clinical trial (see Chapter 21, "Investigational Treatments"). Many new therapies and adjuvant treatments are under investigation. Most involve chemotherapy and radiation therapy and different methods of delivering drugs or radiation directly to the liver.

Several new therapies take advantage of the fact that liver tumors get their blood supply mainly from the hepatic artery. The infusion of various drugs through special catheters placed in the liver allows high concentrations of drugs to reach the cancer. There are many techniques for accomplishing this, and for reducing the dosage of the drug to the rest of the body. The optimal use and effectiveness of this approach is still not established.

Tumor shrinkage and symptom relief have been demonstrated with chemoembolization, in which chemotherapeutic agents are injected into the liver's main artery along with substances that block or slow blood flow. This gives the drugs more time to kill the cancer cells and prevents the cells from receiving oxygen via the hepatic artery. A risk with this approach or any infusion therapy is interruption of the blood supply to the organ. Liver function tests and evaluation for any clots in the major inflow vein, the portal vein, are essential to the pretreatment planning for this therapy.

Another treatment renders liver tumors more susceptible to radiation by infusing radiosensitizers through the hepatic artery. Using special radiologic techniques, the zone of the liver containing the tumor can be more safely irradiated with high doses.

GALLBLADDER AND BILE DUCTS

Gallbladder and bile duct cancers are rare, and together make up only 2 to 3 percent of all cancers. Gallbladder cancers account for two-thirds of these cancers; bile duct cancers are responsible for the rest. An early diagnosis, which is rare, is usually made when the organ is removed because of gallstones.

The causes of gallbladder cancer remain unknown, although 70 to 90 percent of those with the disease have a history of gallstones. Either the gallstones themselves or the irritation, infection, or metabolic changes they cause may be a major factor. (Despite this strong link, most people with gallstones will not develop gallbladder cancer.)

The causes of bile duct cancer are unknown, but exposure to environmental or industrial toxins and infection by certain parasites have been associated with the disease. There also appears to be an association with a chronic inflammatory condition of the colon and rectum known as *colitis*. Other disorders, such as hepatic fibrosis, polycystic disease, and chronic blockage of the bile duct, have been linked to this cancer too.

The *gallbladder* and *bile duct* are part of the body's *biliary system*, a group of organs that store digestive juices from the liver and transport them to the upper small intestine. The gallbladder is a pear-shaped pouch that joins to the bile duct at its neck, or upper end. It lies just under the liver in the upper abdomen and empties its contents into the small intestine in response to the stomach filling with food. The gallbladder stores and transports *bile*, a substance made in the liver that aids fat digestion.

The *common bile duct* connects the gallbladder and the liver and carries bile to the *duodenum*, or upper part of the small intestine, passing through a part of the pancreas. As the common bile duct proceeds toward the liver, it divides into a right and left bile duct and then further divides within the liver. For purposes of treatment, the common bile duct outside the liver is often divided into three sections: the upper third, the middle third, and the lower third.

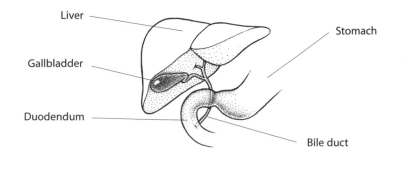

Liver

Stomach

Gallbladder

Duodendum

Bile duct

Who Is at Risk?

- People age 60 to 70;

- People with a history of gallstones;

- Women, who are three times more likely than men to get gallbladder cancer.

Screening Tests

No tests are available.

Types of Gallbladder and Bile Duct Cancer

Gallbladder Cancer

Most gallbladder and bile duct cancers are *adenocarcinomas*, which originate in the *mucosa*, the innermost layer of the organ. Most of those are the *scirrhous*, or hard, type. The *papillary* type is a small, nipplelike projection and is less common.

Spread to the lymph nodes of the bile duct occurs relatively early. From the nodes, the cancer typically spreads to the nodes of the pancreas and small intestine. Involvement of the lymph nodes may occur as the cancer invades the gallbladder bed, the surface of the liver on which the gallbladder rests. In about half of those with gallbladder cancer, tumors extend to the liver.

Bile Duct Cancer

Cholangiocarcinoma, or bile duct cancer, is classified as papillary, nodular, or diffuse types. The *papillary* type appears most often in the lower third of the bile duct and has the best prognosis. A *nodular* bile duct tumor is a mass occurring most commonly in the middle and upper third of the bile duct. The *diffuse* type is a thickening of the duct wall over an extensive area, often intruding into the bile duct channel, blocking the flow of bile. The resulting buildup of *bilirubin*, a derivative of bile, in the blood leads to *jaundice*, a yellowing of the skin, often the first noticeable sign of the cancer.

Signs and Symptoms

A tumor of the gallbladder may be "silent" for a long time, meaning that it doesn't prompt any signs or symptoms that would cause a person to see a doctor until the cancer reaches an advanced stage. Even when symptoms do appear, they may mimic those of other conditions, including other cancers. Consequently, unless this cancer is discovered accidentally (for example, after surgery to remove gallstones), it is usually not diagnosed until it is in an advanced stage.

Bile duct cancer is more likely to be discovered earlier than gallbladder cancer, because a blocked duct obstructs the flow of bile and causes jaundice. Bile duct cancer may involve surrounding structures by the time it is discovered, however.

- Jaundice;

- A lump in upper right part of the abdomen;

- Fever;

- Nausea;

- Weight loss;

- Upper abdominal discomfort;

- Itching;

- Abdominal swelling;

- Dark-colored urine.

Diagnostic and Staging Tests

For more details regarding these tests, see Chapter 8, "Diagnostic Tests."

- Blood tests, including a complete blood count and liver function tests;

- Ultrasound;

- Needle biopsy in some cases;

- CT scan;

- *Endoscopic retrograde cholangiopancreatography* (ERCP). An endoscope is inserted into the mouth and is passed through the upper gastrointestinal tract to the entrance of the bile duct in the small intestine. Then a catheter is threaded through the endoscope, and a dye is infused into the bile duct to outline the duct system and the gallbladder on a series of x-rays. This test will reveal if the gallbladder is filling properly or whether a stone or a tumor is blocking the main bile duct.

Tests Unique to Gallbladder and Bile Duct Cancer

- *Percutaneous transhepatic cholangiogram.* An x-ray of the bile duct system is taken following injection of a contrast dye into these ducts through a needle inserted directly into the liver. Using x-ray guidance, the doctor inserts the needle through the skin and soft tissues over the liver and into the portion of the duct system that is within the liver.

Staging

- Stage 0 gallbladder carcinoma is a small tumor on the surface of the lining, also called carcinoma in situ.

- Stage I cancer refers to tumors that have invaded either the mucosal lining or the muscle layer but that have not spread to lymph nodes or metastasized. This type of tumor often goes undiscovered even by the surgeon performing gallbladder removal; the pathologist may discover the cancer during laboratory analysis of tissues from the removed organ.

- Stage II gallbladder cancer indicates a tumor that has invaded beyond the muscle layer to the connective tissue but that has not gone through the outer layer, the serosa, or extended into the liver.

- Stage III is characterized by a tumor of any size that has gone through the outer layer (serosa), spread to lymph nodes near the liver, and/or invaded an adjacent organ.

- Stage IV cancer indicates that cells have spread to both the nearby and distant lymph nodes and/or the tumor itself has

extended more than 2 centimeters into the liver or to two or more adjacent organs, such as the stomach, colon, pancreas, or small intestine. There may be distant sites of metastasis as well.

Bile Duct Cancer

- Stage 0 is carcinoma in situ (see earlier).

- Stage I describes a tumor that has invaded the mucosal lining or the muscle layer.

- Stage II is a tumor that has extended as far as the connective tissue that surrounds the bile duct.

- Stage III is a tumor that may extend to the connective tissue but that has spread to the local lymph nodes.

- Stage IV indicates lymph nodes are involved and there is distant metastasis or the tumor has invaded adjacent structures.

Treatment

Gallbladder Cancer

Gallbladder cancers are grouped into three categories for purposes of treatment: localized, unresectable, and recurrent. Removal of the gallbladder (*cholecystectomy*) may be the only treatment required if the cancer is found in stage I or II and is confined to the mucosa or muscle layer (see Chapter 15, "Surgery"). In stage II cases, an *extended* cholecystectomy, which includes removal of adjacent portions of the liver and nearby lymph tissue, is usually performed.

Tumors classified as stage III or higher are usually not resectable, because the cancer has spread to lymph nodes and/or adjacent organs. A person may be suitable for surgical removal of the cancer and the involved tissues, but operative treatment is aimed at symptom relief. Often the bile ducts are blocked by the tumor, which causes considerable discomfort in the form of itching or other symptoms of liver dysfunction. This procedure can be accomplished with ERCP (see "Diagnostic and Staging Tests" above).

Palliative surgery—usually an operation called a bypass—is performed to relieve bile duct obstruction. A tube or shunt is inserted between the upper portion of the bile duct (above the obstruction) and the intestine, allowing the bile to drain into the intestine.

Standard chemotherapy usually is not beneficial in advanced cases of gallbladder cancer, although several combination therapies are currently under investigation (see "Ask About" later and Chapter 17, "Chemotherapy").

Local radiation therapy may temporarily diminish the size of the tumor and relieve some symptoms, but it is of limited value (see Chapter 16, "Radiation").

Bile Duct Cancer

The location of the tumor is key when the oncologist plans treatment. Tumors in the upper third of the bile duct are resectable approximately 20 percent of the time. Surgery may involve removing a portion of the liver as well. However, if surgical margins free of tumor cannot be achieved because of the extent of local tumor growth, surgery may be performed to relieve symptoms by removing or bypassing the obstruction. In some instances this approach will allow for postoperative brachytherapy, a treatment that delivers radiation internally through tubes placed into the tumor area.

Tumors in the lower third of the bile duct are close to, or involve, the pancreas, and removal then includes removal of the head of the pancreas, as with pancreatic cancer (see Chapter 16, "Radiation," "Ask About," later, and "Pancreas" in the Encyclopedia).

When tumors are localized but not removable with surgery, as in stage I or II, radiation therapy may slow the tumor growth and produce some benefit.

Adjuvant chemotherapy with fluorouracil (5-FU) and doxorubicin (Adriamycin) may be successful in increasing survival time for people with advanced disease.

Survival

When a previously unsuspected gallbladder or bile duct cancer is discovered during the course of another surgery and the cancer is localized, the five-year survival rate is 80 percent. If the cancer is not resectable because it has spread to the lymph nodes and/or the liver, the five-year survival rate is less than 5 percent.

Special Needs

After the gallbladder is removed, no special medications or diets are necessary. Digestion of fats is not a problem.

If the pancreas has been removed, as with distal bile duct cancer, pancreatic enzymes may be needed to assist in digestion and fat absorption.

Ask About

Because the possibility of cure is slight when the disease has spread beyond the gallbladder and/or the bile duct itself or has recurred, you may want to discuss with your oncologist one of the many clinical trials available for people with these cancers. For example, there has been some success in extending survival time using various combinations of chemotherapy agents or radiation therapy. One form of radiation therapy being investigated is brachytherapy (see Chapter 16, "Radiation"), which allows high doses of radiation to be targeted directly to this area. Drugs that sensitize cells to radiation or heat, which is also a radiosensitizer, are under study.

LUNG

Lung cancer is the second most common cancer, accounting for about one out of five malignancies in men and one out of nine in women. Unfortunately, what those statistics don't reflect is the current reality: Over the past several years, while the incidence of lung cancer has gradually declined in men, it has been rising alarmingly in women. In 1940 only seven women in 100,000 developed the disease; today the rate is 42 in 100,000. And all the evidence points to smoking as the cause. Smokers are about nine times more likely to develop lung cancer than nonsmokers. And as one specialist in the field reports, "How long it takes to get cancer depends on how many cigarettes you smoke a day." The good news is that quitting smoking does lower the risk.

There are two major types of lung cancer: small cell lung cancer (SCLC)—which is also called *oat cell* cancer, because the cells resemble oat grains—and nonsmall cell lung cancer (NSCLC). The aggressiveness of the disease and, therefore, certain treatment decisions, depend on the type of tumor you have. Because many types of lung cancer grow quickly and spread rapidly and because the lungs are vital organs, early detection and prompt treatment—usually surgery to remove the tumor—are critical.

The *lungs*, comprising the major organ of the respiratory system, are divided into sections, or *lobes*. The right lung has three lobes and is slightly larger than the left lung, which has two lobes.

The *mediastinum* separates the lungs. It is the area that contains the heart, trachea, esophagus, and many lymph nodes. The lungs are covered by a protective membrane, the *pleura*, and are separated from the abdominal cavity by the muscular *diaphragm*.

With each inhalation, air is pulled through the windpipe (*trachea*) and the branching passageways of the lungs (the *bronchi*), filling thousands of tiny air sacs (*alveoli*) at the ends of the bronchi. These sacs, which resemble bunches of grapes, are surrounded by small blood vessels (*capillaries*). Molecules of oxygen pass through the thin membranes of the alveoli and into the bloodstream. The red blood cells pick up the oxygen molecules and carry them to the body's organs and tissues.

As the blood cells release the oxygen they pick up carbon dioxide, a waste product of metabolism. They carry the carbon dioxide back to the lungs and release it into the alveoli. With each exhalation, carbon dioxide is expelled from the bronchi out through the trachea.

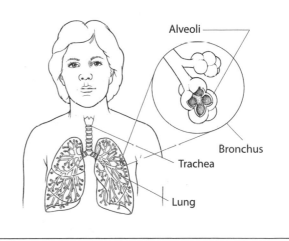

Alveoli

Bronchus

Trachea

Lung

Who Is at Risk?

- Men between 60 and 65 and women about 70;

- Men who smoke, who have a risk of developing lung cancer that is 10 to 17 times higher than that of those who do not smoke; women who smoke, who have a risk that is five to 10 times higher than that of women who do not smoke (the risk increases with the number of cigarettes smoked per day and the number of years the person has smoked; some evidence suggests, however, that women and African-American men are more vulnerable);

- People who do not smoke but who are exposed to smoke in the environment (known as *second-hand, passive,* or *involuntary smoking*), whose risk is as much as 30 percent higher than that of those unexposed to second-hand smoke (the risk is even higher for exposure to *side stream* smoke [from the smoldering end of a cigarette] than for *mainstream* smoke [smoke that has been exhaled by the smoker]);

- Asbestos workers, who have a six- to sevenfold greater risk of death from lung cancer compared to the general population;

- Those exposed to other industrial and atmospheric pollutants, which are responsible for a small percentage of lung cancer.

Screening Tests

There is no routine screening test for lung cancer. Detection at an early stage is possible with an x-ray or sputum analysis; therefore, some doctors order these tests, especially for people who smoke. However, there is no evidence that such attempts at lung cancer screening have a positive impact on treatment or survival. Nevertheless, if a doctor suspects lung cancer, an x-ray is the first step in diagnosis.

Types of Lung Cancer

The information in this section pertains only to *primary* lung cancer, not to *secondary,* or metastatic, cancer that has spread to the lung from another primary site.

Lung cancer often develops at more than one site, but regardless of where it begins, tumor cells spread to nearby lymph nodes in a predictable pattern. Doctors can often determine how advanced the cancer is based on which lymph nodes are involved. Typically, the lymph nodes in the *hilus*, that portion of the lobe nearest the mediastinum, are affected first. From there the cancer may spread to the nodes in the mediastinum and then to the nodes in the neck and/or the abdominal cavity. If the tumor cells enter the bloodstream, they migrate to the liver, other sections of the lung, brain, bone, and/or bone marrow.

Nonsmall Cell Lung Cancer (NSCLC)

Most lung cancers are grouped together as *nonsmall cell lung cancer* (NSCLC). About half of them are *squamous cell carcinomas*. This type of lung cancer, which is sometimes called *epidermoid carcinoma*, usually occurs in men and arises in the lining of the large air passageways, or *bronchi*. Another common type of NSCLC is *adenocarcinoma*, which occurs at the outer edges of the lung. A small percentage of NSCLC are *large-cell carcinomas*, which usually develop in the smaller bronchi. Nonsmall cell lung cancer that begins at the top of the lung sometimes spreads to the nerves and blood vessels leading to the arm.

The three subtypes of NSCLC develop differently. The treatment possibilities your oncologist may discuss are often based on the location of these particular cancers and their rate of spread:

- Squamous cell or epidermoid carcinomas usually occur in the bronchi in the center of the lungs, but about a third of them arise on the periphery. This type of NSCLC is more likely to cause ulcers in the bronchi and bleeding than the other forms. Typically, the cancer cells double every 180 days. Although it often invades nearby tissue, squamous cell carcinoma is less likely to metastasize early than other types.

- Most adenocarcinomas begin in the middle of the lungs; but about 25 percent develop along the lung periphery. These tumors are small, and the cells double about every 180 days. They are likely to metastasize early. The form known as *bronchoalveolar* adenocarcinoma develops in the alveoli and may spread through the airways to other parts of the lung.

- Large cell carcinomas are large, bulky tumors that can arise anywhere within the lung but usually develop on the organ's periphery. The cells double about every 100 days and can invade the mediastinum or the central nervous system early in the course of the disease.

Small Cell Lung Cancer (SCLC)

About one in four malignancies involving the lungs are *small cell lung cancer* (SCLC). There are several types of SCLC or oat cell cancer, including a mix of small cell and other cell types. These cancers grow more rapidly—doubling in cell number about every 30 days—and spread more quickly to lymph nodes and other organs than the nonsmall cell type.

Signs and Symptoms

In many cases symptoms do not appear until the cancer is quite advanced. However, by the time a tumor does cause changes within the lungs, the signs include:

- Difficulty breathing—*stridor* (a harsh sound with each breath), wheezing, labored breathing, shortness of breath;
- Coughing, possibly with blood in sputum;
- Recurring pneumonia or bronchitis;
- Chest, shoulder, or arm pain;
- Loss of appetite;
- Weight loss;
- Bone pain;
- Hoarseness;
- Headaches or seizures;
- Swelling of the face or neck;
- Fatigue.

Diagnostic and Staging Tests

For more details on these tests, see Chapter 8, "Diagnostic Tests."

- Physical examination to detect swollen lymph nodes in the neck or in the region above the collarbones, to determine if the liver is enlarged and/or if any abdominal mass is present;
- Chest examination to reveal breath sounds that are less loud than normal, abnormal breathing noises, or dull sounds when the doctor taps on the chest;
- Needle aspiration of mass in the chest, often involving a CT scan to help guide the needle to the tumor;
- Chest x-rays;
- CT or MRI scans of chest, brain, bone, and abdomen;
- Biopsies of chest lining, lymph nodes, bone, or liver.

Tests Unique to Lung Cancer

- *Microscopic examination*: Sputum or fluid is obtained by needle biopsy (sputum analysis will not reveal abnormal cells if the tumor is on the periphery);
- *Fiber-optic bronchoscopy*: A flexible endoscope is inserted into lungs to see the bronchi and obtain a tissue sample for biopsy. Bronchoscopy is used in all cases involving centrally located tumors and in some cases of peripheral tumors. The test involves mild sedation, which some doctors are equipped to do in their offices.
- *Mediastinoscopy with biopsies*: An endoscope is inserted into the mediastinum through an incision in the neck or chest; a sample of tissue can be obtained for analysis.
- *Thoracotomy*: Small incisions are made in the chest to allow insertion of a miniature video camera and instruments for biopsy. General anesthesia is necessary.

Staging

Nonsmall Cell Lung Cancer

- *Occult* cancer means that cancerous cells are discovered in the sputum but that no tumor can be found in the lung.

- Stage 0, also called carcinoma in situ, describes cancer confined to a local area that has not grown through the top lining of the lung and is incapable of spreading.

- Stage I indicates a tumor of any size that is confined to the lung; T1 tumors are 3 centimeters at their largest dimension; T2 tumors are larger than 3 centimeters or invade nearby tissues regardless of size.

- Stage II indicates a tumor of any size that has spread to lymph nodes in certain regions of the lung: the *hilar* region (the center of the lungs where the blood vessels and nerves enter) or the *peribronchial* nodes (those near the bronchi).

- Stage IIIA refers to any size tumor that has spread to lymph nodes in the mediastinum or near the trachea. Also, regardless of whether lymph nodes are involved, this stage includes any size of tumor that invades other areas adjacent to the lung that can be removed surgically, including the chest wall, the diaphragm, the membrane surrounding the heart (the *pericardium*); or a tumor that obstructs or causes compression (*atelectasis*) of the lung.

- Stage IIIB includes a tumor of any size that has spread to lymph nodes on the opposite lung or to nodes above the collarbone, or a tumor that has invaded a structure that cannot be removed, such as the heart, trachea, esophagus, vertebra, regardless of the extent of lymph node involvement.

- Stage IV refers to lung cancer that has metastasized to a distant location, such as liver or brain, regardless of tumor size or lymph node involvement.

Small Cell Lung Cancer

Instead of the TNM type of staging, SCLCs are often described as either *limited* or *extensive*.

- Limited tumors involve one lung, the mediastinum, and lymph nodes that can be encompassed by a single radiation therapy treatment.

- Extensive tumors (equivalent to stage IV disease, described later) are those that have spread beyond these sites. About one in three people with SCLC have limited disease at the time of their diagnosis.

Treatment

Lung cancer is treated with surgery, radiation therapy, chemotherapy, or some combination of these. However, treatment decisions are always influenced by the type of cancer present (see Chapter 14, "Principles of Treatment").

Nonsmall Cell Lung Cancer

In a very few cases, doctors detect NSCLC before it even shows up on x-ray (occult or stage 0 cancer). Surgery at this stage usually results in complete cure without risk of recurrence of that cancer, although almost half of these patients later develop a new primary cancer elsewhere in the lung.

About one-third of people with lung cancer are diagnosed with early stage I or II disease, when surgery can remove the tumor. A *wedge resection* involves removal of a small part of the lobe containing the tumor. Removing a whole section, or lobe, is called *lobectomy*, and removal of the entire lung is a *pneumonectomy* (see Chapter 15, "Surgery").

If surgery is impossible (for example, in elderly people or those with heart disease, or who for some other reason cannot tolerate an operation), radiation therapy alone can sometimes cure an early-stage cancer (see Chapter 16, "Radiation").

Often people with stage II NSCLC receive both surgery and radiation therapy (see Chapter 20, "Combination Therapy"). Many also enter clinical trials testing adjuvant chemotherapy following surgery (see "Ask About," later).

In most cases, however, the disease is advanced by the time of diagnosis, and surgery is not curative. A few people with stage IIIA disease receive surgery alone. Some receive surgery plus radiation therapy, but most receive only radiation therapy or radiation therapy plus chemotherapy. A recent study found that people who received up to three cycles of chemotherapy before surgery for stage IIIA lung cancer, and another cycle after it, survived up to six times as long as those who received surgery alone. Those with stage IIIB disease cannot be treated successfully by surgery and receive radiation therapy alone.

Stage IV lung cancer involves metastasis to other organs or tissues. Doctors recommend chemotherapy for people who are otherwise functioning well. Radiation therapy may relieve local symptoms and improve quality of life.

Small Cell Lung Cancer

In cases of limited (stages I to IIIB) disease, radiation therapy plus chemotherapy with a combination of several agents are usually recommended. If both methods are used at the same time, your oncologist may avoid prescribing drugs whose side effects get worse with radiation, such as doxorubicin (Adriamycin). Since SCLC spreads so quickly, surgery is often ineffective in controlling the disease.

Chemotherapy. Chemotherapy is the cornerstone of managing SCLC, because it unequivocally improves survival time (see Chapter 17, "Chemotherapy"). Many drugs are available, including carboplatin (Paraplatin), cisplatin (Platinol), cyclophosphamide (Cytoxan), doxorubicin (Adriamycin), etoposide (VePesid), and vincristine (Oncovin). Some of the combinations commonly used include ACE (doxorubicin [Adriamycin], cyclophosphamide [Cytoxan], etoposide [VePesid]), PACE (ACE plus cisplatin [Platinol]), CAV (cyclophosphamide [Cytoxan], doxorubicin [Adriamycin], and vincristine [Oncovin]), and EP (etoposide [VePesid] and cisplatin [Platinol]). Studies do not yet indicate whether any particular combination is significantly better than another. The EP combination is often the choice if the person is also receiving radiation therapy. People usually receive a combination of drugs simultaneously in high doses at frequent intervals (every three to four weeks). Usually combination chemotherapy lasts no more than four to six months. (Twelve to 24 months of treatment does not appear to improve the outcome.) *Partial response* (that is, at least some shrinkage of tumor) occurs in up to 90 percent of people with limited SCLC and 50 to 70 percent of those with extensive disease. *Complete response* rates (disappearance of tumors) can be as high as 50 percent in cases of limited disease, and 20 percent in extensive disease. To reduce the risk of toxicity, elderly people with SCLC often receive less intense therapy; the complete response rate is 17 percent, and the overall response rate (complete or partial response) can be as high as 79 percent.

Regardless of the response to chemotherapy, nine out of 10 people with SCLC will experience recurrence of their disease within two to three years. In most cases the recurrent tumors are highly drug resistant.

Radiation Therapy. People with limited SCLC may receive radiation therapy to the tumor and the nodes in the mediastinum, and in some cases to the nodes above the collarbone. Radiation oncologists also recommend therapy to prevent local recurrence of the tumor.

About 10 percent of people with SCLC have brain metastases at the time of diagnosis, and the chance of developing brain metastasis is as high as 80 percent within two years. As a preventive measure, some oncologists recommend prophylactic radiation therapy directly to the brain, but only if there has been a complete response to other treatment.

Surgery. Because SCLC is such a rapidly growing tumor and there is a high probability that cancer has spread by the time it is diagnosed, the effectiveness of surgery is questionable. Your oncologist may recommend surgery only if your lungs are functioning well and if the tumor is confined either to its primary site or to the involved lung and the lymph nodes in the hilar region on the same side. One possibility to discuss is chemotherapy before surgery to shrink the tumor and then again after the operation.

Survival

Survival rates in people with NSCLC are as follows:

- Five-year survival rate for stage I cancer is 30 to 80 percent.

- Five-year survival rate for stage II cancer is 10 to 35 percent.

- Five-year survival rate for stage IIIA cancer is 10 to 15 percent.

- Five-year survival rate for stage IIIB cancer is less than 5 percent.

- Five-year survival rate for stage IV cancer is less than 5 percent.

Survival rates among those with SCLC are poor; 50 percent of people with limited disease who respond to treatment will live 14 months. The picture for extensive SCLC is even less encouraging. The two-year survival is only 2 percent. Even if the person responds well to treatment, the disease usually recurs, and survival is then only two or three months.

Special Needs

The risk of recurrence of lung cancer is very high. People with the disease need to see their physicians every three months for the first two years, then every six months for two more years, and yearly after that. In the first two years the person receives x-rays and blood tests usually every three or four months or more often if symptoms recur.

People with recurrent cancer need aggressive pain management to maintain the highest possible quality of life (see Chapters 23, "The Pain Challenge," and 24, "Pain Relief").

Ask About

If you have NSCLC, ask your oncologist about entering a clinical trial. Most experimental treatments (see Chapter 21, "Investigational Treatments") involve combinations of the standard treatments: surgery, radiation therapy, and chemotherapy. In some studies, radiation therapy, chemotherapy, or both are used before surgery to remove the tumor.

Because drug therapy is not yet considered a standard treatment of NSCLC, many clinical trials are attempting to determine how chemotherapy can best be used in most stages of this disease. Studies are under way to evaluate new chemotherapy drugs, such as paclitaxel (Taxol); higher doses of currently available drugs, which may involve bone marrow transplant or biological therapy with colony-stimulating factor; or new combinations of standard agents (see Chapters 18, "Biological Therapies," and 19, Bone Marrow Transplant").

Researchers are evaluating different methods of delivering radiation therapy. Studies are being conducted on *accelerated hyperfractionation*, the administration of smaller doses of radiation given more often than usual to increase its effectiveness. Another method being tested is *interdigitation*, which involves manipulating the scheduling of chemotherapy and radiation therapy.

Oncologists are evaluating using lasers in a variety of ways. *Photodynamic therapy* may be an option as an alternative to surgery to remove very-early-stage NSCLC. It involves administering a light-sensitive drug that is absorbed by the cancer cells. When a laser light, directed through a bronchoscope, strikes the tumor, it activates the drug in the cells and they die. Another experimental technique relies on using a laser to destroy a tumor that is blocking the airway.

Finally, if you have been treated for an early-stage lung cancer, you may want to volunteer for a chemoprevention trial where various methods are being tested to prevent a second cancer.

If you have SCLC, ask your oncologist about clinical trials involving new regimens of currently available chemotherapy drugs as well as new agents. Studies are also under way to evaluate surgery and/or radiation therapy combined with chemotherapy. Fractionation of radiation doses is also being tested to treat SCLC.

TESTES

Although cancer of the testes is rare, accounting for only about 1 percent of all cancers in men of all ages and about 5 percent of all male genitourinary system cancers, it is the most common cancer in men between the ages of 15 and 35, and the second most common malignancy in men 35 to 39. Fortunately, testicular cancer is often cured. The treatment success is due to effective diagnostic methods, including identification of tumor markers; effective combinations of chemotherapy drugs; and improved surgical techniques.

Cancer almost always occurs in one testis; about 2 to 3 percent occur in both testes either at the same time or successively. The cancer cells grow rapidly but are very susceptible to chemotherapy and radiation therapy.

Because the incidence of testicular cancer has risen markedly in the past 20 years, numerous studies are exploring possible environmental causes, including the mother's diet during her pregnancy and her use of diethylstilbestrol (DES) to prevent miscarriage. Research is also looking at the increasing presence of estrogen-mimicking pollutants in the environment. The most consistent occupational association has been the elevated rate among men in professional and white-collar occupations, which may be linked to an increased risk observed with lower levels of exercise.

Other possible causes are hereditary factors, genetic abnormalities, congenital defects in the reproductive tract, testicular injury, and atrophy of the testes. Such viral infections as mumps, which cause inflammation of the testes, have not been proved to cause cancer.

The two testicles are egg-shaped male reproductive glands. They hang outside the body in a pouch of loose skin called the *scrotum* below and behind the penis. In maturity, they are usually slightly smaller than golf balls. It is normal for one testicle to be larger than the other.

The testicles produce the hormone *testosterone* as well as *sperm*, the male reproductive cells.

Bladder
Seminal Vesicle
Prostate
Urethra
Penis
Testis
Scrotum

Who Is at Risk?

- Men with cryptorchidism, or undescended testes, which is the failure of one or both testicles to descend from the pelvis (about 10 percent of men with this cancer have a history of cryptorchidism);

- African-Americans (the rate among Caucasians is two-thirds as high);

- Men with a history of hernia;

- Men with extra nipples;

- Men with a history of infertility problems.

Screening Tests

- Monthly testicular self-examination (see Chapter 7, "Examining Yourself");

- Physical examination of the testicles by a physician during regular checkups (see Chapter 4, "The Cancer Checkup").

Types of Testicular Cancer

Ninety-five percent of testicular cancers arise from sperm-forming, or *germ*, cells and are called *germinal tumors*. (The remaining 5 percent are nongerminal tumors.) About 40 percent of germinal tumors are categorized as *seminomas*. Several other types of germinal tumors are referred to collectively as *nonseminomas*.

The distinctions are important because each type grows and spreads differently, which influences treatment.

Seminomas

Germ cells become malignant at a very early stage in their development. They may be *anaplastic, classic* (or typical), or *spermatocytic*, depending on their origin. Eighty-five percent of seminomas are of the classic type. They occur most often in men in their 40s. Anaplastic seminoma is more aggressive and is more likely to metastasize to other parts of the body. Spermatocytic seminoma usually occurs in men over 50. The rate of metastasis for this type of cancer is low.

Nonseminomas

Cells more mature and specialized than the germ cells give rise to nonseminomas. This type

of testicular cancer affects men in their mid-30s; the aggressiveness of the disease varies. Twenty to 25 percent of the tumors are *embryonal carcinomas*, which are aggressive tumors; 25 to 30 percent are *teratoma carcinomas*, which are also aggressive; *yolk-sac tumors*, or *choriocarcinomas*, are extremely rare (about 1 percent of testicular cancers); and some tumors include more than one cell type.

Testicular cancers tend to spread through the spermatic cord and associated blood and lymph vessels into local lymph glands called the *retroperitoneal lymph nodes*. Metastases of the right testis are more likely to affect the lymph nodes near the *aorta*, the major blood vessel supplying the heart, called the *para-aortic lymph nodes*. When metastases beyond the lymph nodes occur, they are most likely to arise in the lungs, liver, bone, or brain.

Signs and Symptoms

- A painless or, less commonly, uncomfortable lump or nodule on a testicle, testicular enlargement, or swelling of the testicles (occurs in more than 90 percent of cases);

- Sensation of heaviness or dragging in the lower abdomen or scrotum;

- Rarely, breast tenderness or enlargement due to high levels of a hormone called human chorionic gonadotropin (HCG) (see "Tests Unique to Testicular Cancer," later);

- Abdominal pain, cough, or bloody sputum if metastasis has occurred.

Diagnostic and Staging Tests

For more detailed information regarding these tests, see Chapter 8, "Diagnostic Tests."

- Ultrasonography;

- Lymphography;

- CT and/or MRI scans of the pelvis and abdomen to evaluate local lymph nodes;

- Urogram to assess further spread;

- Chest x-rays, bone scans, and other tests if metastasis is suspected.

Tests Unique to Testicular Cancer

Blood Tests

Measuring levels of various hormones in the blood may reveal the presence of testicular cancer. Elevations of alpha fetoprotein (AFP), human chorionic gonadotropin, and lactate dehydrogenase (LDH) are tumor markers. In particular, an excess of AFP indicates the presence of a nonseminoma because this protein in the blood rarely rises in seminomas. Monitoring of AFP may also be done to assess response to therapy.

Inguinal Biopsy

An incision is made in the groin at the skin fold where the thigh meets the torso in order to retrieve the suspect testicle. It is brought up and out of the scrotum through the groin and a small tissue sample is taken for biopsy. Depending on the pathology report, the testicle may be returned to the scrotum or surgically removed.

Transscrotal Biopsy

Cutting through the scrotum to obtain a sample of tissue is no longer recommended because of the risk of local spread of malignant cells if any are present.

Staging

- Stage I: Cancer is found only in one or both testicles.

- Stage II: Cancer has spread to abdominal lymph nodes.

- Stage III: Cancer has metastasized beyond the abdominal lymph nodes to distant sites, such as the lungs and liver.

Treatment

Testicular cancers of the seminoma type are very curable in the early stages. Later-stage seminomas and nonseminomas present greater treatment challenges.

Radical inguinal orchiectomy, surgical removal of the affected testicle, is the most common treatment for stage I seminomas (see Chapter 15, "Surgery"). Because seminomas at this stage are likely to recur, the practice of orchiectomy followed solely by surveillance is under study. In some cases, local lymph nodes also may be removed or treated with radiation therapy (see Chapters 16, "Radiation," and 20, "Combination Treatments").

In stage I nonseminomas, some or all the lymph nodes are almost always removed together with the affected testicle.

In stage II seminomas, called nonbulky, because lymph nodes cannot be felt in the abdomen and do not block the *ureters* (the tubes that carry urine from the kidney to the bladder), radical inguinal orchiectomy followed by radiation to the abdominal lymph nodes is often recommended. If the seminoma is very large, orchiectomy is likely to be followed by radiation therapy or systemic chemotherapy. However, some physicians suggest chemotherapy before surgery to reduce the tumor's size. Lymph nodes may also be removed.

In stage II nonseminomas, orchiectomy is likely to include removal of the lymph nodes and may involve subsequent chemotherapy.

Stage III seminomas are treated by orchiectomy followed by chemotherapy, whereas nonseminomas are more likely to be treated with chemotherapy first, followed by surgery to determine whether any cancer cells remain; if they are found, further chemotherapy will be necessary.

Whatever the stage, if malignant cells are found by ultrasonography in the second testicle, treatment may depend on the importance of maintaining fertility and potency. Some physicians recommend simultaneous removal of both testes. Others recommend radiation therapy for the less involved testicle and careful monitoring.

Chemotherapy may include one or more of the following: cisplatin (Platinol), vinblastine (Velban), bleomycin (Blenoxane), actinomycin, and cyclophosphamide (Cytoxan), or, rarely, etoposide (VePesid) or ifosfamide (IFEX) (see Chapter 17, "Chemotherapy").

Survival

Testicular cancer is a highly curable malignancy, especially for patients with seminoma, in which the cure rate exceeds 90 percent in all stages combined. Even situations with widespread metastases may be curable. After treatment:

- Five-year survival for stage I cancer limited to the testicle is greater than 95 percent.

- Five-year survival for stage II with cancerous invasion of the retroperitoneal or para-aortic lymph nodes also is greater than 95 percent. However, the risk of recurrence is increased if more than 5 nodes are involved, if one or more nodes is larger than 2 centimeters, or if there is metastasis beyond the nodes to surrounding fatty tissue.

- Five-year survival for stage III with the spread of cancer beyond the local lymph nodes is 75 percent.

Special Needs

If the chosen therapy poses any potential hazard to fertility and/or potency, men may wish to consider banking their sperm for future parenting before undergoing treatment. However, because those with testicular cancer may already have low sperm counts, it may be impossible to obtain adequate specimens.

After initial treatment of testicular cancer, careful follow-up is essential to detect recurrence or metastasis early. A chest x-ray and blood tests to check AFP and other tumor markers must be done monthly for the first year and at least every two months during the second year. In addition, a CT scan may be done periodically. Although late relapses do occur, most recurrences arise within two years. Therefore, continued screening at various intervals is important. If cancer recurs, chemotherapy will probably be recommended.

Those who have been treated for testicular cancer have about a 1 percent chance of developing cancer in the remaining testicle. Most commonly, this is a new disease rather than a metastasis from the first tumor.

See Chapter 29, "Body Image and Self-Esteem."

Ask About

If your doctor recommends radical retroperitoneal lymph node dissection (removal of the testis and lymph nodes in the area), the surgical method traditionally used in stage I and II cancers, you'll want to discuss the impact of the operation on your fertility. When both testes are removed or when nerve damage occurs, infertility always results because of retrograde ejaculation, so seminal emission during intercourse is reduced or absent. The procedure also can damage nerves required for penile erection and, therefore, result in impotence (see Chapter 30, "Sexuality"). However, some modifications of the surgery are being used to try to avoid nerve damage and preserve the ability to ejaculate.

You may want to consider participating in one of the clinical trials exploring the value of chemotherapy in stage II nonseminomas as a potentially more effective way of retaining fertility and potency than lymph node removal.

If you have a stage III seminoma, you might ask your oncologist about trials evaluating the benefits of radiation therapy in addition to surgery and chemotherapy. New chemotherapy drugs and doses combined with autologous bone marrow transplantation (see Chapter 19, "Bone Marrow Transplant") are being evaluated for treating nonseminomas and recurrent disease.

Clinical trials are exploring the value of chemotherapy in stage II nonseminomas as a potentially more effective way of retaining fertility and potency than lymph node removal (see Chapter 21, "Investigational Treatments").

If chemotherapy is recommended, you may want to discuss the choice of drug(s) or drug combination(s) carefully to compare side effects in the context of other health problems you may have or your parenting plans. Platinum-based treatments may impair fertility, although in 50 percent of cases it returns within three years of therapy.

PROSTATE

Prostate cancer is the second most frequently diagnosed cancer in American men, following only skin cancer. It is estimated that one of every seven African-Americans and one of every eight Caucasians develop the disease. Although prostate cancer is most common in men over 65, it has been diagnosed in men as young as 40.

Prostate cancer is the second most common cause of cancer death in American males and the leading cause of cancer death in males over 55. This high mortality rate may be the result of late detection, because studies show that 87 percent of men treated when their cancer is diagnosed early can expect to be alive in five years. Prostate cancer should not be confused with benign prostate hypertrophy (BPH), a gradual enlargement of the prostate gland that occurs in more than half of men over 45. BPH may cause the prostate to press on the urethra and bladder neck, leading to frequent urination or interference with urinary flow. BPH is not a malignant condition, but prostate cancer is present in about 38 percent of men who undergo surgery to relieve the symptoms caused by an enlarged prostate.

Because the annual incidence of prostate cancer has risen steadily during the past 60 years, epidemiologic studies suggest that environmental factors, such as a high-fat diet, play a role. Because the incidence increases with age, sex hormones and steroid hormones may also be important. (For example, some experts say that prolonged exposure to testosterone, the male hormone, is responsible.)

The prostate is a walnut-sized organ that is one of the accessory glands of the male reproductive system. Its two lobes contain from 30 to 50 glands surrounded by a capsule of fibrous tissue (the *prostatic capsule*). The prostate is located just above the rectum and attached to the neck of the bladder. It surrounds the *urethra,* the muscular tube in the penis that carries urine from the bladder out of the body.

The prostate secretes a slightly milky fluid that is a vehicle for semen ejaculated through the urethra during orgasm. The male hormone *testosterone* regulates the prostate's function.

Who Is at Risk?

- Men over 65;

- Men who eat a high-fat diet, particulary saturated fats;

- Men with a family history of prostate cancer (the risk doubles if a man's father had the disease, and if a brother had it, the risk triples; hereditary prostate cancer typically begins among a cluster of relatives before age 55);

- African-Americans, who have a higher incidence than do black men in Africa;

- Possibly, men exposed to such chemicals as cadmium.

Screening Tests

The following tests and examinations are recommended annually by the American Cancer Society for all men beginning at age 50. Men at higher risk, such as those with a family history of the disease or African-Americans, may start at a younger age.

- *Digital rectal examination (DRE).* The physician inserts a lubricated gloved finger into the rectum to feel the prostate gland. About 12 percent to 15 percent of malignancies arise in the periphery of the gland where they are palpable, but those that arise elsewhere within the gland usually escape detection by DRE (see Chapter 4, "The Cancer Checkup").

- *Prostate-specific antigen (PSA) blood test.* This test evaluates blood levels of a substance called prostate-specific antigen secreted only by the glands in the prostate. Although PSA can rise slightly in the presence of BPH, when the PSA is above 4 ng/ml (nanograms per milliliter of blood), there is a 35–40 percent chance that prostate cancer is present (see Chapter 8, "Diagnostic Tests").

Types of Prostate Cancer

Ninety-five percent of prostate cancers are adenocarcinomas that arise from glandular tissue. More rarely, cancer begins in the tissues surrounding the gland. These types include leiomyosarcoma and rhabdomyosarcoma.

Prostatic intraepithelial neoplasia (PIN) is an abnormal change in prostate cells that eventually become malignant.

Prostate carcinoma usually arises near the surface of the gland, where it may be felt by a doctor during a rectal examination (see "Screening Tests," above).

As the tumor grows, the prostate expands around the urethra and may cause urinary problems similar to BPH (see "Signs and Symptoms," below). By the time the tumor is large enough to cause symptoms, it has often spread beyond its capsule.

Prostate cancer may invade surrounding fat and tissue, the *seminal vesicles* (which carry sperm from the testicles to the urethra), and/or the neck of the bladder. It may invade lymph nodes in the pelvic region. Later, prostate cancer can spread to the bones, primarily those in the spine, hip, pelvis, and chest. Metastasis often occurs in the lungs, liver, and adrenal glands.

Signs and Symptoms

- Weak urinary stream;

- Frequent and/or urgent urination, especially at night;
- Difficulty starting or stopping the urinary stream;
- Incomplete emptying of the bladder;
- Painful or burning urination;
- Blood in the urine or semen;
- Painful ejaculation;
- Pain or stiffness in the lower back, hips, or upper thighs.

Diagnostic and Staging Tests

For more detailed information regarding these tests, see Chapter 8, "Diagnostic Tests."

- Fine-needle aspiration or core needle biopsy. Fifty percent of prostate nodules that can be felt by DRE prove to be malignant on biopsy. Precise insertion of the needle may be guided by ultrasound. The test is relatively painless.

- *Lymphangiogram,* an x-ray of the lymph nodes, and/or lymph node biopsy may be performed before surgery if the doctor suspects advanced disease;

- Chest x-rays, intravenous pyelogram, cystoscopy, CT, MRI and bone scans, and other tests may be done if metastasis is suspected;

- Flow cytometry (see "Cancer Cell Tests" in Chapter 14, "Principles of Treatment").

Tests Unique to Prostate Cancer

- PSA (see "Screening Tests," above);
- *Transrectal ultrasonography* (TRUS) (a probe inserted into the rectum emits sound waves; echoes of the sound are converted by a computer into an image of tissue).

Staging

- Stage I: The cancer cannot be felt by digital rectal examination and causes no symptoms. Usually, it has been found incidentally, such as when surgery is performed to treat benign prostate enlargement. Malignant cells may be found in one or many areas of the gland tissue removed.

- Stage II: The cancer can be felt during a rectal examination or has been discovered because of PSA testing, but malignant cells are found only in the prostate gland.

- Stage III: Malignant cells have spread beyond the prostatic capsule. The seminal vesicles may also have cancerous cells.

- Stage IV: Cancer has spread to adjacent structures, such as the bladder and rectum. It may have invaded local or distant lymph nodes and spread to the bones, liver, or lungs.

Treatment

The subject of when, whether, and how to treat prostate cancer is highly controversial. Certain types of prostate cancer grow very slowly and may not affect life expectancy; other types are fast growing, do spread, and become life-threatening.

Treatment considerations vary enormously from one man to another, depending on the stage of the cancer and its rate of growth. Options vary from "watchful waiting" (see box on page 608), also called *expectant conservative management,* to aggressive treatment to cure the disease. In advanced prostate cancer, therapy may provide comfort but not cure.

The choice of primary treatment—surgery, radiation, and/or hormone therapy—depends on the man's age, stage of disease, speed of cancer growth, physical condition, and personal desires about possible side effects, such as impotence (see Chapter 14, "Principles of Treatment").

Surgery

There are several options for removing the prostate gland (see Chapter 15, "Surgery").

- *Radical prostatectomy* is the removal of the entire prostate and some surrounding tissue through an incision in the abdomen or *perineum,* the area between the scrotum and the anus. This operation can usually cure stage I or II prostate cancer and is often rec-

ommended for men in good health, under age 70, whose life expectancy is more than 10 years. The major risks of radical prostatectomy are urinary incontinence (less than 5 percent of patients), and impotence (30 to 50 percent). Potency returns in 50 to 80 percent of men within a year of surgery. Rectal injury, infection, swollen lymph glands, nerve damage, and ureteral injury are all rare.

- *Radical nerve-sparing retropubic prostatectomy* places the incision in the lower abdomen and removes the gland but preserves the nerves, which can help prevent impotence. Although it allows removal of pelvic lymph nodes, the long-term success of this method is unknown. It is usually recommended only for men with early-stage tumors.

- *Perineal prostatectomy* places the incision in the perineum. Although recovery is quicker than after the abdominal operation, lymph nodes cannot be removed. It is used most often for small tumors when lymph node involvement is unlikely.

- *Transurethral resection* removes only part of the prostate. It is a curative operation in about 15 percent of patients. A very small periscope-like instrument through which the surgeon sees the prostate, a resectoscope, is inserted through the urethra. The surgeon passes a heated wire loop through the resectoscope and scrapes away a large portion of the tumor.

Radiation

The most common alternative to surgery in early prostate cancer is radiation therapy, which can cure early-stage disease and prevents cancer spread. It has slightly less successful survival rates than surgery. Radiation therapy works best when the cancer is confined to a small area, but it may also be recommended for older men, those in poor health, or those with more advanced tumors (see Chapter 16, "Radiation").

External beam radiation therapy is less likely to cause impotence (25 percent of men) than surgery. It does cause inflammation of the bladder, penis, and scrotum, and this can lead to temporary genital swelling, diarrhea, urinary retention, and incontinence in 30 to 50 percent of men. More rarely, these conditions are chronic.

Interstitial radiation therapy is less apt to damage potency, but its long-term effectiveness is unknown. Side effects such as infection, blood clots, urinary retention, genital swelling, rectal discomfort, and ejaculatory abnormalities may occur but are rare. In some cases radiation therapy includes both external and internal radiation.

Hormonal Therapy

Primary hormonal therapy alone—without surgery, radiation, or chemotherapy—may be another option for men with localized disease. If one type of hormonal therapy fails to halt or slow tumor growth adequately, another hormone or combination of hormones may be successful.

Because testosterone stimulates prostate cancer cell growth, various hormones may be given to decrease or counteract its activity. However, hormonal therapies do have risks. Treatment with *luteinizing hormone-releasing hormone* or one of its analogues, which control the production of sex hormones, has side effects similar to surgical removal of the testicles, including decreased libido and potency and hot flashes similar to those experienced by women at menopause. Another disadvantage is that the drug must be given by injection once a month. Diethylstilbestrol (DES), flutamide, and megestrol acetate (estrogen) may cause breast growth (*gynecomastia*), as well as fluid retention and gastrointestinal upset. DES may decrease libido and sexual potency. Flutamide preserves potency in about 75 percent of men; it may damage the liver, but this is rare. Both DES and megestrol may increase the risk of dangerous blood clots.

If hormone therapy has been insufficient to halt or slow tumor growth, the testicles may be surgically removed (*orchiectomy*) to deprive the body of testosterone permanently.

If orchiectomy fails, chemotherapy can be used. Oncologists usually suggest it only for symptom relief in advanced disease.

Survival

When prostate cancer is treated in stages I and II, there is an excellent chance of a full life expectancy; 15-year-survival rates among men with clinically localized disease treated with radical prostatectomy range from 86 to 93 percent. Less than 15 percent of patients with lymph node metastases can be cured, although treatment can prolong life and alleviate symptoms.

- Five-year survival for stage I cancer is 87 percent.

- Five-year survival for stage II cancer is 85 percent. Ten-year survival is 50 percent if cancer occurs in only a single nodule in one lobe of the prostate, but it is 37 percent if involvement is more extensive.

Watchful Waiting

Watchful waiting does not mean doing nothing. Typically it involves periodic monitoring of PSA levels and repeated DREs to track the progression of abnormal cells. These tests are done every three to four months for the first five years, then every six months for five years, and yearly thereafter. At any time, if testing or symptoms suggest that the cancer is becoming more active, therapy can begin.

Because relatively inactive cancers rarely cause problems, some studies have shown that treatment of localized prostate cancer yields little improvement in life expectancy when quality of life issues are considered. For example, with increasing age, men over 60 experience greater problems with treatment side effects, and the potential benefits of treatment in terms of longevity and quality of life decrease.

However, no standard criteria currently exist to identify the potentially insignificant cancers for which treatment can safely be avoided or delayed. So, although some physicians question whether the risks of aggressive treatment for early prostate cancer outweigh the benefits, others believe that watchful waiting carries a substantial risk of delayed intervention.

- Five-year survival for stage III cancer is 48 percent.

- Five-year survival of metastatic stage IV cancer is 21 percent.

If the cancer recurs or continues to progress, renewed therapy can extend life.

Special Needs

If treatment impairs potency, a urologist often can restore the ability to have an erection by using a vacuum erection device, intracorporeal injection of a vasodilator, or implantation of a penile prosthesis (see Chapter 30, "Sexuality").

More than 100 support groups for men who have prostate cancer have formed in recent years. They can be found under such names as Man-to-Man and Us Too (see Appendix I, "Resources").

Ask About

Monitoring cancer growth (see box, "Watchful Waiting") is increasingly recommended for elderly men with a life expectancy of less than 10 years who have low-grade, early-stage prostate cancer discovered while being treated for BPH. If watchful waiting is suggested to you, ask you doctor how often you will need to schedule check-up appointments and which tests will be done at what intervals.

If your doctor suggests surgery to remove pelvic lymph nodes, you might inquire about *laparoscopic lymphadenectomy*, which involves insertion of a periscope-like instrument called an endoscope into the pelvis through a tiny incision in the belly button. The surgeon then retrieves the lymph nodes through the scope, eliminating major surgery.

Another type of surgery under study is *cryosurgery*, in which small incisions are made in the perineum, and small freezing probes are inserted into the prostate for up to 15 minutes. Impotence occurs in 20 to 67 percent of men who undergo cryosurgery, but the nerves may regenerate within a year after the procedure.

Some experts say that cryosurgery often fails to remove all the cancer. However, the importance of this shortcoming varies according to the age and wishes of the man.

If you have stage III or IV disease, you may want to consider entering a clinical trial (see Chapter 21, "Investigational Treatments"). Several studies are evaluating different methods of radiation therapy. Various uses of chemotherapy—including hormonal drugs to relieve symptoms—are also being investigated.

PENIS

Cancer of the penis accounts for 2 to 5 percent of all cancers affecting the male urinary and genital tracts. It affects only one or two American men in 100,000. Virtually all penile carcinomas are of squamous cell (see Chapter 2, "The Language of Cancer") origin and are similar to slow-growing cancers found elsewhere on the skin. Rarely, penile carcinomas are *melanomas*, which usually grow on the glans and spread more rapidly (see "Melanoma" in the Encyclopedia). Even less commonly, *sarcomas* can arise in the deeper tissues of the penis.

Because penile cancer is almost never seen in men who were circumcised in infancy, poor foreskin hygiene is believed to be a critical factor. When circumcision is performed at puberty, the incidence of penile cancer is slightly higher than when it is done in infancy. Men who are circumcised as adults have the same incidence in middle age as those who have not been circumcised.

Recent studies suggest that infection by one of the many types of human papillomaviruses

(HPV) may increase the risk of penile cancer. Recent studies suggest that HPV-16 and HPV-18 may cause up to one-third of penile cancers. These types of HPV cause nearly invisible "flat warts" that are also known to be associated with cervical cancer in women.

The penis is the primary external part of the male reproductive system. The head of the penis is called the *glans*. At birth, the glans is covered by a loose piece of skin called the *foreskin*.

The *corpora cavernosa* are two parallel long and slender cylinders of tissue inside the shaft of the penis that contain spongy tissue and blood vessels that fill with blood and expand to produce an erection.

The *urethra* is a hollow tube, about 8 to 9 inches long, that opens onto the tip of the penis. It carries semen (composed of sperm and fluid) and urine outside of the body.

Who Is at Risk?

- Uncircumcised males;

- Men with a history of genital warts, especially types HPV-16 and HPV-18.

Screening Tests

Men should examine all surfaces of their penis, including retraction of the foreskin to examine its undersurface for nodules or masses in the glans, once a month if they are uncircumcised.

Types of Penile Cancer

Although cancer can occur anywhere in or on the penis, most malignancies arise on the glans or foreskin. This is usually a slow-growing cancer amenable to cure if treated early. Unfortunately, estimates suggest that more than 50 percent of men delay for more than a year after the appearance of a penile sore before seeking medical attention.

Cancer that extends beyond the penis usually affects the groin and pelvic lymph nodes. Distant metastases are most likely to occur in the bones and lungs.

Signs and Symptoms

- Usually a painless ulcer or growth on the penis (this may be hidden if the foreskin is not retracted);

- A reddish, velvety rash, small crusty bumps, or blue-brown flat growths;

- Persistent discharge, possibly foul-smelling, from beneath the foreskin;

- Swollen lymph glands in the groin.

Diagnostic and Staging Tests

For more information regarding these tests, see Chapter 8, "Diagnostic Tests."

- Physical examination;

- Biopsy of the suspicious tissue;

- Chest and skeletal x-rays and CT scan, liver and lymph node scans may be done if metastasis is suspected.

Tests Unique to Penile Cancer

No tests are available.

Staging

- Stage I: Cancer is found only on the surface of the glans and the foreskin.

- Stage II: Cancer is found in the deeper tissues of the glans or in the corpora cavernosa (in the shaft) of the penis.

- Stage III: Cancer found in the penis also has spread to nearby lymph nodes in the groin.

- Stage IV: Cancer is present throughout the penis and the lymph nodes in the groin and/or has spread to other parts of the body.

Treatment

Penile cancer diagnosed in stages I and II is

highly curable with surgery, but the effectiveness of treatment decreases sharply in stages III and IV (see Chapter 15, "Surgery").

In uncircumcised men, if the cancer is limited to the foreskin, simple circumcision under local anesthesia and, possibly, removal of some surrounding skin may remove all the cancer. Penile sensation returns to normal within a month, and the man can resume sexual activity within five or six weeks after surgery.

If carcinoma in situ occurs on penile skin and is very small and superficial, topical chemotherapy may be attempted. Fluorouracil (5-FU) cream is applied to the area twice daily for several weeks (see Chapter 17, "Chemotherapy"). Then another biopsy is done to assess the effects of treatment and determine whether further topical or surgical treatment is necessary.

More extensive stage I cancers may require a combination of surgery and topical chemotherapy. To ensure that all malignant cells are removed with as little damage to the penis as possible, the surgeon may examine cells with a microscope directly during the procedure.

If cancer has infiltrated the glans, at least *partial penectomy*, in which part of the penis is surgically removed, usually is necessary.

In stage II, partial or *total penectomy* (amputation of the penis) is the most frequent treatment. In some cases, radiation therapy may be able to destroy the cancer instead of surgery (see Chapter 16, "Radiation").

In uncircumcised men, circumcision is always performed before radiation therapy. However, because irradiation may destroy so much tissue and cause narrowing of the urethra, subsequent surgery may be required to remove part or all of the penis.

In stage III, total penectomy is the standard treatment. The penis is removed at the base, and the urethra exits in the perineum, the area between the base of the scrotum and the anus. Lymph nodes on both sides of the groin may also be removed. However, if it is suspected that lymph node swelling is due to infection rather than cancer, and swelling persists for a month or so after surgery despite antibiotic treatment, the nodes are removed. Radiation therapy is not often used.

In stage IV, treatment is designed to alleviate symptoms for cancer that cannot be cured. Depending on the discomfort, therapy may be local excision of malignant tissue, partial or total amputation of the penis, radiation therapy, or chemotherapy (see Chapter 20, "Combination Treatments").

Survival

- Five-year survival for stage I cancer limited to the glans and foreskin is 80 percent.

- Five-year survival for stage II with cancerous invasion of the corpora cavernosa but no spread to the lymph nodes is also 80 percent.

- Five-year survival for stage III with cancerous invasion of the local lymph nodes is related to the number and extent of nodes involved. The average is 50 percent.

- Five-year survival for stage IV with metastasis to lymph nodes and/or distant metastases is 20 percent.

Special Needs

Penile cancer can be emotionally devastating and for some men the fear of surgical amputation may outweigh fear of death and cause significant delay in seeking medical care.

Partial penectomy, while disfiguring, usually leaves enough penis structure for urination and sexual intercourse.

After total penectomy, the man must sit to urinate. In such cases, the man and his sexual partner also need to explore other methods of obtaining sexual satisfaction (see Chapter 30, "Sexuality"). However, if total or partial penectomy is necessary, subsequent penile reconstruction is available.

Ask About

If you have stage I or II cancer, you may want to discuss the possibility of laser therapy to vaporize malignant cells. This technique is being studied. In some cases it can preserve the appearance and sexual function of the penis, as long as the lesions are very small.

If you have stage III or IV penile cancer, you may want to volunteer for a clinical trial exploring the value of various combinations of chemotherapy drugs and drugs that make the cancer cells more sensitive to radiation therapy (see Chapter 21, "Investigational Treatments").

ORAL

As a group, cancers of the head and neck (excluding skin cancers) represent 5 percent of the new cancers that occur each year. They affect about 17 people in 100,000. This section focuses on cancer of the mouth and nose. Tumors in other head and neck tissues—the throat and larynx, major salivary glands, brain and spinal cord, eyes, thyroid gland, esophagus, and skin—are discussed in other Encyclopedia sections.

Approximately 40 percent of tumors that originate in the head and neck arise in the mouth. These cancers affect about eight people in 100,000.

Tongue and lip cancers each account for about one in four cases of oral cancer. The next most common sites are the floor of the mouth (13 percent), cheeks (9 percent), and gums (9 percent).

Nasal and paranasal sinus cancers are relatively rare, causing only about 4 percent of head and neck cancers. About 80 percent of these occur in the large maxillary sinus, located in the center of the cheek above the teeth; most of the rest occur in the small ethmoid sinuses in the bone behind the bridge of the nose and next to the eyes.

Most oral cancers are related to smoking and alcohol. Smoking cigarettes, cigars, or pipes (using tobacco or marijuana) and chewing tobacco or using snuff damages the delicate tissues of the mouth. Increasing evidence suggests that smoke causes cancer by removing essential snippets of genetic material from the DNA of cells. Without the full set of genetic instructions to regulate their growth, cells multiply in an uncontrolled way. Inhaling second-hand smoke (tobacco smoke in the environment) can also cause cancer. The role of alcohol is less clear, but apparently heavy drinking can weaken tissue resistance to cancer. People who use both tobacco and alcohol have a risk of developing oral cancer that is 16 to 100 times higher than that of those who do not use these substances.

Radiation can also contribute to cancers in the mouth. People who were treated with radiation therapy during childhood for such conditions as acne or tonsillitis are more prone to develop oral cancers later in life. Rates are also high among Japanese victims of the atomic bomb.

Exposure to environmental irritants such as asbestos, wood dust, chemicals used in metal working, textile processing, or plastics manufacturing may be a contributing factor.

Inadequate nutrition, poor oral hygiene, ill-fitting dental prostheses (dentures or braces, for example), or long-term serious illness such as advanced syphilis or chronic alcoholism are linked to oral cancer.

In women, especially those of northern European ancestry, a chronic iron deficiency (Plummer-Vinson syndrome) is associated with certain oral cancers, especially those of the tongue.

The mouth, or oral cavity, includes the lips, the moist inner lining of the cheek and lips (the *buccal mucosa*), the gums, the jaw bone holding the teeth (the upper and lower *alveolar ridge*), the front two-thirds of the tongue, the floor of the mouth (between the tongue and the alveolar ridge), the roof of the mouth (*hard palate*), and the area along the rising part of the jawbone, or *mandible*, which lies behind the wisdom teeth.

The nose includes the nostrils, the nasal passages and sinuses, and the mucous membranes that line them.

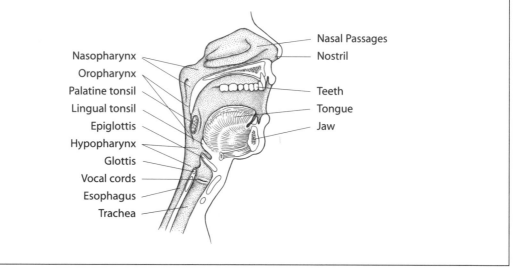

Who Is at Risk?

- Men, who are twice as likely as women to develop oral or nasal cancer;

- People over 40 (the incidence rises over time and reaches a peak around 65);

- People who smoke heavily, chew tobacco, or are exposed to secondhand smoke, especially those who also drink large quantities of alcohol;

- People who have received radiation therapy to the head and neck;

- People exposed to radiation;

- People exposed to excessive amounts of sunlight (lip cancer);

- People exposed to environmental irritants, chemicals, fumes;

- People whose diets are inadequate;

- People who practice poor oral hygiene.

Screening Tests

No tests are available, although careful examination of the mouth during a thorough routine physical or dental examination often reveals the presence of oral cancer or precancerous lesions (see "Types").

Types of Oral and Nasal Cancer

Almost all oral cancers are squamous cell cancers, which means they affect cells in the surface layer of the tissues that line the mouth and nose. The remaining 5 to 10 percent are adenocarcinomas, and they affect the salivary glands in the mouth (see "Salivary Gland," page 618).

Squamous cell carcinoma starts as one or more flat, raised, precancerous patches, or *plaques*, which are either white (*leukoplakia*) or red (*erythroplasia*). Both types of plaque can occur at the same time: Leukoplakia is more often found on the cheeks; erythroplasia is more common on the gums or floor of the mouth. Plaques do not usually cause pain or other symptoms. Unless they are in a very obvious place, like the tip of the tongue, the lesions are only detected by coincidence during a dental examination or a thorough physical examination.

As the plaque becomes cancerous, its cells may grow outward in little bumps like the surface of a raspberry. These are called *exophytic* tumors. Other times, the tumor is *endophytic*, in which dead cells pile up and then slough off, leaving behind a small pit or ulcer. The area may only feel hard, with no visible signs except possibly a slight color change.

The tumor continues to grow both outward and downward, depending on where it is. If it invades surrounding nerves, bone, or muscles, it can cause pain and may interfere with function. Tongue cancer, for example, can affect the tongue muscle and cause slurred speech.

The larger the tumor and the deeper it invades, the more likely it is to spread throughout the lymphatic system. In about 2 percent of cases, cancer cells can also invade blood vessels near an involved lymph node, increasing the risk of metastasis to distant organs such as the liver or lungs. In cases involving tumors more than 4 centimeters in diameter, the risk of metastasis is about 30 percent.

Signs and Symptoms

Oral cancer:

- Raised red or white patches inside the mouth;
- Pain or soreness, especially on the tongue;
- Mouth sores ("canker" sores) that don't heal in two weeks.

Nasal cancer:

- Local dull pain in face or tooth;
- Nasal obstruction;
- Runny nose;
- Nosebleed;
- Numbness in the cheek;
- Muscle spasms;
- Swelling in the mucous membranes.

Diagnostic and Staging Tests

For more information regarding these tests, see Chapter 8, "Diagnostic Tests."

- *Tissue sampling*, which involves painlessly scraping cells from the mucous membranes for laboratory analysis;
- CT scan, which is usually performed before biopsy to detect extent of bone involvement;
- Biopsy—fine-needle, incisional, or excisional.

Tests Unique to Oral and Nasal Cancer

- *In vivo staining*, in which a harmless chemical (toluidine blue) is applied to the suspicious area with a cotton-tipped applicator and then rinsed off. Abnormal cells will hold the dye and appear blue.

- *Indirect laryngoscopy*, in which the physician uses a mirror and a small headlamp to examine the larynx; it is called "indirect" because the doctor studies a reflection in the mirror rather than examining the tissue directly.

- *Direct laryngoscopy* or *endoscopy* using a flexible or rigid scope with a light source directed into the cavities of the mouth, nose, and throat to provide direct view of tissues.

- *Panorex images* use a revolving radiographic camera that produces a panoramic x-ray of the affected area; by seeing the tumor site from different angles, the physician gets a clearer picture of the cancer.

Staging

Oral Cancer

- Stage 0 is a localized, contained tumor.
- Stage I is a tumor less than 2 centimeters.
- Stage II is a 2- to 4-centimeter tumor.
- Stage III is a tumor greater than 4 centimeters. Or stage III may mean that the tumor can be of any size but that it has spread to one node.
- Stage IV varies from any size tumor that invades adjacent structures, with or with-

out node involvement but no spread to distant sites, to any tumor involving one or more nodes, to any tumor involving distant metastasis.

Sinus or Nasal Cancer

The only nasal cancer that uses the TNM system is cancer of the maxillary sinus. Cancers of the other nasal sinuses (ethmoid, frontal, sphenoid) do not have a staging system.

- Stage 0 is tumor in situ.

- Stage I is a tumor limited to the mucous membrane with no bone involvement.

- Stage II indicates the tumor has spread to the hard palate and/or to a nearby nasal cavity.

- Stage III is a tumor that invades the sinus wall, the skin of the cheek, the eye socket, or the nearby sinus cavity, or it is any tumor that has spread to at least one lymph node.

- Stage IV may be of several types: the tumor may have invaded the eye and/or other structures such as the bone beneath the eye, the sinus, nasopharynx, soft palate, or skull. It may involve one or more large nodes but without metastasis, or it may involve distant spread.

Treatment

Most people with oral and nasal cancers of the maxillary sinus have surgery to remove the tumor (see Chapter 15, "Surgery"). Sometimes this is followed by radiation therapy (see Chapters 16, "Radiation," and 20, "Combination Treatments"). Either surgery or radiation therapy alone will cure most stage I and stage II cancers (see later). In stage III or IV disease, which involves spread to other tissues and organs, surgery is more extensive and is usually followed by, and sometimes preceded by, radiation therapy. If the person cannot tolerate an operation or if the tumor cannot be completely excised, radiation therapy or chemotherapy is an option (see Chapter 17, "Chemotherapy"). Chemotherapy is not often used alone or as initial therapy, except to shrink certain large tumors (such as those on the tongue) prior to surgery.

Oral Cancer

The choice of surgery or radiation therapy depends on how accessible the tumor is and the potential functional or cosmetic impact of the treatment. Most cancers in the oral cavity arise on the floor of the mouth or tongue. Small tumors on the floor of the mouth can be removed through the mouth, provided there is a margin of normal tissue between the lesion and the gum. It may be excised with a scalpel or destroyed with either a laser, an electric current (electrocoagulation), or freezing (cryotherapy). Surgical removal of part of the tongue usually cures most tongue cancers that are less than 4 centimeters in their largest dimension. To preserve function and appearance, some oncologists may recommend radiation therapy when the cancer is on the tip of the tongue or the cheek.

Lip cancer is usually easily treated with surgery or radiation; the latter is less likely to produce unacceptable scarring.

Tumors on ridges around the teeth may require removal of some teeth. If the cancer is on the upper gums, surgery may remove part of the nasal cavity or sinus.

When the tumor is large or unreachable through the mouth, or if lymph nodes are involved, treatment usually combines surgery followed by radiation therapy. Surgery may involve an opening in the neck and removal of part of the jawbone. Reconstructive surgery, which may require a bone graft from the person's own tissue, is usually not performed at the time of the cancer surgery because of the infection risk. Instead the surgeon may insert a temporary metal plate to rejoin the jawbone and perform the bone graft at a later time. Other prosthetic devices or reconstructive surgery are sometimes necessary to permit swallowing or eating.

If the cancer has spread to the lymph nodes in the neck, a *radical neck dissection* may be needed in addition to the surgery that removes the primary lesion. This major procedure removes the affected nodes and is sometimes performed to prevent spread to other nodes. Because the surgery often affects the nerves and muscles that control the arms and shoulders, recovery may involve special exercises to strengthen these areas.

Radiation therapy can be given before surgery to shrink the tumor, but in many cases, it is not done because it would interfere with the tissues' ability to heal. Also, using radiation therapy after surgery, rather than before, means there is less diseased tissue to treat, so the radiation doses can be lower. For that reason many oncologists prefer to delay radiation therapy until after surgery if possible.

Chemotherapy has a more limited role. In people who have been treated but whose disease has metastasized or has recurred locally, combination chemotherapy can relieve pain, improve swallowing, and, in 20 to 40 percent of cases, reduce tumor size. Sometimes further surgery may be indicated. Available agents include methotrexate, cisplatin (Platinol), 5–fluorouracil (5–FU), bleomycin (Blenoxane), and vinblastine (Velban).

Nasal Cancer

Squamous cell cancers in the nasal cavity or stage I cancers in the maxillary sinus are treated with surgery, often followed by radiation therapy. People with stage II and III tumors may receive radiation therapy before or after surgery. Stage IV tumors require radiation therapy in combination with surgery or chemotherapy.

Since some nasal locations, such as the sphenoid sinus, are hard to reach, tumors there are more difficult to remove and radiation therapy may be the only treatment option. In some cases surgery may be attempted, with or without radiation therapy later.

Survival

- Five-year survival for stage I oral cancer in any location is 90 to 100 percent.

- Five-year survival for stage II cancer of the lip, cheek, or lower gums is 90 percent.

- Five-year survival for stage II cancer of the tongue or floor of the mouth is 50 to 70 percent.

- Five-year survival for stage III cancer of the lower gums is 50 percent.

- Five-year survival for stage III cancer of the hard palate or upper gums is 30 to 40 percent.

- Five-year survival for stage III cancer of the floor of the mouth is 45 to 50 percent.

- Five-year survival for stage III cancer of the tongue is 25 to 40 percent.

- Five-year survival for stage III cancer of the lip is 75 percent.

- Five-year survival for any stage IV oral cancer is less than 25 percent.

- Five-year survival for stage I and II nasal cancer is 60 to 70 percent.

- Five-year survival for stage III nasal cancer is 25 to 35 percent.

- Five-year survival for stage IV nasal cancer is 10 to 25 percent.

Special Needs

In many cases, treatment of oral cancer sometimes requires removal of part of the jaw. It may be necessary to perform bone grafts or to take other steps to preserve the appearance and function of the affected area as much as possible. Sometimes the head and neck surgeon may work in conjunction with a plastic surgeon to execute the complicated reconstructive process. (See Chapter 29, "Body Image and Self-Esteem.")

Often, too, a number of teeth and/or part of the nasal sinus are removed in surgery. A dental prosthodontist can create a special dental plate to reconstruct the defect in the sinus.

Special therapists can help in the rehabilitation process. A physical therapist can assist with exercises of the head, arms, and shoulders following extensive surgery and reconstruction in the neck. Following surgery on the tongue or jaw, speech therapists can help you learn how to compensate for problems caused by the alterations (see Chapter 28, "Managing Disabilities and Limitations"). Because oral cancer and its treatment affect the ability to chew and swallow, a nutritionist can offer advice on what to eat to ensure a proper diet (see Chapter 26, "Food and Nutrition").

There are support groups and organizations devoted to the needs of people with oral cancer. One such group, called Let's Face It, is designed to serve people with facially disfiguring illnesses (see Appendix I, "Resources").

Ask About

The use of chemotherapy before surgery to shrink larger tumors is increasing. Cisplatin (Platinol) combined with 5-fluorouracil (5-FU) is the approach that may have the most promise.

If you have stage III or IV cancer of the lip or mouth and your cancer is large and/or involves lymph nodes, you may want to discuss volunteering for a clinical trial with your oncologist (see Chapter 21, "Investigational Treatments"). Studies evaluating combination surgery and radiation therapy are under way, as well as the use of radiosensitizers (drugs that are absorbed by the tumor and are activated when exposed to radiation) and combination chemotherapy and surgery and/or radiation therapy.

If you have been treated for this type of cancer and your oncologist feels you are at risk of developing a secondary tumor, as many are, you might want to talk with him or her about the use of retinoids. Studies have shown that a year of therapy lowers the risk of a new, secondary tumor.

If your doctor recommends extensive surgery, you may want to consult with a plastic surgeon about new prosthetic devices and other advances that may make it possible to perform reconstructive surgery either at the time of the initial operation or later.

Induction chemotherapy—use of anticancer drugs to reduce the size of tumor—produces significant tumor regression in 70 to 90 percent of cases and complete disappearance of tumor in 20 to 50 percent of cases (see Chapter 17, "Chemotherapy"). Clinical trials are in progress to determine if chemotherapy used in this way may improve the outcome of treatment.

Immunotherapy—boosting the patient's immune system with biological agents—is being tested for its potential role for widely metastatic or resistant disease.

SALIVARY GLAND

Malignant salivary gland cancers account for approximately 7 percent of head and neck tumors, affecting one person in 100,000. About 90 percent of the tumors develop in one of the parotid glands, the largest salivary glands. Most of the remaining ones arise in submandibular glands, and only a small number affect the sublingual glands. The hard and the soft palates are common locations for cancer in the minor salivary glands.

People who were treated with radiation therapy to the head and neck for such conditions as acne or tonsillitis as children or young adults are five to 11 times more likely to develop cancer in a major salivary gland later in life. Rates are also high among Japanese victims of the atomic bomb, indicating that radiation is involved. Sometimes the cancer does not appear until decades after exposure to radiation.

Use of tobacco is not as clearly linked to salivary gland cancer as it is to other forms of head and neck cancer.

Glands contain several types of specialized cells whose function is to secrete substances necessary for the body. The salivary glands produce *saliva*, a fluid that lubricates the throat and moistens mucous membranes, mixes with and dissolves food to make swallowing and digestion easier, and contains protective natural antibiotics.

There are two groups of salivary glands, *major* and *minor*. The three major glands are the *parotid* glands, the largest salivary glands, extending from the front of the ear down and around the back of the lower jaw; the *submandibular* glands, located below the lower jawbone; and the *sublingual* glands, just below the tongue and behind the teeth. The minor salivary glands are located in several areas throughout the mouth and digestive tract, including the mucous membranes, palate, uvula, floor of the mouth, the rear section of the tongue, and around the tonsils.

Like other glands, the salivary glands have various types of cells: *stromal cells* are found in the tissues that support, protect, or give structure to a gland. These cells do not participate in saliva production. *Epithelial cells* cover the surface of a gland. *Parenchymal cells* actually process and secrete saliva.

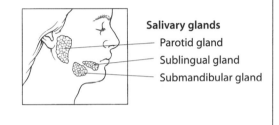

Salivary glands
Parotid gland
Sublingual gland
Submandibular gland

Who Is at Risk?

- People age 49 and older;

- People who have received radiation therapy to the head and neck;

- People who smoke heavily or chew tobacco, especially those who also drink large quantities of alcohol.

Screening Tests

No tests are available.

Types of Salivary Gland Cancer

Cancers arising in glandular tissue are called *adenocarcinomas*. A small percentage develop in squamous cells of the gland's ductal system or in its supportive tissues (the stromal cells).

There are several types of malignant tumors, depending on the cells involved; each behaves differently. The most common type of malignant tumor in the parotid gland is *mucoepidermoid carcinoma*. In the submandibular gland, malignant tumors are more likely to be *adenoidcystic carcinomas*.

Malignant tumors vary in their rate of growth and spread. *Low-grade* mucoepidermoid tumors spread slowly and are easily treated; *high-grade* tumors spread quickly to a number of nearby lymph nodes.

Some malignant tumors, including the adenoidcystic variety, are more likely to spread along nerves. In time the cancer can cause facial paralysis or can involve the skin of the face. Aggressive tumors originating in the submandibular gland are more likely to metastasize to distant organs, such as the liver, and to recur after treatment.

Benign tumors can be dangerous because they sometimes grow aggressively and invade nearby tissue, such as the tongue, and interfere with functioning.

Signs and Symptoms

- Swollen glands;

- Intermittent pain, especially when eating;

- Facial nerve pain;

- Appearance of tumors on skin above the affected area.

Diagnostic and Staging Tests

For more information regarding these tests, see Chapter 8, "Diagnostic Tests."

- Fine-needle biopsy;

- CT scan.

Tests Unique to Salivary Gland Cancer

No tests are available.

Staging

- Stage I is a tumor less than 4 centimeters in diameter.

- Stage II is a tumor less than 4 centimeters in diameter with invasion, or a tumor 4 to 6 centimeters in diameter without invasion.

- Stage III is a tumor 4 to 6 centimeters in diameter with invasion. Or stage II may be described as a tumor larger than 6 centimeters in diameter with no invasion. Stage III may also indicate a tumor of any size with the cancer involving one lymph node.

- Stage IV includes the following: any tumor larger than 6 centimeters with invasion that involves one lymph node but that has not spread to distant sites; any tumor, with or without invasion, that involves one or more large lymph nodes but shows no metastasis; and any tumor that has metastasized.

Treatment

Treatment choices for major salivary gland cancer depend on the gland involved, the stage of the disease, and whether the tumor is aggressive. Surgery to remove the tumor usually cures early-stage, low-grade cancer (see Chapter 15, "Surgery"). A tumor that is large or more aggressive or both may require radiation therapy after surgery (see Chapters 16, "Radiation," and 20, "Combination Therapy").

Some tumors are inoperable, either because complete removal is impossible or because they have metastasized to distant sites. In such cases radiation therapy, with or without chemotherapy, may be the best option.

Chemotherapy is seldom used, except in cases involving tumors that recur and do not respond to other treatments (see Chapter 17, "Chemotherapy"). However, fluorouracil (5-FU), doxorubicin (Adriamycin), or cisplatin (Platinol) produces partial response rates (meaning at least some reduction in tumor size) in 30 to 70 percent of people with advanced local, regional, or metastatic disease. Response to chemotherapy agents, however, is seldom complete, nor is it usually long-lasting. Surgery, or surgery plus radiation therapy, is more likely to be successful.

People with low-grade cancer of the parotid gland receive at least a *superficial parotidectomy*, removal of part of the gland where the majority of tumors are located. The surgeon is careful not to disrupt the facial nerves and muscles.

Larger or more aggressive tumors may require total excision of the gland, which may require removal of part or all of the facial nerve and can cause temporary or permanent paralysis of facial muscles in that area.

The surgeon may perform a *radical neck dissection* to remove any lymph nodes that are involved. This could require removing part of the jawbone and floor of the mouth, particularly when treating submandibular tumors, leading to disfigurement and loss of some of the nerves that control the tongue and jaw.

In addition to surgery, people with advanced disease almost always receive radiation therapy to the affected site or the lymph nodes in the neck or both. There is no known cure for stage IV cancer that has spread to distant organs.

Survival

- Five-year survival for stage I cancer is 90 percent.

- Five-year survival for stage II cancer is 55 percent.

- Five-year survival for stage III cancer is 22 percent.

- Five-year survival for stage IV cancer is 10 percent.

Special Needs

People who have had surgery for salivary gland cancer may need special instructions to help them eat and chew properly, and to make sure they maintain adequate nutrition. Physical therapy and exercises may be necessary to maintain tone in the muscles of the face (see Chapter 28, "Managing Disabilities and Limitations"). In many cases, nerve damage is only temporary, and function gradually returns, although persistent weakness of the lower lip is common. If full movement does not return, the person may have a facial nerve graft that may be at least partially restorative.

Support groups, such as Let's Face It (see Appendix I, "Resources"), are available and are designed to meet the needs of those who are trying to cope with facially disfiguring surgery.

Ask About

If you have stage III or IV salivary gland cancer, you may want to ask your oncologist about participating in a clinical trial (see Chapter 21, "Investigational Treatments"). Various chemotherapeutic agents, including new combinations of standard drugs, and combining chemotherapy with radiation therapy are currently being studied.

Fast neutron beam-radiation therapy, which is available in a few centers, is a relatively new technology that may prove to have greater effectiveness against certain types of salivary gland cancers compared to standard radiation therapy using x-rays. Studies are also exploring whether *hyperfractionated radiation therapy*—administering smaller doses of radiation more often than usual—may be of value. Another approach being evaluated involves the use of *radiosensitizers* (drugs that are absorbed by the tumor and are activated when exposed to radiation).

PHARYNX

Cancer of the larynx accounts for less than 1 percent of malignant tumors. Approximately 25 percent of head and neck cancers develop in the larynx (most of them in the glottis), which means that about one person in 100,000 has this form of cancer. Another 4 percent develop cancer in the nasopharynx, and 15 percent have it in the oropharynx and hypopharynx.

Most of these cancers are related to use of tobacco and alcohol. Smoking cigarettes, cigars, or pipes and chewing tobacco or using snuff can damage the delicate tissues of the throat. Evidence is mounting that tobacco causes cancer by removing essential snippets of genetic material from the DNA of cells. Without the full set of genetic instructions to regulate their growth, cells multiply in an uncontrolled way.

Inhaling second-hand smoke (tobacco smoke in the environment) can also cause these cancers. The role of alcohol is less clear, but many experts believe that heavy drinking weakens the tissue's ability to resist cancer. People who use both tobacco and alcohol are at a higher risk of developing these cancers than those who do not.

The precise cause of cancers of the hypopharynx is unknown, but there is a link to smoking and alcohol use. In women, especially those of northern European ancestry, a chronic iron deficiency (Plummer-Vinson syndrome) is associated with certain types of hypopharyngeal cancer.

Cancers of the nasopharynx are relatively rare in the United States. Infection by the Epstein-Barr virus (EBV) is a suspected cause, because the highest rate of nasopharyngeal cancer (25 times higher than that of any other group) occurs among people in southern China, where EBV infection is high. Incidence of nasopharyngeal cancer is also high where consumption of salted fish is high.

Radiation can also contribute to cancers in the throat. People treated with radiation therapy for such conditions as thyroid disease, acne, or tonsillitis are more prone to develop oral cancers later in life. Rates are also high among Japanese victims of the atomic bomb, indicating that radiation is involved.

Inadequate nutrition, poor oral hygiene, ill-fitting dentures and dental braces, and such long-term serious illness as advanced syphilis or chronic alcoholism can promote these cancers.

Exposure to environmental irritants such as wood dust or fumes from chemicals used in metal working, textile processing, or plastics manufacturing may help cause these cancers. There also appears to be a link between asbestos and cancer of the larynx.

Recent evidence suggests that laryngeal cancer is associated with gastroesophageal reflux, a condition in which the stomach contents rise up the throat. The high acid content of stomach material is very irritating to sensitive tissues in the throat.

The throat, or *pharynx*, is the muscular tube that connects the mouth and nose to the esophagus and *trachea*, or windpipe. It is the passageway, about 5 inches long, for air from the nose, and air and food from the mouth. The pharynx is divided into several distinct regions: the *nasopharynx*, the area behind the nose and above the soft palate containing the nasal tonsils; the *oropharynx*, the region behind the tongue and posterior wall of the throat, including the back third of the tongue and the *pala-* *tine* and *lingual* tonsils; and the *hypopharynx*, which is behind and adjacent to the *larynx*, or voice box, and joins the esophagus.

Below the pharynx is the larynx, which contains the *vocal cords*, membranes that open, close, and vibrate when air passes between them to produce speech. The *vocal cords* and the opening above them are known as the *glottis*. The larynx is covered by a flap of cartilage called the *epiglottis*, which covers the trachea during swallowing to prevent choking.

Who Is at Risk?

- Men, who develop these cancers at higher rates and earlier in life than women do;

- Men 45 to 70;

- Women over 50;

- People who smoke heavily, especially those who also drink large quantities of alcohol;

- People who have received radiation therapy to areas of the head and neck;

- People exposed to environmental irritants (chemicals, fumes, dust);

- People with inadequate nutrition;

- People who practice poor oral hygiene.

Screening Tests

No tests are available, although many pharyn-geal cancers are detected during a thorough physical examination of the oral cavity.

Types of Cancer of the Pharynx and Larynx

Almost all tumors in the oropharynx, hypopharynx, and larynx are *squamous cell cancers*, which means they affect the cells in the uppermost layer of tissue. *Verrucous*, or wartlike, cancers sometimes develop on the vocal cords.

Cancers of the nasopharynx are of a somewhat different nature from those arising in other parts of the throat. Although 50 percent of these tumors are squamous cell cancers, about 30 percent are tumors of the lymph system. These tumors have a distinctive appearance under the microscope. The remainder are lymphomas, melanomas, and minor salivary gland neoplasms.

Cancers that arise in squamous cells in the upper layer of throat tissue start as flat, raised, precancerous patches called *plaques*. They are either white (*leukoplakia*) or red (*erythroplasia*). Both types of plaque can occur at the same time. Usually plaques do not cause pain or other symptoms. Because the structures of the throat are not readily visible, plaques may be detected by coincidence during a dental or thorough physical examination.

As a plaque becomes cancerous, its cells may grow outward in little bumps like the surface of a raspberry. These are called *exophytic* tumors. Other tumors are *endophytic*; in these the dead cells pile up and then slough off, leaving behind a small pit or ulcer. In certain cases the area feels hard but may produce no visible signs, except perhaps a slight color change.

Depending on its location, the tumor continues to grow both outward and downward. If it invades nerves, bone, or muscles, it can cause pain or interfere with function of the affected area of the throat. For example, a tumor the size of a pinhead appearing on the vocal cords is enough to cause a hoarse voice. Left untreated, the cancer will spread to the lymph nodes and eventually metastasize throughout the lymphatic system. Tumors in certain sites of the head and neck usually spread to specific lymph nodes along a predictable path. This is an important feature in the diagnosis and treatment of these cancers, because signs of cancer in a certain node are a valuable clue that helps the doctor locate the original (primary) site of the tumor.

In about 2 percent of cases, cancerous cells also spread into blood vessels near an involved lymph node, increasing the risk of metastasis to distant organs such as the liver or lungs.

Signs and Symptoms

General symptoms:
- Sore throat that persists for two weeks;
- Swollen lymph nodes in the neck;
- Pain in the ear or that shoots into the neck on swallowing;
- Bleeding;
- Pain in the throat;
- Difficult or painful swallowing;
- Difficulty breathing;
- Weight loss.

Specific nasopharyngeal symptoms:
- Nasal obstruction;
- Nosebleed;
- Hearing loss;
- Ringing in the ears (tinnitus);
- Headache, facial pain, or other nerve-related symptoms;

Specific symptoms of the oropharynx and hypopharynx:
- Pain: sore throat, difficulty swallowing, pain radiating to the ear;
- Tongue muscle spasms, slurred speech, hoarse voice;
- Constant clearing of throat;
- Excessive salivation; bloody saliva.

Specific symptoms of the larynx:
- Hoarseness;
- Difficulty swallowing or extremely painful swallowing;
- Coughing up of blood;
- Abnormal breathing;
- Swollen lymph nodes;
- Complete loss of voice (called vocal cord fixation).

Diagnostic and Staging Tests

Also see page 615 for diagnostic and staging tests.

- CT scan.
- Fine-needle biopsy of lymph nodes in the neck (only if no primary tumor in the throat has been found).

Tests Unique to Cancer of the Pharynx and Larynx

No tests are available.

Staging

Cancer of the Nasopharynx and Hypopharynx

Nasopharyngeal Cancer

- Stage 0 is a tumor that has not spread (in situ).

- Stage I is a tumor that is limited to one subsite: the front, rear, or side wall.

- Stage II is a tumor that involves more than one subsite.

- Stage III is a tumor that invades the nasal cavity and/or the oropharynx, without lymph node involvement or metastasis. Or stage III cancer may mean any tumor with lymph node involvement.

- Stage IV varies from a tumor that invades the skull or cranial nerves to a tumor that involves one or more large lymph nodes, or a tumor with distant metastasis.

Cancer of the Hypopharynx

- Stage 0 is a tumor that has not spread.

- Stage I is a tumor limited to one subsite: the junction of the pharynx and esophagus, the rear wall, or the sinus.

- Stage II is a tumor that invades more than one subsite.

- Stage III is a tumor that invades more than one subsite or adjacent site and causes fixation of part of the vocal cords. Or stage III can mean any tumor with lymph node involvement.

- Stage IV varies from a tumor that invades cartilage or soft tissue of the neck, with or without lymph node involvement, with no metastasis, to any tumor involving one or more large lymph nodes or any tumor with distant metastasis.

Cancer of the Oropharynx

- Stage 0 is tumor in situ. The tumor has not invaded any local tissue.

- Stage I means the tumor is less than 2 centimeters in diameter.

- Stage II is a tumor between 2 and 4 centimeters in diameter.

- Stage III is a tumor greater than 4 centimeters in diameter, or any size tumor with spread to one lymph node.

- Stage IV may be one of several types. The tumor may invade an adjacent structure, with or without lymph node involvement. It may also be any tumor that involves at least one large lymph node or any tumor with distant metastasis.

Cancer of the Larynx

Supraglottis

- Stage I means the cancer of the supraglottis is limited to one subsite, with normal vocal cords.

- Stage II means more than one subsite of the supraglottis is involved but the vocal cords remain normal.

- Stage III is a tumor limited to the larynx with fixation of the vocal cords or one that invades nearby structures.

- Stage IV describes a tumor that invades through the thyroid cartilage and/or extends to the oropharynx or the soft tissues of the neck.

Glottis

- Stage I cancer of the glottis is limited to one or both vocal cords, with normal mobility.

- Stage II cancer extends to the supraglottis and/or the subglottis, and/or impairs vocal cord mobility.

- Stage III means the tumor is limited to the larynx and causes vocal cord fixation.

- Stage IV describes a tumor that invades through the thyroid cartilage and/or extends to the oropharynx or the soft tissues of the neck.

Subglottis

- Stage I means the tumor is confined to the subglottis.

- Stage II is a tumor that extends to the vocal cord(s), with normal or impaired mobility.

- Stage III means the tumor is limited to the larynx and causes vocal cord fixation.

- Stage IV describes a tumor that invades through the thyroid cartilage and/or extends to the oropharynx or the soft tissues of the neck.

Treatment

See the section in the Encyclopedia titled "Oral."

Cancer of the Nasopharynx

The nasopharynx is particularly difficult for surgeons to reach. In stage I and II disease, oncologists typically recommend radiation therapy alone (see Chapter 16, "Radiation"). External-beam radiation is aimed both at the tumor and at potentially involved lymph nodes. In some cases the radiologist may use brachytherapy, in which radioactive "seeds" are implanted in or near the tumor, alone or in combination with external-beam radiation. Treatment of stage III and IV disease may be the same as that for stages I and II, but it may also involve *radical neck dissection* (surgical removal of swollen lymph nodes in the neck) if radiation therapy has not controlled the involved nodes (see Chapters 15, "Surgery," and 20, "Combination Treatments"). In addition, the person may receive chemotherapy during or after surgery or radiation therapy.

Cancer of the Oropharynx

Treatment of cancer in the oropharynx usually involves some combination of surgery and radiation therapy. Chemotherapy may also be an option. In stage I and II disease, surgery and radiation therapy are equally successful. Surgery such as removing the tissue near the tonsils is often suggested if it would not seriously impair function of the throat. In contrast, radiation therapy is often a better option for treating cancer of the base of the tongue. More advanced stages of cancer in any part of the pharynx and larynx are more difficult to treat. Surgery combined with radiation may be effective. Many people also receive chemotherapy before surgery or radiation or both (see

Chapter 17, "Chemotherapy"). Because reconstruction and rehabilitation may be necessary, it is important to choose a surgeon who has a great deal of experience operating on the head and neck.

Cancer of the Hypopharynx

Tumors in the hypopharynx often grow for a long time before they are detected, and so tend to reach more advanced stages before treatment begins. Less than 2 percent of cases are diagnosed in stage I, when the tumor is small, protrudes from the surface, and is responsive to radiation therapy alone.

For more involved stage I or II tumors, surgery followed by radiation therapy is the usual approach. The surgeon typically removes the larynx and pharynx (*laryngopharyngectomy*) and does a radical neck dissection. In some cases, only part of the larynx is removed and the voice can be preserved. *Neoadjuvant chemotherapy* (use of drugs before surgery or the start of radiation therapy) can help shrink the tumor and can increase the effectiveness of the other treatments.

Treatment is more complex for stage III disease and involves extensive surgery followed by postoperative radiation therapy. To replace tissue removed during the operation, surgeons sometimes use tissue from the stomach (a procedure called the *gastric pull-up*) or from the small bowel (*jejunal* transfer). Many people also undergo chemotherapy before, along with, or after surgery or radiation. Surgery for stage IV disease is similar to that for stage III. If the tumor is inoperable, oncologists often recommend radiation alone, possibly with chemotherapy.

Cancer of the Larynx

Treatment varies according to whether the cancer is above, on, or below the vocal cords. Small cancers that have not spread have a good prognosis. Radiation therapy is usually the first line of treatment because it offers a better chance of preserving the voice. Surgery may follow if the tumor does not shrink or if it recurs. In advanced laryngeal cancer, chemotherapy is given before radiation therapy in an aggressive effort to preserve the vocal cords. Different surgical techniques include *cordectomy* (removal of the vocal cords); *supraglottic laryngectomy* (removal of supraglottis); partial or *hemilaryngectomy* (removal of part of the larynx); and total *laryngectomy* (removal of the larynx) followed by *tracheostomy* (creation of a hole in the neck for breathing).

Laser surgery has recently become a standard method of excising stage I and certain stage II tumors on the vocal cords. Even in low-stage cancers, however, partial or total laryngectomy may be needed. Cancer that has spread to the lymph nodes requires radical neck dissection.

Survival

- Five-year survival for stage I cancer of the nasopharynx is 65 to 85 percent; cancer of the oropharynx is 60 to 75 percent; cancer of the hypopharynx is 50 to 80 percent; cancer of the larynx is 75 to 95 percent.

- Five-year survival for stage II cancer of the nasopharynx is 35 to 50 percent; cancer of the oropharynx is 45 percent; cancer of the hypopharynx is 50 to 60 percent; cancer of the larynx in the supraglottis is 60 to 75 percent; cancer of the larynx in the glottis is 60 to 80 percent; cancer of the larynx in the subglottis is 30 to 40 percent.

- Five-year survival for stage III cancer of the nasopharynx is 25 percent; cancer of the oropharynx in the tonsil is 30 to 35 percent; cancer of the oropharynx at the base of the tongue is 10 to 20 percent; cancer of the hypopharynx is 25 percent; cancer of the larynx in the supraglottis is 45 to 60 percent; cancer of the larynx in the glottis is 50 percent. (No data are available on five-year survival rates for stage III cancer of the larynx in the subglottis.)

- Five-year survival for stage IV cancer of the nasopharynx is 5 to 10 percent; cancer of the oropharynx in the tonsil is 14 percent; cancer of the oropharynx at the base of the tongue is 10 percent; cancer of the hypopharynx is 5 to 10 percent; cancer of the larynx in the supraglottis is 20 to 30 percent; cancer of the larynx in the glottis is 20 to 30 percent; cancer of the hypopharynx is 5 to 10 percent; few people with stage IV cancer of the larynx in the subglottis survive for five years.

Special Needs

People with pharyngeal cancers require careful follow-up after treatment. This will include an examination of the original tumor site and neck, chest x-rays, CT or MRI scans, and blood work. Tests to evaluate the function of the thyroid and pituitary glands may also be ordered. A new dental and oral hygiene routine may be prescribed, jaw exercises may be recommended to retain mobility, and nerve function will be monitored. In addition, any systemic complaints will be evaluated to rule out the presence of metastasis.

Pharyngeal cancers can seriously affect some of the most basic functions of life, such as eating, breathing, and talking. People attempting to cope with these serious disruptions in basic function and to return to the highest possible quality of life may need special counseling.

Following partial or total laryngectomy, a speech therapist teaches new methods of talking. For example, it is possible to learn how to swallow air and belch it back up so that sounds can be made as air is expelled. Technical devices are also available, including special tubes that carry air from the hole in the trachea up to the corner of the mouth. Microphone-like objects can be held against the neck to amplify sound. Creation of a fistula between the trachea and esophagus can be helpful.

Among the caregivers often involved in post-treatment rehabilitation are speech therapists, dentists, home-care nurses, and other paramedical specialists. The American Cancer Society supports a group called the International Association of Laryngectomees, which has many local chapters and is dedicated to helping people improve their speech. Similar groups include the Lost Cord Clubs (also called New Voice Clubs) and Let's Face It, another international group that provides information and support for people coping with facial disfigurement (see Appendix I, "Resources," and Chapter 28, "Managing Disabilities and Limitations").

Ask About

If a cancer affects any part of your pharynx and/or larynx at almost any stage, a clinical trial is under way that you might consider. Even if you receive standard treatment, you may want to volunteer for a study to determine if retinoids (isotretinoin) taken daily for a year after treatment prevents recurrence or development of new cancers in the nose, mouth, and throat.

Clinical trials are attempting to determine if chemotherapy before, during, or after radiation therapy or surgery (see Chapter 21, "Investigational Treatments") is more effective than postoperative treatment.

Studies are also exploring whether hyperfractionation of radiation—administering smaller doses of radiation more often than usual—may be of value. Drugs that enhance the sensitivity of tumors to radiation, radiosensitizers, are being tested, too.

BASAL CELL AND SQUAMOUS CELL

The statistics of skin cancer are formidable: It is the most common type of cancer in the United States—an estimated one in five Americans who reach age 65 will develop a skin cancer. It has the highest cure rate—almost 100 percent when treated at an early stage. And it is one of the most preventable—90–95 percent of cases are caused by overexposure to the sun and may have been avoided with life-long sun protection.

It is believed that when the ultraviolet (UV) radiation of sunlight bombards the delicate DNA molecules within the nucleus of a skin cell, the molecules fuse into useless fragments. The cell then

The skin, which is the outer covering of the body and is its largest organ, serves many functions. It protects the body from heat, light, injury, and infection, and it regulates body temperature and converts sunlight into vitamin D. Information about the environment—temperature, pressure, pain, vibration—is picked up by nerve cells in the skin and sent to the brain.

Skin consists of several layers. The top one is the epidermis. Beneath its outermost protective coating of dead cells is a thicker layer of flat, scale-like cells called *squamous* cells. Beneath that layer are the *basal* cells. This deepest part of the epidermis also contains *melanocytes*, cells that produce *melanin*, which gives skin its color and protects against UV rays in sunlight. Skin cancer is called *squamous cell carcinoma, basal cell carcinoma*, or melanoma, depending on the kind of cells involved.

Under the epidermis is an inner layer of skin, the dermis, which contains blood and lymph vessels, hair follicles, and two types of glands. Openings in the skin, called pores, allow sweat and sebum to reach the surface.

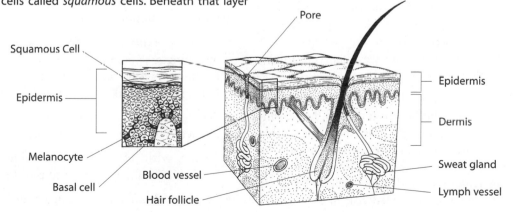

Squamous Cell
Epidermis
Melanocyte
Basal cell
Blood vessel
Hair follicle
Pore
Epidermis
Dermis
Sweat gland
Lymph vessel

secretes enzymes, which act like chemical scissors to snip out the damaged fragments and help generate replacement DNA. The theory is that during the repair process, regrowth can continue unchecked, causing tumors to develop. Genetic factors within the skin cells may also play a role in this process.

The incidence of skin cancer has been steadily rising, in part because people are living more active lives outdoors, and many are purposefully exposing more of their bodies to the sun more often to acquire a tan. Another factor is our changing atmosphere: The ozone layer, which defends the earth from UV radiation, is diminishing.

Melanin, the pigment in skin, offers some natural protection and explains the enormous difference in skin cancer rates between Caucasians (about 250 in 100,000 will get nonmelanoma skin cancer) and African-Americans (about three in 100,000 will have the disease).

There are three common forms of skin cancer: melanoma, the most serious (see "Melanoma" in the next Encyclopedia section); basal cell carcinoma (BCC), the most common; and squamous cell cancer (SCC). This section discusses the latter, nonmelanoma skin cancers.

Basal cell carcinoma accounts for 75 to 90 percent of all nonmelanoma skin cancers and about one-fourth of all cancers detected each year. Squamous cell cancer is the second most common form, causing about 15 percent of all cases of skin cancer (see "Types," later).

Who Is at Risk?

- Men, who are twice as likely to have BCC as women and two to three times as likely to have SCC;

- People who live in regions that get a lot of sun (for example, the rate of nonmelanoma skin cancer in Tucson, Arizona, is 317 per 100,000 population, whereas in Rochester, Minnesota, it is 146 per 100,000);

- People who live in sunbelt states or other regions close to the equator;

- Older people (the incidence among persons 55 to 75 years of age is four to eight times that of people age 35 to 54. SCC is more common in people over age 60, and BCC is more common after the age of 50; however, the incidence of skin cancer among younger people is on the increase, with about 2.6 percent of cases occurring among people in their 30s);

- People who have exposed themselves to UV radiation, whether from the sun, home sunlamps, or tanning salons (the earlier in life exposure begins and the longer it lasts, the greater the risk; chronic sun exposure during childhood and adolescence is directly related to an increased risk of skin cancer in adulthood);

- People who fail to use sunscreens or sun blocks with a high sun protection factor (SPF 15 or greater);

- People with fair skin that burns or freckles easily;

- Children with heavy freckling or moles with a diameter greater than 5 centimeters (such moles are markers of a genetic tendency to develop tumors);

- People who have precancerous conditions, such as *actinic keratosis* (rough, scaly red or brown patches caused by sun exposure), *actinic cheilitis* (sun damage to the lips), *leukoplakia* (white patches on the tongue or inside the mouth), and *Bowen's disease* (persistent, red-brown scaly patches resembling psoriasis or eczema);

- Workers exposed to certain chemicals, including arsenic, tar, coal, paraffin, or oils containing polycyclic aromatic hydrocarbons, such as shale oil or asphalt;

- People taking certain immunosuppressive medications or psoriasis treatments;

- People with HIV infection, which can weaken immune resistance to tumors;

- People with *albinism*, a congenital lack of melanin;

- People with conditions involving chronic inflammation, such as lupus, osteomyelitis, acne, or severe burns, which can weaken skin cell's resistance to skin cancer;

- People who have received radiation therapy.

Screening Tests

- Skin examination, including mouth, behind the ears, nose, scalp, genitals, rectum, palms, and soles, as part of an annual checkup (see Chapters 4, "The Cancer Checkup," and 7, "Examining Yourself").

Types of Nonmelanoma Skin Cancer

A skin cancer occurs most often on parts of the body exposed to sunlight, especially the face, neck, ears, scalp, shoulders, and back.

Squamous Cell Carcinoma

About 75 percent of SCC lesions occur on the head and face, and 15 percent occur on the hands, including the fingernails. But skin cancer can occur anywhere on the body, including the legs, chest, back, and mucous membranes. SCC of the penis is rare, accounting for less than 1 percent of cases among males, and occurs invariably in uncircumcised men, especially those who practice poor hygiene (see "Penis"). SCC lesions typically are firm, reddish, scaly nodules with raised edges that may be well defined or indistinct. Lesions may develop ulcers, a scaly crust, or a wartlike surface. SCC lesions are classified as superficial if they penetrate only to the upper part of the dermis and as infiltrative if the lower dermis or subcutaneous layer is involved.

SCC is more likely to metastasize than BCC. Metastasis occurs in perhaps 3 to 10 percent of cases. The lesions most likely to spread are those on the temple, ear, forehead, hand, or lip, and that are more than 1 centimeter in diameter and 4 millimeters thick. Regional lymph nodes are the site of metastasis in about 85 percent of cases, but distant sites, such as the liver, lung, bone, and brain, may also be involved.

Basal Cell Carcinoma

Approximately 80 percent of BCC tumors occur on the head and neck, most often on the nose, eyelids, and cheeks, although they can also occur on the chest, back, palms, and soles.

There are several types of BCC, each producing lesions with a distinctive appearance.

- Forty-five to 50 percent of cases are *nodular BCC lesions*, translucent, flesh-colored or pink, pearly nodes that can ulcerate and become crusty.

- Fifteen to 35 percent are *superficial lesions,* which are red, scaly patches that resemble psoriasis.

- Four to 17 percent are *morpheaform lesions*, which can be flat, indented, or slightly raised areas, off-white or yellow, that resemble scar tissue.

- One to 2 percent are *pigmented lesions*, which are darker than the surrounding skin, usually appearing blue, brown, or black.

Metastasis of skin cancer is rare. The rate of BCC metastasis is probably less than one case in 4,000, but when it does spread, the most common areas are the head (especially the scalp) and neck.

Signs and Symptoms

- A sore or mark on skin that changes in size, color, shape, or thickness;

- New growth or a sore that doesn't heal within three weeks;

- A spot or sore that continues to itch, hurt, crust, scab, erode, or bleed;

- Persistent skin ulcers not explained by other causes;

- Ulcers in sites of previous radiation treatment.

Diagnostic and Staging Tests

For more information regarding these tests, see Chapter 8, "Diagnostic Tests."

- Biopsy (shave, punch, incisional, or excisional, depending on the size and location of the lesion);

- Chest x-rays and blood tests if metastasis is suspected.

Tests Unique to Skin Cancer

Mohs' micrographic surgery (see "Treatment," later).

Staging

According to the TNM system established by the American Joint Committee on Cancer, the stages of nonmelanoma skin cancer are as follows:

- Stage I: The lesion or tumor is localized and is 2 centimeters or less at its greatest dimension.

- Stage II: The tumor is larger than 2 centimeters but not more than 5 centimeters at its greatest dimension.

- Stage III: The tumor is larger than 5 centimeters at its greatest dimension, or it is of any size and there is lymph node involvement.

- Stage IV: A tumor of any size with lymph node involvement and distant metastasis.

Because metastasis of BCC is rare, staging tests are rarely done following biopsy unless the growth is very large or has been present for a long time.

Treatment

The goal in treating BCC and SCC is to remove or destroy the tumor completely, causing minimal damage to surrounding normal tissue and leaving the smallest scar possible. Surgery is usually the treatment of choice (see Chapter 15, "Surgery"). Following surgery, if the area of cancer is large or is in a part of the body that is usually visible, the physician may also perform a skin graft to minimize the remaining defect. This involves transplanting an area of healthy skin from a less visible part of the person's body, such as the back or the buttocks, to the wound.

Surgery under local anesthesia can remove lesions greater than 3 centimeters (about an inch) in diameter on the scalp, forehead, arms, legs, eyelid, lip, penis, vulva, and anus. In many cases, the biopsy completely excises the cancer and completes treatment. Cosmetic results are good and the wound heals quickly. Lymph nodes near the cancer may be removed at the time of surgery and evaluated. Other nodes are removed if it is suspected that the cancer has spread.

Another surgical technique is curettage. After injecting a local anesthetic to numb the area, the surgeon scrapes away the cancer with a sharp-edged, curved curette. The surgeon then touches the area with an electronic probe to destroy any remaining cancer cells. This process, called *electrodesiccation*, also cauterizes the blood vessels and controls bleeding. Most people who undergo curettage will have flat, white scars after healing. Curettage is only appropriate for certain types of lesions (superficial SCC and superficial and nodular BCC) in areas where risk of recurrence is low. It can take less time and requires somewhat less surgical skill than excision.

Mohs' micrographic surgery (also known as microscopically controlled surgery) is a technique, also performed under local anesthesia, in which a specially trained surgeon removes cancerous tissue by shaving off one layer at a time. After each layer is removed, a pathologist immediately examines the tissue under a microscope. The surgeon stops removing layers of tissue when all the cells appear normal. Surgeons use this technique when they are uncertain about how extensive the cancer is. It is also used when tumors are large, recurring, or located in hard-to-reach places, or when the maximum amount of healthy skin needs to be preserved (such as when cancer is on the eyelid, nose, finger, or genitalia). The degree of scarring that results depends on the location, size, and depth of the lesion.

Cryosurgery involves use of a liquid nitrogen spray or a probe to freeze and kill abnormal cells. Gradually, as the dead tissue thaws, it falls away. This technique is sometimes used to treat precancerous conditions, such as actinic keratosis and small skin cancers. In some cases, several procedures are needed for complete treatment. Cryosurgery is a good choice for BCC of the eyelids because it may preserve normal tissue and avoid the need for reconstructive surgery. (However, it is not used for the morphea form of BCC.) SCC lesions that are less than 2 centimeters in diameter (about the size of a nickel) and that have well-defined borders respond well to cryosurgery. The treated skin turns white and may give the impression that the tumor has been completely destroyed when it has not. Tumors need to be frozen once or twice for 10 to 90 seconds during the same session, depending on their size and depth. Because cryosurgery avoids invasive surgery, it may be a good choice for the elderly or those who have medical conditions or are taking anticoagulants that would make surgery an especially risky procedure. Usually the procedure involves no pain, but some people experience pain and swelling afterward. Blistering, crusting, and swelling may also develop, and the wound can take a few weeks to heal. Loss of skin pigment in the treated area is inevitable, resulting in white scars, but overall cosmetic results are good.

Laser surgery is a relatively new approach and is used after a biopsy confirms the presence of cancer cells. A local anesthetic is used to numb the area; then a highly focused beam of light energy destroys cancer cells. It is especially useful for cancers on the outer layer of skin. Laser surgery is often used to treat large superficial basal cell carcinomas. There is less pain after laser treatment than after other kinds of surgery, but scarring still occurs.

Sometimes radiation therapy or chemotherapy, or both, can shrink tumors or kill cancerous cells when surgery is impossible or would cause unacceptable disfigurement.

Radiation therapy is often the treatment of choice if the tumor is in a spot that is especially prominent (such as the tip of the nose) or difficult to reach surgically (such as the eyelid) (see Chapter 16, "Radiation"). Although treatment with one x-ray dose often cures small lesions (1 centimeter or less), complete therapy usually involves smaller doses given during several sessions over a period of one to four weeks. Radiation also can relieve symptoms of inoperable cancers, thus providing a higher quality of life than would otherwise be possible. It is sometimes a choice for elderly people who may be unwilling or unable to undergo an extensive operation or one that would require reconstruction.

After radiation some people experience a rash, or their skin may become dry or red. Sometimes these changes in skin color or texture do not emerge until several years after treatment, and the changes often become worse with time. About half of people given radiation therapy develop skin changes within nine to 12 years. For this reason, doctors usually do not prescribe radiation therapy for younger people.

Topical chemotherapy employs anticancer drugs applied directly on the skin in lotions, creams, or liquid solutions (see Chapter 17, "Chemotherapy"). For example, 5-fluorouracil (5-FU) applied daily for several weeks will obliterate actinic keratosis and SCC. It is most often used when there are multiple cancers and/or precancerous lesions. 5-FU blocks DNA synthesis, which prevents cell growth and eventually leads to cell death. Most people experience severe inflammation for two to three weeks as a result of this treatment, but scarring is usually not a problem. One concern with topical treatment is that it may control a tumor on the surface of the skin but deeper cells may continue to invade tissue.

Systemic chemotherapy, sometimes used in combination with radiation, is an option when cancer has spread, especially to the bone. Cisplatin (Platinol) produces the best results with the longest remission. The combination of cisplatin (Platinol) and doxorubicin (Adriamycin) and radiation therapy can relieve symptoms in widely disseminated or inoperable BCC.

Survival

Skin cancer is nearly 100 percent curable if it is detected before it spreads. Recurrence and cure rates vary, depending on the type, site, and extent of the lesions, and on treatment. When the tumor is from 2 to 5 millimeters in diameter, the cure rate is 85 to 95 percent; in some reports it is nearly 99 percent after five years. But there is a 50 percent recurrence rate when the tumor is 3 centimeters or larger. Following Mohs' surgery, the cure rate can be higher than

99 percent, again depending on the size, type, and location of the cancer. Cure rates from cryosurgery are as high as 96 to 98 percent.

There is a risk that skin cancer will recur, usually within five years but sometimes even later. In roughly one-third of BCC cases, new primary carcinomas can also appear within a year of treatment of the original lesion.

Special Needs

People who have been treated need to:

- Perform a thorough skin self-examination for signs of new lesions every one to three months, depending on their risk of recurrence.

- Have a checkup every six months for five years.

- Minimize risk by avoiding unprotected exposure to the sun.

Those treated with topical drugs, such as 5-FU, need to be especially vigilant, because the medication may not penetrate all areas of the skin evenly, leading to an increased risk of recurrence.

Ask About

Because many forms of treatment for skin cancer leave scars, you may feel apprehensive about your appearance. Nevertheless, effective treatment requires complete removal of the tumor. Otherwise, the risk of recurrence of the cancer is high. You can discuss with your doctor, perhaps in consultation with a plastic surgeon and/or dermatologist, what form of treatment is most likely to eliminate the cancer, while doing everything possible to preserve normal appearance, including skin grafts and reconstructive surgery.

One promising approach involves *photodynamic therapy*. In this method you take a drug that cancer cells absorb and retain, making them more sensitive to light. When a laser is focused on the lesion, the cells containing the drug absorb the light and are destroyed.

Partial cure of BCC has been seen in a few experiments using drugs derived from vitamin A known as *retinoids*. High doses of systemic isotretinoin given in pills or in a lotion applied to the skin, for example, can cause the tumors to regress and may prevent their recurrence, but the side effects, including uncomfortable chapping of the lips, can be so serious that people stop therapy. If you are at high risk of developing skin cancer, you may want to discuss volunteering for a clinical trial testing the effectiveness of retinoids for prevention (see Chapter 21, "Investigational Treatments").

Biological therapy, or immunotherapy, involving injections of interferon directly into the tumor three times a week for three weeks, can result in a cure rate of 81 percent after one year. However, the side effects, although manageable, are difficult to live with. They include fever, malaise, aches, chills, lower white blood cell count, and itching at the site of injection. Both alpha interferon and gamma interferon are being investigated in clinical trials. (See Chapter 18, "Biological Therapies).

MELANOMA

Melanoma is less common than other forms of skin cancer, accounting for about 5 percent of them, but its incidence is rising more rapidly than any other cancer. This may be due to the increase in detection as a result of public education and screening, but it may also reflect the habit of sunbathing. The American Cancer Society estimates that by the year 2000, one in 75 Americans will be diagnosed with melanoma.

Melanoma arises in pigment-producing cells called *melanocytes*, which occur singly or in clusters throughout the top layer of the skin, the *epidermis*. It is not known what causes these cells to proliferate uncontrollably, but a genetic link appears to be involved, and sun exposure—particularly sunburning in childhood—seems related. More rarely, melanoma can occur in the eye, mouth, rectum, and vagina.

Although the cancer often occurs in people at the prime of their lives, melanoma is exceptional in that it is one of the easiest to detect. And if it is diagnosed early, cure is likely. However, if not treated early, melanoma is one of the most lethal cancers (see "Survival," later).

When the tumor penetrates the lower layers of skin that contain blood and lymph vessels, the risk that the cancer will spread to other parts of the body increases dramatically. Melanoma can spread to virtually any organ and tissue within the body, but the liver, lungs, bones, brain, and spinal cord are particularly vulnerable. Melanoma is also the form of cancer most likely to pass to the fetus of a pregnant woman, although such spread is quite rare.

Who Is at Risk?

- Caucasian people with fair complexions, especially those with red hair and a tendency to sunburn after brief exposure in sunlight (two to three times more likely to develop melanoma than others);

- People between the ages of 40 and 60;

- Women in their 20s, who develop melanoma at a rate twice that of men (the incidence among women between the ages of 30 and 39 is 1.5 times that of men; after age 40, it is about the same in men and women).

Having one or two of the following risk factors increases the risk of melanoma three or four times; having three or more increases the risk almost 20 times.

- Red or blond hair;

- Personal or family history of melanoma;

- *Actinic keratoses*, which are rough, scaly red or brown patches caused by sun exposure;

- Susceptibility to freckling, especially on the upper back;

- Three or more blistering sunburns before age 20;

- Three or more years with outdoor summer jobs during the teen years.

Other risk factors include:
- Blue eyes;

- Excessive exposure to sunlight;

- Residence in the sunbelt states, Hawaii, or other regions near the equator;

- Multiple large brown moles at birth;

- Presence of atypical moles (*dysplastic nevi*), which are larger than 0.25 inch, irregularly shaped, multicolored, especially in a person with a family history of atypical moles;

- Indoor work (office jobs or school) alternating with intensive exposure to sunlight on days off;

- Treatment with immunosuppressive drugs, which weaken resistance to tumors.

Screening Tests

- Skin examination, including mouth, behind the ears, nose, scalp, genitals, rectum, palms, and soles, as part of an annual checkup (see Chapter 4, "The Cancer Checkup").

People can also check themselves by watching all moles and birthmarks on their bodies for any changes in shape, size, color, or location (see the box entitled "Looking for Skin Cancer" in Chapter 7, "Examining Yourself").

Types of Melanoma

Cutaneous melanoma involves the skin and grows in one of four patterns:
- *Superficial spreading melanoma.* Seventy percent of cutaneous melanomas begin as flat moles that may expand slowly outward

or rise quickly vertically or both. The edges of the lesion are irregular and the surface may be uneven. It ranges in color from black to brown or reddish pink to white. This type of melanoma is usually easily treated and has a relatively good prognosis.

- *Nodular melanoma.* Twenty percent of cutaneous melanomas grow vertically and are often blue, black, or without abnormal pigmentation.

- *Lentigo malignant melanoma.* Five percent of cutaneous melanomas slowly expand outward and are black and tan. They typically arise on the face and neck of older Caucasian people who have deep tans. About one in 20 of these tumors becomes invasive.

- *Acral lentiginous melanoma.* Five percent of cutaneous melanomas among Caucasians and 35 to 60 percent of cutaneous melanomas among African-Americans are of this type. It begins as a flat tumor that later rises vertically. This may happen gradually or quickly. The most common sites are the palms, soles, and areas underneath the fingernails.

Signs and Symptoms

There is usually a delay of 10 to 20 years between exposure to sunlight and the appearance of melanoma. However, in many cases the lesion may begin to change over one to five years, followed by a period of rapid growth.

Common moles and malignant melanomas do not look alike. Look at your moles and pay attention to characteristics that are easily summarized using the formula "ABCD":

- Asymmetry;

- Border irregularity;

- Color variety;

- Diameter greater than 6 millimeters or about the width of a pencil eraser).

Any change in a new or existing pigmented (tan, brown) area of the skin or in a mole indicates a melanoma. These include changes in the following:

- Size, especially sudden or continuous enlargement;

- Color, especially multiple shades of tan, brown, dark brown, black; the mixing of red, blue, and white; or the spreading of color from the edge into the surrounding skin;

- Shape, especially the development of an irregular, notched border that used to be regular;

- Elevation, especially in a part of a pigmented area that used to be flat or only slightly elevated;

- Surface, especially scaliness, erosion, oozing, crusting, ulceration, or bleeding;

- Surrounding skin, especially redness, swelling, or the development of colored blemishes next to but not part of the pigmented area;

- Sensation, especially itchiness, tenderness, or pain;

- Consistency, especially softening or hardening.

Diagnostic and Staging Tests

For more information regarding these tests, see Chapter 8, "Diagnostic Tests."

- Excisional or core-punch biopsy of the entire lesion, including a rim of normal-looking skin and some of the subcutaneous fat, if the lesion is less than 1.5 centimeters in diameter;

- Incisional biopsy if the tumor is larger than 1.5 centimeters.

- A new process, *dermoscopy*, shows promise. Using a small, hand-held, magnifying microscope, the physician can look through the upper layers of skin directly to the pigmented layer and study any suspicious lesions. A similar experimental process, computerized dermoscopic imaging, creates a digital image of the lesion.

Tests Unique to Melanoma

No tests are available.

Staging

A biopsy is needed for accurate staging of the tumor. Because staging depends on how thick the tumor is and how deeply it extends into surrounding tissue, the physician usually removes the entire tumor when obtaining a biopsy, rather than just a portion of it. According to the TNM system established by the American Joint Committee on Cancer, the stages of malignant melanoma of the skin (except of the eyelids) are as follows:

- Stage I: A tumor on the outer layer of skin up to 1.5 millimeters in thickness, which has not spread on the surface but which may have penetrated to the upper part of the inner layer of skin (the dermis).

- Stage II: A localized melanoma that is between 1.5 and 4 millimeters in diameter and/or that invades more deeply into dermis.

- Stage III: One or more of the following:
  - The tumor is more than 4 millimeters thick.

  - The tumor has spread to the body tissue below the skin.

  - There are additional tumor growths within 1 inch of the original tumor (satellite tumors).

  - The tumor has spread to nearby lymph nodes or there are additional tumor growths between the original tumor and the lymph nodes in the area.

- Stage IV: The tumor has spread to other organs or to lymph nodes at some distance from the original tumor.

Treatment

Surgery

Because it is necessary to remove a wider margin around a melanoma than other kinds of skin cancer, surgery is usually more extensive than for the same size squamous or basal cell carcinoma, the other type of skin cancers (see

"Basal Cell and Squamous Cell" and Chapter 15, "Surgery").

- Stage I and II melanomas are treated through surgery, using a wide excision of normal tissue and a skin graft, if necessary, to cover the wound.

- Stage III melanoma without lymph node involvement is also treated with surgery and skin grafts. If any lymph nodes are enlarged, they are removed.

- Stage IV melanoma treatment may include surgical excision of the primary tumor and other tumors that result from metastasis plus removal of affected lymph nodes.

It is unclear whether removing all lymph nodes near the site of the tumor, even if those nodes do not seem enlarged, will prevent the spread of melanoma and improve the outlook for survival.

Radiation

Most melanomas do not respond to radiation treatment, but it can temporarily relieve symptoms, such as bleeding or ulceration of the skin, especially in cases of spread to the brain, bones, or abdominal organs. Radiation therapy can also shrink lesions that are too large to excise or in a location where they cannot be removed easily (see Chapter 16, "Radiation").

Chemotherapy

Systemic chemotherapy may be an option. Single-drug chemotherapy with dacarbazine (DTIC) shrinks tumors in about 20 percent of cases of advanced disease and provides complete remission in less than 5 percent of patients. Drug combinations with dacarbazine (DTIC), carmustine (BiCNU), cisplatin (Platinol), and tamoxifen (Nolvadex) may shrink tumors by more than 50 percent in about half of cases; complete remission occurs in about 15 percent of cases, but the cancer usually recurs in a few months (see Chapters 17, "Chemotherapy," and 20, "Combination Treatments").

Survival

Melanoma is nearly 100 percent curable if it is

detected early. The thickness of a lesion is the most important factor in determining the survivability of the disease. Lesions less than 0.75 millimeter thick have a survival rate of nearly 100 percent. But survival at five years decreases to 20 to 50 percent when lesions are 3 millimeters or more thick, or if the cancer has spread to the lymph nodes. Five-year survival of stage IV melanoma is less than 10 percent.

Malignant melanoma is the tumor most often reported to disappear, although the incidence of spontaneous remission is less than 1 percent.

Special Needs

Careful follow-up is essential, because a person who has had one malignant melanoma has a 6 percent risk of developing another one. People with melanoma should check themselves for changes in skin growths. With training they can learn to recognize lumps under the skin and swollen lymph nodes under the arms or in the groin.

Liver function tests and chest x-rays every three months, and CT or MRI scans every six months are done in cases of advanced melanoma to monitor spread of the disease.

Ask About

If you have a stage I melanoma, talk with your doctor about how much tissue he or she will remove around the skin cancer. Typically, surgeons excise a wide margin of normal-looking tissue to make sure the whole tumor has been removed. But National Institutes of Health/U.S. government guidelines now advocate taking a narrower margin if the tumor is 1 millimeter or less in thickness. This minimizes disfigurement without affecting recurrence, metastasis, or mortality. There is some controversy about this method, but a growing body of scientific literature supports the approach.

Because patients who have had surgery for melanoma are at risk of recurrence, adjuvant therapy is often given to kill cancer cells remain-ing in the body for stage II or higher disease.

Isolated limb perfusion (also called *arterial perfusions*) is being evaluated when melanoma is in an arm or leg. This procedure involves giving high doses of anticancer drugs only to the affected limb. The technique stops blood flow to the limb temporarily, "detours" the blood through a machine that adds oxygen and the drug [usually melphalan (Alkeran)], and then returns it to the body. Sometimes the blood is heated during this process to enhance the drug's effectiveness. This method reduces the risk of systemic side effects. A similar investigational technique, intra-arterial regional infusion, involves stopping the blood circulation in the limb and infusing the drug (usually dacarbazine [DTIC] or cisplatin [Platinol]) directly into the main artery supplying the arm or leg.

Dacarbazine (DTIC) is being studied as a systemic chemotherapy for melanoma that has spread to lymph nodes and other sites. So far chemotherapy of melanoma with single drugs or drug combinations has not produced a significant impact on long-term survival.

Because some melanoma cells depend on estrogen for growth, the estrogen-blocking drug tamoxifen may prove to have a role in the treatment of melanoma. Clinical trials are currently under way to evaluate this therapy.

If you have stage III melanoma you may want to consider entering a clinical trial exploring one of several methods of boosting the immune response in advanced melanoma (see Chapter 18, "Biological Therapies"). The following are among the strategies: vaccines made of inactivated melanoma cells, either alone or in combination with the bacillus Calmette-Guerin (BCG); interferon, either alone or in combination with other biological agents or anticancer drugs; interleukin-2 and tumor-infiltrating leukocytes (TIL), sometimes used in combination with the anticancer drug cyclophosphamide (Cytoxan); and genetic therapy (see Chapter 21, "Investigational Treatments").

KIDNEY

Kidney cancer, also known as renal cell cancer, is the eleventh most common cancer, accounting for about 2 percent of adult cancers. About seven people in 100,000 are diagnosed with this type of cancer each year. The incidence has increased enormously since the 1950s, which may be due to greater exposure to various carcinogens in the environment and in certain occupations. It may also be the result of improved diagnostic methods.

Eighty-five percent of primary kidney cancers are *adenocarcinomas* that start in the lining of the tubules. Less common are *fibrosarcomas*, which start in the cells of the shell that encloses the kidney (see "Types," later). A small percentage of kidney malignancies are transitional cell cancers that arise in the renal pelvis, which has the same lining that the ureters and bladder have.

Located on either side of the backbone just above the waist, the two kidneys are bean-shaped organs about 3 inches wide, 5 inches long, and 1 inch thick. Each has a *ureter*, a muscular tube, about 10 inches long that carries urine to the bladder, a saclike structure low in the pelvic cavity.

The kidney is an organ of the urinary system. The renal artery brings blood to the kidney, where it is filtered through tiny tubules. Cleansed blood returns to the body through the renal vein; and the waste, mixed with water, drains into the hollow kidney pelvis, where it flows into the ureter. The kidneys also regulate the delicate balance of electrolytes such as sodium and potassium, and they produce a hormone that facilitates red blood cell formation.

If one kidney is damaged, missing, or must be removed, the other can handle its tasks. If both are only partly damaged, they often can still function adequately.

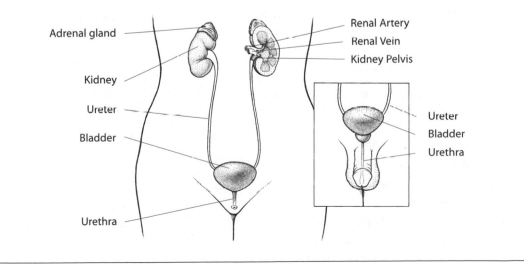

Adrenal gland
Kidney
Ureter
Bladder
Urethra

Renal Artery
Renal Vein
Kidney Pelvis

Ureter
Bladder
Urethra

There is no known cause of kidney cancer, but some experts believe it may be linked to chemical carcinogens that enter the body through the air or are ingested, such as nitrosamines, aflatoxins, asbestos, lead acetate, and potassium bromate. Because the kidney filters wastes, it is assumed that if these carcinogens enter the body, the kidney will eventually be exposed to them. Some experts believe that inherited factors make people less able to detoxify these carcinogens. Thus far, though, no direct link has been proved in humans. One exception is the analgesic phenacetin. Because it has been implicated in some cases of renal cell carcinoma, phenacetin is no longer approved by the U.S. Food and Drug Administration for use in pain-relieving products.

Some experts believe that benign tumors in the kidney called *adenomas* may become malignant and might be considered cancer *precursors*.

Certain inherited disorders—such as, von Hippel-Lindau's disease, Sturge-Weber syndrome, and neurofibromatosis—put a person at risk for kidney cancer, but familial cancers are quite rare.

Who Is at Risk?

- Women, who are twice as likely to get cancer of the kidney as men;

- Caucasian men, who are at somewhat higher risk than African-American men (transitional cell carcinoma is twice as common among Caucasian men as among African-American men);

- People between the ages of 50 and 70 (transitional cell carcinoma occurs primarily after the age of 65);

- People living in urban, industrialized areas;

- People whose jobs expose them to trace metals such as cadmium;

- People who used the analgesic phenacetin—once widely used in over-the-counter products such as APC (aspirin, phenacetin, and caffeine)—for a prolonged time;

- People exposed to certain chemicals such as nitrosamines, aflatoxins, lead acetate, and potassium bromate;

- People exposed to asbestos;

- Coke oven workers (workers in the rubber, leather, petroleum, dye, textile, and plastic industries may have an increased risk of transitional cell carcinoma);

- People who are obese, especially women, and possibly those who consume a diet high in animal fat;

- People with a family history of kidney cancer, especially when other inherited disorders are present, such as tuberous sclerosis, von Hippel-Laundau's disease, Sturge-Weber syndrome, neurofibromatosis, and ataxia telangiectasia;

- People who have undergone long-term hemodialysis treatment;

- Smokers, who are four times as likely to develop transitional kidney cancer as nonsmokers.

Screening Tests

No tests are available.

Types of Kidney Cancer

- Renal cell cancer (adenocarcinoma, or hypernephroma, and fibrosarcoma);

- Transitional cell cancer of the renal pelvis and/or ureter;

- Wilms' tumor, which occurs in children (see Chapter 35, "Cancer in Children").

Kidney cancer usually affects only one of the body's two kidneys. When cancer in one kidney has been successfully treated by surgery, the odds of it developing in the other are only 20 percent. If cancer occurs in the untreated kidney within the first year after surgery, the original cancer was probably bilateral but simply not detected earlier. If cancer develops more than a year after the first surgery, it is presumed to be a metastasis of the primary tumor. Differentiating between the two circumstances may affect subsequent treatment decisions.

Kidney cancer is most apt to spread first to lymph nodes in the pelvic region. Later, it may spread to the lungs, liver, bone, or brain.

Signs and Symptoms

- Most commonly, gross or microscopic blood in the urine;

- Pain in the side or one side of lower back;

- Less commonly, a smooth, hard lump at the side of the abdomen;

- Fever;

- High blood pressure;

- Fatigue and loss of appetite and weight.

Diagnostic and Staging Tests

For more information regarding these tests, see Chapter 8, "Diagnostic Tests."

- Urinalysis to detect blood in the urine;

- Urine cytology to detect abnormal cells in the urine;

- Ultrasound;

- Arteriogram;

- CT or MRI scan;

- Needle biopsy;

- Chest and skeletal x-rays, liver function studies, and bone scan if metastasis is suspected.

Tests Unique to Kidney Cancer

Intravenous pyelography (IVP) is a series of x-rays of the kidney taken five, 10, and 15 minutes after a special dye has been injected into the bloodstream. As the dye circulates through the kidney, the structure and function of the kidneys, ureters, and bladder can be evaluated. Some people complain of a brief, generalized burning sensation and a metallic taste when the dye is injected. The only other discomfort arises from having to maintain a still position during the x-ray. It is necessary to fast for eight hours prior to the test.

A *nephrotomogram* is a series of x-rays of cross sections of the kidney. These x-ray views are taken from several angles, before and after injection of a contrast dye that helps visualize the kidney.

Ureteroscopy may be recommended to aid in staging cancer of the ureters or renal pelvis. After a local anesthetic has been instilled into the urethra to numb the area, a narrow flexible tube is passed through it, into the bladder, and into a ureter. The tube, fitted with a magnifying lens and light source, is a variation on an endoscope and is called a *ureteroscope*. If any abnormal tissue is observed, small instruments may be inserted through the scope to retrieve samples for biopsy. The procedure may be repeated in the other ureter. There is little discomfort, because the patient receives a sedative, but during the procedure, which takes less than 30 minutes, there may be an urge to urinate.

Be sure to drink plenty of fluids for several hours before and after ureteroscopy. This helps maintain a good flow of urine, which may prevent infection by bacteria that enter the urinary tract during the examination. Further, diluted urine will decrease burning during urination that may occur after the test.

Staging

Renal Cell Cancer

- Stage I: A tumor of 2.5 centimeters or less is found only in the kidney.

- Stage II: A tumor of more than 2.5 centimeters is found and has spread into the fat surrounding the kidney but has not spread to or through the capsule that contains the kidney.

- Stage III: The cancer has spread beyond the kidney in one of three ways: to the main vein that carries blood from the kidney, to the blood vessel that carries blood from the lower part of the body to the heart (inferior vena cava), or to lymph nodes immediately in the vicinity of the kidney, but it has not extended beyond the fibrous membrane that encapsulates the kidney.

- Stage IV: Cancer has spread to nearby organs such as the bowel or pancreas or has spread to other places in the body, such as the lungs.

Transitional Cell Cancer

The American Joint Committee on Cancer has established four stages for cancer of the renal pelvis and ureter, which is similar to bladder cancer. However, cancer may also be described in the following way:

- *Localized*: The cancer is limited to the collection system or pelvis of the kidney and has not spread outside the kidney or ureter. Within this category are:
  - Group 1, low-grade tumors described as of *papilloma* quality, meaning they are pendulous, mushroomlike growths that are very superficial;
  - Group 2, grade I to II carcinomas, which have not significantly invaded underlying tissue but not through the kidney pelvis;
  - Group 3, high-grade tumors, which have entered the renal pelvic wall or passed through it.
- *Regional*: Group 4, tumors that have spread to pelvic lymph nodes or other tissue around the kidney;
- *Metastatic*: Tumors that have spread to other parts of the body.

Treatment

Surgery—radical nephrectomy—is often curative when cancer is limited to the kidney. This is the mainstay of treatment (see Chapter 15, "Surgery").

In stage I renal cell cancer, *simple nephrectomy* removes the whole kidney. More commonly, depending on the surgical findings, a *radical nephrectomy* is done to remove tissue around the kidney, including the adrenal gland and the encapsulating fascia, and neighboring lymph nodes.

A *partial nephrectomy* may be done to remove only the low-grade and early-stage cancer and some of the tissue surrounding it, if the other kidney has been removed, is damaged, and/or is affected by the cancer.

In stage II or III renal cell cancer, radiation therapy may be given before or after nephrectomy (see Chapter 16, "Radiation"). Although this may improve survival results compared with surgery alone in selected individuals, there has not been conclusive evidence of radiotherapy's general benefit. Chemotherapy is used infrequently.

Total nephroureterectomy is removal of the kidney, ureter, and a portion of the bladder. It is indicated in transitional cell cancer if the renal pelvis or ureter or both are involved with transitional cancer.

Survival

Renal cell cancer can often be cured if it is confined to the kidney and immediately surrounding tissue when it is diagnosed. Even when lymph glands or blood vessels in the area are affected, a significant number of people can have prolonged survival and possibly be cured.

Renal Cell Cancer

After treatment:

- Five-year survival rate for stages I and II, with cancer confined to the kidney, is 70 percent.
- Five-year survival rate for some stage III cancers, when some tissues around the kidney and even the adrenal gland may be involved but the tumor is still contained within the capsule, is 50 percent.
- Five-year survival rate for stage III cancers involving the renal vein, inferior vena cava, and/or regional lymph nodes, or both, is 35 percent.
- Five-year survival for stage IV cancers with metastases to adjacent organs other than the adrenals or to distant sites is 5 percent.

Transitional Cell Cancer

Treatment can have a very positive outcome when diagnosed and treated early.

- Five-year survival for localized group 1 and 2 cancers is nearly 100 percent after nephroureterectomy.

- Five-year survival for localized group 3 cancers is 10 to 20 percent after nephroureterectomy because of the greater risk of distant spread.

- Five-year survival for regional cancers is 10 to 20 percent.

- Five-year survival for transitional cell cancer of the ureters is generally 10 to 20 percent lower than that of renal pelvic tumors, depending on the extent to which the cancer has penetrated the ureteral wall.

Special Needs

Smokers should quit immediately to reduce the risk of kidney cancer recurrence.

Those whose work involves electroplating, alloy making, or welding should consider a job with less hazardous tasks. In any circumstance, exposure to cadmium must be scrupulously avoided. Use all available personal protective equipment properly.

A posttreatment checkup is recommended every three months for the first five years, every six months for the next five years, and annually thereafter. It will likely include a physical examination, blood tests, and a CT scan of the abdomen; further tests may be required if there are any signs of metastasis.

Those who have had transitional cell cancer of the ureters should have periodic cystoscopies because these tumors tend to recur in the bladder. However, such bladder cancers can usually be very easily treated and cured if detected promptly (see "Bladder").

Ask About

Renal Cell Cancer

If you have stage II renal cell cancer you may want to discuss radiation therapy before or after surgery. In some selected people it may be helpful, but in many it does not improve survival. If the tumor is inoperable or it has significantly enlarged the kidney, you may want to inquire about *arterial embolization* to alleviate symptoms. This procedure involves the injection of small pieces of a special gelatin sponge into the main blood vessel that enters the kidney. This blocks the blood cells that feed the tumor, preventing the cancer cells from getting oxygen and other substances they need to grow.

You may also want to consider entering one of the clinical trials evaluating interferon (see Chapters 18, "Biological Therapies," and 21, "Investigational Treatments") and various combinations of chemotherapy drugs.

Transitional Cell Carcinoma

You may want to investigate several different approaches to treating transitional cell carcinoma before embarking on a course of therapy. Clinical trials are evaluating the use of electrofulguration and laser surgery, for example, which is done through an instrument inserted into the ureter. Some studies are evaluating direct introduction of chemotherapy drugs. Various biological therapies are also being tested to determine if the body's immune system can be stimulated to fight the cancer.

BLADDER

Bladder cancer is the fourth most common cancer in men and the eighth most common in women. The incidence rate is about four times greater among men than among women. It accounts for 7 percent of all cancers in men and 2 percent of those in women.

Carcinogens and inherited factors that make people less able to detoxify them seem to play a role in causing bladder cancer. For example, cigarette smokers develop bladder cancers four times as often as nonsmokers. Chronic irritation due to urinary stones and parasitic infection also are predisposing factors.

The most common type of bladder tumor is shaped like a tiny mushroom, with its stem attached to the inner lining of the bladder. Several of these *papillary* tumors may occur at once, and they are most likely to be malignant. Less common are solid tumors that grow directly in the lining of the bladder and can invade its muscular wall.

The empty *bladder* is about the size and shape of a pear. It is located in the lower pelvic cavity. Urine drains from the kidneys into the bladder through the *ureters*. From the bladder, urine is excreted through a tube called the *urethra*. In women, this tube is about 1.5 inches long and exits the body at the upper aspect of the vaginal opening. In men the urethra is about 8 inches long and passes through the penis, opening at its tip.

The bladder has flexible muscular walls three layers thick. As urine fills the bladder, these walls expand; they contract to expel urine. Although the bladder can hold about a pint of urine, the urge to urinate usually starts when it is about half full.

Who Is at Risk?

- People who smoke;

- People between the ages of 60 and 80;

- People who have taken certain chemotherapy drugs, such as cyclophosphamide (Cytoxan) or who have had radiation therapy to the pelvic area;

- Workers exposed to industrial chemicals, such as benzidine and beta-naphthylamine, aniline dyes, and organic chemicals used or produced in rubber manufacture, leather treatment, and paint production.

Screening Tests

No tests are available. However, smokers and people who have been exposed to industrial carcinogens associated with the risk of bladder cancer should consider annual testing for blood or abnormal cells in the urine.

Types of Bladder Cancer

Transitional Cell Carcinoma

Transitional cell carcinoma accounts for more than 90 percent of all bladder cancers. Early ones most commonly occur as one or more superficial papillary tumors that are easily treated. More advanced cases can invade the bladder's muscular wall.

Squamous Cell Cancer

About 8 percent of bladder cancers are the squamous cell type and usually have infiltrated the bladder wall at the time of diagnosis.

Adenocarcinoma

Adenocarcinomas account for about 2 percent of all bladder cancers. This type is likely to have spread from a primary cancer in the bowel.

Cancer may recur in the bladder or metastasize to other sites, such as the lymph nodes in the pelvis and groin, liver, lungs, and bones.

Carcinosarcoma

Carcinosarcoma is a very rare type of bladder cancer.

Signs and Symptoms

- Occasional to frequent blood in the urine, which appears smoky, rusty, or deep red. This is the only symptom in about 80 percent of people.

- Increased frequency of urination;

- Burning sensation during urination;

- Urge to urinate but nothing passes;

- Rarely, incontinence;

- Pain, which may occur in more advanced bladder cancers.

Diagnostic and Staging Tests

For more information regarding these tests, see Chapter 8, "Diagnostic Tests."

- Urinalysis to detect blood;

- Urine cytology to detect abnormal cells;

- Intravenous pyelography (IVP) (see "Kidney" in the Encyclopedia);

- Biopsy, in which a sample of suspicious tissue may be removed from the bladder during *cystoscopy*;

- Chest and skeletal x-rays, liver function studies, CT scan and bone scan if metastasis is suspected.

Tests Unique to Bladder Cancer

Cystoscopy involves insertion of a narrow, flexible tube, fitted with a magnifying lens and light source, through the urethra and into the bladder. If any abnormal tissue is observed, small instruments may be inserted through the cystoscope to retrieve tissue samples for biopsy. A local anesthetic instilled into the urethra numbs the area.

> Be sure to drink plenty of fluids for several hours before and after cystoscopy. This helps maintain a good flow of urine, which may prevent an infection by bacteria that can enter the tract during examination. Medication is given following the procedure to prevent any burning during urination that would occur after the test.

Staging

- Stage 0: This is very early cancer, found only on the inner lining of the bladder. It includes noninvasive papillary carcinoma and carcinoma in situ, which can be slow growing and cover a large area. It is also known as *flat tumor*.

- Stage I: Cancer extends into the bladder's inner lining but has not reached the muscular wall.

- Stage II: Cancer has spread to the inside lining of the bladder's muscular wall or beyond to the muscle or the perivesical fat.

- Stage III: Cancer has invaded the perivesical fat and possibly the prostate, uterus, or vagina.

- Stage IV: A tumor of any size with lymph node involvement or metastasis. In some cases, cancer may have spread to distant lymph nodes and other organs further removed from the bladder.

Treatment

Transurethral resection (TUR), removal or destruction of the tumor through a cystoscope, is the most common treatment when bladder cancer is diagnosed early. One or more papillary tumors can be surgically removed with an instrument that passes through the cystoscope, or the tumor(s) can be vaporized with a laser or burned away with electricity (*fulguration*).

Surgery involving an external incision is needed if the cancer is more extensive (see Chapter 15, "Surgery"). If the cancer is in only one area, particularly the dome of the bladder, only part of the organ is removed in a *segmental cystectomy*. *Total cystectomy* removes the entire bladder. A radical cystectomy removes the bladder and tissue surrounding it, which in women may include the uterus, ovaries, fallopian tubes, the urethra, and part of the vagina. In men, it may include the prostate, seminal vesicles, and sometimes the urethra. Lymph nodes in the pelvis are also taken out.

When the bladder is removed, the surgeon creates a new conduit to carry urine from the ureters to an opening, or *stoma*, in the abdominal wall (a *urostomy*) using a section of the small intestine or the colon. A bag fitted over the stoma collects the urine, and it is emptied periodically. Sometimes part of the small intestine can be used to make a new storage pouch inside the body, which is then drained at intervals with a catheter. Newer techniques may enable an inside pouch to be connected to the urethra for normal urine passage.

In very advanced cancer, the bladder may not be removed but, to relieve symptoms, an ostomy may be created so urine can pass out of the body.

Chemotherapy drugs may be instilled directly into the bladder to treat early-stage and low-grade lesions (see Chapter 17, "Chemotherapy"). This is called *intravesical therapy*. A narrow tube is inserted into the bladder, and the medication is instilled through it. Urination is avoided for at least one hour. Treatment is repeated once a week for about six weeks. Two weeks later a cystoscopy is done and possibly another biopsy.

Intravesical therapy may also follow surgery in an attempt to prevent recurrence.

Radiation therapy is sometimes used alone or in addition to surgery to help shrink tumors. It may be delivered by an external beam, or radioisotopes may be surgically implanted in the pelvic cavity (see Chapters 16, "Radiation," and 20, "Combination Treatments").

When bladder cancer is more advanced and widespread in the body, in addition to radical cystectomy, chemotherapy may include drugs such as methotrexate, vinblastine (Velban), doxorubicin (Adriamycin), and cisplatin (Platinol) (known as MVAC).

Survival

If diagnosed early, bladder cancer is one of the most easily treated malignancies.

- Five-year survival for stage 0 noninvasive papillary carcinoma and carcinoma in situ is 90 percent.

- Five-year survival for stage I without deep cancerous invasion is 75 percent.

- Five-year survival for stage II with invasion of the deep muscle of the bladder is 35 percent.

- Five-year survival for stage III with cancerous invasion through the bladder wall and into the perivesical fat is 20 percent.

- Five-year survival for stage IV with metastasis to distant lymph nodes or organs is 9 percent.

Special Needs

Smokers should quit immediately to reduce the risk of bladder cancer recurrence.

Those whose work requires exposure to chemicals associated with bladder cancer should consider a job with less hazardous tasks. If this is not possible, all available personal protective equipment should be used.

The Ostomy Rehabilitation Program of the American Cancer Society and the United Ostomy Association can provide help in living with a urinary ostomy (see Appendix I, "Resources").

In men, if cancer has spread beyond the bladder and removal of the prostate is necessary, impotence may result; in women, if part of the vagina must be removed, sexual difficulties also may arise. Special counseling can assist in developing new ways of expressing sexual intimacy (see Chapter 30, "Sexuality").

After pelvic radiation therapy, women may develop a dry, inelastic vagina. Use of a water-based lubricant or a prescribed estrogen cream may be helpful.

All bladder cancer patients require ongoing checkups by their urologist. Even in the earliest cases treated with TUR followed by six weeks of intravesical therapy, cystoscopy and biopsy are repeated a few weeks after the last treatment; urine evaluation is usually done every three months and cystoscopy every six months. After a period of time, if no changes are seen, cytology of urine is negative, and the patient is not smoking, checkups are reduced to annual visits. However, urine cytology may be done every three to four months.

> Avoid drinking any fluids for several hours before intravesical therapy. This will decrease the urge to urinate, permitting the medicated fluid to be retained in the bladder for a longer time, preferably at least one to two hours.

Ask About

If you have a cancer that cannot be cured with surgery and intravesical chemotherapy (see "Treatment," earlier)—and most superficial cancers can be effectively treated this way—you may want to discuss participating in one of the clinical trials designed to evaluate a range of treatments. These include studies of new chemotherapy drugs and combinations of standard ones; radiologic techniques; and biological therapies, such as intravesical therapy with bacillus Calmette-Guernin (BCG) and interferon (see Chapter 18, "Biological Therapies").

Clinical trials are evaluating whether chemotherapy or radiation therapy may be more effective before or after cystectomy in advanced cases of bladder cancer (see Chapter 21, "Investigational Treatments"). For stage I cancer, clinical trials are being conducted to evaluate chemoprevention as a means of avoiding recurrence.

RESOURCES

Listings in this chapter represent organizations that operate on a national level or local organizations that provide services in other parts of the country as well. However, there are local or regional resources too numerous to mention that help people only in their area. This list is designed to give you a starting point for seeking information. If you have a question that cannot be answered by one of the sources listed here, do not give up. Many of these organizations provide referrals, and your questions may be directed to other organizations or individuals.

You will note that e-mail (electronic mail) or Internet addresses (beginning with http) are listed for some of the following organizations. Consult Appendix II, "Cancer Information On Line," for resource listings and instructions for communicating with individuals and cancer organizations electronically, including how to obtain Internet addresses that may not be listed here.

American Cancer Society

The American Cancer Society (ACS) provides educational material and information on cancer, maintains several rehabilitation and support programs, and directs people to services in their community. (Individual programs are listed throughout this appendix.) Contact the division office for your state or region to find your local office, or call 800-ACS-2345.

National Office

1599 Clifton Road NE
Atlanta, GA 30329-4251
800-ACS-2345
800-227-2345
http://www.cancer.org

Chartered Divisions

There are forty-nine ACS chartered divisions and over 3,400 regional offices throught the United States and Puerto Rico. They are responsible for providing cancer control programs and activities to the communities in their area. Note that the following division listings are organized by state. If you live in Kansas, Nebraska, Missouri, or Oklahoma, see the Heartland Division listing in Missouri.

Mid-South Division, Inc.
504 Brookwood Boulevard
Homewood, AL 35209
205-879-2242
205-870-7436 Fax

Alaska Division, Inc.
406 West Fireweed Lane, Suite 204
Anchorage, AK 99503
907-277-8696
907-263-2073 Fax

Southwest Division, Inc.
2929 East Thomas Road
Phoenix, AZ 85016
602-224-0524
602-381-3096 Fax

Mid-South Division, Inc.
901 North University
Little Rock, AR 72203
501-664-3480
501-666-0068 Fax

California Division, Inc.
1710 Webster Street
Oakland, CA 94612
510-893-7900
510-835-8656 Fax

Colorado Division, Inc.
2255 South Oneida
Denver, CO 80224
303-758-2030
303-758-7006 Fax

Connecticut Division, Inc.
Barnes Park South
14 Village Lane
Wallingford, CT 06492
203-265-7161
203-265-0281 Fax

Delaware Division, Inc.
92 Read's Way, Suite 205
New Castle, DE 19720
302-324-4227
302-324-4233 Fax

District of Columbia Division, Inc.
1875 Connecticut Avenue NW,
Suite 730
Washington, DC 20009
202-483-2600
202-483-1174 Fax

Florida Division, Inc.
3709 West Jetton Avenue
Tampa, FL 33629-5146
813-253-0541
813-254-5857 Fax

Georgia Division, Inc.
Lenox Park
2200 Lake Boulevard
Atlanta, GA 30319
404-816-7800
404-816-9443 Fax

Hawaii Pacific Division, Inc.
Community Services Center Building
2370 Nuuanu Avenue
Honolulu, HI 96817
808-595-7500
808-595-7502 Fax

Idaho Division, Inc.
2676 Vista Avenue
Boise, ID 83705-0836
208-343-4609
208-343-9922 Fax

Illinois Division, Inc.
77 East Monroe Street
Chicago, IL 60603-5795
312-641-6150
312-641-6588 Fax

Indiana Division, Inc.
8730 Commerce Park Place
Indianapolis, IN 46268
317-872-4432
317-879-4114 Fax

Iowa Division, Inc.
8364 Hickman Road, Suite D
Des Moines, IA 50325-4300
515-253-0147
515-253-0806 Fax

Kentucky Division, Inc.
701 West Muhammad Ali
Boulevard
Louisville, KY 40203-1909
502-584-6782
502-584-8946 Fax

Mid-South Division, Inc.
2200 Veteran's Memorial
Boulevard, Suite 214
Kenner, LA 70062
504-469-0021
504-469-0033 Fax

Maine Division, Inc.
52 Federal Street
Brunswick, ME 04011
207-729-3339
207-729-0635 Fax

Maryland Division, Inc.
8219 Town Center Drive
Baltimore, MD 21236-0026
410-931-6868
410-931-6875 Fax

Massachusetts Division, Inc.
247 Commonwealth Avenue
Boston, MA 02116
617-267-2650
617-536-3163 Fax

Michigan Division, Inc.
1205 East Saginaw Street
Lansing, MI 48906
517-371-2920
517-371-2605 Fax

Minnesota Division, Inc.
3316 West 66th Street
Minneapolis, MN 55435
612-925-2772
612-925-6333 Fax

Mid-South Division, Inc.
1380 Livingston Lane
Lakeover Office Park
Jackson, MS 39213
601-362-8874
601-362-8876 Fax

Heartland Division, Inc.
1100 Pennsylvania Avenue
Kansas City, MO 64105
816-842-7111
816-842-8828 Fax

Montana Division, Inc.
17 North 26th Street
Billings, MT 59101
406-252-7111
406-252-7112 Fax

Southwest Division, Inc.
1325 East Harmon
Las Vegas, NV 89119
702-798-6857
702-798-0530 Fax

New Hampshire Division, Inc.
Gail Singer Memorial Building
360 State Route 101, Suite 501
Bedford, NH 03110-5032
603-472-8899
603-472-7093 Fax

New Jersey Division, Inc.
2600 US Highway 1
North Brunswick, NJ 08902-0803
908-297-8000
908-297-9043 Fax

Southwest Division, Inc.
5800 Lomas Boulevard NE
Albuquerque NM 87110
505-260-2105
505-266-9513 Fax

New York City Division, Inc.
19 West 56th Street
New York, NY 10019
212-586-8700
212-237-3852 Fax

New York State Division, Inc.
6725 Lyons Street
East Syracuse, NY 13057
315-437-7025
315-437-0540 Fax

Queens Division, Inc.
112-25 Queens Boulevard
Forest Hills, NY 11375
718-263-2224
718-261-0758 Fax

Long Island Division, Inc.
75 Davids Drive
Hauppauge, NY 11788
516-436-7070
516-436-5380 Fax

Westchester Division, Inc.
30 Glenn Street
White Plains, NY 10603
914-949-4800
914-949-4279 Fax

North Carolina Division, Inc.
11 South Boylan Avenue, Suite 221
Raleigh, NC 27603
919-843-8463
919-839-0551 Fax

North Dakota Division, Inc.
1005 Westrac Drive
Fargo, ND 58102
701-232-1385
701-232-1109 Fax

Ohio Division, Inc.
5555 Frantz Road
Dublin, OH 43017
614-889-9565
614-889-6578 Fax

Oregon Division, Inc.
0330 SW Curry Street
Portland, OR 97201
503-295-6422
503-228-1062 Fax

Pennsylvania Division, Inc.
Route 422 and Sipe Avenue
Hershey, PA 17033-0897
717-533-6144
717-534-1075 Fax

Philadelphia Division, Inc.
1626 Locust Street
Philadelphia, PA 19103
215-665-2900
215-985-5406 Fax

Puerto Rico Division, Inc.
Calle Alverio #577
Esquina Sargento Medina
Hato Rey, PR 00918
809-764-2295
809-764-0553 Fax

Rhode Island Division, Inc.
400 Main Street
Pawtucket, RI 02860
401-722-8480
401-727-9449 Fax

South Carolina Division, Inc.
128 Stonemark Lane
Columbia, SC 29210-3855
803-750-1693
803-750-4000 Fax

South Dakota Division, Inc.
4101 South Carnegie Place
Sioux Falls, SD 57106-2322
605-361-8277
605-361-8537 Fax

Tennessee Division, Inc.
1315 Eighth Avenue South
Nashville, TN 37203
615-255-1227
615-255-1230 Fax

Texas Division, Inc.
2433 Ridgepoint Drive
Austin, TX 78754
512-928-2262
512-929-9243 Fax

Utah Division, Inc.
941 East 3300 South
Salt Lake City, UT 84106
801-483-1500
801-483-1558 Fax

Vermont Division, Inc.
13 Loomis Street
Montpelier, VT 05602
802-223-2348
802-223-2818 Fax

Virginia Division, Inc.
4240 Park Place Court
Glen Allen, VA 23060
804-527-3700
804-527-3792 Fax

Western Pacific Division, Inc.
2120 First Avenue North
Seattle, WA 98209-1140
206-283-1152
206-283-3469 Fax

West Virginia Division, Inc.
2428 Kanawha Boulevard East
Charleston, WV 25311
304-344-3611
304-343-6549 Fax

Wisconsin Division, Inc.
N19 W24350 Riverwood Drive
Waukesha, WI 53188
414-523-5500
414-523-5533 Fax

Wyoming Division, Inc.
4202 Ridge Road
Cheyenne, WY 82001
307-638-3331
307-638-1199 Fax

National Cancer Institute

The National Cancer Institute (NCI) has a toll-free telephone service for people with cancer and their families, the public, and health care professionals. You can access the latest information about cancer and local resources by calling 800-4-CANCER. You may also be connected to the regional NCI center that serves your area.

National Cancer Institute
National Institutes of Health
Bethesda, MD 20892
301-496-4000
800-4-CANCER
800-422-6237
http://wwwicic.nci.gor/nci-icic.html

Comprehensive Cancer Centers

Comprehensive Cancer Centers have been designated as such by the National Cancer Institute. They are required to have basic laboratory research in several fields; to be able to transfer research findings into clinical practice; to conduct clinical studies and trials; to research cancer prevention and control; to offer information about cancer to patients, the public, and health care professionals; and to provide community service related to cancer control. See Chapter 11.

University of Alabama at
Birmingham
Comprehensive Cancer Center
Basic Health Sciences Building
1824 Sixth Avenue South
Birmingham, AL 35294-3300
205-934-5077
http://www.ccc.uab.edu

University of Arizona Cancer
Center
1501 North Campbell Avenue
Tucson, AZ 85724
602-626-7925

Jonsson Comprehensive Cancer Center
University of California at Los Angeles
10833 Le Conte Avenue
Los Angeles, CA 90095-1781
800-825-2631
310-825-5268

USC/Norris Comprehensive Cancer
Center
University of Southern California
1441 Eastlake Avenue
Los Angeles, CA 90033-0800
213-764-0816

Yale Comprehensive Cancer Center
Yale University School of Medicine
333 Cedar Street
New Haven, CT 06520-8028
203-785-4095

Lombardi Cancer Research Center
Georgetown University Medical
Center
3800 Reservoir Road NW
Washington, DC 20007
202-687-2110

Sylvester Comprehensive Cancer
Center
University of Miami Medical School
1475 Northwest 12th Avenue
Miami, FL 33136
305-548-4918

The Johns Hopkins Oncology Center
600 North Wolfe Street
Baltimore, MD 21287-8943
· 410-955-8822

Dana-Farber Cancer Institute
44 Binney Street
Boston, MA 02115
617-632-2223
http://www.dfci.harvard.edu

University of Michigan
Comprehensive Cancer Center
102 Observatory
Ann Arbor, MI 48109-0724
313-936-1831
http://www.cancer.med.umich.edu:8
0/cancen.html

Barbara Ann Karmanos Cancer
Institute
110 East Warren Avenue
Detroit, MI 48201
313-833-1146

Norris Cotton Cancer Center
Dartmouth-Hitchcock Medical
Center
One Medical Center Drive
Lebanon, NH 03756
603-650-4141

Roswell Park Cancer Institute
Elm and Carlton Streets
Buffalo, NY 14263
800-767-9355
213-845-5770
http://rpci.med.buffalo.edu/index.html

Columbia-Presbyterian
Comprehensive Cancer Center
College of Physicians and Surgeons
701 West 168th Street
New York, NY 10032
212-305-6921
http://cpmcnet.columbia.edu

Memorial Sloan-Kettering Cancer
Center
1275 York Avenue
New York, NY 10021
800-525-2225
212-639-6561
http://www.mskcc.org

UNC Lineberger Comprehensive
Cancer Center
University of North Carolina
School of Medicine
Chapel Hill, NC 27599
919-966-3036

Duke Comprehensive Cancer
Center
Duke University Medical Center
Durham, NC 27710
919-684-5613

Comprehensive Cancer Center of
Wake Forest University at Bowman
Gray School of Medicine
Medical Center Boulevard
Winston-Salem, NC 27157
919-716-7971

Ohio State University
Comprehensive Cancer Center
Arthur G. James Cancer Hospital
300 West 10th Avenue
Columbus, OH 43210
800-638-6996
614-293-4878
http://www.cancer.med.ohio-
state.edu

Fox Chase Cancer Center
7701 Burholme Avenue
Philadelphia, PA 19111
215-728-2781
http://www.fccc.edu

University of Pennsylvania Cancer
Center
3400 Spruce Street
Philadelphia, PA 19104
215-662-6334

University of Pittsburgh Cancer
Institute
200 Meyran Avenue
Pittsburgh, PA 15213-2592
800-537-4063
412-692-4670

The University of Texas
M.D. Anderson Cancer Center
1515 Holcolmbe Boulevard
Houston, TX 77030
713-792-7500
http://utmdacc.uth.tmc.edu

San Antonio Cancer Institute
8122 Datapoint Drive
San Antonio, TX 78229
210-616-5580

Vermont Regional Cancer Center
University of Vermont
1 South Prospect Street
Burlington, VT 05401
802-656-4414

Fred Hutchinson Cancer Research
Center
1124 Columbia Street
Seattle, WA 98104
206-667-5000
206-667-4302

University of Wisconsin
Comprehensive Cancer Center
600 Highland Avenue
Madison, WI 53792
608-263-8610

Clinical Cancer Centers

Clinical Cancer Centers have support from the National Cancer Institute for programs that investigate new treatments or research programs. For information on a clinical cancer center in your area, call the National Cancer Institute's Cancer Information Service at 800-4-CANCER. See also Chapter 11.

City of Hope National Medical
Center
Beckman Research Institute
1500 East Duarte Road
Duarte, CA 91010
818-359-8111
818-301-8164
http://www.cityofhope.org

University of California at Irvine
Cancer Center
101 The City Drive
Orange, CA 92668
714-456-6310

University of California at San
Diego Cancer Center
200 West Arbor Drive
San Diego, CA 92103
619-543-3325

University of Colorado Cancer Center
4200 East 9th Avenue
Denver, CO 80262
303-270-3007

University of Chicago Cancer
Research Center
5841 South Maryland Avenue
Chicago, IL 60637
312-702-6180

Robert H. Lurie Cancer Center
Northwestern University
303 East Chicago Avenue
Olson Pavilion, Room 8250
Chicago, IL 60611
312-908-5250
http://www.nums.nwu.edu/lurie/index.
html/

Mayo Cancer Center
Mayo Foundation
200 First Street SW
Rochester, MN 55905
507-284-3753

Albert Einstein College of Medicine
Cancer Research Center
Chanin Building
1300 Morris Park Avenue
Bronx, NY 10461
718-430-2302

Kaplan Cancer Center
New York University Medical
Center
550 First Avenue
New York, NY 10016
212-263-5349

University of Rochester Cancer
Center
601 Elmwood Avenue
Rochester, NY 14642
716-275-6292

Case Western Reserve University
Cancer Research Center
11100 Euclid Avenue
Cleveland, OH 44106
216-844-8652

Jefferson Cancer Center
Thomas Jefferson University
233 South 10th Street
Philadelphia, PA 19107
215-503-4645

St. Jude Children's Research
Hospital
332 North Lauderdale
Memphis, TN 38105
901-495-3301

Vanderbilt Cancer Center
Vanderbilt University
649 Medical Research Building II
Nashville, TN 37232
615-936-1782

Huntsman Cancer Institute
University of Utah Health
Sciences Center
Building 533
Salt Lake City, UT 84112
801-581-4048
801-581-4330

Cancer Center
University of Virginia Health
Sciences Center
Charlottesville, VA 22908
804-924-2562

Massey Cancer Center
Medical College of Virginia
1200 East Broad Street
Richmond, VA 23298
804-828-0450

Clinical Trials Cooperative Groups

The Clinical Trials Cooperative Group Program is a major component of the National Cancer Institute's (NCI) effort to generate and conduct clinical trials. It was started in 1955—after Congress approved a proposal to increase support for the study of chemotherapy in the treatment of cancer. The program is composed of academic institutions and cancer treatment centers throughout the United States. Some groups concentrate on the treatment of a single kind of cancer, others study a specific type of therapy, and still others focus on a variety of cancers. You may contact a clinical trials cooperative group or ask your physician to contact an appropriate one for you.

Brain Tumor Cooperative Group
William R. Shapiro, M.D., Chair
Barrow Neurological Institute
St. Joseph Hospital and Medical Center
350 West Thomas Road
Phoenix, AZ 85013

Eastern Cooperative Oncology Group
Douglass Tormey, M.D., Chair
AMC Research Center
1600 Pierce Street
Denver, CO 80214

Pediatric Oncology Group
Sharon P. Murphy, M.D., Chair
645 North Michigan Avenue, Suite 910
Chicago, IL 60611

Intergroup Rhabdomyosarcoma Study
Harold M. Maurer, M.D., Chair
Dean's Office
University of Nebraska College of Medicine
600 South 42nd Street
Omaha, NE 68198-6545

Cancer and Leukemia Group B
O. Ross McIntyre, M.D., Chair
Central Office of the Chair
444 Mount Support Road, Suite 2
Rural Route 3, Box 750
Lebanon, NH 03766

National Wilms' Tumor Study Group
Daniel M. Green, M.D., Chair
Roswell Park Cancer Institute
Elm and Carlton Streets
Buffalo, NY 14263

North Central Cancer Treatment Group
Michael J. O'Connell, M.D., Chair
Mayo Foundation
200 First Street, SW
Rochester, NY 55905

Gynecologic Oncology Group
Robert C. Park, M.D., Chair
GOC Central Office
Suite 1945
1234 Market Street
Philadelphia, PA 19107

National Surgical Adjuvant Breast and Bowel Project
Ronald Heberman, M.D., Interim Chair
University of Pittsburgh
914 Scaife Hall

3550 Terrace Street
Pittsburgh, PA 15261

Quality Assurance Review Center
Arvin S. Glicksman, M.D., Chair
Roger Williams General Hospital
825 Chalkstone Avenue
Providence, RI 02908

Children's Cancer Group
W. Archie Bleyer, M.D., Chair
Department of Pediatrics, Box 87
University of Texas Medical Department
Anderson Cancer Center
1515 Holcolmbe Boulevard
Houston, TX 77030

Radiation Therapy Oncology Group
James Cox, M.D., Chair
University of Texas M.D. Anderson Cancer Center
1515 Holcolmbe Boulevard
Houston, TX 77030

Southwest Oncology Group
Charles A. Coltman, M.D., Chair
14980 Omicron Drive
San Antonio, TX 78245-3217

Community Clinical Oncology Programs

Community Clinical Oncology Programs link community-based doctors with the Clinical Trials Cooperative Group Program, cancer centers, and public health departments for participation in National Cancer Institute-approved treatment and clinical trials. These programs promote participation by people with cancer in clinical trials and disperse the latest research findings to the community level.

University of South Alabama
Minority-Based CCOP
USA Cancer Center, Room 414
307 University Boulevard
Mobile, AL 36688
205-460-7194

Greater Phoenix CCOP
925 East McDowell Road, 2nd floor
Phoenix, AZ 85006-2726
602-239-2413

Scottsdale CCOP Mayo Clinic
13400 East Shea Boulevard
Scottsdale, AZ 85259
602-301-8294

Bay Area Tumor Institute CCOP
2844 Summit Street, Suite 204
Oakland, CA 94609-3637
510-465-8570

Central Los Angeles CCOP
St. Vincent Medical Center
P.O. Box 57992
2131 West Third Street
Los Angeles, CA 90057
213-484-7086

San Diego Kaiser Permanente CCOP
Department of Oncology
4647 Zion Avenue
San Diego, CA 92120
619-528-5888

Medical Center of Delaware CCOP
P.O. Box 1668
Wilmington, DE 19899
302-731-8116

Florida Pediatric CCOP
Florida Association of Pediatric Tumor Programs, Inc.

P.O. Box 17757
Tampa, FL 33682-7757
813-632-1310

Mount Sinai Community Clinical Oncology Program
Mount Sinai Medical Center
4300 Alton Road
Miami Beach, FL 33140
305-674-2625

Atlanta Regional CCOP
St. Joseph's Hospital
5665 Peachtree Dunwoody Road NE
Atlanta, GA 30342-1701
404-851-7114

Grady Hospital Minority-Based CCOP
P.O. Box 26149
Atlanta, GA 30335-3801
404-616-5975

University of Illinois Minority-
Based CCOP
Section of Medical Oncology
Room 720N CSB
840 South Wood Street
Chicago, IL 60612
312-996-5958

Kellogg Cancer Care Center CCOP
Evanston Hospital
2650 Ridge Avenue
Evanston, IL 60201
708-570-2109

Illinois Oncology Research
Association CCOP
Suite 780
900 Main Street
Peoria, IL 61602
309-672-5783

Central Illinois CCOP
Memorial Medical Center
800 North Rutledge Street
Springfield, IL 62781-0001
217-788-4178

Carle Cancer Center CCOP
Carle Clinic Association
602 West University Avenue
Urbana, IL 61801
217-383-3010

Cedar Rapids Oncology Project
CCOP
525 10th Street SE
Cedar Rapids, IA 52403
319-363-8303

Iowa Oncology Research
Association
1223 Center Street, Suite 19
Des Moines, IA 50309-1014
515-244-7586

Wichita CCOP
P.O. Box 1358
929 North Saint Francis Street
Wichita, KS 67201
316-262-5784

Ochsner CCOP
Ochsner Cancer Institute
1514 Jefferson Highway
New Orleans, LA 70121
504-838-3708

Grand Rapids Clinical Oncology
Program CCOP
Butterworth Hospital
100 Michigan Street NE
Grand Rapids, MI 49503
616-774-1230

Kalamazoo Community Clinical
Oncology Program of Metropolitan
Detroit
27211 Lahser Road, Suite 200
Southfield, MI 48034-9998
313-356-2828

Duluth CCOP
400 East Third Street
Duluth, MN 55805
218-772-8364, ext. 3308

Metro-Minneapolis CCOP
5000 West 39th Street
Minneapolis, MN 55416-2699
612-928-1517

Scottsdale CCOP
Mayo Foundation
200 First Street SW
Rochester, MN 55905
507-284-2511

Kansas City CCOP
Baptist Medical Center
6601 Rockhill Road
Kansas City, MO 64131
816-276-7834

St. Louis-Cape Girardeau CCOP
Mercy Doctors Building
Suite 3018, Tower B
621 South New Ballas Road
St. Louis, MO 63141
314-569-6959

Ozarks Regional CCOP
1235 East Cherokee Street
Springfield, MO 65804-2263
417-883-2610

Southern Nevada Cancer Research
Foundation CCOP
501 South Rancho Drive, Suite C-14
Las Vegas, NV 89106
702-384-0013

Bergen-Passaic CCOP
Northern New Jersey Cancer Center
5 Summit Street
Hackensack, NJ 07601
201-996-5900

South Jersey Oncology Group CCOP
3 Cooper Plaza, Suite 220
Camden, NJ 08103
609-693-3572

Saint Michael's Medical Center Tri-
County CCOP
268 Dr. Martin Luther King
Boulevard

Newark, NJ 07102
201-877-5000

Brooklyn CCOP
Cancer Institute of Brooklyn
927 49th Street
Brooklyn, NY 11219
718-972-5816

Kings County Minority-Based
CCOP
SUNY Health Science Center,
Brooklyn
450 Clarkson Avenue, Box 55
Brooklyn, NY 11203
718-780-1419

North Shore University Hospital
CCOP
300 Community Drive
Manhasset, NY 11030
516-562-8910

Syracuse Hematology-Oncology
CCOP
100 East Genessee Street
Syracuse, NY 13210
315-472-7504

Southeast Cancer Control
Consortium CCOP
2150 Country Club Road, Suite 220
Winston-Salem, NC 27104-4241
919-777-3036

Merit-Care Hospital CCOP
820 4th Street North
Fargo, ND 58122
701-234-2397

Columbus CCOP
1151 South High Street
Columbus, OH 43206
614-443-2267

Dayton Clinical Oncology Program
Cox Heart Institute
3525 Southern Boulevard
Kettering, OH 45429
513-296-7278

Toledo Community Clinical
Oncology Program
3314 Collingwood Boulevard
Toledo, OH 43610
419-255-5433

St. Francis Hospital/Natalie Warren
Bryant CCOP
6161 South Yale Avenue
Tulsa, OK 74136
918-494-5139

Columbia River CCOP
4805 Northeast Glisan Road
Portland, OR 97213
503-230-6008

Geisinger Clinical Oncology
Program
Department of
Hematology/Oncology
Geisinger Medical Center
North Academy Avenue
Danville, PA 17822-2001
717-271-6544

Allegheny CCOP
Allegheny General Hospital
320 East North Avenue
Pittsburgh, PA 15212-9986
412-359-6191

Mercy Hospital CCOP
General Services Building, Suite 205
743 Jefferson Avenue
Scranton, PA 18501
717-342-3675

San Juan City Minority-Based CCOP
G.P.O. Box 70344
Centro Medico Mail Station 54
San Juan, PR 00936-7344
809-758-7348

Spartanburg CCOP
Spartanburg Regional Medical Center
101 East Wood Street
Spartanburg, SC 29303
803-560-6812

Sioux Community Cancer
Consortium CCOP
Central Plains Clinic, Ltd., Suite 2000
1000 East 21st Street
Sioux Falls, SD 57105
605-331-3160
605-331-3150

San Antonio Minority-Based CCOP
Santa Rosa Hospital
519 West Houston Street
San Antonio, TX 78215
210-224-6531

South Texas Pediatric Minority-
Based CCOP
Department of Pediatrics
Division of Hematology/Oncology
University of Texas Health Science
Center
7703 Floyd Curl Drive
San Antonio, TX 78284-7810
210-567-5265

Green Mountain Oncology Group
Rutland Regional Medical Center
160 Allen Street
Rutland, VT 05701
802-747-1655

Fairfax CCOP
Fairfax Hospital, Suite 206
3301 Woodburn Road
Annandale, VA 22003
703-560-7210

Medical College of Virginia
Minority-Based CCOP
Box 37, MCV Station
Richmond, VA 23298-0037
804-786-0450

Virginia Mason Medical Center
CCOP
1100 9th Avenue
Seattle, WA 98111
206-223-7507

Northwest CCOP
Tacoma General Hospital
314 Martin Luther King Lane,
Suite 204
Tacoma, WA 98405-0986
206-552-1461

Marshfield Medical Research
Foundation CCOP
Marshfield Clinic
1000 North Oak Avenue
Marshfield, WI 54449
715-387-5134

Cancer Registries

Registry for Research on Hormonal
Transplacental Carcinogenesis
University of Chicago
5841 South Maryland Avenue
MC2050
Chicago, IL 60637
312-702-6671
312-702-0840 Fax to general
department (indicate that you want
to contact the registry)
A registry for women with clear-cell
adenocarcinoma of the genital
tract, with or without diethylstilbestrol (DES) exposure.

Hereditary Colorectal Cancer
Polyposis Registry
Johns Hopkins Hospital
550 North Broadway, Suite 108
Baltimore, MD 21205
410-955-3875

410-614-9544 Fax
Provides an opportunity to participate in research on hereditary colon
cancer.

Hereditary Cancer Institute
Creighton University
2500 California Plaza
Omaha, NE 68178
402-280-1746
402-280-1734 Fax
Evaluates families in order to identify possible hereditary cancer syndromes. Will send educational
material upon request. Provides
recommendations for surveillance.

Gilda Radner Familial Ovarian
Cancer Registry
Roswell Park Cancer Institute
Elm and Carlton Streets
Buffalo, NY 14263
800-682-7426
716-845-7608 Fax
A registry for women with two or
more first-degree relatives with
ovarian cancer, for research purposes. The registry is also a source of
public education and information
regarding diagnostic tests, risk factors, and warning signs.

Intestinal Multiple Polyposis and
Colorectal Cancer (IMPACC)
Box 908
Conynghan, PA 18219
717-788-1818
Clearinghouse of registries, support
groups, and information for those
affected by polyposis. Genetic
counseling is available. When calling, indicate that you wish to reach
IMPACC.

Children's Cancers

Make-A-Wish Foundation of
America
100 West Clarendon, Suite 2200
Phoenix, AZ 85013-3518
602-279-9474
800-722-9474
602-278-0855 Fax
Grants wishes to children with life-
threatening illnesses between the
ages of 2–18.

Starlight Foundation International
12424 Wilshire Boulevard, Suite
1050
Los Angeles, CA 90025

310-207-5558
800-274-7827
310-207-2554 Fax
Provides entertainment and recreational activities for seriously ill children age 4–18 through a mobile "fun center" containing a TV, VCR, and video games, and wish-granting activities in chapter areas.

Hole in the Wall Gang Camp
565 Ashford Center Road
Ashford, CT 06278
860-429-3444
860-429-7295 Fax
A free, ten-day summer camp for children age 7–15 with cancer or other serious blood or immunologic disorders.

Children's Hospice International
1850 M Street NW, Suite 900
Washington, DC 20036
703-684-0330
800-242-4453
703-684-0226 Fax
Creates hospice support for children and provides medical and technical assistance, research, and education to their families and health care professionals.

Sunshine Foundation
P.O. Box 255
Loughman, FL 33858
941-424-4188
800-457-1976
941-424-4360 Fax
Grants wishes to chronically or terminally ill and handicapped children age 3–21 whose families are under a financial strain due to their child's illness.

Ronald McDonald House Charities
Department 014
1 Kroc Drive
Oakbrook, IL 60521
708-575-7418
708-575-7488 Fax
Supports temporary lodging facilities for the families of seriously ill children being treated at nearby hospitals.

Children's Oncology Camps of America (COCA)
2309 West White Oaks Drive
Springfield, IL 62704
301-402-0271
Provides annual national directory of oncology camps.

The Children's Organ Transplant Association (COTA)
2501 COTA Drive
Bloomington, IN 47403
812-336-8872
800-366-2682
812-336-8885 Fax
Helps families and communities raise funds for children needing transplants and transplant-related expenses.

Association for the Care of Children's Health
7910 Woodmont Avenue, Suite 300
Bethesda, MD 20814
301-654-6549
800-808-ACCH
301-986-4553 Fax
internet acch@clark.net
Promotes interdisciplinary collaboration among professionals and families in order to humanize children's health care. Family-centered care emphasizes informed choices and views the health care experience as a transformational opportunity for physical, psychosocial, and spiritual growth.

Candlelighters Childhood Cancer Foundation
7910 Woodmont Avenue, Suite 460
Bethesda, MD 20814
301-657-8401
800-366-2233
Provides information, support, and advocacy to families of children with cancer, survivors of childhood cancer, and professionals who work with them.

Federation for Children with Special Needs
95 Berkeley Street, Suite 104
Boston, MA 02116
617-482-2915
800-331-0688 toll-free in MA only
617-695-2939 Fax
An information and referral agency, providing training for parents on understanding their rights under special education laws, and helping parents become health-care advocates.

Chai Lifeline/Camp Simcha
48 West 25th Street
New York, NY 10010
212-255-1160
800-343-2527
212-255-1495 Fax

Provides a kosher camp for children with cancer or hematological conditions, free of charge, including transportation from anywhere in the world. Open to children of any religion who meet the medical approval of the director.

Sunshine Kids
2902 Ferndale Place
Houston, TX 77098
713-524-1264
800-594-5756
713-524-7165 Fax
Offers sports, cultural events, and group activities, free of charge, to children receiving cancer treatment.

Special Love, Inc. (Camp Fantastic)
117 Youth Development Court
Winchester, VA 22602
540-667-3774
540-667-8144 Fax
Provides recreational programs for children with cancer and their families.

Diethylestilbestrol (DES)

DES Action USA
Long Island Jewish Medical Center
New Hyde Park, NY 11040
516-775-3450
800-337-9288 (CA)
800-DES NEWS (NY)
Publishes information and a newsletter about the effects of DES exposure.

DES Cancer Network
P.O. Box 10185
Rochester, NY 14610
716-473-6119
800-DES-NET4
800-337-6384
716-473-4979 Fax
A network for women and men exposed to DES (diethylstilbestrol), with a special focus on cancer. Supports referrals, education, research advocacy, and an annual conference for cancer survivors and publishes a newsletter.

Family Support

Bone Marrow Transplant Family Support Network
P.O. Box 845
Avon, CT 06001
800-826-9376
Telephone support network for

bone marrow transplant patients and their families.

Sibling Information Network
A. J. Pappanikou Center
University of Connecticut
249 Glenbrook Road, Box U64
Storrs, CT 0626-2064
860-486-4985
860-486-5037 Fax
Publishes a newsletter about issues of importance to people with developmental disabilities and their families.

Centering Corporation
1531 North Saddle Creek Road
Omaha, NE 68104
402-553-1200
402-553-0507 Fax
Offers resources for bereavement and coping with loss.

Compassionate Friends
P.O. Box 3696
Oakbrook, IL 60522-3696
708-990-0010
708-990-0246 Fax
Offers support for bereaved parents and siblings.

National Association of Hospital Hospitality Houses, Inc.
4013 West Jackson Street
Muncie, IN 47304
317-883-2226
800-542-9730
317-287-0321 Fax
Membership organization of facilities that coordinate lodging and accommodations for people receiving medical care.

National Family Caregivers Association
9621 East Bexhill Drive
Kensington, MD 20895
301-942-6430
800-896-3650
301-942-2303 Fax
Provides research, education, support, advocacy, and respite care to caregivers.

VHL Family Alliance
171 Clinton Road
Brookline, MA 02146
617-232-5946
800-767-4VHL
617-734-8233 Fax
http://132.183.1.64/vhl-fa
Provides literature and information, referrals, and research resources to von Hipple-Lindau (VHL) syndrome patients and their families.

Families Against Cancer (FACT)
P.O. Box 588
Dewitt, NY 13214
315-446-5326
315-446-6385
Advocacy agency and source of information on how to support increasing federal dollars for cancer research as well as educational materials on cancer prevention and intervention.

Well Spouse Foundation
610 Lexington Avenue, Suite 814
New York, NY 10022-6005
212-644-1241
800-838-0879
212-644-1338 Fax
Offers support to husbands, wives, and partners of people who are chronically ill and/or disabled.

Cancer Family Care
Central Office
7162 Reading Road, Suite 1050
Cincinnati, OH 45237
513-731-3346
513-731-3424
A psychosocial counseling agency for people with cancer and their families.

Home Health Care

Visiting Nurse Association of America (VNAA)
National Office
3801 East Florida Avenue, Suite 900
Denver, CO 80210
800-426-2547
303-753-0218
303-753-0258 Fax
Organization of visiting nurse associations. Members provide highly skilled nursing and assistance with bathing, dressing, and eating. Call for an association that serves your area.

National Association for Home Care
519 C Street NE
Washington, DC 20002
202-547-7424
202-547-3540 Fax
Represents the interests of Americans who need home care and caregivers. Please request information in writing.

Amherst H. Wilder Foundation
919 Lafond Avenue
St. Paul, MN 55104
612-642-4000
642-4068 Fax
Offers services such as psychiatric clinics for children and the elderly, community services, and senior housing.

Oley Foundation
214 Hun Memorial
Albany Medical Center A-23
Albany, NY
518-262-5079
800-776-OLEY
518-262-5528 Fax
Support for home parenteral and/or enteral nutrition therapy through a newsletter, conferences, meetings, and outreach activities.

Olsten Kimberly QualityCare
Headquarters
175 Broadhollow Road
Melville, NY 11747
516-844-7800
800-66-NURSE
The largest provider of community home health care services, including chemotherapy, nutrition and hydration therapies, pain management, physical therapy, and general nursing services.

Hospice and Supportive Services

National Institute for Jewish Hospices
8723 Alden Drive, Suite 219
Los Angeles, CA 90048
310-854-3036
213-HOSPICE
800-446-4448
310-854-5683 Fax; call before faxing.
Provides hospice care, counseling, and referrals with a Jewish perspective.

Hospice Education Institute (HOSPICELINK)
190 Westbrook Road
Essex, CT 06426-0713
800-331-1620
Provides general information about hospice care and referrals to the hospice nearest you.

Foundation for Hospice and Home Care
513 C Street NE
Washington, DC 20002
202-547-6586

202-547-6586 Fax
Diverse organization with a broad array of programs to serve the dying, disabled, and disadvantaged.

Hospice Association of America
519 C Street NE
Washington, DC 20002
Membership organization for all hospices that offers addresses of local hospice organizations.

Choice in Dying
200 Varick Street, Suite 1001
New York, NY 10014
212-366-5540
800-989-WILL
Concerned with protecting the rights and serving the needs of people who are dying of any illness and their families. Choice in Dying distributes free information on living will and power of attorney and offers a free counseling service on end-of-life issues.

National Hospice Organization
1901 North Moore Street, Suite 901
Arlington, VA 22209
703-243-5900
800-658-8898
703-525-5762 Fax
Provides educational services and publications regarding hospice and referrals to hospices throughout the country.

Money and Insurance

Civilian Health and Medical Programs of the Uniformed Services (CHAMPUS)
Information Office of CHAMPUS
Aurora, CO 80045
303-361-1000

Disabled American Veterans
807 Main Avenue SW
Washington, DC 20024
202-554-3501
202-554-3581 Fax

Group Health Association of America
Membership Department
129 20th Street NW, Suite 600
Washington, DC 20036
202-778-3200
202-331-7487 Fax

Health Insurance Association of America (HIAA)
1025 Connecticut Avenue NW,

Suite 1200
Washington, DC 20036
The National Insurance Consumer
202-824-1600

Pension and Welfare Benefits Administration
U.S. Department of Labor, Room N-5669
200 Constitution Avenue NW
Washington, DC 20210
202-523-8521

Blue Cross and Blue Shield Association
676 North St. Clair Street
Chicago, IL 60601
312-440-6000

United States Department of Health and Human Services
Medicare
Social Security Administration
Baltimore, MD 21235
800-772-1213

Hill-Burton Program
Health Resources and Services Administration
Bureau of Health Resources Development
5600 Fishers' Lane, Room 731
Rockville, MD 20857
800-492-0359—Maryland residents
800-638-0742
A noncost or reduced-cost program for those within the poverty guidelines as defined by the federal government. Hotline gives information defining the guidelines and fulfills requests for local Hill-Burton facilities.

Medical Information Bureau, Inc. (MIB)
Consumer Information Office
P.O. Box 105
Essex Station
Boston, MA 02112
617-426-3660
Aims to prevent insurance fraud. Write to request a copy of your MIB file and, if necessary, request corrections.

Communicating for Agriculture, Inc.
2626 East 82nd Street, Suite 325
Bloomington, MN 55425
800-445-1525
612-854-9005
Organization of ranchers, farmers, and self-employed people that

offers many services that do not relate to cancer. However, each year it publishes the *Guide to Comprehensive Health Insurance for High-risk Individuals: A State by State Analysis*, which may be useful to people with cancer.

National Underwriter Company
505 Gest Street
Cincinnati, OH 45203
513-721-2140

Pain

American Academy of Pain Medicine
4700 West Lake Avenue
Glenville, IL 60025
708-966-9510
708-375-4777 Fax
internet: aapm@dial.cic.net
Supports quality care to patients suffering with pain through the education and training of physicians, research, and the advancement of the specialty of pain medicine. Also provides information regarding specific pain medications.

American Society of Clinical Hypnosis
2200 East Vine Ave Suite 291
Des Plaines, IL 60018
847-297-3317
847-297-7309 Fax
Maintains a list of licensed hypnotists that work with people in pain. Send request in writing and include a self-addressed, stamped envelope.

American Pain Society
4700 West Lake Avenue
Glenville, IL 60025
847-966-5595
847-966-9418 Fax
An organization of clinicians and researchers that serves people in pain by advancing research, education, treatment, and professional practice.

American Society of Anesthesiologists
Wood Library and Museum of Anesthesiology
515 Busse Highway
Park Ridge, IL 60068
847-825-5586
Distributes patient education brochures. The Wood Library will research your questions regarding anesthesia and pain management free of charge.

National Chronic Pain Outreach
Association
7979 Old Georgetown Road,
Suite 100
Bethesda, MD 20814-2429
301-652-4948
301-907-0745 Fax
Educates patients, health care professionals, and the public about
chronic pain and its treatment.

Agency for Health Care Policy and
Research
Publications Clearinghouse
P.O. Box 8547
Silver Spring, MD 20907-8547
800-358-9295
301-594-2800 Fax
Offers a free publication on cancer
pain.

Patient Education, Support, and Advocacy

Cancervive
6500 Wilshire Boulevard, Suite 500
Los Angeles, CA 90048
213-655-3758
Offers several services to people
with cancer, including telephone
counseling, referrals, and education.

The Wellness Community–National
2716 Ocean Park Boulevard, Suite
1040
Santa Monica, CA 90405-5211
310-314-2555
310-314-7586 Fax
Offers support to adult cancer
patients and their families at no
charge as an adjunct to conventional medical treatment in 13 U.S.
cities. Support groups are led by
licensed psychotherapists.

The Mautamar Project for Lesbians
with Cancer
1707 L Street NW, Suite 1060
Washington, DC 20036
202-332-5536
202-265-6854 Fax
Provides vital services and support,
including education, information,
and advocacy for health issues
relating to lesbians with cancer and
their families.

National Coalition for Cancer
Research (NCCR)
426 C Street NE
Washington, DC 20002
202-544-1880

Cancer survivors and researchers
track cancer research and monitor
legislation and funding.

National Women's Health Network
1325 G Street NW
Washington, DC 20005
202-628-7814
202-347-1168 Fax
Provides advocacy and maintains a
clearinghouse on women's health
issues.

National Coalition for Cancer
Survivorship (NCCS)
1010 Wayne Avenue, Suite 300
Silver Spring, MD 20910
301-650-8868
Serves as a clearing house for information, publications, and programs
for organizations that work on survivorship issues. Promotes study of
problems and potentials of survivorship, and advocates interests
of cancer survivors to secure their
rights and combat prejudice.

Make Today Count
Mid-America Cancer Center
1235 East Cherokee
Springfield, MO 65804-2263
417-885-3234
800-432-2273
417-888-7426 Fax
Brings together persons affected by
a life-threatening illness so they
may help each other.

American Self-Help Clearinghouse
Northwest Covenant Medical Center
25 Pocono Road
Denville, NJ 07834-2995
201-625-7101
800-367-6274 (New Jersey only)
201-625-8848 Fax
e-mail:njshc@bc.cybernex.net
http://www.cmhc.com/selfhelp
Maintains a list of self-help groups
in the New Jersey area, provides a
referral service, and helps people
form their own groups. Publishes a
directory of statewide and national
self-help groups.

People Living Through Cancer, Inc.
323 8th Street SW
Albuquerque, NM 87102
505-242-3263
505-842-6658 Fax
Programs and activities to help members make informed choices and
interact with other people who have

been treated for cancer. Services
include a publication, one-to-one
matching, support groups and individual counseling, and training for
Native Americans who would like to
start their own groups.

Cancer Care, Inc.
National Cancer Care Foundation
1180 Avenue of the Americas
New York, NY 10036
212-221-3300
800-813-HOPE (counseling line)
212-719-0263 Fax
e-mail: cancercare@aol.com
Provides emotional and financial
support for people with cancer and
their families and educational programs for the general public. Free
bereavement counseling, outreach
programs, information and referrals
to home care and child care, hospice,
and other services are also available.

Cancer Research Institute
681 5th Avenue
New York, NY 10022
212-688-7515
800-99-CANCER
212-832-9376 Fax
e-mail: cancerres@aol.com
Supports clinical research and has a
free public education service. Offers
a cancer help book free of charge,
which includes a resource directory.
They will also search Physician's
Data Query (see Public
Information) for protocols that
may be appropriate for your cancer.

CanSurmount
American Cancer Society
800-ACS-2345
Trained volunteers offer one-on-one
support through visits to people
with cancer and their families.
Volunteers are knowledgeable
about resources that may help people cope with cancer.

I Can Cope
American Cancer Society
800-ACS-2345
An education program for people
with cancer and their families. In a
series of classes, health care
providers present information on
diagnosis, treatment, communication skills, community resources,
and self-care strategies.

Burger King Cancer Caring Center
4117 Liberty Avenue
Pittsburgh, PA 15224
412-622-1212
Dedicated to providing psychological support to people diagnosed with cancer and their families and friends. The Cancer Caring Center is now handling calls for the Cancer Guidance Hotline.

Coping Magazine
P.O. Box 682268
Franklin, TN 37068-2268
615-790-2400
615-794-0179 Fax
e-mail: copingmag@aol.com
A bimonthly publication that is the only nationally distributed consumer magazine for people whose lives have been touched by cancer.

Public Information

National Council Against Health Fraud Resource Center
Main Office
P.O. Box 1276
Loma Linda, CA 92354
909-824-4690
909-824-4838 Fax
Focuses on health misinformation, fraud and quackery and provides information on unusual methods of cancer management. Can refer people to lawyers and help those who have had negative experiences to share their story.

American Association of Retired Persons
601 E Street NW
Washington, DC 20049
202-434-3525 (Washington area)
800-424-3410
e-mail: aarp.bil2
Gives information regarding AARP insurance, Social Security, and Medicare. Research specialists available.

American Institute for Cancer Research (AICR)
1759 R Street NW
Washington, DC 20009
202-328-7744
800-843-8114 Hotline
202-328-7226 Fax
Focuses on the relationship between diet and nutrition and cancer prevention and treatment. Creates public health education

programs, funds research, and provides information to the public and health care professionals.

Cancer Information Service
800-4-CANCER
800-422-6237
Offers free publications, lists FDA-certified mammography centers, and has cancer information specialists that will tell you where clinical trials are taking place and answer your questions in English or Spanish.

CancerFax
National Cancer Institute
301-402-5874
301-496-7403 for technical assistance
CancerFax provides treatment guidelines, with current data on prognosis, staging, and histologic classifications, news and announcements of important cancer-related issues. Call CancerFax from your fax machine, not your telephone.

Consumer Products Safety Commission
5401 Westbard Avenue
Washington, DC 20207
800-638-2772
Releases information about unsafe products and product recall lists.

National Consumers League
1701 K Street NW, Suite 1200
Washington, DC 20006
202-835-3323
202-835-0747 Fax
Provides consumer protection and advocacy, with experts in law, business, and labor. Publishes education brochures about general health issues, including cancer screening tests.

National Library of Medicine
8600 Rockville Pike
Bethesda, MD 20894
800-638-8480
800-272-4787 (MEDLARS)
The online database of National Library of Medicine is called MEDLARS. See Appendix II.

National Institutes of Health Consensus Program
P.O. Box 2577
Kensington, MD 20891
800-644-2271
Voice Mail: 800-NIH OMAR
301-816-2494 Fax

http://text.nom.nih.govstp://public.nih.gov/hstit
Updates practicing physicians and the public with current responsible information on the pros and cons of various medical technologies.

Food and Drug Administration
Office of Consumer Affairs
HFE-88
5600 Fishers Lane
Rockville, MD 20857
The Breast Implant Information Hotline
800-532-4440
Women considering or who have had breast reconstruction using implants can obtain an information package.

MedWatch Program
800-332-1088
Maintains adverse event and product reporting program for professionals, but will accept reports of problems with food, drugs, or devices from the general public.

Mammography Hotline
800-4-CANCER
The FDA in cooperation with the National Cancer Institute provides information on mammography and refers women to an FDA-certified facility in their area.

Consumer Health Information Research Institute
300 East Pink Hill Road
Independence, MO 64057-3223
816-228-4595
816-228-4995 Fax
e-mail: drrenner@msn.com
Helps access information on and investigates medical quackery and fraud. Evaluates unusual treatments, and provides an integrity index, a credibility of publication index, including one which rates cancer books.
http://www.reutershealth.com (click on Internet Health Watch)

Physicians Data Query (PDQ)
800-4-CANCER
PDQ is the National Cancer Institute's computerized listing of up-to-date and accurate information for people with cancer and health care professionals on the latest treatments, research studies, and clinical trials. See also Appendix II.

Rehabilitation

See also specific cancers, below.

National Lymphedema Network
2211 Post Street, Suite 404
San Francisco, CA 94115
415-921-2911
800-541-3259
415-921-4284 Fax
http://www.primenet.com/dean/lymph.html.
Gives practical education, emotional support, and referrals to people with cancer who have lymphedema. Quarterly newsletter lists local support groups.

Look Good, Feel Better
American Cancer Society
800-395-LOOK
Founded in partnership with the National Cosmetology Association, and the Cosmetic, Toiletry, and Fragrance Association (CTFA) Foundation as a free national public service program dedicated to teaching women with cancer how to restore a healthy appearance and self-image during and after chemotherapy and radiation therapy.

Patient Referral Service
American Society of Plastic and Reconstructive Surgeons
444 East Algonquin Road
Arlington Heights, IL 60005
708-228-9900
800-635-0635
708-228-0117 Fax
Will provide list of five board-certified plastic surgeons to women interested in breast reconstruction.

United Ostomy Association
36 Executive Park, Suite 120
Irvine, CA 92714
714-660-8624
800-826-0826
714-660-9262 Fax
Assists people who have or will have intestinal or urinary tract diversions (ostomies) with psychological and family support and educational services.

Ostomy Rehabilitation Program
American Cancer Society
800-ACS-2345
The ACS and the United Ostomy Association jointly produce educa-

tional materials for people with ostomies. Trained volunteers who have ostomies visit patients for one-on-one support.

Wound Ostomy and Continence Nurses Society
2755 Bristol Street, Suite 110
Costa Mesa, CA 92626
714-476-0268
714-545-3643 Fax
Refers patients to enterostomal nurses in their area.

Smoking

Office on Smoking and Health
Center for Disease Control
4770 Buford Highway NE
Mail Stop K50
Atlanta, GA 30341-3724
404-488-5705
800-CDC 1311
Offers public education and information on smoking and how to stop.

American Lung Association
National Office
1740 Broadway
New York, NY 10019-4374
212-315-8700
800-LUNG USA to reach your local office
212-265-5642 Fax
Helps people stop smoking and provides information about lung disease.

Specific Cancers/Diseases

AIDS

PWA Coalition Hotline
50 West 17th Street, 8th floor
New York, NY 10011
800-828-3280
Offers counseling for people with HIV or AIDS, referral to support groups and other organizations, and information about entitlements. Provides information regarding treatments, medication, and opportunistic infections upon request.

National AIDS Hotline
800-342-2437 (24-hours)
800-344-7432 (Spanish)
800-243-7889 (hearing-impaired)

Educates people regarding HIV and AIDS, and operates a large database listing educational resources, testing centers, and treatment facilities.

Public Health Service AIDS Hotline
800-342-AIDS
800-342-2437
Gives general information regarding AIDS, referrals, and educational pamphlets. The hotline operates 24 hours a day, 7 days a week, in English or Spanish.

Brain Tumor

National Brain Tumor Foundation
785 Market Street, Suite 1600
San Francisco, CA 94103
415-284-0208
415-284-0209 Fax
800-934-CURE
e-mail: ssts39b@prodigy.com
Raises funds for research and provides information and support services to people with brain tumors and their families.

American Brain Tumor Association
2720 River Road, Suite 146
Des Plaines, IL 60018
800-886-2282
847-827-9910
847-827-9918 Fax
e-mail: abta@aol.com
Offers publications and services to people with brain tumors and their families, including information about treatments, coping mechanisms, a book for children, a list of support groups, a pen pal program, and a newsletter.

Breast Cancer

Reach to Recovery
American Cancer Society
800-ACS-2345
Offers support and information about breast cancer and its treatment. The program is designed to help people deal with the physical, emotional, and cosmetic needs related to breast cancer.

ENCORE Plus
YWCA
Office of Women's Health Initiatives
624 9th Street NW
Washington, DC 20001
202-628-3636

800-953-7587
202-783-7123 Fax
Promotes breast health through education, clinical service delivery, and patient advocacy. Community-based programs target women over 50 in need of breast and cervical cancer screening and support services. It also provides women treated for breast cancer with a combined support group and exercise program.

The National Breast Cancer Coalition
1707 L Street NW, Suite 1060
Washington, DC 20036
202-296-7477
800-935-0434
202-265-6854 Fax
Strives to involve women with breast cancer and those that care about them in changing public policy. Goals include increasing breast cancer research funding and improving access to screening, increasing the influence that breast cancer survivors have over research, clinical trials, and national policy.

Y-ME National Breast Cancer Organization
212 West Van Buren
Chicago, IL 60607
800-221-2141
312-926-8228-24-hour hotline (emergency only)
312-986-0020 Fax
Provides information, referrals, and emotional support to individuals concerned about or diagnosed with breast cancer

Rose Kushner Breast Cancer Advisory Center
5450 Whitley Park Terrace, Unit 613
Bethesda, MD 20814
301-897-3445
301-897-3444 Fax
Publishes "If you've thought about breast cancer...," which includes information on treatment and diagnosis to help women save their breasts as well as their lives.

National Alliance of Breast Cancer Organizations (NABCO)
9 East 37th Street, 10th floor
New York, NY 10016
212-719-0154
800-719-9154
212-689-1213 Fax

e-mail: nabcoinfo@aol.com
http://www.nabco.org
A network of 370 organizations that provides information, assistance, and referral to anyone with questions about breast cancer. Acts as a voice for interests and concerns of breast cancer survivors and women at risk of the disease. Publishes quarterly newsletter; provides updates on search, treatment, and policy; annual Breast Cancer Resource List.

The Susan G. Komen Breast Cancer Foundation
Occidental Tower
5005 LBJ Freeway, Suite 370
Dallas, TX 75244
214-450-1777
214-450-1710 Fax
800-I'M-AWARE (800-462-4273) (National Helpline)
http://www.komen.com
Funds research dedicated solely to breast cancer, breast cancer education, and screening and treatment projects for the medically underserved. Maintains a Breast Care Helpline to provide infromation to callers with breast health and cancer concerns.

Gynecologic Cancers

Hysterectomy Educational Resources and Services (HERS)
422 Bryn Mawr Avenue
Bala Cynwyd, PA 19004
610-667-7757
610-667-8096 Fax
Provides information about hysterectomy alternatives, risks of those alternatives, and consequences of surgery. Telephone counseling is available by appointment. HERS gives referrals to specialists, publishes a newsletter, provides medical journal articles, and holds semiannual conferences.

Head and Neck

International Association of Laryngectomees (IAL)
American Cancer Society
Atlanta, GA 30329
800-ACS-2345
A voluntary organization dedicated to the total rehabilitation of laryngectomees. Promotes exchange and dissemination of ideas and informa-

tion to laryngectomee clubs and to the public.

Let's Face It
P.O. Box 711
Concord, MA 01742
508-371-3186
Information and support network for people with head and neck cancer and others with facial disfigurement.

The Lost Chord
See International Association of Laryngectomees

Support for People with Oral and Head and Neck Cancer (SPOHNC)
P.O. Box 53
Locust Valley, NY 11560-0053
516-759-5333
Fax to number; call first
Patient-directed, self-help organization dedicated to meeting the needs of people with oral and head and neck cancer. Includes a networking program and newsletter, support group in Long Island, and referral to additional resources.

Kidney Cancer

National Kidney Cancer Association
1234 Sherman Avenue, Suite 200
Evanston, IL 60202
708-332-1051
708-328-4425 Fax
708-332-1052 computerized information system (24 hours)
e-mail:
nkca@merle@acsns.nwuu.edu
Provides information to patients and physicians, sponsors research on kidney cancer, gives referrals to physicians, publishes a newsletter, and acts as a patient advocate.

Leukemia

National Leukemia Association, Inc.
Children's Leukemia Research
585 Stewart Avenue, Suite 536
Garden City, NY 11530
516-222-1944
516-222-0457 Fax
Provides financial assistance to people with leukemia.

Leukemia Society of America, Inc.
National Office
600 Third Avenue, 4th Floor
New York, NY 10016

212-573-8484
800-955-4LSA
Publishes educational material and a newsletter, and offers a patient financial aid program. Contact the national office for a listing of your local chapter.

Lymphoma

Lymphoma Research Foundation of America, Inc.
2318 Prosser Avenue
Los Angeles, CA 90064
310-470-4912
310-470-8502 Fax
Funds medical research devoted to improving lymphoma treatments. Offers a newsletter and support system to patients and their families.

Skin Cancer and Melanoma

American Melanoma Foundation
Center for Biological Therapy and Melanoma Research
University of California, San Diego
9500 Gilman Drive
La Jolla, CA 92093
619-534-3713
619-534-3940
Supports research and patient education programs about melanoma, its treatment, biological therapies, and prevention strategies.

Skin Cancer Foundation
245 Fifth Avenue, Suite 2402
New York, NY 10016
212-725-5176
800-SKIN-440
212-725-5751 Fax
Conducts educational programs for the public and medical communities; supports medical training, cancer screening, and prevention programs; provides information about safe sun exposure for children and adults; and publishes a journal.

Myeloma

International Myeloma Foundation
2120 Stanley Hills Drive
Los Angeles, CA 90046
213-654-3023
800-452-CURE
213-656-1182 Fax
e-mail: IMF@aol.com
http://www.comed.com./IMF/imf.html
Dedicated to improving quality of life for myeloma patients, while working toward prevention and a cure.

Prostate Cancer

Man-To-Man
American Cancer Society
800-ACS-2345
An educational and support program for men with prostate cancer and their families. Health professionals make presentations relevant to men followed by a question and answer period and support session.

The Mathews Foundation for Prostate Cancer Research
1010 Hurley Way, Suite 195
Sacramento, CA 95825
916-567-1400
800-234-6284
916-567-1415 Fax
Supplies individual answers to questions about prostate cancer, its treatment, and symptoms.

US-TOO
930 North York Road, Suite 50
Hinsdale, IL 60521-2993
800-82-US-TOO
708-323-1002
708-323-1003 Fax
Provides prostate cancer survivors and their families emotional and educational support.

American Foundation for Urologic Disease, Inc.
300-West Pratt Street, Suite 401
Baltimore, MD 21201
Supports medical research and education of medical professionals and the public about urological diseases and dysfunction, including prostate and bladder cancer. Sponsors a prostate cancer support group network (See Us-Too) and a research scholars program, publishes a quarterly magazine and patient education materials. Contact them in writing.

Patient Advocates for Advanced Cancer Treatments
1143 Parmelee NW
Grand Rapids, MI 49504
616-453-1477
616-453-1846 Fax
616-453-1351 voice mail
Distributes updated literature about prostate cancer, including information about treatments, how to get them, complimentary therapies, support group listings, advanced biopsy procedures, and phone numbers for Medicare to help cover costs.

Transportation Services

AirLifeLine
6133 Freeport Boulevard
Sacramento, CA 95822
916-429-2500
800-446-1231
916-429-2166 Fax
Provides emergency medical transportation for financially needy people who are ambulatory. The organization requires at least ten days' notice to assess need and make arrangements.

National Patient Air Transport Hotline
800-296-1217
Gives information on all volunteer groups, known airline specials, and medical escort and air ambulance services.

Corporate Angel Network, Inc.
Westchester County Airport
Building 1
White Plains, NY 10604
914-328-1313
800-328-4246 Fax
Provides free transportation to or from a hospital or treatment center for people with cancer and family members, using corporate airlines. Travelers must be ambulatory and self-sufficient. People who are donating bone marrow or blood to the cancer patient may also travel free.

Road To Recovery
American Cancer Society
800-ACS-2345
Some ACS units have trained volunteers to transport people with cancer to and from medical treatments in their own vehicles at no charge.

Air Care Alliance
P.O. Box 1940
Manassas, VA 22110
800-296-1217
Provides a flight to the ambulatory and medically stable person who is unable to travel on public transportation. Call for your local organization.

Mercy Medical Airlift (MMA)
P.O. Box 1940
Manassas, VA 22110
703-361-1191
800-296-1191
Helps those in financial need with transportation. Also provides an air

ambulance service and referrals to medical escorts on commercial airlines, transportation for someone in a stretcher, and nursing en route.

Treatments

BMT/Transplants

Bone Marrow Transplant
Newsletter
1985 Spruce Avenue
Highland Park, Il 60035
847-831-1913
http://nysernet.org/bcic/bmt/bmt.news.html
Bimonthly newsletter for people with cancer, their families and friends, medical professionals, and support organizations that work with people undergoing bone marrow transplant. Maintains an attorney referral service for those who have insurance problems. Links prospective patients and others who have been through the BMT experience.

National Bone Marrow Transplant
Link
29209 Northwestern Highway, #624
Southfield, MI 48034
800-LINK-BMT
Provides resources, peer support, and information about bone marrow transplant. Clearinghouse for BMT patients and their families.

National Marrow Donor Program
3433 Broadway Street NE, Suite 400
Minneapolis, MN 55413
612-627-5800
800-526-7809
800-MARROW2 for donor information
612-627-5899 Fax
Registry matches donors and patients. Patient advocacy department is a source of information regarding insurance, choosing a hospital, and other concerns. The MARROW line answers general calls and explains how to become a marrow donor.

The Organ Transplant Fund
1027 South Yates
Memphis, TN 38119
901-684-1697
800-489-3863
Provides health care support services, financial services, and advocacy programs for transplantation candidates, recipients, and their families.

Living Bank
4545 Post Oak Place, Suite 315
Houston, TX 77027
800-528-2971
713-528-2971 (Houston area)
713-961-0979 Fax
Attempts to motivate and facilitate organ and tissue donor commitment.

Chemotherapy

ChemoCare
231 North Avenue West
Westfield, NJ 07090
800-55-CHEMO
908-233-1103
908-233-0228 Fax
Offers one-to-one emotional support to people with cancer and their families by matching patients to cancer survivors.

The Chemotherapy Foundation
183 Madison Avenue, Suite 403
New York, NY 10016
212-213-9292
212-689-5164 Fax
Supports laboratory and clinical research to develop more effective methods of cancer diagnosis and therapy. Conducts professional and public education programs and publishes free patient/public information booklets.

CANCER INFORMATION ON LINE

The amount of cancer information available on the Internet, already enormous, is multiplying daily. This appendix briefly explains what the Internet is, what's available on it, and how to get connected; it then follows with lists of many cancer-related Internet resources and locations.

On-Line Basics

The *Internet* is a vast network of computers around the world linked together by satellite and accessed through telephone lines. Part of the Internet is the *World Wide Web* (*WWW*, or simply the *Web*), which includes not just text but pictures, sounds, and other advanced features. To publish information on the Web, a person or an organization creates a collection of specially designed and programmed pages (files). This collection of files, commonly known as a *Web site* or *home page*, is stored on a *server*, which is a sophisticated computer designed to interact and communicate with the Internet. Each Web site or home page, when added to a server, is assigned a specific address, known as a *URL (Universal Resource Locator)*. By typing in a particular URL, a user can locate a Web site anywhere on the Internet. To access the Internet, your computer (which must be equipped with a *modem*) dials a telephone number that connects it to an Internet computer. Then, using a software program called a *browser* (such as Netscape or Mosaic), you can look up the Web site's address, find the home page, and display it on your monitor.

Electronic mail (e-mail) is a popular Internet feature that lets you send messages instantly to any person or organization that is on line. *Newsgroups* are another way in which people with a shared interest can communicate. Messages sent to the newsgroup are stored in a central location, which can be accessed at any time and displayed as a list. Not only can you read and write messages, but you can also post a response to a particular message.

You can use e-mail to subscribe to *mailing lists* (sometimes called *listservers*). On a regular basis, like digital newsletters, these free information services automatically send you a complete collection of e-mail correspondence from fellow subscribers. Most people who correspond via the cancer-related mailing lists are usually patients or their families, although anyone can participate.

What's Available

Cancer-related Web sites are produced and maintained by a variety of individuals and groups: agencies of the federal government such as the National Cancer Institute (NCI), nonprofit organizations such as the American Cancer Society (ACS), university teaching hospitals, comprehensive cancer centers, pharmaceutical companies, research facilities, and others. Many other useful sites are created by computer-literate cancer survivors who volunteer their time and expertise. Depending on their origin and focus, Web sites offer:

- basic facts about all forms of cancer;

- updates on current clinical trials and protocols;

- sources of psychological and social support;

- articles from newspapers, magazines, and journals;

- information about hospitals and physicians;

- alternative therapies.

To find Web information on cancer or any topic or the Web site of a particular organization, you can use a *search engine* (see the listing at the end of this appendix). With lively names like Yahoo and Excite, these indexes are powerful programs that scan thousands of Web sites around the world. When you type in the subject, keywords, or organization you're looking for, the search engine acts like an efficient librarian, rummaging through a vast collection of information, finding files or terms that match the request, and displaying a list of the results. If you see something of interest, you can click on the highlighted text and you will be connected directly to that Web site. Then you can proceed to read the pages, print particular sections, or save the information on your hard disk for later use. If you can't find what you are looking for with one search engine, try another.

Many of the cancer-related Web sites or information sources provide direct links to one another through the click of a mouse. For example, from the American Cancer Society (ACS) home page, you can move to National Cancer Institute (NCI) resources and to excellent sites of information maintained by cancer survivors such as Cansearch and CancerGuide (all these sites are detailed later in this chapter). Many of the groups can also be accessed directly through their own URLs or by using one of the search engines.

A number of the same sources of information can be accessed in other ways, although some are more readily used by those who are skilled at computer data searches. For example, depending on your Internet connection and your ability to conduct a search, there are many ways you can tap into the National Library of Medicine and its vast archive of scientific articles known collectively as MEDLARS (Medical Literature Analysis and Retrieval System) and (usually for a fee) search for articles by title, author, or subject. Most of the articles include an abstract (brief summary of the contents), which you can download, or you can request that a copy of the full text be printed and sent to your local library for an additional charge. The two most pertinent divisions of MEDLARS are:

- MEDLINE (MEDLARS Online), with 8 million articles published in the last three decades from thousands of medical journals worldwide.

- CancerLit (Cancer Literature), a collection of more than 1 million articles, reports, and monographs. You can access abstracts of CancerLit articles free via the OncoLink Web site, maintained by the University of Pennsylvania (see page 671). If you have a Compuserve account, you can search all of MEDLINE by accessing the very user-friendly Paper Chase (GO PCH). The charge is added to your monthly Compuserve bill. If you are adept at searching, it is also possible to set up your own MEDLINE direct account that works through your Internet connection. You need to apply for your own user ID code and password; for information, contact MEDLARS at the National Library of Medicine (800-638-8480). You can conduct a literature search using your Web browser (such as Netscape) by entering the URL (http://igm.mlm.nih.gov). Or you might want to use special software called Internet Grateful Med, which costs around $30. This program lets you write out your search request before dialing into the MEDLARS system, thus saving you time on line (and reducing costs). With a MEDLARS account, you do not pay long-distance charges or monthly fees; you pay only for the time connected to the computer (plus the cost of retrieving any full-text articles you request).

- The Physicians Data Query (PDQ), a very important source of information maintained by the NCI, is a series of fact-filled, no-nonsense, up-to-date publications that come in two varieties, one for lay readers and one for health care professionals, although both are available to anyone. They explain the cancer staging system, treatments, and survival rates. PDQ is accessible free via the NCI International Cancer Information Center and for a fee from the Compuserve service (all detailed later in this appendix), among others.

- The CancerNet, maintained by the NCI and available from its Web site, provides access to the PDQ and offers fact sheets on more than 100 topics from the NCI's Office of Cancer Communications plus news, abstracts from medical articles, and tips on supportive care.

Some Caveats

The information offered by Web sites, on-line support groups, or mailing lists can be very helpful, but it varies widely in quality and accuracy. The most reliable sources are major organizations, such as the ACS, government agencies, hospitals, or universities, whose information is reviewed by noted experts and updated frequently. Less reliable are anecdotal reports or unsubstantiated claims about various alternative therapies. Use good judgment and common sense when evaluating the advice you read in Web sites or mailing list archives. Since Web sites are largely unregulated, don't accept any information as authoritative just because it appears on the Internet. Ask your caregivers for their opinions of what you find. The Consumer Health Information Research Institute (see Appendix I, "Resources") monitors the Internet and constantly updates its list of "unscientific" medical Web sites. Its URL is: http://www.reutershealth.com (click on Internet Health Watch).

Be aware, too, that because the Internet is expanding and changing so rapidly, and chaotically, any descriptions provided here, though accurate as this book goes to press, may no longer be valid by the time you read it.

Getting Connected

There are two basic ways to connect to the Internet. The simplest is to subscribe to one of the major commercial on-line services, listed later. These companies provide free software and technical support, and their programs are designed to make it easy to find your way on the Web.

These on-line services also offer collections of information not available elsewhere, such as magazine or newspaper archives, and they provide "chat rooms," forums, and bulletin boards where people with a common interest can "meet" and exchange information. Forums are highly popular among people who have cancer or who are caring for someone with cancer. However, you can access certain forums only if you belong to that particular on-line service. For example, the Prodigy prostate cancer bulletin board is available only to Prodigy subscribers. On-line services typically charge $10 and up monthly for a fixed number of hours, plus an additional hourly fee (around $3) and surcharges for using certain features or for *downloading* (copying to your own computer) various articles or programs.

The second way to connect is through an *Internet service provider (ISP)*. An ISP provides you direct access to the Internet—direct because you don't have to go through a "gateway" such as Compuserve. Depending on the type of account, ISPs usually charge a flat monthly fee (typically $20 to $30) with no additional hourly charges; some ISPs also charge for setting up the account. ISPs provide technical support, but unlike the commercial services, they usually do not offer extra services or flashy features. Once you sign on and install your Internet software, you're basically on your own. The advantage, however, is cost. If you are on line more than 15 hours or so a month, it will probably be cheaper to use an ISP.

If you are already a member of a commercial on-line service, you can locate the names of ISPs in your area by conducting a database search. If you are not on line, check the Yellow Pages, ask your local computer store or librarian for a suggestion, consult the ads in computer magazines and newspapers, or ask a computer-savvy friend or neighbor.

When selecting any on-line service, find out whether your connection will be through a local or a toll-free call. Having to pay long-distance charges while on line can increase the cost significantly. Also, if you want to join a specific newsgroup, ask your prospective on-line provider if that group is available before you sign up.

On-Line Services and Selected Relevant Features

- America Online: 800-827-6364
    American Cancer Society: Keyword: ACS
    Scientific American Cancer Journal: Keyword: Cancer J SciAm
    On-line support groups (select Health and Medical Chat icon): Living with Cancer, Cancer Survivors, Loved Ones of Cancer Survivors

- Compuserve: 800-848-8990
    Cancer Forum: GO CANCER
    Consumer Reports Drug Database: GO DRUGS
    Health Database Plus: GO HTLDB
    Knowledge Index: GO KI
    MEDLINE (Paperchase): GO PCH
    MedSig Forum: GO MEDSIG
    NORD Services/Rare Disease Database: GO NORD
    Physician's Data Query: GO PDQ

- Prodigy: 800-PRODIGY (800-776-3449)
    Medical Support Bulletin Boards

- Microsoft Network: 800-386-5550
    Cancer Awareness
    Cancer Support Bulletin Board
    Leukemia Support Bulletin Board
    Childhood Cancers
    Women and Cancer

Cancer-Related Web Resources

Be aware that new Web sites appear daily while old ones expand, move, or disappear entirely. It's worth mentioning again that some of the URLs given below or their content may be different by the time you read this book.

When typing the URL into your Web browser, use the exact punctuation as shown (including slashes), but delete the parentheses. If you can't access the specific sites with these URLs, use a search engine (entering the name of an organization or keywords such as "Cancer" or "Cancer Treatment") to locate what you're looking for.

Major Sources of Information

Many of these large Web sites offer access to some of the same sources of information or direct links to one another.

American Cancer Society (http://www.cancer.org). Information about cancer, including statistics, advice, patient and family counseling, diet, home health care, getting help with medical costs, pain control, and other subjects. Also data about local ACS divisions, publications, meetings, programs, events, and links to other cancer resources on the Web, plus an on-line form to order selected ACS publications.

Canadian Cancer Society (http://www.ncf.carleton.ca/freeport /health/ccs/menu). Facts about cancer, treatment, prevention, and Canadian units of the CCS, in English and French.

National Cancer Institute International Cancer Information Center (http://wwwicic.nci.nih.gov/). The federal government's on-line cancer resource, offering a wide range of information and news reports, texts of articles from the *Journal of the National Cancer Institute*, plus bibliographies of NCI publications for lay readers and health professionals, information about using CancerFax and the Cancer Information Service, and updates on clinical trials, drug testing protocols, and research projects. The site also offers a resource for children, including pictures, stories, and poems by kids with cancer.

CenterWatch Clinical Trials Listing Service (http://www.centerwatch.com/). International listing of over 1,400 current trials, with information about the researchers and the medical facilities. Offers an electronic mailing list so you can be notified about future studies.

Medicine On Line (http://www.meds.com/mol/welcome.html). Health information service with cancer-related topics, discussion groups, and links to other Web sites.

MedWeb: Oncology (http://neuro-www.mgh.harvard.edu/hospital-web.nclk). Very thorough directory of Web links to cancer databases, documents, treatment facilities,

handbooks, electronic newsletters and journals, and patient guides.

National Alliance of Breast Cancer Organizations (http://www.nabco.org/). Nonprofit central resource, a network of more than 370 organizations providing detection, treatment, and care. Site offers fact sheets, updates on clinical trials, information about support groups.

National Comprehensive Cancer Center Network (http://www.cancer.med.umich.edu/NCCN/NCCN.html). More than a dozen Comprehensive Cancer Centers provide information about their treatment guidelines and philosophy and links to the hospital's home pages.

OncoLink (http://cancer.med.upenn.edu/). Sponsored by the University of Pennsylvania Cancer Center Resource, this Web site offers detailed descriptions of various cancers and medical specialties; news developments; stories by cancer survivors; information about causes and prevention of cancer; current clinical trials; answers to FAQs (Frequently Asked Questions); and information about insurance and financial assistance.

Some Other Sources

Bone Marrow Donors Worldwide (http://BMDW.LeidenUniv.NL). A worldwide genetic registry of over three million volunteer bone marrow donors in 27 countries.

Bone Marrow Transplant Newsletter (http://nysernet.org/bcic/bmt/bmt.news.html). Archives of back issues, plus text of a thorough book on the subject for patients and families.

Breast Cancer Information Clearinghouse (http://nysernet.org/bcic/). From the New York State Education and Research Network, information for patients and families about detection, treatment, and health care resources.

The Cancer FAQ (Frequently Asked Questions)

(http://www.cancercare.org/faq/cancer_faq.html). Thorough and thoughtful answers about finding cancer information on the Internet. Subjects include breast cancer, lymphomas, gynecologic oncology, leukemias, grief.

CancerGuide (http://cancerguide.org/). Information about cancer assembled by a computer-literate layperson: cancer fundamentals, recommended books, clinical trials, how to research medical literature, alternative therapies.

Cancer Information from Gray Laboratory Cancer Research Center, UK (http://www.graylab.ac.uk/cancer.html). From a facility in Britain, links to Web information, including several dozen medical journals.

Cansearch: National Coalition for Cancer Survivorship Guide to Cancer Resources (http://www.access.digex.net/~mkragen/cansearch.html). Excellent, user-friendly guide to Web information written by a long-term survivor of colon cancer. Overview of sources, information on specific cancers, and survivors' stories.

GriefNet (http://www.rivendell.org/). Support for people experiencing loss and grief.

Hospital Web (http://neuro-www.mgh.harvard.edu/hospitalweb.nclk). Indexes of hospitals that have home pages on the Internet.

International Cancer Alliance (http://www2.ari.net/icare/). A nonprofit organization dedicated to improving survival by increasing awareness of treatment options and providing information to patients and physicians.

Med Help International (http://medhlp.netusa.net/). Nonprofit organization providing medical information in easy-to-understand language.

Roxane Pain Institute (http://www.Roxane.COM/Roxane/RPI/). Information for professionals and patients, newsletters, and links to other Web sites.

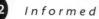

Selected Home Pages of Cancer Treatment Centers

The following URLs are the Web sites of some major cancer hospitals. Each of these home pages contains different features: information about the facilities, staff, physician referrals, types of treatment offered, patient educational materials, prevention, clinical trials, support services, ongoing research, and so on. (Many are also accessible through the National Comprehensive Cancer Center Network, listed earlier.) If a center is not listed here, you can do a search on one of the Web indexes or consult Hospital Web (described earlier).

Cedars-Sinai Comprehensive Cancer Center, Los Angeles CA (http://www.csccc.com)

City of Hope National Medical Center, Duarte CA (http://www.cityofhope.org/)

The Cleveland Clinic Foundation, Cleveland OH (http://www.ccf.org)

Columbia-Presbyterian Medical Center, New York NY (http://cpmc-net.columbia.edu/)

Dana-Farber Cancer Institute, Boston MA (http://www.dfci.harvard.edu/)

Fox Chase Cancer Center, Philadelphia PA (http://www.fccc.edu/)

Fred Hutchinson Cancer Research Center, Seattle WA (http://www.fhcrc.org)

Johns Hopkins Oncology Center, Baltimore MD (gopher://jhuniverse.hcf.jhu.edu/)

Memorial Sloan-Kettering Cancer Center, New York NY (http://www.mskcc.org/)

Northwestern University/Lurie Cancer Center, Chicago IL (http://pubweb.acns.nwu.edu/~dtn307/lurie.html)

Ohio State University Comprehensive Cancer Center, Columbus OH (http://www-cancer.med.ohio-state.edu/)

Roswell Park Cancer Institute, Buffalo NY (http://rpci.med.buffalo.edu/)

St. Jude's Children's Research Hospital, Memphis TN (http://www.stjude.org)

Stanford University Medical Center, Palo Alto CA (http://www-med.stanford.edu/)

University of Michigan Comprehensive Cancer Center, Ann Arbor MI (http://www.cancer.med.umich.edu:80/cancen.html)

University of Nebraska Medical Center, Omaha NE (http://www.unmc.edu/unmc.html)

University of Texas M. D. Anderson Cancer Center, Houston TX (http://utmdacc.uth.tmc.edu)

Newsgroups

Among the cancer-related newsgroups on the Internet at the time of this writing are the following:

alt.grief
alt.health.policy.drug-approval
alt.image.medical
alt.support.cancer
alt.support.ostomy

alt.support.cancer.prostate
sci.med
sci.med.diseases.cancer
sci.med.prostate.cancer

Be aware that some commercial services or ISPs may not make all newsgroups available to their subscribers. If one of these is of interest to you, check with the provider before setting up your account.

Internet Mailing Lists

Medinfo.Org (http://cure.medinfo.org/) is a central archive containing all the messages from all the cancer mailing lists and discussion groups. You can browse or search these archives to find answers to specific questions or to determine whether you would like to subscribe to the list.

To subscribe to an individual mailing list, send an e-mail message to the following addresses. Do not enter any information in the "Subject" line of your e-mail header. On the first line of the message, insert the information shown. For the words *your name*, substitute your first and last name, separated by a space.

Bone Marrow Transplant Discussion Mailing List
Address: bmt-talk-request@ai.mit.edu
Message: subscribe
(This list also has a Web page at http://www.ai.mit.edu/people/laurel/Bmt-talk/bmt-talk.html.)

Brain Tumor Discussion Mailing List
Address: listserv@mitvma.mit.edu
Message: subscribe BRAINTMR *your name*

Breast Cancer Discussion Mailing List
Address: listserv@morgan.ucs.mun.ca
Message: subscribe breast-cancer *your name*

CANCER-L (a general support group)
Address: listserv@wvnvm.wvnet.edu
Message: subscribe CANCER-L *your name*

Clinical Trial Finder List
Address: listserv@garcia.com
Message: subscribe ctf *your name*

Clinical Trials Mailing List
Address: majordomo@world.std.com
Message: subscribe Clinical_Trials

Colon Cancer Mailing List
Address: listserv@sjuvm.stjohns.edu
Message: colon *your name*

Drug Information Consumer Discussion Group
Address: majordomo@lists.kbt.com
Message: subscribe mol-cancer

Esophageal Cancer Mailing List
Address: listserv@sjuvm.stjohns.edu
Message: sub ec-group *your name*

Hematology-Oncology (HEM-ONC) Mailing List
(leukemia, lymphoma, multiple myeloma, and related conditions)
Address: listserv@sjuvm.stjohns.edu
Message: subscribe hem-oncology *your name*

Hodgkin's Disease Mailing List
Address: listserv@solar.org
Message: subscribe hodgkins
Note: Do not include your name

Ovarian Cancer Mailing List
Address: listserv@sjuvm.stjohns.edu
Message: subscribe ovarian *your name*

Prostate Mailing List
Address: listserv@sjuvm.stjohns.edu
Message: subscribe prostate *your name*

Radiation Oncology Listserve
Address: biosci-server@net.bio.net
Message: subscribe radoncjc

Transplant Mailing List
Address: listserv@wuvmd.wustl.edu
Message: subscribe transplnt *your name*

(Note: the second *a* in transplant is omitted.)

Web Search Engines

Use these on the Internet in search of information on cancer or any subject. They operate with varying degrees of efficiency. If you can't find what you want on one, try another.

Alta Vista (http://altavista.digital.com)

DejaNews (http://dejanews.com/)

Electric Library (http://www.elibrary.com/id/2525)

Excite (http://www.excite.com)

Lycos (http://www.lycos.com/)

Magellan (http://www.mckinley.com)

Open Text Index (http://www.opentext.com/omw/f-omw.html)

WhoWhere (http://www.whowhere.com)

Yahoo (http://www.yahoo.com)

ABOUT THE EDITORS

Gerald P. Murphy, M.D.
Medical Editor

Chief medical officer for the American Cancer Society from 1988 to 1993, Gerald P. Murphy is currently director of research at the Northwest Hospital and Pacific Northwest Cancer Foundation in Seattle, Washington. A urologist and surgical oncologist, Dr. Murphy headed the research team that discovered and developed the prostate specific antigen (PSA) test for prostate cancer. He is author or co-author of over 1,100 scientific publications and more than 15 books, and he is currently editor in chief of four distinguished medical journals. Dr. Murphy is the recipient of national and international awards and honorary degrees for his research and leadership in cancer detection and control.

Lois B. Morris
Executive Editor

Lois B. Morris is a New York–based author and journalist whose work appears frequently in magazines and newspapers. She has written or co-authored seven books on health and behavior, and she served as editorial director of *The Columbia University College of Physicians and Surgeons Complete Home Guide to Mental Health*. She writes the "Mood News" column for *Allure* magazine.

Dianne Lange
Editorial Director

Trained as a nurse, Dianne Lange is a medical journalist and author currently residing in Santa Monica, California. She has been the editor in chief of *Health* magazine and award-winning health editor for *Self, Mirabella,* and *Allure* magazines. She is a contributing editor and "Body News" columnist for *Allure*.